# PHARMACOPŒIA OF INDIA

# PHARMACOPŒIA OF INDIA,

PREPARED UNDER THE AUTHORITY OF
HER MAJESTY'S SECRETARY OF STATE FOR INDIA
IN COUNCIL.

**EDWARD JOHN WARING, M. D.**

GYAN

*Published by*

Gyan Publishing House
5, Ansari Road
Daryaganj, New Delhi-110002
Phone: 011-47034999, 9811692060
E-mail: books@gyanbooks.com

*Distribution Network*
gyanbooks.com
India, USA, Canada, UK, Australia, France



ISBN: 978-81-212-8350-2 (PB)
First Published, 1868

2nd Impression 2023

*Printed at:* Gyan Press, Delhi.



**PHARMACOPŒIA OF INDIA**
Author: EDWARD JOHN WARING

# PHARMACOPŒIA OF INDIA,

PREPARED UNDER THE AUTHORITY OF

HER MAJESTY'S SECRETARY OF STATE FOR INDIA IN COUNCIL.

BY

EDWARD JOHN WARING, M.D.,

MEMBER OF THE ROYAL COLLEGE OF PHYSICIANS OF LONDON,
SURGEON IN HER MAJESTY'S INDIAN ARMY,

ASSISTED BY A COMMITTEE APPOINTED FOR THE PURPOSE.

INDIA OFFICE:
1868.

---

LONDON:
W. H. ALLEN & CO., 13, WATERLOO PLACE,
PUBLISHERS TO THE INDIA OFFICE.

# CONTENTS.



Y 9439. Wt. P. 717. I. 891.

# PREFACE.

TWENTY-FOUR years have elapsed since the Bengal Pharmacopœia was issued in Calcutta, "by order of Government." Since then great advances have been made in our knowledge of the medicinal properties and therapeutic uses of the drugs indigenous to our Eastern Empire. Some of them have already been admitted into the British Pharmacopœia; whilst many others, having been subjected to the test of clinical observation, have been found to possess considerable value as therapeutic agents, and to be well worthy of the attention of the medical profession in India. The information relating to them, however, is scattered through a large number of periodical and standard works, which are inaccessible to the great mass of medical officers serving in India, and therefore unavailable for general reference.

The British Pharmacopœia issued by the Medical Council of England in 1865 authorized great changes in the nomenclature and composition of many important preparations; and still greater changes have been effected in the edition of 1867. As the use of that work is enjoined by Government authority, all pre-existing pharmacopœias, and other works having special reference to pharmacy and materia medica in use in Great Britain, unless brought up to that standard, are rendered, to a certain extent, valueless to the British practitioner.

Under these circumstances, with the view, firstly, of bringing to the notice of the profession in India those indigenous drugs which European experience has proved to possess value as medicinal agents, and which may be employed as efficient substitutes for imported articles; and, secondly, of re-modelling the Bengal Pharmacopœia of 1844, Her Majesty's Secretary of State for India in Council was pleased to sanction the publication of a Pharmacopœia for India based upon the British Pharmacopœia, which, while affording all the information contained in that work of practical use in India, would embody and combine with it such supplementary matter of special value in that country as should adapt it to meet the requirements of the Indian Medical Department.

In order to carry out these views, and to superintend the preparation of the work, Her Majesty's Secretary of State for India in Council organized a Committee composed of the following members:—

Inspector-General of Hospitals Sir J. Ranald Martin, C.B., F.R.S., late Bengal army, *President*.

Sir William O'Shaughnessy Brooke,* M.D., F.R.S., late Bengal army.

Alexander Gibson,† Esq., F.L.S., late Bombay army.

Daniel Hanbury, Esq., F.R.S., F.L.S.

Thomas Thomson, M.D., F.R.S., late Bengal army.

John Forbes Watson, M.D., M.A., F.L.S., late Bombay army.

Robert Wight, M.D., F.R.S., late Madras army.

Edward John Waring, M.D., M.R.C.P., Lond., F.L.S., Madras army, *Editor*.

---

* Formerly Sir W. B. O'Shaughnessy. He assumed by royal licence the surname of Brooke in 1861. With his sanction, his former name, so well known in the records of Indian Materia Medica, has been retained in the following pages.

† Deceased January 16th, 1867.

Much important assistance has been rendered by Professor Christison, of Edinburgh, who perused the sheets as they passed through the press, and offered many valuable suggestions. In the latter portion of the work, much valuable aid has been afforded in the same way by Dr. Albert J. Bernays, of St. Thomas's Hospital.

The Committee held their first meeting at the India Board Office, Cannon Row, March 15th, 1865, and proceeded to the consideration of the most effectual means of carrying out the work entrusted to them.

To this end it was resolved, in the first instance, to prepare lists of the principal drugs and medicinal plants of India, for distribution in that country, with the view of obtaining from medical officers serving there, any information they might have acquired from personal experience, which would enable the Committee to assign with greater precision an approximate value to each article. By means of the information thus collected, superadded to that obtained from an exhaustive examination of the principal English works on Indian Materia Medica, especially the Bengal Dispensatory, the Committee have the satisfaction of feeling that there will be found embodied in the following pages, in a condensed form, the principal part of the information which, up to the present day, exists relative to the indigenous drugs of India. The reports received from India have contributed in no small degree to whatever value the present volume may possess. Some of them, in addition to the record of personal experience, contain much matter relative to the use of the different drugs by the natives, and other particulars, of which the Committee were unable to avail themselves; but, in order that the information should not be lost, the documents have been deposited in the India Museum, where they are available for reference.

The best mode of arranging the materials at command received at the outset, the most careful consideration, and it was ultimately decided to divide the articles into two classes, viz. "Officinal" and "Non-officinal;" the first to include those articles officinal in the British Pharmacopœia, together with those indigenous products of India whose claims as medicinal agents are established on a solid basis; the second or "Non-officinal" list to comprise a large number of articles whose reputation is not so well established, but which, possessing considerable activity, are deemed worthy of attention. In addition to these, there have been included a few drugs respecting which, either from their high repute amongst the natives, or from marked physical characters, it is desirable to obtain further information. Some of the articles in this class will doubtless, on trial, prove worthless, and will justly be discarded in future editions; whilst others, it is expected, will prove valuable remedial agents, and worthy of being eventually transferred to the officinal class.

After much deliberation it was likewise determined to depart from the alphabetical arrangement usually employed in pharmacopœias, and to adopt one based on a scientific classification, as being better adapted for bringing to notice the numerous articles of materia medica to which it was deemed desirable to call attention.

It was further resolved to depart from the old Pharmacopœia routine of furnishing a simple list of articles of materia medica, with their physical characters and preparations, and to supply information with regard to their medical properties, therapeutic uses, and doses; to form, in fact, a Text Book which might prove useful to the medical student, and, it was hoped, also, though perhaps in a minor degree, to the practitioner in remote stations where works on materia medica are not always available for reference.

In accordance with these views, it was deemed expedient to place under each individual drug the preparations of which it forms the active ingredient. By this arrangement it is obvious that the various preparations are presented to view more conveniently than if they were inserted in detached portions of the work, under the separate headings of Infusions, Tinctures, Extracts, and so forth. All difficulties with regard to reference are obviated by a carefully prepared and extensive Index.

It was also decided to include in the present work, *all* the drugs which are officinal in the British Pharmacopœia. Some of these, which require to be used in the fresh state, are, of course, unavailable in India; others, from readily undergoing decomposition at high temperatures, are unsuited for use in the tropics. These, together with a few minor articles for which India yields efficient substitutes, it was at first thought might safely be omitted without detracting from the utility of the work to the Indian practitioner. But it was decided not to omit any of them; so that the student in India, where this work may be adopted as a Text Book, will have brought before him, in due course, all the articles which are officinal in Great Britain, while the notes appended will indicate their value and applicability to Indian practice.

In endeavouring to impart an educational character to the Indian Pharmacopœia, the Committee feel that they have taken the surest mode of carrying into effect one of the primary objects of the work, namely, the introduction of the indigenous products of India into European practice in that country. If they are ever to come into general use in hospitals and dispensaries throughout India, it is to the medical colleges and schools that we must look in the first instance. It is there that a correct knowledge of them should be first instilled; that the student should become familiarized with the articles themselves; that he should be made acquainted with their physical characters and medicinal properties; and it is there, during the period of student life, that he should become practically instructed in their employment in the treatment of disease. On the value of knowledge thus gained, it is impossible to place too high an estimate, familiarizing, as it will, the embryo practitioner with remedies which are at hand in the remotest corners of our Indian empire, rendering him in a great measure independent of costly imported articles, and effecting a considerable annual saving to the State.

Amongst the returns received from India was one from Native Surgeon Moodeen Sheriff, of Madras, containing the vernacular names of indigenous plants and drugs, in twelve of the native languages of India, a work of immense labour, reflecting the greatest credit on the intelligence and industry of the compiler. This Catalogue, having been submitted to eminent Oriental scholars at home, and pronounced generally correct, it was resolved to append to the Pharmacopœia. It was accordingly forwarded to Madras, for the purpose of being printed under Mr. Moodeen Sheriff's superintendence. Unexpected circumstances, however, having arisen there to delay its publication, it has been deemed advisable, rather than to defer the publication of this work, to issue the Catalogue in a separate or supplementary volume.

In connexion with this branch of the subject, much valuable assistance has been rendered by Col. W. H. Sykes, M.P., Sir Walter Elliot, K.S.I., Dr. Fitzedward Hall, Mr. C. P. Brown, and Mr. G. H. K. Thwaites, of Ceylon.

The processes employed in the manufacture of chemical preparations have generally been omitted. To have inserted them would have tended materially to increase the size of the volume without any corresponding advantage, seeing that such articles could only be prepared at the Government Medical Stores, and perhaps in the laboratories of a few of the larger private firms in the Presidency towns, the needful appliances not existing elsewhere; and at these establishments the British Pharmacopœia will of course be available, and the directions contained in that work should always be followed, excepting in those cases where experience has shown that, owing to difference of climate or other circumstances, a modification of the directions is requisite.

The double system of chemical notation adopted in the British Pharmacopœia has been followed; and, in accordance with the plan pursued in that work, the formulæ according to the old system are printed in the lighter Roman type (Al), and those according to the new system in the heavier Egyptian type (**Al**); when, however, the notation under the new, agrees with that under the old system, only that in the lighter Roman type has been inserted.

With regard to weights and measures, it has not been deemed advisable to depart from the standard adopted by the British Medical Council. For the higher denominations of weights and fluid measures, the avoirdupois weight and imperial measure are respectively employed. The following are the weights and measures adopted in the Pharmacopœia of India:—

*Weights.*

| | | | |
|---|---|---|---|
| 1 grain | - - | gr. | |
| 1 scruple | - | ℈i | = 20 grains. |
| 1 drachm | - - | drm. (ʒi) | = 60 grains. |
| 1 ounce | - - | oz. (℥i) | = 437·5 grains. |
| 1 pound | - - | lb. | = 7000 grains. |

*Measures of Capacity.*

| | | | |
|---|---|---|---|
| 1 minim | - - | min. (♏). | |
| 1 fluid drachm | - | fl. drm. (fʒi) | = 60 minims. |
| 1 fluid ounce | - | fl. oz. (f℥i) | = 8 fluid drachms. |
| 1 pint | - - - | O. | = 20 fluid ounces. |
| 1 gallon | - - - | C. | = 8 pints. |

The doses named are the average ones for adults, excepting when otherwise expressly noted; these, however, are liable to considerable modification, according to circumstances; and their regulation in each individual case must be left to the discretion of the practitioner.

The Appendix contains numerous bibliographical references, extracts from the Reports received from India, and other information connected chiefly with Indian Materia Medica, which would have been less appropriately placed in the body of the work.

In conclusion, the Committee desire to record the high sense they unanimously entertain of the liberal spirit in which Her Majesty's Secretary of State for India in Council has on all occasions treated their suggestions and requirements. Their best thanks are likewise due to the other Authorities at the India Office, including the Officers of the India Museum and Library, for the cordial aid which, in their respective departments, they have afforded to the Committee during the progress of the work.

## List of Medical Officers and others in India from whom reports have been received.

### *Bengal.*

Surgeon R. F. Hutchinson, M.D.
„ W. B. Beatson, M.D.
Assistant Surgeon C. F. Oldham, M.D.
„ T. E. B. Brown.
„ J. Newton.
„ E. Bonavia, M.D.
„ S. Delpratt.
„ G. A. Watson.
„ J. M. Coates, M.D.
„ Bholanauth Bose, M.D.
Uncovenanted ditto W. C. Kiernander, M.D.
„ J. A. Green, M. D.
„ N. Jackson.
„ H. C. Bowser.
Sub-Assistant Surgeon Roma Chuer Bose.
„ Odoy Chund Dutt.
„ Sudrul Huq.
„ Gopaul Chuder Pauttuck.
„ Unnoda Churn Custogery.
„ Dinnonauth Doss.
„ Tara Chund Banjoorjee.
„ Obhoy Churn Newgee.
„ Turruck Chunder Lahory.
„ Bhoobun Mohun Chatterjee.
„ Kanny Lall Dey.
„ A. J. Meyer.
„ Raheem Khan.

### *Madras.*

Surgeon-Major A. Hunter, M.D.
„ G. Smith, M.D.
„ W. J. Van Someren, M.D.

Surgeon L. W. Stewart.

„ H. R. Oswald, M.D.

„ W. H. Rean, M.D.

„ G. Marr, M.D.

Assistant-Surgeon J. Shortt, M.D.

„ H. King, M.D.

„ H. E. Busteed.

„ J. Kees, M.D.

„ Æ. Ross, M.D.

„ W. R. Grylls.

Apothecary J. J. Wood.

Native Surgeon Moodeen Sheriff.

„ M. Iyasawmy.

---

S. Pulney Andy, M.D.

D. R. Thomson, M.D.

*Bombay.*

Surgeon-Major D. Wyllie, M.D.

Surgeon H. V. Carter, M.D.

„ R. Haines, M.B.

Assistant Surgeon W. Dymock, M.D.

---

G. Birdwood, M.D.

N. A. Dalzell, Esq., M.A.

---

In addition to the above, communications have been received from Clements R. Markham, Esq., of the India Office, Dr. W. C. B. Eatwell, Dr. Alexander Grant, and Dr. William Wright, of the Bengal Medical Service; Dr. James Winchester, late Bombay Medical Service; and Drs. Hugh Cleghorn, George Bidie, and Francis Day, of the Madras Medical Service.

## Articles Officinal in the Pharmacopœia of India not contained in the British Pharmacopœia.

*Distinguished from British officinal articles by an asterisk.*

Aconitum ferox, *Wall.* Root.
Aconitum heterophyllum, *Wall.* Root.
Coptis Teeta. *Wall.* Root.
Tinospora cordifolia, *Miers.* Root and stems.
Berberis Asiatica, *D. C.*; *B.* aristata, *D.C.*; and B. Lycium, *Royle.* Root-bark.
Narcotine.
Sinapis juncea, *Linn.* Seeds.
Gynocardia odorata, *R. Br.* Seeds.
Garcinia pictoria, *Roxb.* Gum-resin.
Garcinia purpurea, *Roxb.* Oil of the seeds.
Dipterocarpus lævis, *Ham.* Balsamic exudation.
Hibiscus esculentus, *Linn.* Capsules.
Citrus Bergamia, *Risso.* Juice of the fruit.
Toddalia aculeata, *Pers.* Root.
Boswellia floribunda, *Endl.* Gum-resin.
Azadirachta Indica, *Juss.* Bark and leaves.
Soymida febrifuga, *Juss.* Bark.
Mucuna pruriens, *D.C.* Legumes.
Acacia Catechu, *Willd.* Extract of the wood.
Cæsalpinia (Guilandina) Bonducella, *Linn.* Seeds.
Butea frondosa, *Roxb.* Inspissated juice.
Abrus precatorius, *Linn.* Root.
Arachis hypogæa, *Linn.* Oil of seeds.
Carum (Ptychotis) Ajowan, *D.C.* Fruit.
Hydrocotyle Asiatica, *Linn.* Leaves.
Diospyros Embryopteris, *Pers.* Fruit.
Punica granatum, *Linn.* Rind of fruit.
Alstonia scholaris, *R. Br.* Bark.
Calotropis gigantea, *R. Br.*; and C. procera, *R. Br.* Root-bark.

Tylophora asthmatica, *W. et A.* Leaves.
Pharbitis Nil, *Choisy.* Seeds.
Andrographis paniculata, *Nees.* Stalks and roots.
Datura alba, *Linn.* Leaves and seeds.
Plantago Ispaghula, *Roxb.* Seeds.
Crinum Asiaticum, *Herb.* Bulbs.
Oryza sativa, *Linn.* Seeds.
Andropogon citratum, *D.C.*; *A.* Nardus, *Linn.*; and A. pachnodes, *Trin.* Volatile oil.
Gracilaria lichenoides, *Greville,* and other species. Dried plant.
Mylabris Cichorii, *Fabr.* Dried insect.
Squalus Carcharias, *Linn.* Oil obtained from the liver.

# VEGETABLE MATERIA MEDICA.

## Class 1. Dicotyledones *vel* Exogenae.

### RANUNCULACEÆ.

#### ACONITUM NAPELLUS, *Linn.* ACONITE OF MONKSHOOD.

(*Engl. Bot.*, t. 2730; *ed. Syme*, t. 48.)

*Habitat.*—Mountainous parts of Central Europe and Asia, extending to Northern India.

*Officinal Parts.*—1. The dried root (*Aconiti Radix*) collected in the winter or early spring before the leaves have appeared. (1) It has the following characters: Usually from one to three inches in length, seldom thicker than the middle finger at the crown, tapering, blackish brown, internally whitish. A minute portion cautiously chewed causes prolonged tingling and numbness. 2. The fresh leaves (*Aconiti Folia*) and flowering tops, gathered, when about one-third of the flowers are expanded, from plants cultivated in Britain. The leaves are smooth, palmate, divided into five deeply cut wedge-shaped segments; exciting, when chewed, a sensation of tingling. Flowers numerous, irregular, deep blue, in dense racemes. *Active principle*, an Alkaloid, *Aconitia*.

*Properties.*—Powerfully sedative, anodyne, and antiphlogistic. In large doses a virulent poison.

*Therapeutic Uses.*—In various forms of neuralgia, tetanus, acute and chronic rheumatism, gout, erysipelas, and in affections of the heart characterised by increased action, it is a remedy of established value, but its operation on the system requires to be carefully watched.

*Preparations of the Root.*—**Tincture of Aconite** (*Tinctura Aconiti*). Take of Aconite Root, in coarse powder, two ounces and a half; Rectified Spirit, one pint. Macerate the aconite root for forty-eight hours in fifteen fluid ounces of the spirit, in a closed vessel, agitating occasionally; then transfer to a percolator; and when the fluid ceases to pass, continue the percolation with the remaining five ounces of spirit. Afterwards subject the contents of the percolator to pressure, filter the product, mix the liquids, and add sufficient rectified spirit to make one pint.

This tincture has one fourth of the strength of Tinctura Aconiti, *Dubl. Ph.*, and one third of that of Tinctura Aconiti, *Lond. Ph.* Each fluid ounce represents 54½ grains of the dried root.

*Dose.*—From five to fifteen minims.

**Liniment of Aconite** (*Linimentum Aconiti*). Take of Aconite Root, in coarse powder, twenty ounces; Camphor, one ounce; Rectified Spirit, a sufficiency. Moisten the aconite with some of the spirit, and macerate in a closed vessel for three days; then transfer to a percolator; and, adding more spirit, percolate slowly into a receiver containing the camphor, until the product measures one pint.

This preparation is intended only for external use, and proves valuable in rheumatic and neuralgic affections, care being taken not to apply it to mucous or abraded surfaces. One fluid ounce represents one ounce of the dried root.

**Aconitia** (*Aconitia*). An alkaloid, obtained from Aconite Root. A white, usually amorphous solid, soluble in 150 parts of cold, and 50 of hot water; much more soluble in alcohol and in ether; strongly alkaline to reddened litmus, neutralising acids, and precipitated from them by the caustic alkalies, but not by carbonate of ammonia or the bicarbonates of soda or potash. It melts with heat, and burns with a smoky flame, leaving no residue when burned with free access of air. When rubbed on the skin it causes a tingling sensation, followed by prolonged numbness. It is a very active poison. Not administered internally.

**Aconitia Ointment** (*Unguentum Aconitiæ*). Take of Aconitia, eight grains; Olive Oil, half a fluid drachm; Prepared Lard, one ounce. Rub the aconitia with the oil, add the lard, and mix thoroughly.

A useful application in neuralgic affections.

*Preparation of the Leaves and Flowering Tops.*—**Extract of Aconite** (*Extractum Aconiti*). Take of the fresh Leaves and Flowering Tops of Aconite, one hundred and twelve pounds. Bruise in a stone mortar, and press out the juice; heat it gradually to 130°, and separate the green colouring matter by a calico filter. Heat the strained liquor to 200° to coagulate the albumen, and again filter. Evaporate the filtrate by a water-bath to the consistence of a thin syrup; then add to it the green colouring matter previously separated, and stirring the whole together assiduously, continue the evaporation at a temperature not exceeding 140°, until the extract is of a suitable consistence for forming pills.

*Dose.*—From one to two grains. An uncertain preparation, readily spoiling in hot climates.

## *ACONITUM FEROX, *Wall.* BIKH or BISH.

(*No plate: that in Wallich's Plant. Asiat. Rar.*, t. 41, *is A. napellus.*)

*Habitat.*—Temperate and Sub-Alpine Himalaya, at 10,000 to 14,000 feet elevation, from Gurhwal to Sikkim.

*Officinal Part.*—The dried root (*Aconiti ferocis Radix*), in common with those of other Himalayan species, viz., *Aconitum Napellus*, Linn., *A. palmatum*, Don, and *A. luridum*, H. et T., constitutes the drug well known in the bazaars of Upper India under the Hindústani name of *Bish* or *Bikh.*(2) It occurs in the form of tuberous roots of a more or less conical form, from two to three inches in length, and from half an inch to one inch in thickness at their upper end. They have usually a shrunken appearance, and are covered with a dark shrivelled bark; fracture shining and resinous, sometimes waxy, varying in colour from pale to deep brown. Some specimens are white and spongy; and these, it is asserted, are superior in activity to the more compact kinds.(3) Inodorous; taste at first slightly bitter, leaving a peculiar sense of numbness on the tongue and fauces. Active principle, *Aconitia.*

*Medical Properties and Uses.*—Similar to those of *Aconitum Napellus* of Europe. (4)

*Preparations.*—This root may be advantageously used for the manufacture of Aconitia, the proportion of this alkaloid being much larger than in the European drug, and also for the preparation of Linimentum Aconiti. From its greater activity, however, it is unsuited for the preparation of the tincture, which is intended for internal use.

## *ACONITUM HETEROPHYLLUM, *Wall.* ATÍS.

(*Royle, Illust.*, t. 13.)

*Habitat.*—Western temperate Himalaya, at 8,000 to 13,000 feet elevation; from the Indus to Kumaon.

*Officinal Part.*—The dried root (*Aconiti heterophylli Radix*). Ovoid tuberous roots, tapering downwards to a point, from one to one and a half inches or more in length, and from three eighths to half an inch in thickness. The surface, which is covered with a thin greyish epidermis, is slightly wrinkled longitudinally, and marked here and there with rootlet-scars. A transverse section shows it to consist of a pure white friable amylaceous substance, marked by five or six concentrically arranged dots, the terminations of threads of woody fibre traversing the root longitudinally. It is inodorous, and of a bitter taste, devoid of acridity. Does not contain aconitia. It may be readily distinguished from other roots sold in the bazaars under the same vernacular name (*Atís*) by its characteristic bitterness.

*Properties.*—Tonic and antiperiodic. In consequence of the absence of aconitia or other poisonous principle, it may be administered internally with safety.

*Therapeutic Uses.*—In convalescence after debilitating diseases, and in intermittent and other paroxysmal fevers, it has been found an efficient remedy. (5)

*Dose.*—As a tonic, from five to ten grains thrice daily; as an antiperiodic, from twenty to thirty grains of the powdered root every three or four hours, irrespective of the presence of pyrexia. This is the best form of administration.

## *COPTIS TEETA, *Wall.* COPTIS, or MISHMI TITA.

*Habitat.*—Mishmee Mountains, east of Assam.

*Officinal Part.*—The dried root (*Coptidis Radix*), imported into Bengal from Assam in small rattan baskets, each containing from one to two ounces of the drug. This consists of pieces of a woody rhizome, of the thickness of a small goose-quill, and from one to two inches in length, often contracted at one extremity into a short woody stem; the surface is usually rough, irregular, more or less annulated, and marked with the remains of rootlets in the shape of short spiny points. Externally it is of a yellowish-brown colour, internally much brighter, frequently of a golden yellow colour, exhibiting on fracture a radiated structure. Taste persistently bitter, and when chewed tinges the saliva yellow. It contains neither tannic nor gallic acid, but abounds with a yellow bitter principle soluble in water and in alcohol,

*Properties.*—Pure bitter tonic.

*Therapeutic Uses.*—In debility, convalescence after fevers and other debilitating diseases, atonic dyspepsia, and in mild forms of intermittent fevers, it has been found to produce excellent effects. (6)

*Dose.*—From ten to fifteen grains of the powdered root thrice daily.

*Preparations.*—**Tincture of Coptis** (*Tinctura Coptidis*). Take of Coptis Root, in coarse powder, two ounces and a half; Proof Spirit, two pints. Macerate for seven days in a closed vessel, with occasional agitation; strain, press, filter, and add sufficient proof spirit to make one pint.

*Dose.*—From one half to two fluid drachms.

**Infusion of Coptis** (*Infusum Coptidis*). Take of Coptis Root, in coarse powder, five drachms; Boiling Water, a pint. Infuse in a covered vessel for two hours, and strain.

*Dose.*—From one to two fluid ounces thrice daily.

(*Non-officinal.*)

**Thalictrum foliolosum,** *D.C.*—The root of this plant, common throughout temperate Himalaya, is called by the Hill people *Pila jari*, i.e. *Yellow Root*, and is exported from the Kumaon mountains under the name of *Momeeree* (Madden). It occurs in pieces about the thickness of a crow-quill, fibrous, fasciculate, dark brown externally, yellow internally; contains a yellow bitter extractive, which it yields to alcohol and to water; a watery solution is not blackened by a persalt of iron. It combines tonic and aperient properties, and has been found useful in convalescence after acute diseases, in mild forms of intermittent fevers, and in atonic dyspepsia. *Dose* of the powdered root, from five to ten grains; of the Extract (prepared as Extract of Gentian, *q.v.*), from two to three grains, thrice daily. (*Bengal Disp.*, p. 161.)

**Nigella sativa,** *Lin.* (*Sibthorp Flora Græca*, t. 511).—The seeds of this plant are procurable in most parts of India, and may be resorted to as a carminative in the absence of other remedies of the same class. A tincture (Nigella seeds four ounces and a half, Proof Spirit two pints,) was officinal in the Bengal Ph. under the name of Tincture of Mugrela. It is there described as an excellent adjunct to purgative draughts, in doses of half a drachm to a drachm.

## MAGNOLIACEÆ.

### ILLICIUM ANISATUM, *Linn.* STAR ANISE.

(*Nees, Plant. Med.*, t. 371.)

*Habitat.*—China.

*Officinal Part.*—The fruit (*Star Anise,*) which is an inch and a quarter or more in diameter, consists of about eight follicles arranged in a radiate form, compressed, externally rugose, internally smooth, opening by their upper margin, and containing solitary, polished, ovate seeds. They have an agreeable aromatic odour, resembling that of aniseed, and a sweetish, acidulous, aromatic taste. Star Anise is officinal only on account of its volatile oil (*Oleum Illicii Anisati*), obtained by distillation, which constitutes a great portion of the oil of anise met with in commerce. The oil is colourless, or pale yellow, with the odour of anise and a warm sweetish taste; concretes at 50°.

*Medical Properties and Uses.*—Stomachic and carminative, proving serviceable in flatulent and spasmodic affections of the intestinal canal.

*Dose.*—From two to five minims of the volatile oil.

(*Non-officinal.*)

**Michelia Champaca**, *Linn.* (*Rheede, Hort. Mal.*, vol. i. t. 19)—The bitter aromatic bark of this tree approximates in properties to that of the *Magnolia glauca* of North America (*Bengal Disp.*, p. 193). It has been successfully employed in the Mauritius by Dr. H. Lolliot in the treatment of the low intermittent fevers of that island. He administered it in infusion (one ounce, water one pint), or in decoction (one ounce, water two pints boiled to one pint), in doses of a wineglassful every hour for three hours preceding, and for the same period following, a paroxysm. (Bouton, *Med. Plants of Mauritius*, p. 3.) Further trials with this bark appear desirable. It is easily procurable in all parts of India, the tree being extensively cultivated for the sake of its fragrant flowers.

## MENISPERMACEÆ.

### JATEORHIZA COLUMBA, *Miers*, and J. MIERSII, *Oliver*. CALUMBA.

*Cocculus palmatus*, D.C., *Brit. Pharm.*, 1864. (*Bot. Mag.*, t. 2970, 2971.)

*Habitat.*—Forest of Eastern Africa between Ibo and the Zambezi.

*Officinal Part.*—The root (*Calumbæ Radix*). It occurs in transverse slices, flat, circular, or oval, about two inches in diameter, and from two to four lines thick, softer and thinner towards the centre; greyish yellow; odour faint; taste very bitter. A decoction when cold is blackened by a solution of iodine. Sulphate of iron, tartar emetic, and gelatine produce no obvious change in an infusion, showing the absence of tannic and gallic acids. Contains a bitter crystallizable principle, *Calumbin*, and a bitter neutral principle, *Berberina*.

*Medical Properties.*—Valuable tonic and stomachic.

*Therapeutic Uses.*—In general debility, atonic dyspepsia, gastric irritability, vomiting attendant on pregnancy, and in the advanced stage of diarrhœa and dysentery, it has been found of great value.

*Dose.*—From five to twenty grains of the powdered root twice or thrice daily.

*Preparations.*—**Infusion of Calumba** (*Infusum Calumbæ*). Take of Calumba Root, cut small, half an ounce; cold Water, ten fluid ounces. Macerate in a covered vessel for one hour, and strain.

*Dose.*—From one to two fluid ounces.

**Tincture of Calumba** (*Tinctura Calumbæ*). Take of Calumba Root, cut small, two ounces and a half; Proof Spirit, one pint. Macerate the calumba for forty-eight hours in fifteen fluid ounces of the spirit, in a closed vessel, agitating occasionally; then transfer to a percolator, and when the fluid ceases to pass, continue the percolation with the remaining five ounces of spirit. Afterwards subject the contents of the percolator to pressure, filter the product, mix the liquids, and add sufficient proof spirit to make one pint.

*Dose.*—From thirty minims to two fluid drachms.

**Extract of Calumba** (*Extractum Calumbæ*). Take of Calumba Root, cut small, one pound; Water, four pints. Macerate the calumba with two pints of the water for twelve hours, strain and press. Macerate again with the same quantity of water, strain and press as before. Mix and filter the liquors, and evaporate them by the heat of a water bath until the extract is of a suitable consistence for forming pills.

*Dose.*—From three to ten grains.

## CISSAMPELOS PAREIRA, *Linn.* PAREIRA BRAVA.

(*Woodville, Med. Bot.*, t. 82.)

*Habitat.*—Common throughout the tropics of both hemispheres.

*Officinal Part.*—The dried root (*Pareiræ Radix*). It occurs in the form of cylindrical, oval or compressed pieces entire or split longitudinally, half an inch to four inches in diameter, and from four inches to four feet in length. Bark greyish-brown, longitudinally wrinkled, crossed transversely by annular elevations; interior woody, yellowish-grey, porous, with well marked, often incomplete, concentric rings and medullary rays. Taste at first sweetish and aromatic, afterwards intensely bitter.†

*Medical Properties.*—Mild tonic and diuretic, exercising apparently an astringent and sedative action on the mucous membranes of the genito-urinary organs.

*Therapeutic Uses.*—Advanced stages of acute and chronic cystitis, catarrhal affections of the bladder and cystirrhæa.

*Preparations.*—**Decoction of Pareira** (*Decoctum Pareiræ*). Take of Pareira Root, sliced, one ounce and a half; Water, one pint. Boil for fifteen minutes in a covered vessel, then strain, and pour as much water over the contents of the strainer as will make the strained product measure a pint.

*Dose.*—From one to three fluid ounces.

**Extract of Pareira** (*Extractum Pareiræ*). Take of Pareira Root, in coarse powder, one pound; Boiling Water, one gallon, or a sufficiency. Digest the pareira with a pint of the water for twenty-four hours, then pack in a percolator, and, adding more of the water, allow the liquor slowly to pass until a gallon has been collected, or the pareira is exhausted. Evaporate the liquor by a water bath until the extract has acquired a suitable consistence for forming pills.

*Dose.*—From ten to twenty grains.

**Liquid Extract of Pareira** (*Extractum Pareiræ Liquidum*). Take of Pareira Root, in coarse powder, one pound; Boiling Water, one gallon, or a sufficiency; Rectified Spirit, three fluid ounces. Digest the pareira with a pint of the water for twenty-four hours, then pack in a percolator, and, adding more of the water, allow the liquor slowly to pass until a gallon has been collected, or the pareira is exhausted. Evaporate the liquor by a water bath to thirteen fluid ounces, and, when it is cold, add the spirit and filter through paper.

*Dose.*—From half a fluid drachm to two fluid drachms.

---

† The drug thus described, and to which the name *Pareira Brava* is commonly attributed, is regarded by Mr. Hanbury as not afforded by *Cissampelos Pareira*, L., but by some other menispermaceous plant of Brazil. A sample of the drug, actually derived from *Cissampelos Pareira*, L., in the possession of Mr. Hanbury, consists of long cylindrical stems, some of them terminating in roots, and some bearing here and there roots emitted at intervals. They vary in diameter from $\frac{1}{4}$ of an inch to an inch or more, but have mostly a diameter of about half an inch, exhibiting, when cut transversely, conspicuous medullary rays, but not the concentric zones so evident in the so-called *Pareira Brava* of commerce. The colour of the wood is pale greyish brown; its bark is of the same hue, but darker. It has a bitter taste, but is neither sweetish nor aromatic.

## *ANAMIRTA COCCULUS, *W. et A.* Cocculus Indicus.

(*Wallich, Asiat. Res.*, vol. xiii. t. 15, 16.)

*Habitat.*—Mountain forests of Ceylon, Malabar, Travancore, the Concans, and Orissa, extending to Khasia and Assam.

*Officinal Part.*—The fruit dried (*Cocculus Indicus*); rather larger than a full-sized pea, somewhat kidney-shaped, blackish brown, wrinkled, containing a yellowish, oily, bitter, reniform seed, inclosed in a two-valved shell. The seed contains a crystallizable principle, *Picrotoxine,* which is powerfully poisonous.

*Medical Properties, &c.*—Not administered internally. As an insecticide it proves very effectual, and hence forms the active ingredient in the following ointment, employed for the destruction of pediculi.

**Ointment of Cocculus Indicus** (*Unguentum Cocculi*). Take of the seeds of Cocculus Indicus, eighty grains; Prepared Lard, one ounce. Beat the seeds well in a mortar, and incorporate thoroughly with the lard.

In applying this ointment care should be taken to avoid abraded surfaces on account of the danger of absorption.

## * TINOSPORA CORDIFOLIA, *Miers.* Gulancha.

(*Cocculus cordifolius,* D.C.)

(*Wight, Icones,* vol. ii. t. 485, 486.)

*Habitat.* — Bengal, Assam, Bahar, Deccan, Orissa, the Carnatic, Malabar, Mysore, and other parts of tropical India.

*Officinal Part.*—The root and stems (*Tinosporæ Radix et Caules*), collected during the hot season, when the bitter principle is most abundant and concentrated. As met with in the bazaars, it consists of dried transverse segments of a cylindrical woody stem. These segments vary in diameter from ¼ of an inch to 2 inches (averaging about ½ an inch), and are from ½ an inch to 2 inches in length. They exhibit a shrunken appearance, especially those derived from the younger stems, and are covered with a smooth translucent, shrivelled bark, which becomes dull and rugose with age. Many of the pieces are marked on their surface with warty prominences. The transverse section shows a radiated structure, with conspicuous medullary rays traversing a very porous tissue. It is inodorous, but has a very bitter taste. Its infusion is not blackened by a persalt of iron.

*Medical Properties.*—Tonic, antiperiodic, and diuretic.

*Therapeutic Uses.*—In mild forms of intermittents, in general debility after fevers and other exhausting diseases, and in secondary syphilitic affections and chronic rheumatism, it has been employed with good results. (7)

*Preparations.*—**Tincture of Gulancha** (*Tinctura Tinosporæ*). Take of Gulancha, cut small, four ounces; Proof Spirit, one pint. Macerate for seven days in a closed vessel, with occasional agitation, filter, and add sufficient spirit to make one pint.

*Dose.*—From one to two fluid drachms.

**Infusion of Gulancha** (*Infusum Tinosporæ*). Take of Gulancha, cut small, one ounce; Cold Water, ten fluid ounces. Macerate in a covered vessel for two hours, and strain.

*Dose.*—From one to three fluid ounces thrice daily.

**Extract of Gulancha** (*Extractum Tinosporæ*). Take of Gulancha, cut small and bruised, one pound; Water, four pints. Macerate the gulancha with two pints of the water for twelve hours, strain and press. Macerate again with the same quantity of water, strain and press as before. Mix and filter the liquors, and evaporate them by the heat of a water-bath until the extract is of a suitable consistence for forming pills.

*Dose.*—From ten to thirty grains daily, in divided doses. This corresponds with an impure extract prepared by the natives, called *Palo*, which, in doses of one to three drachms, is highly esteemed by them as a tonic in convalescence after fevers, spleen affections, &c.

(*Non-officinal.*)

**Coscinium fenestratum**, *Colebr.* (*Miers, in Bot. Mag.*, t. 4658.)—A native of the forests of Ceylon and Malabar. It is met with in the bazaars of Southern India, under the Tamul name of *Mara Munjil.* It occurs in the form of cylindrical woody stems of variable length, having a diameter of from one to four inches, covered with a thin pale corky bark. A transverse section shows the wood to consist of very porous tissue, traversed by conspicuous medullary rays, but without concentric zones. The wood has a bright greenish-yellow colour, and pure bitter taste. It was a few years since imported into England from Ceylon, under the name of *Calumba Wood*, and, analysed by Mr. Perrins (*Pharm. Journ.*, 1853, vol. xii. pp. 180, 500), was found to contain Berberine. An extensive trial with it was instituted by the Editor, at the Trevandrum Charity Hospital, and the conclusion arrived at was, that, in all cases requiring a pure bitter tonic, and where Calumba was not available, it might be resorted to with manifest advantage. It was prescribed in the form of infusion and tincture of the same strength as the corresponding preparations of Calumba. It is well worthy of the attention of practitioners in the East, as a cheap and efficient tonic (*Indian Ann. of Med. Science*, 1858, vol. v. p. 610).

**Cissampelos hernandifolia,** *Wall.*—Sir W. O'Shaughnessy (*Bengal Disp.*, p. 201) speaks highly of this plant, under the Bengali name of *Neemooka;* but it has been shown by Drs. Hooker and Thomson in their Flora Indica that the plant so called by Dr. Wallich is the Pareira Brava, which is extremely common throughout India.

**Cocculus villosus,** *D.C.*, **Tinospora crispa,** *Miers*, and some other allied species inhabiting various parts of India, possess the bitterness and probably the tonic properties of Gulancha.

## BERBERIDEÆ.

### PODOPHYLLUM PELTATUM, *Linn.* PODOPHYLLUM.
(*Bot. Mag.*, t. 1819; *Gray, Genera*, t. 35, 36.)

*Habitat.*—Throughout the United States of North America.

*Officinal Part.*—The dried rhizome (*Podophylli Radix, Podophyllum Root*). It occurs in pieces of variable length, about two lines thick, mostly wrinkled longitudinally, dark reddish-brown externally, whitish within, breaking with a short fracture; accompanied with pale brown rootlets. Powder yellowish-grey, sweetish in odour, bitterish, subacrid and nauseous in taste. It is officinal solely as the source of its resin.

*Preparation.*—**Resin of Podophyllum** (*Podophylli Resina, Podophyllin*). Take of Podophyllum Root, in coarse powder, one pound; Rectified Spirit, three pints, or a sufficiency; Water, a sufficiency; Hydrochloric Acid, a sufficiency. Exhaust the podophyllum with the spirit by percolation; place the tincture in a still, and draw off the greater part of the spirit. Acidulate the water with one twenty-fourth of its bulk of hydrochloric acid, and slowly pour the liquid which remains after the distillation of the tincture into three times its volume of the acidulated water, constantly stirring. Allow the mixture to stand for twenty-four hours to deposit the resin. Wash the resin on a filter with distilled water, and dry it in a stove. *Characters.*—A pale greenish-brown amorphous powder, soluble in rectified spirit and in ammonia; precipitated from the former solution by water, from the latter by acids. Almost entirely soluble in pure ether.

*Medical Properties.*—Purgative and cholagogue; alterative in small continued doses.

*Therapeutic Uses.*—In constipation, chronic hepatic affections, especially congestion and torpor of the liver, in gouty, rheumatic, and syphilitic affections, it has been used with advantage.

*Dose.*—As a cholagogue and cathartic, from one to two grains; as an aperient, from half a grain to one grain; as an alterative, from one twelfth to one eighth of a grain, twice or thrice daily.

[One species of **Podophyllum** (**P. Emodi,** *Wall*), (*Jacquemont, Voyage*, t. 9) is indigenous to the Himalaya; its properties may be deserving of investigation.]

## *BERBERIS ASIATICA, *D.C.* BERBERIS ARISTATA, *D.C.* BERBERIS LYCIUM, *Royle.* — INDIAN BARBERRY.

(*Wight, Illust.*, vol. i. t. 8.)

*Habitat.*—All those species are common throughout the drier temperate Himalaya, and *B. aristata* extends thence to the higher mountains of the Madras Peninsula.

*Officinal Part.*—The root-bark (*Berberis Cortex*), collected at the fall of the year, as it then most abounds in the bitter principle. The bark should be stript off whilst fresh, and then dried. It is light-coloured, corky, almost inodorous, with a bitter mucilaginous taste. Contains a bitter crystallizable principle, *Berberine.*

*Medical Properties.*—Tonic, antiperiodic, diaphoretic. (8)

*Therapeutic Uses.*—In intermittent and remittent fevers, and in general debility, especially in that consequent on fevers, it is a remedy of great value. The extract (*Rusot*) is applied locally in ophthalmia and other affections of the eyes.

*Preparations.* — **Tincture of Indian Barberry** (*Tinctura Berberis*). Take of the Root-bark of Indian Barberry, cut small, twelve ounces; Proof Spirit, two pints. Macerate for seven days in a closed vessel, with occasional agitation. Strain, press, filter, and add sufficient proof spirit to make two pints. It may also be prepared by percolation in the same manner as Tincture of Calumba, *q.v.*

*Dose.* — As an antiperiodic, from three or four to six fluid drachms immediately before the accession of the cold stage; (9) as a tonic, from thirty minims to two fluid drachms twice or thrice daily.

**Infusion of Indian Barberry** (*Infusum Berberis*). Take of the Root-bark of Indian Barberry, cut small, half an ounce; Boiling Water, ten fluid ounces. Infuse in a covered vessel for one hour, and strain.

*Dose.* —From one and a half to three fluid ounces twice or thrice daily.

**Extract of Indian Barberry** (*Extractum Berberis*). Take of the Root-bark of Indian Barberry, cut small, one pound; Proof Spirit, four pints. Macerate the root-bark in two pints of the spirit for twenty-four hours; pack in a percolator, and pass the remainder of the spirit slowly through it; distil off the spirit, and evaporate the residue until the extract is of a suitable consistence for forming pills.

*Dose.*—From twenty to thirty grains daily.

[A watery extract from the wood and bark of several species of Berberis, sold in the bazaars under the name of *Rasot* or *Rusot*, has long been held in high esteem by the natives as a febrifuge, and as a local application in eye diseases. (10) It generally contains a large proportion of impurities, and in this state may be resorted to, in the absence of purer forms, in doses of half a drachm to a drachm; but it is safer to treat bazaar Rusot with alcohol, which dissolves the pure extract, and leaves the impurities behind. The alcoholic solution can then be evaporated to a pillular consistence.]

## PAPAVERACEÆ.

### PAPAVER RHŒAS, *Linn.* RED POPPY.

(*Engl. Bot.*, t. 645; *ed. Syme*, t. 58.)

*Habitat.*—Europe and temperate Asia.

*Officinal Part.*—The petals (*Rhœados Petala*). Scarlet, and with a heavy poppy odour.

*Preparation.* — **Syrup of Red Poppy** (*Syrupus Rhœados*). Take of fresh Red Poppy Petals, thirteen ounces; Refined Sugar, two pounds and a quarter; Water, one pint, or a sufficiency; Rectified Spirit, two fluid ounces and a half. Add the petals gradually to the water heated in a water bath, frequently stirring; and afterwards, the vessel being removed, infuse for twelve hours. Then press out the liquor, strain, add the sugar, and dissolve by means of heat. When nearly cold, add the spirit, and as much water as may be necessary to make up for loss in the process, so that the product shall weigh three pounds ten ounces. It should have the specific gravity 1·330.

*Dose.* — One fluid drachm. It is only employed as a colouring agent. From the fact of its readily fermenting at high temperatures, it is unsuited for use in tropical climates, excepting when freshly prepared.

### PAPAVER SOMNIFERUM, *Linn.* WHITE POPPY.

(*Engl. Bot.*, t. 2145; *ed. Syme*, t. 57.)

*Habitat.*—South-eastern Europe and Western Asia.

*Officinal Part.*—The nearly ripe capsules (*Papaveris Capsulæ*), dried and deprived of the seeds. They are globular or ovoid, from one to two or more inches in diameter, crowned by a sessile, stellate stigma; of an opiate taste. From the capsules of the growing plant opium is obtained.

*Medical Properties.*—Sedative and anodyne.

*Therapeutic Uses.*—Externally applied in the form of fomentation in various external inflammations, bruises, sprains, and other painful affections.

*Preparations.*—**Decoction of Poppies** (*Decoctum Papaveris*). Take of Poppy Capsules, bruised, two ounces; Water, one pint and a half. Boil for ten minutes in a covered vessel; then strain, and pour as much water over the contents of the strainer as will make the strained product measure a pint.

Employed externally as a sedative fomentation.

**Extract of Poppies** (*Extractum Papaveris*). Take of Poppy Capsules, dried, freed from the seeds and coarsely powdered, one pound; Rectified Spirit, two ounces; Boiling Water, a sufficiency. Mix the poppy capsules with two pints of the water, and infuse for twenty-four hours, stirring them frequently; then pack them in a percolator, and, adding more of the water, allow the liquor slowly to pass until about a gallon has been collected, or the poppies are exhausted. Evaporate the liquor by a water bath until it is reduced to a pint, and, when cold, add the spirit. Let the mixture stand for twenty-four hours; then separate the clear liquor by filtration, and evaporate this by a water bath until the extract has acquired a suitable consistence for forming pills.

*Dose.*—From two to five grains.

**Syrup of Poppies** (*Syrupus Papaveris*). Take of Poppy Capsules, dried, freed from the seeds and coarsely powdered, thirty-six ounces; Rectified Spirit, sixteen fluid ounces; Refined Sugar, four pounds; Boiling Water, a sufficiency. Mix the poppy capsules with four pints of the water, and infuse for twenty-four hours, stirring them frequently; then pack them in a percolator, and, adding more of the water, allow the liquor slowly to pass until about two gallons have been collected, or the poppies are exhausted. Evaporate the liquor by a water bath until it is reduced to three pints. When quite cold, add the spirit, let the mixture stand for twelve hours, and filter. Distil off the spirit, evaporate the remaining liquor to two pints, and then add the sugar. The product should weigh six pounds and a half, and should have the specific gravity 1·320.

*Dose.*—A fluid drachm or more. It readily ferments at high temperatures, and is unsuited for use in tropical climates, unless freshly prepared.

**Opium.**—The inspissated juice obtained by incision from the capsules of the growing plant. It has the following characters: irregular lumps, weighing from four ounces to two pounds, enveloped in poppy leaves, and generally covered with the chaffy, seed-like fruits of a species of Rumex. When fresh, plastic, tearing with an irregular, slightly moist, chesnut-brown surface, shining when rubbed smooth with the finger, having a peculiar odour and nauseous bitter taste.

The preceding characters have reference to Smyrna, or Turkey, Opium, which is the kind chiefly employed in Great Britain; but they are inapplicable to Indian Opium, employed by practitioners in the East, and which is rarely met with in European commerce. There are several kinds of Indian Opium. Of these, the chief are,—

1. * *Patna Garden Opium;* and 2. **Malwa Opium.*—The former, prepared exclusively for medicinal purposes. occurs in square packages of from two to four pounds weight, covered with layers of talc, and further defended by a case of brown wax about half an inch in thickness. It is solid, brittle in the cold season, of a brown colour and well marked (opiate) odour; it yields a large proportion (7 to 8, or even 10, per cent.) of Morphia. Of Malwa Opium there are many varieties. Of these, the two principal are, first, that in flat circular cakes, of about a pound and a half in weight, without any exterior covering; dull opaque, blackish-brown, externally; internally somewhat darker and soft; odour resembling that of Smyrna Opium, but less powerful, and combined with a slight smoky smell; taste, intensely and permanently bitter: it yields only from 3 to 5 per cent. of Morphia. The other, a superior kind of Malwa Opium, occurs in balls or cakes of smaller size, about ten ounces in weight, covered with a coarse dust composed of broken poppy petals; colour internally, dark brown; texture, homogeneous; odour and taste similar to the other variety; it yields from 7 to 8 per cent. of Morphia. The other varieties of Indian Opium, the Himalayan or "Hill Opium,"(11) and the

opium collected in Kandeish, Kutch, &c., are less applicable than the preceding to medicinal purposes, on account of their varying strength. The only sure test for Opium is the determination of the amount of Morphia which it contains. (12) The British Pharmacopœia indicates from 6 to 8 per cent. as the proportion of morphia in soft opium suitable for medicinal purposes.

*Chemical Composition.*—Opium contains a peculiar acid, *Meconic Acid;* four alkaloids, viz., *Morphia, Codeia, Papaverina,* and *Thebaia* or *Paramorphia*; and several neutral crystallizable bodies, viz., *Narcotine, Narceia, Meconine* or *Opianyl, Opianine* and *Porphyroxine.* It also contains several resins, gummy, fatty, and extractive matters, caoutchouc, a trace of volatile oil and inorganic salts. Of these principles Morphia and Codeia are narcotic and sedative, and Narcotine tonic and anti-periodic. The action of the other principles is unknown, but the resinous matter appears to possess considerable power.

*Properties.*—The primary effect of opium in medicinal doses is stimulant; its secondary effect, narcotic, anodyne, and anti-spasmodic. It operates chiefly on the cerebro-spinal system, and, through the nerves arising therefrom, it affects more or less every organ of the body. It tends to diminish every secretion of the body, excepting that of the skin, which increases under its use. In over-doses it is a powerful poison.

*Therapeutic Uses.*—These are multifarious and important. In inflammation, especially of serous membranes, it has been employed extensively, either alone, or in combination with calomel, antimony, and other remedies. As a general rule it is less applicable to inflammatory, and other diseases, in which the tendency to death is by coma or by apnœa, than to those which produce death by asthenia. In the latter, as in peritonitis, it holds the first place as a remedial agent. In fevers, especially in the advanced stages, it is of the highest value, either alone, or in combination with antimony, camphor, &c., allaying vascular and nervous excitement, and procuring sleep; but, as a general rule, it is inadmissible when contraction of the pupil is strongly marked. In painful spasmodic affections, opium in large and repeated doses often affords immediate relief. In various morbid states of the abdominal viscera, *e.g.*, simple or cancerous ulceration of the stomach, chronic gastritis, gastrodynia, nervous and sympathetic vomiting, diarrhœa, dysentery, colica pictonum, strangulated hernia, visceral obstructions, &c., it is often given with the best results. In diseases of the genito-urinary system, *e.g.*, cystitis, cystirrhœa, spasmodic stricture of the urethra, also in menorrhagia, dysmenorrhœa, irritable states of the uterus, metritis, &c., it is a remedy of the highest value. Tetanus, acute rheumatism, and delirium tremens are amongst the other diseases in which opium has been employed as a sheet anchor. In cholera it has been used, but with doubtful results. In cancerous and gangrenous ulceration, opium, by allaying constitutional disturbances, often exercises a favourable influence on the local symptoms. As an external application, opium proves valuable in various rheumatic, neuralgic, and other painful affections; also in ophthalmia and other diseases of the eye.

*Dose.*—From a quarter of a grain to two grains or more, according to circumstances. In many painful affections the sole criterion for the regulation of the dose is the amount of relief afforded. In some cases very large quantities are borne without inconvenience.

*Preparations of Opium.*†—**Extract of Opium** (*Extractum Opii*). Take of Opium, in thin slices, one pound; Water, six pints. Macerate the opium in two pints of the water for twenty-four hours, and express the liquor. Reduce the residue of the opium to a uniform pulp, macerate it again in two pints of the water for twenty-four hours, and express. Repeat the operation a third time. Mix the liquors, strain through flannel, and evaporate by a water bath until the extract has acquired a suitable consistence for forming pills.

*Dose.*—From half a grain to two grains. This preparation is believed to be less stimulant than powdered opium, and preferable to it as a sedative.

**Liquid Extract of Opium** (*Extractum Opii Liquidum*). Take of Extract of Opium, one ounce; Water, sixteen fluid ounces; Rectified Spirit, four fluid ounces. Macerate the extract of opium in the water for an hour, stirring frequently; then add the spirit, and filter. The product should measure one pint.

*Dose.*—From ten to forty minims. It contains twenty-two grains of extract of opium, nearly, in each fluid ounce. It is one-eighth part stronger than the Tincture of Opium.

**Tincture of Opium** (*Tinctura Opii, Laudanum*). Take of Opium, in coarse powder, one ounce and a half; Proof Spirit, one pint. Macerate for seven days in a closed vessel, with occasional agitation, then strain, press, filter, and add sufficient proof spirit to make one pint.

*Dose.*—From five to forty minims. It contains the soluble matter of thirty-three grains of opium, nearly, in one fluid ounce; about one grain to every fifteen minims. This, as well as all preparations of opium, requires to be given with great caution to infants and young children.

---

† In these formulæ, taken from the British Pharmacopœia, the Opium to be used is that of Turkey. Experience may show that some of them require to be modified in order to adapt them to the Opium of India.

**Ammoniated Tincture of Opium** (*Tinctura Opii Ammoniata*). Take of Opium, in coarse powder, one hundred grains; Saffron, cut small, Benzoic acid, of each one hundred and eighty grains; Oil of Anise, one fluid drachm; Strong Solution of Ammonia, four fluid ounces; Rectified Spirit, sixteen fluid ounces. Macerate for seven days in a well closed vessel, with occasional agitation, then strain, press, filter, and add sufficient rectified spirit to make one pint.

*Dose.*—From one half to one fluid drachm. It contains about five grains of opium in each fluid ounce.

**Wine of Opium** (*Vinum Opii*). Take of Extract of Opium, one ounce; Cinnamon Bark, bruised, Cloves, bruised, of each, seventy-five grains; Sherry, one pint. Macerate for seven days in a closed vessel, with occasional agitation, and filter.

*Dose.*—From ten to forty minims or more. It contains about twenty-two grains of the extract of opium in each fluid ounce. It is about one-fourth stronger than Vinum Opii of the *Brit. Pharm.* 1864, and also of the *Edin.* and *Dubl. Pharm.* It is about one-fifth weaker than Vinum Opii, *Lond.*, and corresponds in strength with Extractum Opii Liquidum. It is employed as a local application in ophthalmia and other affections of the eyes.

**Compound Powder of Opium** (*Pulvis Opii Compositus*). Take of Opium, in powder, one ounce and a half; Black Pepper, in powder, two ounces; Ginger, in powder, five ounces; Caraway Fruit, in powder, six ounces; Tragacanth, in powder, half an ounce. Mix them thoroughly, pass the powder through a fine sieve, and finally rub it lightly in a mortar. Keep it in a stoppered bottle.

*Dose.*—From two to five grains. Ten grains contain about one grain of opium.

**Confection of Opium** (*Confectio Opii*). Take of Compound Powder of Opium, one hundred and ninety-two grains; Syrup, one fluid ounce. Mix.

*Dose.*—From five to twenty grains. One part of opium is contained in about forty of the confection.

**Opium Lozenges** (*Trochisci Opii*). Take of Extract of Opium, seventy-two grains; Tincture of Tolu, one-half fluid ounce; Refined Sugar, in powder, sixteen ounces; Gum Acacia, in powder, two ounces; Extract of Liquorice, six ounces; Water, a sufficiency. Add the extract of opium, first softened by means of a little water, and the tincture of tolu, to the extract of liquorice heated in a water bath. When the mixture is reduced to a proper consistence, remove it to a slab, add the sugar and gum, previously rubbed together, and mix thoroughly. Divide the mass into 720 lozenges, and dry these in a hot-air chamber with a moderate heat.

*Dose.*—From one to six lozenges. Each lozenge contains one-tenth of a grain of extract of opium.

**Enema of Opium** (*Enema Opii*). Take of Tincture of Opium, half a fluid drachm; Mucilage of Starch, two fluid ounces. Mix.

**Liniment of Opium** (*Linimentum Opii*). Take of Tincture of Opium and Liniment of Soap, of each, two fluid ounces. Mix.

A very useful external application in rheumatic and other painful affections.

**Opium Plaster** (*Emplastrum Opii*). Take of Opium, in fine powder, one ounce; Resin Plaster, nine ounces. Melt the resin plaster by means of a water bath; then add the opium by degrees, and mix thoroughly.

Applicable to the same class of cases as Linimentum Opii.

In addition to the above, Opium enters into the following preparations:—Pilula Ipecacuanhæ cum Scillâ, Pilula Plumbi cum Opio, Pilula Saponis composita, Pulvis Cretæ Aromaticus cum Opio, Pulvis Ipecacuanhæ compositus, Pulvis Kino compositus, Tinctura Camphoræ compositâ, Unguentum Gallæ cum Opio, and Suppositoria Plumbi composita.

*Other Medicinal Preparations of Opium.*—**Hydrochlorate of Morphia** (*Morphiæ Hydrochloras, Morphiæ Murias, Edin. et Dubl. Ph.*) $C_{34}H_{19}NO_6,HCl+6HO$ or $\mathbf{C_{17}H_{19}NO_3.HCl.3H_2O}$. It occurs in white flexible acicular prisms of a silky lustre, not changed by exposure to the air, and soluble in water and spirit. The aqueous solution gives a white curdy precipitate with nitrate of silver, and if of the strength of 1 part in 200 it becomes intense, but fugacious indigo-blue with solution of perchloride of iron. Moistened with strong nitric acid it becomes orange-red, and, with solution of perchloride of iron, greenish-blue. Entirely destructible by heat, leaving no residue. Twenty grains of the salt dissolved in half an ounce of warm water, with ammonia added in the slightest possible excess, give on cooling a crystalline precipitate, which, when washed with a little cold water, and dried by exposure to the air, weighs 15·18 grains.

*Medical Properties and Uses.*—The same as Tincture of Opium, over which it is considered to possess the advantages of producing a less degree of vascular and arterial excitement, less headache and vertigo, less subsequent depression, and less constipation. Notwithstanding, opium in many cases proves effectual when morphia and its salts fail. It is chiefly adapted for allaying nervous irritability, and inducing tranquillity of the system. In large doses it is a powerful narcotic poison. Its full physiological effects are speedily induced if it be introduced into the system by the hypodermic method.

*Dose.*—From one-eighth of a grain to one grain.

*Preparations.*—**Solution of the Hydrochlorate of Morphia** (*Liquor Morphiæ Hydrochloratis*). Take of Hydrochlorate of Morphia, four grains; Dilute Hydrochloric Acid, eight minims; Rectified Spirit, two fluid drachms; Water, six fluid drachms. Mix the hydrochloric acid, the spirit, and the water, and dissolve the hydrochlorate of morphia in the mixture.

*Dose.*—From ten to sixty minims. Half a grain of the hydrochlorate of morphia is contained in each fluid drachm. It is one half the strength of the Liquor Morphiæ Hydrochloratis of the London Pharmacopœia.

**Morphia Lozenges** (*Trochisci Morphiæ*). Take of Hydrochlorate of Morphia, twenty grains; Tincture of Tolu, half a fluid ounce; Refined Sugar, in powder, twenty-four ounces; Gum Acacia, in powder, one ounce; Mucilage of Gum Acacia, a sufficiency; Distilled Water, half a fluid ounce. Dissolve the hydrochlorate of morphia in the water; add this solution to the tincture of tolu, previously mixed with the mucilage; and with the gum and the sugar, also previously well mixed, form a proper mass. Divide into 720 lozenges, and dry these in a hot-air chamber with a moderate heat.

Each lozenge contains one thirty-sixth of a grain of hydrochlorate of morphia.

**Morphia and Ipecacuanha Lozenges** (*Trochisci Morphiæ et Ipecacuanhæ*). Take of Hydrochlorate of Morphia, twenty grains; Ipecacuanha, in fine powder, sixty grains; Tincture of Tolu, half a fluid ounce; Refined Sugar, in powder, twenty-four ounces; Gum Acacia, in powder, one ounce; Mucilage of Gum Acacia, a sufficiency; Distilled Water, half a fluid ounce. Dissolve the hydrochlorate of morphia in the water; add this solution to the tincture of tolu, previously mixed with the mucilage; and with the ipecacuanha, the gum, and the sugar, also previously well mixed, form a proper mass. Divide into 720 lozenges, and dry these in a hot-air chamber with a moderate heat.

Each lozenge contains one thirty-sixth of a grain of hydrochlorate of morphia, and one-twelfth of a grain of ipecacuanha.

This and the preceding preparation allowed to dissolve in the mouth, prove serviceable in allaying cough and irritation of the throat and fauces. From ten to twenty lozenges may be taken daily, as circumstances may require.

**Morphia Suppositories** (*Suppositoria Morphiæ*). Take of Hydrochlorate of Morphia, six grains; Benzoated Lard, sixty-four grains; White Wax, twenty grains; Oil of Theobroma, ninety grains. Melt the wax and oil of theobroma with a gentle heat, then add the hydrochlorate of morphia and benzoated lard previously rubbed together in a mortar, and mix all the ingredients thoroughly. Pour the mixture while it is fluid into suitable moulds of the capacity of fifteen grains; or the fluid mixture may be allowed to cool, and then be divided into twelve equal parts, each of which shall be made into a conical or other convenient form for a suppository.

Each suppository contains half a grain of hydrochlorate of morphia. Introduced into the rectum, it acts as a valuable local means of relief in painful affection of that viscus, as well as of the uterus, bladder, and contiguous parts. Care should be taken that it is well introduced beyond the sphincter ani.

**Acetate of Morphia** (*Morphiæ Acetas*). $C_{34}H_{19}NO_6, C_4H_3O_3+HO$ or $\mathbf{C_{17}H_{19}NO_3.C_2H_4O_2}$. A white powder, soluble in water and in spirit. From its solution potash throws down a precipitate which is dissolved by excess of the alkali. It is affected by nitric acid and perchloride of iron in the same way as hydrochlorate of morphia is. When sulphuric acid is added to the salt, acetous vapours are evolved.

*Dose.*—From one eighth to one half of a grain or more.

*Preparation.*—**Solution of the Acetate of Morphia** (*Liquor Morphiæ Acetatis.*) Take of Acetate of Morphia, four grains; Diluted Acetic Acid, eight minims; Rectified Spirit, two fluid drachms; Water six fluid drachms. Mix the acid, the spirit, and the water, and dissolve the acetate of morphia in the mixture

*Dose.*—From ten to sixty minims. One grain of the acetate is contained in two fluid drachms of the solution. This solution contains half as much morphia as the Liquor Morphiæ Acetatis, *Lond. Pharm.*

* **Narcotine** (*Narcotina, Anarcotina*). A neutral crystalizable body contained in Opium in the proportion of from 1 to 8 per cent. It occurs in colourless, flat prisms, pearly in lustre, inodorous, insipid, insoluble in water or potash solution, soluble in rectified spirit, and more so in ether. With diluted acids it forms very bitter solutions, which do not yield crystalline salts, or become blue with perchloride of iron.

*Properties.*—Tonic and antiperiodic. When pure, it is wholly devoid of narcotic properties. In large doses diaphoretic.

*Therapeutic Uses.*—In intermittent fevers, in general debility, especially in that produced by prolonged lactation, and in convalescence after acute febrile and inflammatory diseases, it has been used with excellent effect in the East. (13)

*Dose.*—As a tonic, from half one grain to a grain thrice daily; as an antiperiodic, from two to three grains dissolved in water by the addition of hydrochloric or sulphuric acid, repeated thrice daily.

(*Non-officinal.*)

**Argemone Mexicana**, *Linn.* (*Wight, Illust.*, vol. i. t. 11.) A tropical American plant, now a common weed throughout India. The seeds yield on expression a fixed oil, which has long been in use amongst West Indian practitioners as an aperient.(14) The unfavorable report of Sir W. O'Shaughnessy (*Bengal Disp.*, p. 183) led to it being neglected; but more recent trials of its properties by several medical officers in Bengal serve to prove that in half drachm doses it acts as a gentle aperient, and at the same time allays, apparently by a sedative action, the pain in colic. The smallness of the dose, and the mildness of its operation, are recommendations to its employment. Age apparently affects its activity, the freshly prepared oil proving more energetic and uniform in operation than that which has been long on hand. Applied to herpetic eruptions and other forms of skin disease, it is reported to exercise a well-marked soothing influence, according to Dr. Bonavia and others (*Indian Med. Gaz.*, 1866, vol. i. p. 206). As a local application to indolent and ill-conditioned ulcers, the expressed yellow glutinous juice of the plant is held in much esteem by the natives. Dr. W. Dymock, of Bombay, reports having used it thus with good effect. The native practice of applying this juice to the eye in ophthalmia is dangerous. Both in a chemical and therapeutical point of view this plant appears worthy of investigation.

**Meconopsis aculeata**, *Royle* (*Illust.*, t. 15†), and **M. Nipalensis**, *D.C.*, (*Hooker, fil., Illust. of Himal. Plants*, t. 9,) both Himalayan species, have had powerfully narcotic and poisonous properties attributed to them, especially to the roots; but Sir W. O'Shaughnessy (*Op. cit.*, p. 184) administered a drachm of the alcoholic extract of the root of *M. aculeata* to a dog, without producing any sensible effect. The subject, however, is still open for investigation.

---

† The flowers are purple, and not red, as those represented in the plate.

**Corydalis Govaniana,** *Wall.* A Himalayan plant (Bhútkis, *Vern.*), in the roots of which Sir W. O'Shaughnessy detected a crystallizable principle, *Corydalia.* It occurs in pearly crystals, is soluble in acids with which it forms salts, which do not crystallize, and which are intensely bitter to the taste. Twenty grains in solution were given to dogs without inconvenience. Sir W. O'Shaughnessy expresses a hope that further trials will be made with this article as a tonic and antiperiodic.

## CRUCIFERÆ.

### COCHLEARIA ARMORACIA, *Linn.* HORSERADISH.

(*Engl. Bot.*, t. 2323; *ed. Syme*, t. 123.)

*Habitat.*—Cultivated in all parts of Europe and North America.

*Officinal Part.*—The fresh root (*Armoraciæ Radix, Horseradish Root*). A long cylindrical fleshy root, half an inch to one inch in diameter, expanding at the crown into several very short stems; internally white, of a pungent taste and smell. By distillation it yields a volatile oil of exceedingly powerful scent and taste.

*Properties.*—Stimulant, sudorific, and diuretic. Externally applied, irritant and vesicant; sialagogue when chewed.

*Therapeutic Uses.*—In atonic dropsical affections, chronic rheumatism, scurvy, &c., it has been given internally. Locally it has been used, chewed in substance, in toothache; in hoarseness arising from relaxation, in the form of gargle; and in paralysis &c., as a stimulant embrocation or cataplasm.

*Preparations.*—**Compound Spirit of Horseradish** (*Spiritus Armoraciæ Compositus*). Take of Horseradish † scraped, Bitter Orange Peel bruised, of each, twenty ounces; Nutmeg, bruised, half an ounce; Proof Spirit, one gallon; Water, two pints. Mix, and distil a gallon with a moderate heat.

*Dose.*—From one to two fluid drachms.

[† The fresh root of *Moringa pterygosperma, Gærtn.*, forms an efficient substitute.]

### SINAPIS ALBA, *Linn.* WHITE MUSTARD.

(*Engl. Bot.*, t. 1677; *ed. Syme*, t. 84.)

### SINAPIS NIGRA, *Linn.* BLACK MUSTARD.

(*Engl. Bot.*, t. 969; *ed. Syme*, t. 85.)

(Brassica, *Bentham et Hooker.*)

*Habitat.*—Europe; extensively cultivated in many parts of the globe.

*Officinal Part.*—A mixture of the seeds of both species reduced to powder (*Sinapis, Mustard*). It is of a greenish yellow colour; of an acrid, bitterish, oily, pungent taste; inodorous when dry, but exhaling, when moist, a pungent, penetrating, peculiar odour, very irritating to the nostrils and eyes. A decoction cooled is not made blue by tincture of iodine.

*Properties.*—Externally applied, rubefacient; and vesicant if kept long in contact with the skin. In moderate quantities, taken with food, it acts as a digestive; in doses varying from one to three teaspoonfuls in a tumblerful of water, it operates as a speedy and safe emetic.

*Therapeutic Uses.*—Applied externally, Mustard Poultices (*infra*) prove highly serviceable in the advanced stages, or low forms, of febrile and inflammatory diseases, in internal congestions, in spasmodic, neuralgic, and rheumatic affections, and in those morbid states of the cerebro-spinal system, &c. in which counter-irritants and derivatives are requisite. As an emetic, mustard is indicated in ebrietas and other cases where it is desirable simply to empty the stomach without inducing a depressing influence on the system.

*Preparation.*—**Mustard Poultice, Sinapism** (*Cataplasma Sinapis*). Take of Mustard in powder, and of Linseed Meal, of each two ounces and a half; Cold or Tepid Water, ten fluid ounces. Mix gradually the linseed meal with the water, and add the mustard, constantly stirring.

In the absence of linseed meal, rice flour may be substituted, or it may be omitted altogether; the rule being, in all cases, to remove the poultice either when it causes much pain or well-defined redness of the cuticle.

**Oil of Mustard** (*Oleum Sinapis*). The oil distilled with water from the seeds of Black Mustard after the expression of the fixed oil. It is colourless or pale yellow; Sp. gr. 1·015; dissolves readily in alcohol and ether, and to a slight extent in water; odour intensely penetrating, taste very acrid and burning; applied to the skin it produces almost instant vesication.

**Compound Liniment of Mustard** (*Linimentum Sinapis Compositum*). Take of Oil of Mustard one fluid drachm; Ethereal Extract of Mezereon, forty grains; Camphor, one hundred and twenty grains; Castor Oil, five fluid drachms; Rectified Spirit, four fluid ounces. Dissolve the extract of mezereon and camphor in the spirit, and add the oil of mustard and castor oil.

A stimulant embrecation for rheumatic and paralytic cases.

### * SINAPIS JUNCEA, *Linn.* RAI OF INDIAN MUSTARD PLANT.

(Brassica juncea, *Hooker, fil., et Thomson.*)

*Habitat.*—Cultivated in all parts of India.

*Officinal Part.*—The seeds (*Sinapis Indica*), commonly met with in the bazaars of India, which from their colour may be denominated *Brown Mustard seed,* possess properties similar to those of the Black and White Mustard seed, for which they may be employed as an efficient substitute, especially in the preparation of Mustard Poultices (*ante*). If previously deprived of their fixed oil by expression, their activity is increased. By long keeping they lose much of their pungency; hence fresh seeds should be employed.

## CAPPARIDEÆ.

(*Non-officinal.*)

**Gynandropsis pentaphylla,** *D. C.* (*Rheede, Hort. Mal.,* vol. ix. t. 24.)—A common Indian plant, of which Sir W. Jones observes that its sensible qualities seem to promise great antispasmodic virtues, it having a scent much resembling assafœtida, but comparatively delicate. According to Dr. Wight (*Illust.* i. p. 34), the bruised leaves are rubefacient and vesicant, producing a very copious exudation, and affording in many cases the relief obtained from a blister, without its inconveniences. The expressed juice is a popular remedy, in high repute as a local application in otalgia, both amongst the natives of India and the settlers in the West Indies, where the plant is also indigenous. Dr. J. Shortt states that the seeds are used as a substitute for mustard, and yield a good (fixed?) oil.

**Cratæva religiosa,** *Forst.* (*Hooker, Icon. Plant,* t. 178), is in common use amongst the natives as a stomachic and tonic. An infusion (fresh or recently dried Leaves two ounces, Boiling Water one pint) was officinal in the Bengal Ph. It is there described as slightly bitter and aromatic, and the dose placed at from two to four fluid ounces thrice daily. Its virtues are doubtful.

## CANELLACEÆ.

### CANELLA ALBA, *Murray.* WHITE CANELLA.

(*Woodville, Med. Bot.,* t. 237.)

*Habitat.*—West Indies.

*Officinal Part.*—The bark (*Canellæ Albæ Cortex*). It occurs in quills or broken pieces; hard, of a yellowish-white or pale orange colour, somewhat lighter on the internal surface; of an aromatic clove-like odour and an acrid peppery taste. Its activity resides in a volatile oil, bitter extractive and resin.

*Properties.*—Aromatic stimulant.

*Therapeutic Uses.*—Very limited, used chiefly in combination with other articles in constitutional debility, dyspepsia, scurvy, &c.

*Dose.*—From ten to thirty grains in powder.

*Preparations.*—It forms an ingredient in Vinum Rhei.

## BIXINEÆ.

### * GYNOCARDIA ODORATA, *R. Br.* CHAULMÚGRA.

(*Roxb., Corom. Plants*, t. 299.)

*Habitat.*—Forests of the Malayan Peninsula and Eastern India as far north as Assam, extending thence along the base of the Himalaya as far west as Sikkim.

*Officinal Part.*—The seeds (*Gynocardiæ Semina, Chaulmúgra Seeds*), about an inch in length, of an ovoid form, rendered more or less irregular by mutual compression. Each seed has a grayish brown, smooth and fragile testa, within which is a mass of oily albumen, enclosing an embryo with large heart-shaped three-nerved cotyledons. They yield by expression a fixed oil (*Oleum Gynocardiæ* which has a peculiar and slightly unpleasant smell and taste. The oil procured from the bazaar is usually impure.

*Properties.*—Alterative tonic; in large doses, emetic.

*Therapeutic Uses.*—In leprosy it has been used with excellent effects: it has also been advantageously employed in scrofula, skin diseases, and rheumatism. [15]

*Dose.*—Of the seeds coarsely powdered about six grains, thrice daily, in the form of a pill; gradually increased to three or four times that amount, or until it causes nausea, when the dose may be diminished, or the use of the remedy suspended for a time. This is the best form of administration. The dose of the oil is from five to six drops gradually increased, as in the case of the seeds. The oil is also used as a local stimulant, or the seeds may be used in the following form, officinal in the Bengal Pharmacopœia.

**Chaulmúgra Ointment** (*Unguentum Gynocardiæ*). Take of Chaulmúgra seeds a sufficiency, remove the husks, and beat the seed into a paste with as much Simple Ointment as is requisite to give it proper consistence.

Used in many skin diseases, especially in herpes and tinea.

(*Non-officinal.*)

**Hydnocarpus inebrians**, *Vahl*, (*Wight, Illust.*, vol. i. t. 16,) a tree of Malabar, Travancore, and Ceylon. The seeds, the *Neeradimootoo* of Ainslie (*Mat. Ind.* ii. p. 235,) resemble those of the Chaulmúgra, but are of smaller size; they are somewhat pointed at one extremity, and covered with a testa, rough, with coarse, irregular longitudinal striæ. In the fresh state the seed has a nauseous smell and unctuous slightly acrid taste. The expressed oil of the seeds is held in much repute amongst the natives as a remedy in leprosy; and considering the success which has attended the use of the Chaulmúgra, to which it is nearly allied, there appear to be good grounds for giving it a trial, especially in those parts of India where Chaulmúgra is not procurable. The dose is placed by Ainslie at half a teaspoonful twice daily. It would probably be better to commence with a smaller dose, and gradually to increase it.

**Flacourtia Cataphracta**, *Roxb.* (*Corom. Plants*, t. 222.) The small leaves and tender shoots of this shrub constitute the *Talisputrie* of the Indian Materia Medica. In doses of about half a drachm it is much used as a remedy in diarrhœa, general debility, &c. Its virtues, if any, rest solely on native testimony.

**Cochlospermum Gossypium**, *D.C.* (*Wight, in Hooker Bot. Misc.*, vol. ii. t. 18.) Yields the *Kutira* or *Kuteera Gum* of the bazaars; used as a substitute for Tragacanth in the North-western Provinces (Royle). It is an article of very minor importance.

## POLYGALEÆ.

### POLYGALA SENEGA, *Linn.* SENEGA OR SENEKA.

(*Bot. Mag.*, t. 1051.)

*Habitat.*—United States of North America.

*Officinal Part.*—The dried root (*Senegæ Radix*): a knobby root-stock with a branched tap-root, of about the thickness of a quill, twisted and keeled; bark yellowish brown; odour peculiar and nauseous; taste sweetish, afterwards acrid and pungent, exciting salivation; interior woody, tasteless, and inert. Activity depends upon an acrid principle, *Polygalic Acid.*

*Properties.*—Stimulant, expectorant, diuretic, and emmenagogue; in large doses, emetic and cathartic.

*Therapeutic Uses.*—In sub-acute and chronic affections of the lungs, in functional derangements of the heart characterised by irregular action, in dropsy supervening on fevers, and in amenorrhœa and dysmenorrhœa, it has been successfully employed.

*Dose.*—From ten to twenty grains of the powdered root.

*Preparations.*—**Infusion of Senega** (*Infusum Senegæ*). Take of Senega bruised, half an ounce; boiling Water, ten fluid ounces. Infuse in a covered vessel for an hour, and strain.

*Dose.*—From one to two fluid ounces twice daily, or oftener.

**Tincture of Senega** (*Tinctura Senegæ*). Take of Senega, in coarse powder, two ounces and a half; Proof Spirit, one pint. Macerate the senega for forty-eight hours, with fifteen ounces of the spirit, in a closed vessel, agitating occasionally; then transfer to a percolator, and when the fluid ceases to pass, continue the percolation with the remaining five ounces of the spirit. Afterwards subject the contents of the percolator to pressure, filter the product, mix the two liquids, and add sufficient proof spirit to make one pint.

*Dose.*—From one half to two fluid drachms. An excellent adjunct to stimulant, expectorant, and diuretic mixtures.

## KRAMERIA TRIANDRA, *Ruiz et Pavon.* KRAMERIA, RHATANY.

(*Woodville, Med. Bot.*, t. 35.)

*Habitat.*—Peru and Bolivia.

*Officinal Part.*—The dried root (*Krameriæ* vel *Rhataniæ Radix*): consists of numerous long woody cylindrical branches, about an inch in diameter, brownish red and rough externally, reddish-yellow internally, strongly astringent, tinging the saliva red. Properties due to Tannin, which ranges from 38 to 42 per cent.

*Properties.*—Powerfully astringent; tonic.

*Therapeutic Uses.*—It has been successfully employed in chronic diarrhœa, also in passive or atonic hæmorrhages, and locally in leucorrhœa, ozœna, ophthalmia, fissures of the anus, &c.

*Dose.*—From ten to twenty grains of the powdered root.

*Preparations.* — **Infusion of Rhatany** (*Infusum Krameriæ*). Take of Rhatany Root, bruised, half an ounce; Boiling Water, ten fluid ounces. Infuse in a covered vessel for an hour, and strain.

*Dose.*—From one to two fluid ounces twice or thrice daily.

**Tincture of Rhatany** (*Tinctura Krameriæ*). Take of Rhatany Root, bruised, two ounces and a half; Proof Spirit, one pint. Macerate the rhatany root for forty-eight hours in fifteen fluid ounces of the spirit, in a closed vessel, agitating occasionally; then transfer to a percolator, and when the fluid ceases to pass continue the percolation with the remaining five ounces of spirit. Afterwards subject the contents of the percolator to pressure, filter the product, mix the liquids, and add sufficient proof spirit to make one pint.

*Dose.*—From one half to two fluid drachms.

**Extract of Rhatany** (*Extractum Krameriæ*). Take of Rhatany Root, in coarse powder, one pound; Distilled Water, a sufficiency. Macerate the rhatany in a pint and a half of the water for twenty-four hours; then pack in a percolator, and add more distilled water, until twelve pints have been collected, or the rhatany is exhausted. Evaporate the liquor by a water bath to dryness.

*Dose.*—From five to twenty grains.

[Savanilla Rhatany, the produce of *Krameria Ixina*, Linn., inhabiting New Grenada and Brazil, is regarded by some as superior to officinal Rhatany, the produce of *K. triandra* (*ante*).]

(*Non-officinal.*)

**Polygala crotalarioides** (*Ham*), and **P. telephioides** (*Willd*). The former inhabits the Himalaya, and the latter the Madras Peninsula. They are used medicinally in catarrhal affections by the natives of the localities they respectively inhabit, and may be deserving of further attention.

## TAMARISCINEÆ.

(*Non-officinal.*)

**Tamarix Gallica,** *Linn.*, (*Wight, Illust.*, vol. i. t. 24.) A small shrub common throughout India; yields a kind of galls (*Sumrat-úl-túrfa*, Arab.; *Bara mai*, Hind.) employed medicinally by the natives as an astringent. The late Dr. Stocks, in a letter to Dr. J. Forbes Watson (13th January 1852), speaks highly of the astringent properties of the Tamarix Gall, and from personal experience recommends a strong infusion of them as a local application to foul, sloughing ulcers and phagedenic buboes. They act in virtue of the tannic and gallic acid which they contain. By the natives they are also administered internally in dysentery and diarrhœa. The shrub yields also a kind of manna, called *Gazanjabin* (the *Guz-ungu-been* of the Ulfaz Udwiyeh, No. 1296), which, however, is not produced in India, nor is it met with in the bazaars.

**Tamarix Orientalis,** *Vahl.* (*T. Furas, Ham*), also yields galls similar to, but of smaller size than the preceding. Their native names are *Sumrat-úl-asl* (Arab.) and *Chota mai* (Hind.) They are also employed as an astringent (Royle). The bark is bitter, astringent, and probably tonic. (Walker, *Bombay Med. Phys. Trans.*, 1840, p. 66.)

# GUTTIFERÆ

## GARCINIA MORELLA, *Desv.*, var. PEDICELLATA. (16)
### GAMBOGE TREE OF SIAM.

(*Hanbury, Linn. Trans.*, vol. xxiv. t. 50.)

*Habitat.*—Siam.

*Officinal Part.*—The gum-resin (*Cambogia, Gamboge*) occurs in cylindrical pieces, breaking easily with a smooth conchoidal glistening fracture of a tawny colour, changing to yellow when it is rubbed with water; inodorous, of an acrid taste. An emulsion made with boiling water and cooled does not become green with the solution of iodine. It contains a resin (*Cambogic acid*), on which its activity principally depends. The best kinds contain from 71 to 74 per cent. of this principle.

*Properties.*—Valuable hydragogue, cathartic, and anthelmintic.

*Therapeutic Uses.*—In dropsical affections it is a remedy of established value; it has also been used in obstinate constipation, amenorrhœa, and as a vermifuge.

*Dose.*—From one to four grains finely powdered. To obviate the vomiting and griping, which it is apt to occasion when given alone in this state, it should be combined with carbonate of potash, hard soap, or calomel.

*Preparations.*—**Compound Gamboge Pill** (*Pilula Cambogiæ Composita*). Take of Gamboge, one ounce; Barbadoes Aloes,† one ounce; Compound Powder of Cinnamon, one ounce; Hard Soap, in powder, two ounces, Syrup, a sufficiency. Pulverise the gamboge and aloes separately, mix them with the aromatic powder, and afterwards the syrup, and beat the whole into a uniform mass.

*Dose.*—From five to ten grains.

[† Indigenous (Indian) aloes may be substituted for the Barbadoes aloes ordered above.]

## * GARCINIA PICTORIA, *Roxb.* INDIAN GAMBOGE TREE.

(*Wight, Icones,* vol. i. t. 102.)

*Habitat.*—Mysore, Canara, and other parts of the Madras Peninsula.

*Officinal Part.*—The Gum-resin (*Cambogia Indica* vel *Mysoriensis*) resembles Siam Gamboge in all its physical characters, excepting that it occurs in irregular masses of various sizes, in place of cylindrical pieces. It readily forms an emulsion with water; and, analyzed by Prof. Christison, has been found to contain from 77 to 80 per cent. of the resin (*Cambogic acid*), in which the principal activity of the drug appears to reside.

*Properties and Uses.*—Are identical with those of the Siam Gamboge, for which it forms an excellent substitute in the treatment of dropsical affections, obstinate constipation, &c. ([17]).

*Dose.*—From three to four grains, best given in combination with the bitartrate of potash.

## * GARCINIA PURPUREA, *Roxb.* KOKUM BUTTER TREE.

*Habitat.*—Forests of Malabar, the Concans, and other parts of the Madras Peninsula.

*Officinal Part.*—The oil of the seeds (*Garciniæ purpureæ Oleum, Kokum Butter*), obtained by the following process. The seeds are first exposed for some days to the action of the sun to dry; they are then bruised and boiled in water; the oil collects on the surface, and on cooling concretes into a solid cake. When purified it is rather brittle, of a pale yellowish colour, bland and mild to the taste, melting in the mouth like butter, and leaving an impression of cold on the tongue, not unlike that experienced on allowing a small piece of ice to dissolve in the mouth. It melts at 98° F. The seeds yield about 10 per cent. of the oil.

*Properties and Uses.*—This concrete oil is introduced here chiefly with the view of bringing it into use for the preparation of ointments, suppositories, and for other pharmaceutical purposes. It has been used as a local application to ulcerations, fissures of the lips, hands, &c. It is described by Dr. W. Dymock as an excellent substitute for spermaceti ointment. ([18])

(*Non-officinal.*)

**Garcinia Mangostana,** *Linn.* (*Bot. Mag.*, t. 4847.)—The thick fleshy pericarp of the delicious fruit of this tree, the Mangosteen, is an astringent of considerable value. Analyzed by Schmidt (*Chemist*, 1855, vol. ii. p. 475), it has been found to contain tannin, resin, and a crystallizable principle, *Mangostine.* In the advanced stages of dysentery, and in the chronic diarrhœa of natives, the Editor has employed the following formula with manifest advantage: Take of dried Mangosteen rind, two ounces; Coriander fruit and Cummin fruit, of each, one drachm and a half; Water, two pints, and boil slowly to one pint. *Dose.*—Four ounces twice daily, with or without Tr. Opii. Dr. Rean reports that he has found the effect of this remedy very decided in simple diarrhœa. In dysentery it is thought less favourably of by Sub-Assistant Surgeon Odoy Chun Dutt. Dr. Waitz (*Diseases of Children in Hot Climates*, p. 164) recommends a strong decoction as an external astringent application.

**Calophyllum Inophyllum,** *Linn.* (*Wight, Icones*, vol. i. p. 77.) —The kernels of this tree, which is widely distributed over India, yield a grateful smelling fixed oil, held by the natives in high esteem as an external application in rheumatism. From the bark exudes a resinous substance, which has been thought, apparently erroneously, to be the *Tacamahaca* of old pharmacologists. It is stated in the Bengal Dispensatory (p. 238) to resemble myrrh, and to be a useful application to indolent ulcers. True East Indian Tacamahaca is said by Lindley (*Veg. Kingdom*, p. 401) to be the produce of *Calophyllum Calaba*, Linn., a tree indigenous in Malabar and other parts of the Madras Peninsula.

**Mesua ferrea,** *Linn.*, (*Wight, Icones*, vol. i. t. 118,) and **Calysaccion longifolium** (*Wight, Icones*, t. 1999.) — The fragrant flowers of these trees, dried, constitute the *Nagesur* or *Nag-Kesar* sold in the bazaars. They are supposed to possess mild stimulant properties, but are chiefly valued as a perfume, and in the arts for dyeing silks. They are of little medicinal importance. (See Pereira, *Pharm. Journ.*, vol. x. p. 449; Cleghorn, *Ibid.*, p. 597; and B. Seemann, *Ibid.*, vol. xii. p. 62.) Dr. Æ. Ross reports that the expressed oil of the seeds of *Mesua ferrea* is much employed by the people of North Canara as an embrocation in rheumatism; he also speaks of the bark and roots as being, in infusion or decoction, an excellent bitter tonic.

# DIPTEROCARPEÆ.

## * DIPTEROCARPUS LÆVIS, *Ham.*, and other species of DIPTEROCARPUS. GURJUN OR WOOD OIL TREE. (*Roxb.*, *Corom. Plants*, t. 213.)

*Habitat.*—Forests of Eastern India from Bengal to Tenasserim.

*Officinal Part.*—Balsamic exudation (*Dipterocarpi Balsamum, Gurjun Balsam, Wood Oil*), obtained from the trunk by incision and the application of heat. It is an oleo-resin, constituting a transparent liquid, lighter than water, of a dark-brown sherry colour, slightly fluorescent, and consequently presenting a greenish opalescence on the surface; it has the consistence of olive oil, with an odour and taste resembling copaiba, but less powerful. Heated in a vial to 270°, it becomes turbid and gelatinous. It affords a turbid solution when shaken with an equal volume of benzole.

*Properties.*—Stimulant of mucous surfaces, particularly that of the genito-urinary system; diuretic.

*Therapeutic Uses.*—In gonorrhœa and other affections in which copaiba is generally employed, it has proved an effectual remedy. (19)

*Dose.*—From half a drachm to a drachm twice or thrice daily, uncombined or in emulsion.

*(Non-officinal.)*

**Shorea robusta**, *Roxb.* (*Corom. Plants*, t. 212).—The resinous exudation of this tree constitutes the *Dammar* of the Bengal bazaars. Specimens examined by Sir W. O'Shaughnessy were perfectly transparent and colourless, but that generally sold in the bazaars ranges from pale amber to dark brown. It is devoid of taste and smell, sparingly soluble in alcohol, almost entirely so in ether, and perfectly so in turpentine and the fixed oils. It unites with the fixed oils, and forms plasters. The superior kinds are efficient substitutes for the Pine resins of the European Pharmacopœias (*Bengal Disp.*, p. 221). A portion of the Black Dammar met with in the bazaars is said to be the produce of **Vatica Tumbugaia,** W. et A., (*Wight, Icones*, vol. i. t. 2,) another tree of this Natural Order; but the ordinary source is *Canarium strictum*, Roxb., Nat. Ord. Burseraceæ.

**Vateria Indica**, *Linn.* (*Wight, Illust.*, vol. i. t. 36), is the principal source of the White Dammar met with in the bazaars of Southern India. Specimens differ much in colour, fragrance, and density; some being of a light greenish colour, dense, homogeneous, and vitreous on fracture, whilst others are yellow-amber coloured, and vesicular. These differences apparently arise from the mode of collection, and the age of the trees producing them. It burns with a clear steady light, giving off a pleasant smell, but very little smoke. With the aid of heat, and the addition of a small portion of camphor, it is soluble in spirit. Under the influence of gentle heat it combines with wax and oil, and forms an excellent resinous ointment; it forms a good substitute for officinal Resin (*Dr. G. Bidie*). From the fruit, bruised and subjected to boiling, is obtained a solid fatty oil, named *Piney-tallow* or *Vegetable Butter of Canara*, which has obtained considerable repute as a local application in chronic rheumatism and some other painful affections. It might be employed as a basis for ointments, &c.

**Hopea odorata**, *Roxb.* (*Corom. Plants*, t. 210,) yields a fragrant resin, which, reduced to powder, forms a popular styptic amongst the Burmese; its action is probably purely mechanical.

## MALVACEÆ.

GOSSYPIUM HERBACEUM, *Linn.*
GOSSYPIUM ARBOREUM, *Linn.* } COTTON PLANT.
GOSSYPIUM BARBADENSE, *Linn.*

(*Royle, Illust.*, t. 23. *Wight, Illust.*, vol. i. t. 27, 28.)

*Habitat.*—Extensively cultivated within the tropics, and in the hot temperate zone in both hemispheres.

*Officinal Part.*—The hairs of the seeds of the different species of Gossypium (*Gossypium, Cotton*). It consists of white tubular hairs, which by drying become flattened: if in this state they are immersed in water and examined by the microscope, they appear like distinct flattened narrow ribands, with only occasional appearances of joints, which are indicated by a line at a right angle, or nearly so, to the side of the tube.

*Properties and Uses.*—The chief use made of cotton in medicine is as a local application to burns, in which it proves serviceable chiefly by excluding the air and maintaining an equable temperature. It has, on this principle, been applied to erysipelatous and inflamed surfaces.

*Preparations.*—**Gun-Cotton** (*Pyroxylin*). Take of Cotton, one ounce; Sulphuric Acid, Nitric Acid, of each, five fluid ounces. Mix the acids in a porcelain mortar, immerse the cotton in the mixture, and stir it for three minutes with a glass rod, until it is thoroughly wetted by the acids. Transfer the cotton to a vessel containing water; stir it well with a glass rod; decant the liquid; pour more water upon the mass; agitate again, and repeat the affusion, agitation, and decantation, until the washing ceases to give a precipitate with chloride of barium. Drain the product on filtering paper, and dry in a water bath. *Tests.*—Readily soluble in a mixture of ether and rectified spirit; leaves no residue when exploded by heat.

**Collodion** (*Collodium*). Take of Pyroxylin, one ounce; Ether, thirty-six fluid ounces; Rectified Spirit, twelve fluid ounces. Mix the ether and the spirit, and add the pyroxylin. Set aside for a few days, and should there be any sediment, decant the clear solution. Keep it in a well corked bottle. It is a colourless, highly inflammable, liquid, with ethereal odour; it dries rapidly on exposure to the air, leaving a thin transparent film, insoluble in water or rectified spirit.

Collodion has been extensively used as a local application to incised wounds, ulcers, skin diseases, fissures of the lips and nipples, burns, erysipelas, &c. A great objection to its application in its pure state is its liability to crack. This is remedied in a great measure by the use of the following:—

*Preparation.*—**Flexible Collodion** (*Collodion flexile*). Take of Collodion, six fluid ounces; Canada Balsam, one hundred and twenty grains; Castor Oil, one fluid drachm. Mix and keep in a well corked bottle.

## HIBISCUS ESCULENTUS, *Linn* EDIBLE HIBISCUS, OKRA.

*Habitat.*—West Indies; cultivated extensively throughout the tropics as an article of diet.

*Officinal Part.*—The fresh immature capsules (*Hibisci Capsulæ*), from 4 to 6 inches in length, about an inch in diameter at the base, tapering, furrowed; somewhat bristly, particularly at the ridges, which correspond in number with that of the cells and valves, viz., from five to eight, with a single row of smooth round seeds in each cell; abounding in a copious bland viscid mucilage, which exists more or less in all parts of the plant.

*Properties.*—Valuable emollient and demulcent; diuretic.

*Therapeutic Uses.*—In catarrhal affections, ardor urinæ, dysuria, gonorrhœa, and other cases requiring demulcent and emollient remedies, it may be resorted to with confidence.

*Preparation.*—**Decoction of Hibiscus** (*Decoctum Hibisci*). Take of the fresh immature Capsules, sliced transversely, three ounces; Water, a pint and a half. Boil to a pint, and strain; sweeten to taste.

*Dose.*—From three to six ounces, or *ad libitum*, as an ordinary drink. The inhalation of the vapour of the hot decoction has been found very serviceable in allaying cough, hoarseness, irritation of the glottis, and other affections of the throat and fauces. The dried capsules may be employed when they are not procurable in a fresh state.

According to the testimony of Dr. Gibson and others, the fresh capsules bruised form an efficient emollient poultice.

(*Non-officinal.*)

**Sida acuta,** *Burm.* (*Wight, Icones*, vol. i. t. 95.)—The root of this plant combines mucilaginous and bitter properties. In some trials made with it in Calcutta, it was found, when given in the form of infusion, to promote perspiration, to increase the appetite, and in many respects to be a useful substitute for more costly bitters (*Bengal Disp.*, p. 215). It seems worthy of further trials. The roots of other species of *Sida,* especially **S. retusa,** are held in great repute by the natives in the treatment of rheumatism.

**Thespesia populnea,** *Corr.* (*Wight, Icones*, vol. i. t. 8.)—The fruit abounds with a yellow viscid juice, which is a valued local application in scabies and other cutaneous diseases amongst the natives of Southern India, the affected parts being at the same time washed daily with a decoction of the bark of the tree. Several trials with this remedy were made by the Editor; in some cases it exercised a favorable influence, but in the majority it was productive of little or no benefit.

**Hibiscus Rosa-sinensis,** *Linn.* (*Rheede, Hort. Mal.*, vol. ii. t. 17.)—The expressed juice of the dark red petals of this species communicates a bluish-purple tint to paper, which, thus prepared, forms, according to Dr. Wight (*Illust.* vol. i. p. 57), an excellent substitute for litmus paper as a chemical test. To act efficiently, however, in this character, it should be prepared fresh each time it is required for use, as, after a very short period, acids, even of moderate strength, totally fail to affect it. Mr. Moodeen Sheriff reports favourably of an infusion of the petals as a demulcent refrigerant drink in fevers.

**Bombax Malabaricum**, *D.C.* (*Wight, Illust.*, vol. i. t. 29.)—To this tree, which is common in some parts of India, two drugs which hold a prominent place in the Native Materia Medica have been usually but erroneously referred. 1. An astringent gummy exudation, *Múcherus* (Hind.) It occurs in opaque, dark brown, knotty pieces, some presenting a remarkable gall-like appearance, inodorous, of a strongly astringent taste. It contains a large proportion of tannic and gallic acids, and might doubtless be serviceably employed in cases requiring astringents. In this character Mr. Odoy Chund Dutt, however, pronounces it inferior to the Butea Kino. Its botanical source is unknown. 2. Dried roots, well known as *Saféd Músli* (Hind.), commonly sold in the bazaars in the form of shrivelled tubers, of the thickness of a small quill, and from one to two inches in length, externally of a dirty buff colour, inodorous, and of insipid mucilaginous taste. Their structure, however, shows them to belong to a Monocotyledonous plant; hence they cannot be the produce of this tree. See also *Curculigo Orchioides*. Though held in high repute by the natives, these roots probably possess no special virtues, at least none are known to exist on reliable authority.

**Adansonia digitata**, *Linn.* (*Bot. Mag.*, t. 2791, 2792),—*Baobab*, an African tree, now domesticated in many parts of India, deserves notice from the repute it has obtained as a remedy in dysentery. This chiefly rests on the testimony of Dr. Louis Frank, who has recorded his personal experience as to its efficiency. (See Merat et de Lens, *Dict. Mat. Med.*, vol. i. p. 73.) The part employed is the pleasantly acid farinaceous pulp surrounding the seeds. Should benefit not soon be evidenced, it is recommended that the rind or cortex of the fruit, beaten up into a paste with water, be substituted. Dr. R. F. Hutchinson, from trials made with the farinaceous pulp, considers that its action is not due, as is generally thought, to any astringent property it possesses, but to its virtues as a refrigerant and diuretic. The bark has been proposed as a substitute for quinine in the treatment of intermittent fevers by Dr. Duchassaing (*Ann. de Thérap.* 1849, p. 222). He prescribed it in decoction (Bark, bruised, one ounce; Water, one pint boiled to a third). He found this effectual in some cases in which quinine in large doses had previously failed. Dr. Gibson considers that the properties of this tree are well deserving of attention.

## STERCULIACEÆ.

### THEOBROMA CACAO, *Linn.* THEOBROMA, CACAO.

(*Lodd., Bot. Cat.*, t. 545.)

*Habitat.*—Tropical America.

*Officinal Part.*—A concrete oil (*Theobromæ Oleum, Oil of Theobroma*) obtained by expression and heat from the ground seeds. It is of the consistence of tallow, of a yellowish colour, odour resembling that of chocolate, taste bland and agreeable; fracture clean, presenting no appearance of foreign matter. Does not become rancid from exposure to the air. Melts at a temperature of 122° Fahr.

*Properties and Uses.*—Emollient; employed chiefly for pharmaceutical purposes. It enters into the composition of Suppositoria Acidi Tannici, Sup. Hydrargyri, Sup. Morphiæ, and Sup. Plumbi composita.

## LINEÆ.

### LINUM USITATISSIMUM, *Linn.* COMMON FLAX.

(*Engl. Bot.* t. 1357; *ed. Syme*, t. 292.)

*Habitat.*—Southern Europe; cultivated extensively in many parts of Europe, Asia, and North America.

*Officinal Part.*—The seeds (*Lini Semina, Linseed*), small, oval, oblong, flattened, sharp-edged, pointed at one extremity, smooth, shining, brown externally, yellowish white internally, inodorous, of a mucilaginous oily taste.

*Properties.*—Emollient and demulcent; nutritive.

*Therapeutic Uses.*—In irritable and inflamed states of the pulmonary, genito-urinary, and other mucous membranes.

*Preparations.*—**Infusion of Linseed** (*Infusum Lini*). Take of Linseed, bruised, one hundred and sixty grains; Liquorice Root, sliced, one drachm; Boiling Water, ten fluid ounces. Infuse in a covered vessel for four hours, and strain.

*Dose.*—From two to four fluid ounces, or *ad libitum*. The addition of sliced lemon and sugar renders it more palatable.

**Linseed Poultice** (*Cataplasma Lini*). Take of Linseed Meal (the seeds ground, and deprived of their fixed oil by expression), four ounces; Olive Oil, half a fluid ounce; Boiling Water, ten fluid ounces. Mix the linseed meal gradually with the water, and then add the oil, constantly stirring.

A valuable emollient application.

**Linseed Oil** (*Oleum Lini*), expressed from the seeds without heat. Viscid, yellow, with faint odour and oleaginous taste.

Linseed oil obtained after the seeds have been subjected to a heat of 200°, as usually met with, is of a darker colour and more marked odour and taste. In doses of from half a fluid ounce to an ounce it proves aperient; it is, however, rarely administered internally. Its chief medicinal use is in the preparation of a liniment for burns.

## ZYGOPHYLLEÆ.

### GUAIACUM OFFICINALE, *Linn.* GUAIACUM OR LIGNUM-VITÆ TREE.

(*Woodville, Med. Bot.*, t. 200.)

*Habitat.*—West Indies.

*Officinal Parts.*—1. The Wood (*Guaiaci Lignum, Guaiacum Wood*), which is imported in large logs, is extremely hard, presenting, when examined as a transverse section, only indistinct traces of concentric zones. The outer or sap wood is of a pale brown; the inner or heart wood is of a dark greenish brown. For medicinal purposes Guaiacum wood is generally met with in the shape of turnings or raspings, which may be distinguished from those of other wood by the blue colour imparted to them by nitric acid. 2. The Resin (*Guaiaci Resina, Guaiacum Resin*) obtained from the stem by natural exudation, by incisions, or by heat. It occurs in large masses of a brownish or greenish-brown colour; fractured surface, resinous, translucent at the edges. Taste at first slightly bitter, but afterwards acrid, leaving a burning sensation on the fauces; odour slightly balsamic; evolves a fragrant odour when heated or pulverized. A solution in rectified spirit strikes a clear blue colour when applied to the inner surface of a paring of raw potato.

*Properties.*—Stimulant, diaphoretic, and alterative; emmenagogue.

*Therapeutic Uses.*—In syphilitic, rheumatic, and gouty affections it has long been an esteemed remedy; in dysmenorrhœa, amenorrhœa, and other uterine affections it has been found effectual; also in cynanche tonsillaris, diphtheria, bronchorrhœa, cutaneous diseases, &c. it has been used with alleged benefit.

*Dose.*—Of the Resin, from ten to thirty grains in bolus or emulsion.

*Preparations of the Resin.*—**Guaiacum Mixture** (*Mistura Guaiaci*). Take of Guaiacum Resin, in powder, half an ounce; Refined Sugar, half an ounce

Gum Acacia, powdered, a quarter of an ounce; Cinnamon Water, one pint. Triturate the guaiacum with the sugar and the gum, adding gradually the cinnamon water.

*Dose.*—From one half to two fluid ounces twice or thrice daily. Each fluid ounce contains eleven grains of the resin.

**Ammoniated Tincture of Guaiacum** (*Tinctura Guaiaci Ammoniata*). Take of Guaiacum Resin, in powder, four ounces; Aromatic Spirit of Ammonia, one pint. Macerate for seven days in a well-closed vessel, and filter; then add sufficient aromatic spirit of ammonia to make one pint.

*Dose.*—From one half to one fluid drachm, made into an emulsion by the aid of mucilage, twice or thrice daily. This is the best form for administration as a sudorific and emmenagogue.

The Resin also enters into the composition of Pilula Hydrargyri Sub-chloridi composita.

*Preparations of the Wood.*—The only preparation into which Guaiacum Wood enters is Decoctum Sarsæ compositum.

(*Non-officinal.*)

**Tribulus lanuginosus,** *Linn.* (*Wight, Icones,* vol. i. t. 98.)—All parts of this plant, but especially the fruit, are held in high repute in Southern India as a diuretic. In trials made with it by the Editor it was found, in some instances, materially to increase the urinary secretion, but in others it exercised no perceptible effect. The formula employed was as follows: Tribulus (Nerinji) fruit, bruised, two ounces; Coriander fruit, two drachms; Water, one pint; boiled to one half. This quantity was given in divided doses during the day. Another favourite mode of administration adopted by the natives is to boil the fruit and root with rice, so as to form a medicated congee water, which is taken in large quantities. Here the amount of fluid may serve to act as a diuretic, irrespective of the presence of any medical agent.

## RUTACEÆ.

### RUTA GRAVEOLENS, *Linn.* COMMON RUE.

(*Woodville, Med. Bot.*, t. 174.)

*Habitat.*—South of Europe; cultivated in America and elsewhere.

*Officinal Part.*—The herb, (*Ruta, Rue,*) which has a very disagreeable odour and bitter nauseous taste. Its active principles are a volatile oil and a bitter extractive.

*Properties.*—Stimulant, its action being chiefly directed to the uterine and nervous systems. Anthelmintic. In over-doses it is an acro-narcotic poison.

*Therapeutic Uses.*—In hysteria, amenorrhœa, and other uterine affections it was formerly held in high popular repute; it has likewise been employed in epilepsy, infantile convulsions, flatulent colic, &c.; but its uses at the present day are very limited.

*Preparation.*—**Oil of Rue** (*Oleum Rutæ*), distilled from the fresh leaves and unripe fruit. It is of a pale yellow colour, disagreeable odour, and acrid bitter taste.

*Dose.*—From two to five drops rubbed down with sugar and water.

[In most parts of India **Ruta angustifolia**, *Pers.* (*Bot. Mag.*, t. 2311), a closely allied species, is cultivated in gardens, and is held in high esteem by the Mahomedan doctors in the same class of affections that *R. graveolens* has been in Europe. It forms a perfect substitute for the officinal article.]

## GALIPEA CUSPARIA, *St. Hil.* CUSPARIA, or ANGUSTURA BARK TREE.

(Bonplandia trifoliata; *Woodville, Med. Bot.*, vol. v. t. 33.)

*Habitat.*—Woods of tropical South America.

*Officinal Part.*—The bark (*Cuspariæ Cortex, Cusparia Bark*). It occurs in straight pieces, more or less incurved at the sides, from half a line to a line in thickness, pared away at the edges; epidermis mottled, brown or yellowish-grey; inner surface yellowish-brown, flaky; breaks with a short fracture; bitter and slightly aromatic. The cut surface, examined with a lens, usually exhibits numerous white points or minute lines. The inner surface touched with nitric acid does not become blood-red.

*Properties.*—Aromatic tonic, antiperiodic.

*Therapeutic Uses.*—In low adynamic malarious fevers it has been much used, but with doubtful advantage. It proves, however, very serviceable in the debility consequent on these and other exhausting diseases. In atonic dyspepsia, the advanced stages of diarrhœa and dysentery, and in general debility, it proves useful.

*Dose.*—From ten to forty grains of the powdered bark. It is best administered in the form of infusion.

*Preparation.*—**Infusion of Cusparia** (*Infusum Cuspariæ*). Take of Cusparia Bark, in coarse powder, half an ounce; Water at 120°, ten fluid ounces. Infuse in a covered vessel for two hours, and strain.

*Dose.*—From one to two fluid ounces.

(*Diosmeæ, Juss.*)

1. BAROSMA BETULINA, *Bart. et Wendl.*
2. BAROSMA CRENULATA, *Hook.*
3. BAROSMA SERRATIFOLIA, *Willd.*

} BUCHU.

(*Bot. Mag.*, t. 3413.)

*Habitat.*—Southern Africa.

*Officinal Part.*—The dried leaves (*Barosmæ* vel *Buchu Folia, Buchu Leaves*). They have the following characters:—Smooth, marked with pellucid dots at the indentations and apex, having a powerful odour and a warm camphoraceous taste. 1. About three quarters of an inch long, coriaceous, obovate, with a recurved truncated apex and sharp cartilaginous spreading teeth. 2. About an inch long, oval-lanceolate, obtuse, minutely crenated, five-nerved. 3. From an inch to an inch and a half long, linear-lanceolate, tapering at each end, sharply and finely serrated, three-nerved. Active principles, a volatile oil and a bitter extractive (*Diosmin*).

*Properties.*—Aromatic stimulant, and tonic, apparently exercising a specific influence on the urinary system.

*Therapeutic Uses.*—In renal affections, irritable states of the urethra, chronic cystitis, prostatic affections, rheumatism, and dyspepsia.

*Dose.*—Of the powdered leaves from twenty to thirty grains. It is best given, however, in one of the subjoined forms.

*Preparations.*—**Infusion of Buchu** (*Infusum Buchu*). Take of Buchu leaves, bruised, half an ounce; Boiling Water, ten fluid ounces. Infuse in a covered vessel for one hour, and strain.

*Dose.*—From one to four fluid ounces twice or thrice daily.

**Tincture of Buchu** (*Tinctura Buchu*). Take of Buchu leaves, in coarse powder, two ounces and a half; Proof Spirit, one pint. Macerate the buchu for forty-eight hours, with fifteen ounces of the spirit, in a closed vessel, agitating occasionally; then transfer to a percolator; and when the fluid ceases to pass, continue the percolation with the remaining five ounces of the spirit

Afterwards subject the contents of the percolator to pressure, filter the product, mix the liquids, and add sufficient proof spirit to make one pint.

*Dose.*—From one to two fluid drachms.

(*Aurantiaceæ, D.C.*)

CITRUS AURANTIUM, *Linn.* THE SWEET AND BITTER ORANGE TREE.

(*Woodville, Med. Bot.*, t. 188.)

*Habitat.*—India and China; extensively cultivated for its fruit.

*Officinal Part.*—The dried outer portion of the rind of the fruit (*Aurantii Cortex*). It occurs in thin slices, of a dark orange colour, nearly free from the white inner part of the rind, having an aromatic bitter taste and fragrant odour. These properties are more marked in the rind of the Bitter Orange, which is to be preferred for medicinal purposes.

*Properties.*—Stomachic and tonic.

*Therapeutic Uses.*—In atonic dyspepsia, anorexia, general debility, &c. it is employed, though rarely alone.

*Preparations.*—**Infusion of Orange Peel** (*Infusum Aurantii*). Take of Bitter Orange Peel, cut small, half an ounce; Boiling Water, ten fluid ounces. Infuse in a covered vessel for fifteen minutes, and strain.

*Dose.*—From one to four fluid ounces.

**Compound Infusion of Orange Peel** (*Infusum Aurantii compositum*). Take of Bitter Orange Peel, cut small, a quarter of an ounce; Fresh Lemon Peel, cut small, sixty grains; Cloves, bruised, thirty grains; Boiling Water, ten fluid ounces. Infuse in a covered vessel for a quarter of an hour, and strain.

*Dose.*—From one to two fluid ounces. This and the preceding are agreeable stomachics, and good vehicles for the exhibition of other medicines, as saline purgatives.

**Tincture of Orange Peel** (*Tinctura Aurantii*). Take of Bitter Orange Peel, cut small and bruised, two ounces; Proof Spirit, one pint. Macerate for seven days in a closed vessel, with occasional agitation, then strain, press, and filter, and add sufficient proof spirit to make one pint.

*Dose.*—From one to two fluid drachms.

**Syrup of Orange Peel** (*Syrupus Aurantii*). Take of Tincture of Orange Peel, one fluid ounce; Syrup, seven fluid ounces. Mix.

*Dose.*—One fluid drachm.

**Orange Flower Water** (*Aqua Aurantii floris*). The water distilled from Orange flowers is employed in doses of one to two fluid ounces, as an antispasmodic and sedative in nervous and hysterical cases. When pure it is nearly colourless, and is unaffected by sulphuretted hydrogen.

**Syrup of Orange Flower** (*Syrupus Aurantii floris*). Take of Orange Flower Water, eight fluid ounces; Refined Sugar, three pounds; Water, sixteen fluid ounces, or a sufficiency. Dissolve the sugar in the water by means of heat; strain, and when nearly cold add the orange-flower water, with a sufficient quantity of water, if necessary, to make the product four pounds and a half. The specific gravity should be 1·330.

Chiefly used as a flavouring agent.

In addition to the above, Bitter Orange Peel is an ingredient in Infusum Gentianæ compositum, Mistura Gentianæ, and Tinctura Gentianæ composita.

## CITRUS LIMONUM, *Risso*. THE LEMON TREE.

(*Woodville, Med. Bot.*, t. 189.)

*Habitat.*—India and China; extensively cultivated in warm countries.

*Officinal Parts.*—1. The outer part of the rind of the ripe fruit (*Limonis Cortex*); 2. The essential oil of the rind (*Limonis Oleum*); and, 3. The expressed juice of the ripe fruit (*Limonis Succus*).

*Properties of the Rind.*—Stomachic and carminative.

*Therapeutic Uses.*—Similar to those of Cortex Aurantii (*ante*); it is, however, principally employed as a flavouring agent.

*Preparations.*—**Tincture of Lemon Peel** (*Tinctura Limonis*). Take of fresh Lemon Peel, sliced thin, two ounces and a half; Proof Spirit, one pint. Macerate for seven days in a closed vessel with occasional agitation, strain, press, and filter, and add sufficient proof spirit to make one pint.

*Dose.*—From one to two fluid drachms.

**Oil of Lemon** (*Oleum Limonis*). Obtained either by distillation or by simple expression of the finely grated rind. It is of a pale yellow colour, agreeable odour, warm and bitter taste.

It is carminative in doses of from two to four drops, but is rarely employed in this character. It forms an ingredient in Spiritus Ammoniæ aromaticus, and in Linimentum Potassii Iodidi cum Sapone. It has been used as a local application in some forms of ophthalmia, but with doubtful results.

**Lemon Juice** (*Succus Limonis*). The expressed strained juice of the ripe fruit. It is a slightly turbid yellowish liquid, possessing a sharp acid taste and grateful odour. Average specific gravity 1·039.

Lemon juice contains citric acid in the proportion of about 32 grains to each fluid ounce, with mucilage and extractive. To prevent its undergoing decomposition, which it is apt to do by keeping, a proportion of about 10 per cent. of spirits of wine or strong brandy may be added, and the mucilage separated by filtration. Another effectual plan is to allow the juice to stand for a short time after expression, till the coagulable matter separates, then to filter and put into bottles with a stratum of almond or other sweet oil upon its surface.

*Properties.*—Valuable anti-scorbutic and refrigerant; primarily, antalkaline; secondarily, antacid.

*Therapeutic Uses.*—In scurvy it is one of the best remedies we possess, both as a prophylactic and as a curative. In febrile and inflammatory affections the diluted juice, sweetened, forms an excellent refrigerant drink. In acute rheumatism and rheumatic gout, in some forms of acute tropical dysentery and diarrhœa, &c., it has been successfully employed. As an antidote to some acro-narcotic poisons, it often proves effectual.

*Dose.*—From two fluid drachms to one ounce or more; in acute rheumatism one to two fluid ounces every four or six hours.

*Preparation.* — **Syrup of Lemons** (*Syrupus Limonis*). Take of Fresh Lemon Peel, two ounces; Lemon Juice, strained, one pint; Refined Sugar, two pounds and a quarter. Heat the lemon juice to the boiling point, and, having put it into a covered vessel with the lemon peel, let them stand until they are cold, then filter and dissolve the sugar in the filtered liquid with a gentle heat. The product should weigh three pounds and a half, and should have the specific gravity 1·34.

*Dose.*—From one to two fluid drachms. It is little adapted for use in tropical countries from its readily fermenting at high temperatures. When required, it should be freshly prepared.

**Citric Acid** (*Acidum Citricum*). A crystalline acid $3HO,C_{12}H_5O_{11} + 2HO$ or $\mathbf{H_3C_6H_5O_7.H_2O}$., prepared from

Lemon or Lime Juice. It occurs in colourless crystals, of which the right rhombic prism is the primary form; very soluble in water, less soluble in rectified spirit, and insoluble in pure ether. The crystals dissolve in three-fourths of their weight of cold, and in half their weight of boiling water. The diluted aqueous solution has an agreeable acid taste. When the solution is made by dissolving thirty-four grains of the acid in one ounce of water, it resembles lemon-juice in strength and in the nature of its acid properties, and, like lemon-juice, it undergoes decomposition and becomes mouldy by keeping. The aqueous solution is not darkened by sulphuretted hydrogen, gives no precipitate when added in excess to solution of acetate of potash, or of chloride of barium, and if sparingly added to cold lime-water it does not render it turbid. The crystals leave no ash when burned with free access of air. Seventy grains of the acid dissolved in distilled water are neutralised by 1000 grain-measures of the volumetric solution of soda.

*Dose.*—From ten to thirty grains.

The chief use of citric acid in medicine is in the preparation of effervescing draughts and refrigerant drinks. An artificial lemon juice may be prepared by dissolving eight drachms of citric acid in sixteen ounces of water, and flavouring with a few drops of the Oil of Lemon. In preparing effervescing draughts, the following are the relative proportions of acid and base required to form a neutral compound:—

| *Citric Acid* | or | *Lemon juice* | | *will saturate grs.* xx. *of* |
|---|---|---|---|---|
| Grs. xiv. | - | fl. drs. iiiss. | - | Bicarbonate of Potash. |
| Grs. xxiv. | - | fl. drs. vi. | - | Carbonate of Ammonia. |
| Grs. xvij. | - | fl. drs. iv. | - | Bicarbonate of Soda. |

## *CITRUS BERGAMIA, *Risso.* THE LIME TREE.

(*Risso et Poit. Hist. des Oranges*, t. 53.)

*Habitat.*—Commonly cultivated in India and other tropical countries.

*Officinal Part.*—The fruit (*Lime*): closely resembles the lemon, but is smaller in size, with a smoother, thinner rind, and of somewhat less fragrant odour. Its juice (*Lime juice*) has the same pungent acid taste, and contains the same ingredients, as lemon juice, though in somewhat different proportions, that of the citric acid being larger, and that of the mucilage less in quantity. Much of the article imported into England under the name of lemon juice is obtained from the lime.

*Properties and Uses.*—Very similar to those of the lemon, the juice being equally refrigerant and anti-scorbutic; indeed, it is preferred by many tropical practitioners. The fresh juice of the lime is procurable in almost every portion of the tropics, and is considered more effectual than preserved lemon juice.

Lime juice may be advantageously employed in the manufacture of citric acid, the proportion of this acid being larger than in lemon juice.

## ÆGLE MARMELOS, *Correa*. BELA, BAEL.

(*Roxb., Corom. Plants*, t. 143.)

*Habitat.*—Common in dry forests throughout India; often cultivated near pagodas, being one of the sacred trees of the Hindús.

*Officinal Part.*—The half-ripe fruit (*Belæ Fructus, Bael*). Roundish or sub-spherical, about the size of a large orange, smooth, with a hard woody rind; from 10 to 15 celled, the cells containing, besides the seeds, a large quantity of an exceedingly tenacious transparent mucus. It has a mild terebinthinate, not ungrateful smell and taste. It contains tannic acid, an essential oil, a bitter principle, and a balsamic principle resembling in odour balsam of Peru. ([20]) It is imported into England in dried slices, or in fragments consisting of portions of the rind and adherent dried pulp and seeds. Rind about a line and a half thick, covered with a smooth pale-brown or greyish epidermis, and internally, as well as the dried pulp, brownish orange, or cherry red. The moistened pulp is mucilaginous.

*Properties.*—Astringent? It is not improbable that its action is that of a mild stimulant of the intestinal mucous membrane, as experience has shown that whilst it tends to arrest diarrhœa when present, it no less certainly acts as a laxative when constipation exists. Under each circumstance it seems to give tone to the intestinal tube.([21])

*Therapeutic Uses.*—In atonic diarrhœa and dysentery, and in the advanced stages of those diseases, in irregularity of the bowels, and in habitual constipation, it is a remedy of much value.

*Preparations.*—***Bael Mixture** (*Mistura Belæ*). Take of the soft tenacious fluid of the interior of the fruit, two fluid ounces; Water, four ounces. Mix thoroughly and add sugar, two ounces, or sufficient to render it palatable.

This, especially if artificially cooled by the addition of ice or otherwise, forms an agreeable draught which possesses the aroma of the fruit, and may be repeated twice or thrice daily. When prepared with the ripe fruit it is not only astringent when diarrhœa exists, but possesses the singular property of being aperient, if the bowels be irregular or costive. When the patient is much reduced in strength, and the stomach irritable, the above mixture sometimes disagrees; it ought then to be given in small and repeated doses, and if these also are rejected the extract may be tried.

***Extract of Bael** (*Extractum Belæ*). Select such fruits as have thin and even shells, and are perfectly matured. Extract the pulp, place it in a vessel, add water sufficient to cover it; stir for two hours, and strain through stout calico. Repeat this process until the fluid which passes through the strainer is tasteless. Evaporate over a water bath to the consistence of a soft extract.

This preparation, which is favourably reported of, retains all the peculiar aroma of the fruit. If prepared with the unripe fruit it is stated to keep better than when made from the mature fruit, as ordered above.

*Dose.*—From half a drachm to one drachm twice or thrice daily, or oftener.

**Liquid Extract of Bael** (*Extractum Belæ Liquidum*). Take of Bael Fruit, one pound; Water, twelve pints; Rectified Spirit, two fluid ounces. Macerate the Bael for twelve hours in one-third of the water; pour off the clear liquor; repeat the maceration a second and third time for one hour in the remaining two-thirds of the water; press the marc; and filter the mixed liquors through flannel. Evaporate to fourteen fluid ounces, and, when cold, add the rectified spirit.

*Dose.*—From one to two fluid drachms. This Extract, prepared from the dried Bael imported into England, appears to possess much less medicinal power than the extract and mixture prepared from the fresh fruit in India.

### *TODDALIA ACULEATA, *Pers.* TODDALIA.

(*Wight, Illust.*, vol. i. t. 66.)

*Habitat.*—Hedge-rows and jungles of Malabar, Coromandel, Mysore, the Concans, and other parts of the Madras Peninsula.

*Officinal Part.*—The root-bark (*Toddaliæ Radix*): a solid heavy branching root, attaining some inches in diameter, covered with a bitter, pungent, aromatic bark, having a suberous, velvety, yellowish epidermis. The interior consists of a hard whitish wood, which in the dry state is nearly tasteless and inodorous.

*Properties.*—Aromatic tonic, and stimulant; antiperiodic?

*Therapeutic Uses.*—In constitutional debility, and in convalescence after febrile and other exhausting diseases, it is apparently a remedy of great value. Under the name of *Lopez Root*, it once enjoyed some celebrity in Europe as a remedy for diarrhœa, but has fallen into disuse. It is, however, worthy of further trials in India, where it can be obtained in the fresh state. (22)

*Preparations.* — **Tincture of Toddalia** (*Tinctura Toddaliæ*). Take of the Root-bark of Toddalia, bruised, two ounces and a half; Proof Spirit, one pint. Macerate for seven days in a closed vessel, with occasional agitation; strain, press, filter, and add sufficient proof spirit to make one pint. It may also be prepared in the same manner as Tincture of Calumba.

*Dose.*—From one and a half to three fluid drachms twice or thrice daily.

**Infusion of Toddalia** (*Infusum Toddaliæ*). Take of the Root-bark of Toddalia, in coarse powder, one ounce; Boiling Water, ten fluid ounces. Infuse in a covered vessel for one hour, and strain.

*Dose.*—From one to two fluid ounces twice or thrice daily.

(*Non-officinal.*)

**Feronia Elephantum**, *Corr.* (*Roxb.*, *Corom. Plants*, t. 141.)—*Wood-apple Tree.* A widely distributed tree throughout India, which yields, in considerable quantities, a gum which Pereira (*Mat. Med.*, vol. ii. P. ii. p. 550) regards as probably constituting a portion of the East Indian Gum Arabic imported into England. It occurs in the form of irregular, semi-transparent, reddish-brown tears. Treated with water, it affords a brownish tasteless mucilage, not less adhesive than that of Gum Arabic, for which it may be used as a substitute. Mr. J. Wood describes the unripe fruit, in decoction, as a powerful astringent, the ripe fruit as an antiscorbutic. In its action it appears to assimilate very closely to Bael, but, being more terebinthinate, it is less grateful to the palate. The young leaves, which possess an agreeable aroma resembling aniseed, are much employed by the natives as a stomachic and carminative.

**Zanthoxylum alatum**, *Roxb.*, **Z. hastile**, *Wall*, and **Z. Budrunga**, *D.C.* Natives of the Himalaya and Khasia Hills, whose fruits constitute articles in the Native Materia Medica. Judging from their aromatic pungency, it is probable that they possess stomachic and carminative properties. On analysis, Dr. Stenhouse detected in the fruit of *Z. alatum* an aromatic essential oil (*Xanthoxylene*), which, when pure, is a hydrocarbon isomeric with oil of turpentine, and likewise a stearopten (*Xanthoxylin*), found floating on the water distilled from the fruits, and also separable from the crude essential oil.

**Peganum Harmala**, *Linn.* (*Lam. Illust.*, t. 401.) This plant, common in Scinde and the Punjaub, has a strong disagreeable odour and bitter taste, and is thought by Dr. Landerer (*Pharm. Journ.*, vol. xiv. p. 369) to approximate in its action to *Cannabis Indica.* The seeds (*Harmul*, Hind.) have long held a place in Eastern Materia Medica as a stimulant, emmenagogue, and anthelmintic. Mild narcotic properties have also been assigned to them, and, according to Käempfer, delirium characterised by cheerfulness follows their use in some cases. Further investigations as to the properties of these seeds are desirable.

**Murraya (Bergera) Königii**, *Linn.* (*Wight, Icones*, vol. i. t. 13.) The bark, root, and leaves of this small tree, common in many parts of India, are much employed in native practice as a tonic and stomachic, and they are favourably reported of in these characters by Dr. Æ. Ross and Dr. J. Shortt. The young leaves are often added to curries with the view of aiding their digestibility.

## SIMARUBEÆ.

### PICRÆNA EXCELSA, *Lindl.* The Officinal or Jamaica Quassia Tree.

(Quassia excelsa, *in Steph. et Church, Med. Bot.* t. 173.)

*Habitat.*—West Indies.

*Officinal Part.*—The wood (*Quassiæ Lignum, Quassia*) is imported in billets varying in size, seldom thicker than the thigh, covered externally with a smooth brittle bark. The wood is dense, tough, yellowish-white, intensely and purely bitter. It is also met with in shops in the form of chips, which may be distinguished from those of other woods by their intensely bitter taste. A watery infusion is not blackened by the addition of a persalt of iron. It contains a bitter neutral principle, *Quassine.*

*Properties.*—A pure bitter tonic and stomachic.

*Therapeutic Uses.*—In debility, in convalescence after febrile diseases, and in atonic dyspepsia it is a remedy of established value, In paroxysmal fevers it exercises some power, but not more than is possessed by other bitter tonics. An enema of the infusion is effectual in dislodging ascarides vermiculares (thread worms) from the rectum.

*Preparations.* — **Infusion of Quassia** (*Infusum Quassiæ*). Take of Quassia, in chips, sixty grains; Cold Water, ten fluid ounces. Infuse in a covered vessel for half an hour, and strain.

*Dose.*—From one to two fluid ounces twice or thrice daily. A good vehicle for the salts of iron.

**Tincture of Quassia** (*Tinctura Quassiæ*). Take of Quassia Wood, in chips, three quarters of an ounce; Proof Spirit, one pint; macerate for seven days in a closed vessel with occasional agitation; then strain, press, filter, and add sufficient spirit to make one pint.

*Dose.*—From thirty minims to two fluid drachms.

**Extract of Quassia** (*Extractum Quassiæ*). Take of Quassia Wood, rasped, one pound; Distilled Water, a sufficiency. Macerate the quassia with eight fluid ounces of the water for twelve hours; then pack in a percolator, and, adding more of the water, allow the liquor slowly to pass until the quassia is exhausted. Evaporate the liquor; filter before it becomes too thick; and again evaporate by water-bath until the extract is of a suitable consistence for forming pills.

*Dose.*—From three to five grains, either alone or combined with metallic tonics.

(*Non-officinal.*)

**Brucea (Nima) Quassioides,** *Ham.*—A Himalayan species, the root of which, according to Royle (*Illust.* p. 158), is as bitter as the quassia of the West Indies. It would, doubtless, prove an excellent substitute for it. The bark is imported into Bengal from the Hills. and is sold under the name of *Bharangi* (Hind.) (the *Bharingee* of the Taleef Shereef, p. 48). It partakes of the bitterness of the root, and appears worthy of further attention.

**Ailanthus Malabarica,** *D.C.* (*Wight, Icones*, vol. iv. t. 1604.)—A large tree of Ceylon, Malabar, and Concan. The bark, on incision, yields an aromatic, gum-resinous substance, known by the Tamul name of *Matti-pawl*, which is used medicinally, especially in dysenteric cases, and as incense. Dr. Gibson regards it as a good stimulant in bronchitic affections. The bark is rough and very thick, with a pleasant and slightly bitter taste. Dr. Wight found it studded with bright garnet-looking grains, apparently of a resinous nature; but as they did not burn like resin, nor dissolve either in spirit or in water, he infers that they are of a peculiar chemical composition yet to be ascertained. A further knowledge of this bark and its exudation is desirable.

**Ailanthus excelsa,** *D.C.* (*Wight, Illust.*, vol. i. t. 67.)—A large tree, found in dry forests from the Carnatic to the base of the Himalaya. Its pleasantly tasted aromatic bark, according to Ainslie, is used by the natives in dyspeptic complaints. Dr. Wight (*Illust.* i. p. 169) mentions that in the Circars the bark is regarded as a powerful febrifuge, and as a tonic in cases of debility.

**Eurycoma longifolia,** *Jack.*—A small tree of the Malayan Peninsula and Archipelago, where it is known by the name of *Penwar pait*. Mr. Oxley, writing in 1850, (*Journ. Agri.-Hort. Soc. of India*, vol. vii. P. ii. p. 56,) states that for three or four years previously he had been in the habit of using a decoction of the root of this tree as a remedy in intermittent fevers; and that, with the exception of quinine, he knows not of a more certain remedy.

## BURSERACEÆ.

### BALSAMODENDRON MYRRHA, *Ehrenb.* THE MYRRH TREE.

(*Nees, Düsseldorf*, t. 357.)

*Habitat.*—Arabia.

*Officinal Part.*—The gum-resinous exudation from the stem (*Myrrha, Myrrh*); occurs in irregular-shaped tears or masses, varying much in size, somewhat translucent, of a reddish-yellow or reddish-brown colour; fractured surface, irregular and somewhat oily; odour, agreeable and aromatic; taste, acrid and bitter. Only partially soluble in water, alcohol, or ether. The first of these takes up the gum principally; the two latter, the resin and the oil.

*Properties.*—Stimulant, expectorant, and emmenagogue.

*Therapeutic Uses.*—In amenorrhœa, chlorosis, and other uterine affections characterised by atony, in pulmonary affections, especially in the asthma of the aged, and in some disordered conditions of the digestive organs, it is a remedy of value. As a local or external agent it is much used in affections of the mouth and fauces, indolent ulceration, &c.

*Dose.*—From ten to twenty grains in powder or pill.

*Preparation.* — **Tincture of Myrrh** (*Tinctura Myrrhæ*). Take of Myrrh, in coarse powder, two ounces and a half; Rectified Spirit, one pint. Macerate the myrrh for forty-eight hours in fifteen ounces of the spirit, in a closed vessel, agitating occasionally; then transfer to a percolator, and, when the fluid ceases to pass, continue the percolation with the remaining five ounces of the spirit. Afterwards subject the contents of the percolator to pressure, filter the product, mix the two liquids, and add sufficient rectified spirit to make one pint.

*Dose.*—From half a fluid drachm to a drachm. Chiefly used diluted, in gargles, &c.

Myrrh enters also into the following preparations: Decoctum Aloes compositum, Pilula Aloes et Myrrhæ, Pilula Assafœtidæ composita, Pilula Rhei composita, and Mistura Ferri composita.

### CANARIUM COMMUNE, *Linn.* ? THE ELEMI TREE.

(*Rumph. Amb.*, vol. ii. t. 47. *Lam. Encyc.*, t. 812.)

*Habitat.*—Continent of India, Ceylon, Eastern Archipelago.

*Officinal Part.*—The concrete resinous exudation (*Elemi*). Chiefly imported into England from Manilla. It occurs in the form of a soft unctuous adhesive mass, becoming harder and more resinous by age; of a yellowish-white colour, with a rather fragrant fennel-like odour; almost entirely soluble in rectified spirit.

The above description has reference to the so-called "East India or Manilla Elemi," the probable source of which is *Canarium commune*, Linn. It differs in some respects from Brazilian Elemi, the produce of *Icica Icicariba*, Marcgr, and from Mexican Elemi, the produce of *Elaphrium elemiferum*, Royle.

*Properties.*—Mild terebinthinate stimulant; not administered internally.

*Therapeutic Uses.*—To indolent and ill-conditioned ulcerations the following ointment forms a good application.

*Preparation.*—**Ointment of Elemi** (*Unguentum Elemi*). Take of Elemi, a quarter of an ounce; Simple Ointment, one ounce. Melt, strain through flannel, and stir constantly until the ointment solidifies.

[The kernels of *Canarium commune* (*Java almonds*) yield a bland oil, which may be substituted for almond oil. Dr. Waitz (*Diseases of Children in Hot Climates*, p. 290) speaks favourably of the kernels in emulsion, as a substitute for the corresponding European preparation (*Mistura Amygdalæ*), to which he considers it preferable for Indian practice, not only on account of its mild laxative action, but because the almonds imported from Europe are often spoilt by long keeping.]

## *BOSWELLIA FLORIBUNDA, *Endl.* THE OLIBANUM OR FRANKINCENSE TREE. †

*Habitat.*—Somali Coast, westward of Cape Guardafui.

*Officinal Part.*—The gum-resin (*Olibanum*); occurs in the form of round, oblong, or ovate tears, semi-opaque, fragile, of a pale yellowish colour, pungent, slightly aromatic taste and balsamic resinous odour, especially when subject to heat; becomes opaque when immersed in alcohol.

*Properties.*—Terebinthinate stimulant; its action, when taken internally, being chiefly directed on the mucous membrane, especially of the lungs.

*Therapeutic Uses.*—In subacute bronchitis, in chronic pulmonary affections, bronchorrhœa, and chronic laryngitis, it has been advantageously employed both internally and in the form of fumigation. Locally as a stimulant in carbuncle, ulcerations, boils, &c. [23]

*Dose.*—From fifteen grains to two drachms.

---

† *Boswellia thurifera, Colebr.*, a tree of the mountainous tracts of Central India and the Coromandel Coast, has been thought to yield East Indian Olibanum, but there is no reliable evidence of its so doing. *Ganda-birosa* (*Hind.*), is applied equally to Olibanum and to the resinous exudation of *Pinus longifolia, Lam.*

*Preparations.*—**Olibanum Ointment** (*Unguentum Olibani*). Take of Olibanum, Sesamum or Poppy Oil, and White Wax, of each an ounce. Melt together with a gentle heat and strain.

(*Non-officinal.*)

**Balsamodendron Mukul,** *Hook*, and **B. pubescens,** *Stocks*. (*Hooker, Kew Journ.*, 1849, vol. i. t. 8, 9.)—These two species, indigenous in Scinde, yield the gum resin, *Bdellium*, the *Gúgul* of the Indian Materia Medica. It occurs in roundish pieces, of a dull dark-red colour, more moist than myrrh, and not brittle like it, softening even with the heat of the hand; bitter and slightly acrid in taste, with a less agreeable odour (*Royle*). The medicinal properties of bdellium approximate closely to those of myrrh, and, as it is much cheaper, it may be substituted for it in dispensary practice (*Beng. Disp.*, p. 288). Dr. J. Newton reports very favourably of it in the form of ointment for cleansing and stimulating indolent and ill-conditioned ulcers. It is a favourite application in Delhi sores, combined with sulphur, catechu, and borax; it is reported to stimulate to healthy action.

**Canarium strictum,** *Roxb.*, only deserves notice in this place as one, if not the principal, source of the Black Dammar of Southern India. This substance occurs in stalactitic masses of a bright shining colour when viewed *en masse*, but translucent and of a deep reddish-brown colour when held between the eye and the light; homogeneous, with a vitreous fracture; partially soluble in boiling alcohol, and completely so in oil of turpentine. Dr. G. Bidie, whose description has been followed, speaks of its use as a substitute for Burgundy Pitch, and furnishes some formulæ into which it enters. (*Madras Quart. Med. Journ.*, 1862, vol. v. p. 292.)

## MELIACEÆ.

### *AZADIRACHTA INDICA, *Juss.* NIM OR MARGOSA TREE.

(*Rheede, Hort. Mal.*, vol. iv. t. 52. *Wight, Icones*, vol. i. t. 17.)

*Habitat.*—Common throughout India; often cultivated in gardens.

*Officinal Parts.*—1. The bark (*Azadirachtæ Cortex, Nim Bark*). It varies much in appearance, according to the size and age of the tree producing it. The bark from the trunk of a tree above three or four years of age, is covered with a thick scaly epidermis, and varies in thickness from ¼ to ½ inch. That from the smaller branches is smooth, of a dullish purple colour, marked by longitudinal lines of ash-coloured epidermis, from one-eighth to one-twelfth of an inch apart. The inner layer of the bark, of a whitish colour in the fresh state, is powerfully bitter, far more so than the outer dark-coloured layer, which, however, possesses a greater amount of astringency. It contains a crystallizable principle (*Margosine*), and an astringent principle (*Catechin*).[24] 2. The fresh leaves (*Azadirachtæ Folia, Nim Leaves*).

*Properties.*—Bark, astringent tonic, and antiperiodic. Leaves stimulant.

*Therapeutic Uses.*—In intermittent and other paroxysmal fevers, in general debility, and convalescence after febrile and other diseases, the bark has been employed with success.[25] The leaves form a useful local application to ulcers, and obstinate skin disease when a mild stimulant is required.

*Dose.*—Of the powdered bark, a drachm three or four times a day.

*Preparations.*—**Decoction of Nim Bark** (*Decoctum Azadirachtæ*). Take of the inner layer of Nim Bark bruised, two ounces; Water, a pint and a half. Boil for fifteen minutes, and strain whilst hot.

*Dose.*—As an antiperiodic, from one and a half to three fluid ounces every second hour previous to an expected paroxysm. As a tonic, one to two fluid ounces twice or thrice daily. As this decoction soon decomposes in hot weather, it should be prepared fresh for use when required.

**Tincture of Nim Bark** (*Tinctura Azadirachtæ*). Take of the inner layer of Nim Bark bruised, two ounces and a half; Proof Spirit, one pint. Macerate for seven days in a closed vessel with occasional agitation; strain, press, filter, and add sufficient proof spirit to make one pint. It may also be prepared by percolation in the same manner as Tincture of Calumba, *q.v.*

*Dose.*—From one half to two fluid drachms as a tonic.

**Poultice of Nim Leaves** (*Cataplasma Azadirachtæ.*) Take of fresh Nim Leaves a sufficiency; bruise, and moisten with tepid water.

A good stimulant application to indolent and ill-conditioned ulcers.[26] Should it cause pain and irritation, as it sometimes does, equal parts of rice flour or linseed meal may be added.

[The bitter oil of the seeds is well deserving of investigation as an external application in rheumatism, and as an anthelmintic, in both of which characters it is held in high repute by the natives. It is reported by Dr. A. Hunter to be an insecticide.]

## *SOYMIDA FEBRIFUGA, *Juss.* ROHUN TREE.
(*Roxb. Corom. Plants*, t. 17.)

*Habitat.*—Mountain forests of Malabar, Concan, and Central India.

*Officinal Part.*—The bark (*Soymidæ Cortex, Rohun Bark*); occurs in compact thick pieces, fibrous, of a rusty colour, and bitter astringent taste. It contains a large proportion of tannic and gallic acids, and a bitter amorphous principle. (27) *Test.*—Nitric acid applied to the inner surface of the bark does not cause a bright red stain.†

*Properties.*—Astringent, tonic, and antiperiodic.

*Therapeutic Uses.*—In intermittent fevers and general debility, in the advanced stages of dysentery, in diarrhœa, and in other cases requiring the use of astringents, it has been used with success. (28)

*Dose.*—Of the powdered bark, a drachm twice daily. This is the best form of administration.

*Preparations.*—**Decoction of Rohun** (*Decoctum Soymidæ*). Take of Rohun Bark bruised, one ounce and a half; Water, one pint. Boil for fifteen minutes in a covered vessel; then strain, and pour as much water over the contents of the strainer as will make the strained product measure a pint.

A good substitute for decoction of oak bark; well adapted for gargles, vaginal injections, and enemas.

(*Non-officinal.*)

**Melia Azedarach,** *Linn.* (*Wight, Icones*, vol. i. t. 160.)—The root-bark of this small tree, a native of America, cultivated in many parts of India, enjoys in America considerable repute as an anthelmintic, and enters into the Secondary List of the United States Ph. It has a bitter, nauseous taste, and yields its virtues to boiling water. It is administered in the form of decoction (four ounces of the fresh root-bark, water two pints, boil to one pint), of which the dose for a child is a tablespoonful repeated every third hour until it sensibly affects the bowels or stomach. Another mode of administration is to give a dose morning and evening for several successive days, and then to administer an active cathartic. In large doses it is reported to produce narcotic effects, but these, when they occur, pass off without perceptible injury to the system. By drying, the bark loses much of its activity. Poisonous properties have been attributed to the fresh berries and leaves.

**Cedrela Toona,** *Roxb.* (*Wight, Icones*, vol. i. t. 161.)—The bark of this tree is a powerful astringent, and may be resorted to when other

† *Note.*—This test is given to distinguish Soymida bark from that of the Strychnos Nux Vomica, which in the Bengal bazaars is sometimes substituted for it,—a substitution which once nearly led to most serious consequences.

remedies of the same class are not available. Dr. Waitz (*Dis. of Children in Hot Climates*, p. 225) used with success an extract of the bark in chronic infantile dysentery. Blume attributes valuable antiperiodic virtues to it, and in this character it is favourably noticed by Dr. J. Kennedy (*Ann. of Med.* 1796, vol. i. p. 387). Dr. Æ. Ross speaks of it as a reliable antiperiodic, and Dr. J. Newton as a good substitute for cinchona. The dose of the dried bark is about an ounce daily in the form of infusion. The powder of the bark was found by Dr. Kennedy to be of great service as a local astringent application in various forms of ulceration.

**Xylocarpus Granatum,** *Kon.* Common in low, swampy sites in all parts of the East. The bark, in common with other parts of the tree, possesses extreme bitterness, conjoined with astringency; it may probably prove a good astringent tonic. It is much employed by the Malays in cholera, colic, diarrhœa, and other abdominal affections.

## CELASTRINEÆ.

(*Non-officinal.*)

**Celastrus paniculata,** *Willd.* (*Wight, Icones,* vol. i. t. 158.)—The seeds of this shrub (*Malkungi,* Hind.), as met with in the bazaars, are of a rusty brown color, of an ellipsoid form, about ⅛ of an inch in length, leaving when crushed on paper an oily stain. Remains of the globular three-valved fruit, which is of the size of a pea, are usually found mixed with them. By a rude form of distillation, the natives obtain from them a black empyreumatic oil, which, under the name of "Oleum nigrum," was brought forward by the late Dr. Herklots as a sovereign remedy in Beri-beri. In doses of from ten to fifteen drops, twice daily, it is a powerful stimulant. Its action in this character is generally followed in a few hours by free diaphoresis unattended by subsequent exhaustion. Though it has failed to realize Dr. Herklots' encomiums, yet, in some cases treated with it detailed by Dr. Malcolmson, its beneficial effects were unequivocally evidenced; in others, however, it failed. It appears to be chiefly adapted for recent cases, and for those in which the nervous and paralytic symptoms predominate. (*See* Malcolmson, *On Beri-beri, &c.*, p. 311, *seq.*)

## RHAMNEÆ.

### RHAMNUS CATHARTICUS, *Linn.* COMMON OR PURGING BUCKTHORN.

(*Engl. Bot.*, t. 1629; *ed. Syme*, t. 318.)

*Habitat.*—Great Britain and other parts of Europe.

*Officinal Part.*—The recently expressed juice of the ripe berries (*Rhamni Succus, Buckthorn juice*).

*Properties.*—Hydragogue cathartic.

*Therapeutic Uses.*—Dropsical affections, obstinate constipation, and other cases requiring active catharsis.

*Preparation.*—**Syrup of Buckthorn** (*Syrupus Rhamni*). Take of Buckthorn juice, four pints; Ginger sliced, and Pimento bruised, of each three quarters of an ounce; Refined Sugar, five pounds or a sufficiency; Rectified Spirit, six fluid ounces. Evaporate the juice to two pints and a half, add the ginger and pimento, digest at a gentle heat for four hours, and strain; when cold, add the spirit; let the mixture stand for two days, then decant off the clear liquor, and in this dissolve the sugar with a gentle heat so as to make the specific gravity 1·32.

*Dose.*—One fluid drachm.† From the readiness with which it ferments at high temperatures it is little adapted for use in tropical countries.

## AMPELIDEÆ.

### VITIS VINIFERA, *Linn.* THE GRAPE VINE.
(*Woodville, Med. Bot.*, t. 57.)

*Habitat.*—Temperate Asia; cultivated in all the temperate regions of the globe.

*Officinal Part.*—The ripe fruit dried in the sun or with artificial heat (*Uvæ, Raisins*). Fruit shrivelled and compressed, smooth, and free from sugary or saline incrustation, agreeably fragrant, pulp soft, very sweet.

*Properties and Uses.*—Demulcent, principally employed as a flavouring agent.

*Preparations.*—Raisins form an ingredient in Tinctura Cardamomi composita, Tinctura Sennæ composita, &c.

**Tartaric Acid** (*Acidum Tartaricum*). A crystalline Acid, $2HO,C_8H_4O_{10}$ or $\mathbf{H_2C_4H_4O_6}$. obtained from the Acid Tartrate of Potash deposited during fermentation from the juice of the grape. It occurs in the form of colourless oblique rhombic prisms, of a strongly acid taste, readily soluble in water and in rectified spirit. When to either solution a little acetate of potash is

---

† This is the dose given in the British Pharmacopœia. Pereira, Christison, and other standard authorities, place the dose at from one half to one fluid ounce.

added, a white crystalline precipitate forms. Seventy-five grains dissolved in water require for neutralization 1000 grain measures of the volumetric solution of soda. Its aqueous solution is not affected by sulphuretted hydrogen, and gives no precipitate with the solution of sulphate of lime, or of oxalate of ammonia. It leaves no residue, or only a mere trace, when burned with free access of air.

*Properties and Uses.*—Refrigerant, sometimes employed as a substitute for Citric Acid in the preparation of refrigerant drinks in fevers, &c. Its more common use, however, is in the formation of "effervescing draughts":—

Twenty grains of the Crystals of Tartaric Acid are saturated by—

| | |
|---|---|
| Crystallized Bicarbonate of Potash | 27 grains. |
| Carbonate of Potash of Commerce | 22 ,, |
| Hydrated Sesquicarbonate of Ammonia | 15½ ,, |
| Crystallized Carbonate of Soda | 38½ ,, |
| Bicarbonate of Soda of Commerce | 22 ,, |

These draughts are not only refrigerant, serving to allay thirst, but by the disengagement of carbonic acid gas, when taken in a state of effervescence, they tend to allay nausea and gastric irritability.

*Dose.*—From ten to thirty grains.

**Alcohol.**
**Wine.**
**Vinegar.** } See Products of Fermentation.

## ANACARDIACEÆ.

### PISTACIA LENTISCUS, *Linn.* THE MASTICH TREE.

(*Woodville, Med. Bot.*, t. 11; *Bot. Mag.*, t. 1967.)

*Habitat.*—Southern Europe, Northern Africa, and the Levant.

*Officinal Part.* — The resinous exudation (*Mastiche, Mastich*) obtained from the stem by incision. It occurs in the form of small irregular yellowish tears, brittle, of a vitreous fracture, becoming soft and ductile when chewed, having a faint agreeable odour increased by the application of heat or by friction. It contains a minute portion of volatile oil, about 90 per cent. of a resin soluble in alcohol (*Mastichic Acid*), and about 10 per cent. of a resin (*Masticine*) insoluble in cold, but soluble in hot, alcohol.

*Properties.*—Terebinthinate stimulant, and diuretic.

*Therapeutic Uses.*—Rarely administered internally. Water in which it has been boiled is said to be useful in infantile diarrhœa.

Cotton saturated with an ethereal solution introduced into a carious tooth, is often successful in relieving toothache.

*Dose.*—From ten to thirty grains.

---

(*Non-officinal.*)

**Pistacia Khinjuk,** *Stocks*, and **P. Cabulica,** *Stocks*, two small trees of Beloochistan and Affghanistan, closely allied, if not identical with, *P. Terebinthus*, Linn., and *P. atalantica*, Desf., yield a resin which, in those countries and likewise in Scinde and Persia, is employed as a succedaneum for mastich. By Persian writers it is designated *Kúndarún* or *Sakir-shirin* (Sweet Mastich), to distinguish it from Olibanum, which is called *Kúndar* or *Sakir-talkh* (Bitter Mastich), and from Mastich itself, which is called *Kúndar-rúmí* or *Sakir-rúmí* (Royle). *P. Khinjuk* yields curiously shaped galls, which enter into the Native Materia Medica under the name of *Gúl-i-pista.* These are fig-shaped, spherical or ovoid excrescences, about half an inch in length and of a reddish brown colour. They are hollow, the walls being thin, fragile, and translucent; taste acidulous, astringent, and slightly terebinthinous.

**Rhus succedanea,** *Linn.* (*Wight, Icones*, vol. iii. t. 560,) a tree of the sub-tropical and temperate Himalaya; known by the name of *Kakra-singhi*, from the horn-like excrescences borne on its branches, caused by insects (*Royle*). These excrescences, the *Kakra-singie* of the Taleef Shereef (p. 112), are large, hollow, thin-walled, generally cylindrical, tapering to either extremity. They are often of the length and thickness of the forefinger, contorted and irregular. Astringent and tonic properties are assigned to them by the natives.

**Mangifera Indica,** *Linn.* (*Rheede, Hort. Mal.*, vol. iv. t. 1, 2; *Bot. Mag.*, t. 4510.)—*Mango tree*, common throughout India. The only part which claims notice in this place is the kernel, which, not only in India but also in Brazil (*Martius' Syst. Mat. Med. Braz.*, p. 64,) is employed as an anthelmintic. Dr. Kirkpatrick (*Cat. of Mysore Drugs*, No. 472) states that, in his own practice, he has frequently employed powdered mango seed in this character (for lumbrici) in doses of twenty to thirty grains, and found it effectual. He adds that it contains a large proportion of gallic acid, and that he has administered it with great success in bleeding piles and in menorrhagia. This remedy appears deserving of further trials.

**Anacardium occidentale,** *Linn.* (*Rheede, Hort. Mal.*, vol. iii. t. 54) —*Cashew tree*, abounds on the sea-coasts of India and other tropical countries. It yields a large supply of gum, which, however, is of little use either in medicine or the arts. Between the laminæ of the shell of the kernel there is a black, caustic fluid, which contains an acrid oily principle, *Cardol*, and a peculiar acid, *Anacardic Acid.* It possesses powerful rubefacient and vesicant properties, but is apparently open to the same objections as the corresponding product of *Semecarpus Anacardium* (*infra*). The seeds, on expression, yield a bland oil, which might be used for pharmaceutical purposes. From the expressed juice of the fruit a spirit is distilled on the Malabar Coast, which is procurable in Bombay (*Dr. Dymock*) and elsewhere. It is described as a good spirit, but with a somewhat peculiar flavour, and might be used as a stimulant in the absence of other remedies of the same class.

**Semecarpus Anacardium,** *Linn.* (*Wight, Icones,* vol. ii. t. 558.)—This tree is generally known as the *Marking-nut tree,* from the fact of the black viscid juice contained between the laminæ of the shell being in common use as marking ink. This juice possesses powerfully caustic properties, and is employed by the natives as a vesicant. Its use in this character is only mentioned here to be condemned, very serious effects having followed, even when it has been accidentally applied to a very circumscribed surface. (*See* Sir W. O'Shaughnessy, *Bengal Disp.*, p. 280, and Dr. Gibson, *Bombay Med. Phys. Trans.*, vol. i. p. 332.) A fatal case of ulceration resulting from blistering with this fluid is on record (*Bombay Med. Phys. Trans.*, vol. iii. p. 45). Much caution is requisite even in handling the juice for domestic purposes, erysipelatous inflammation of the face, &c., having, in some instances, followed too free exposure to its irritating vapour. Some constitutions are more readily affected by it than others. Dr. Grylls reports that the swelling and febrile symptoms following its application are best relieved by the internal administration of salines and the local application of Liquor Plumbi. Dr. J. Newton mentions that the bruised nut applied locally to the os uteri, is one of the means in use amongst native women for procuring abortion.

**Melanorrhœa usitatissima,** *Wall.* (*Plant. Asiat. Rar.*, t. 11, 12.) —A large tree, a native of trans-gangetic India, from Munipur to Tavoy. Every part of it abounds with a thick, viscid, greyish, terebinthinate fluid, which soon assumes a black colour on exposure to the air. This is the *Black Varnish* or *Thit-tsi,* of the Burmese, by whom it is employed extensively, not only in the arts, but as an anthelmintic in cases of Ascarides lumbricoides. In the latter character it is possessed of considerable power. It is administered in the form of electuary, prepared with an equal proportion of honey, the mixture having been subjected for some hours to the action of heat. The dose of this electuary is one, two, or three tablespoonfuls, according to the age of the patient, and is followed in a few hours by a dose of castor oil, which causes the expulsion of the worms in a lifeless state, thus showing that the remedy exercises a specific effect on the entozoa. The extremely nauseous taste of the remedy, and the largeness of the dose required, are great objections to its employment. It appears probable, however, that its activity resides in a volatile oil, which, if procurable in a pure state, would be well worthy of an extended trial. Handling the fresh juice causes, in some constitutions, erysipelatous swellings, which, however, are effectually removed by the local application of an infusion of Teak-wood (*Tectona grandis,* Linn.) See also *Indian Ann. of Medical Science,* vol. vi. 1959.

**Odina Wodier,** *Roxb.* (*Royle, Illust.*, t. 31; *Wight, Icones,* vol. i. t. 60) —*Jiol,* Beng., *Jingan,* Hind., a large tree common throughout India. The bark is very astringent, and in the form of decoction is employed by Dr. Kirkpatrick in the Pettah Hospital, Bangalore, as a lotion in impetiginous eruptions and obstinate ulcerations (*Dr. Oswald*). Dr. Bholanauth Bose speaks of this decoction as forming an excellent astringent gargle. It yields also a large quantity of gum (*Jingam* vel *Kanni ki gond*), which in some parts of India is collected for export. It appears to be possessed of astringent properties. Dr. J. L. Stewart (*Technologist,* April 1st, 1866, p. 388) furnishes a good account of this gum.

# MORINGEÆ.

(*Non-officinal.*)

**Moringa pterygosperma,** *Gærtn.* (*Wight, Illust.*, vol. i. t. 77)—*Sohunjuna*, Hind., the *Horseradish tree* of the Anglo-Indians, so called from its roots possessing the pungent taste and smell of the Horse-radish of Europe. Locally applied, the fresh root acts as a rubefacient and vesicant, but the great pain it causes is an objection to its use. Dr. Wight (*Illust.*, vol. i. p. 187) suggests the addition of the expressed juice of the root to sinapisms, to render their action more energetic; and a similar suggestion is made by Dr. Waitz (*Dis. of Children in Hot Climates*, p. 207). As an internal remedy, stimulant and diuretic properties have been assigned to it; and Dr. G. Bidie (*Madras Quart. Med. Journ.*, 1862, vol. v. p. 279) is probably correct in regarding it as a perfect substitute for armoracia. Dr. J. Shortt reports having found a decoction of the root serviceable as a gargle in hoarseness. The Bengal Ph. furnishes two formulæ for its administration:—1. *Compound Spirit.* Take of Moringa root, sliced, and Orange peel, of each, twenty ounces; Nutmegs, bruised, five drachms; Proof Spirit, one gallon; Water, two pints; Mix and distil a gallon. Stimulant in doses of from two to four fluid drachms. 2. *Compound Infusion.* Take of Moringa root and Mustard seed, bruised, of each, one ounce; Boiling Water, one pint. Infuse for two hours in a covered vessel, strain, and add one ounce of the Compound Spirit (*ante*). Described as a valuable stimulant in doses of from one to two fluid ounces. The seeds yield by expression a bland fixed oil, approximating to the Oil of Ben, the produce of *Moringa aptera*. In native practice, other parts of this tree, *e.g.* the leaves, bark, flowers, and soft reddish gummy exudation, are employed for various purposes, but nothing trustworthy is known concerning them. The wood has been supposed to constitute the *Lignum nephriticum* of the old pharmacologists, but this is very doubtful.

# LEGUMINOSÆ.

## ACACIA VERA, *Willd.*, AND OTHER UNDETERMINED SPECIES OF ACACIA YIELDING GUM ARABIC.—GUM ARABIC TREE.

(*Hayne*, vol. x. t. 34.)

*Habitat.*—Arabia, and Africa from Senegal to Egypt.

*Officinal Part.*—The gummy exudation from the stem (*Acaciæ Gummi, Gum Acacia, Gum Arabic*), collected chiefly in Cordofan in Eastern Africa, and imported into England from Alexandria. It occurs in the form of spheroidal tears from half an inch to an inch in length, nearly colourless, and opaque from numerous minute cracks, or in shining fragments; brittle, bland, and mucilaginous in taste; insoluble in alcohol, soluble in water. The solution forms with subacetate of lead an opaque white jelly. The powder does not become blue on the addition of an aqueous solution of iodine.

Several kinds of Gum Acacia, chiefly named after the locality in which they are produced, e. g. *Barbary* or *Morocco, Senegal, East Indian*, &c., are met with in commerce: they are mostly of inferior quality, and their respective botanical sources are as yet undetermined.

*Properties.*—Demulcent and emollient. Chiefly used as an adjunct to other medicines, and especially for the purpose of suspending heavy powders.

*Therapeutic Uses.*—In catarrhal affections, in pulmonary irritation, in irritable states of the genito-urinary system, in diarrhœa, &c., it proves a valuable auxiliary to other remedies.

It forms an ingredient in Mistura Cretæ, Mistura Guaici, Pulvis Amygdalæ compositus, Pulvis Tragacanthæ compositus, and all the officinal lozenges.

*Preparations.*— **Mucilage of Gum Acacia** (*Mucilago Acaciæ*). Take of Gum Acacia, in small pieces, four ounces; Water, six fluid ounces. Put the gum and water into a covered earthen jar, and stir them frequently until the gum is dissolved. If necessary strain the solution through muslin.

*Dose.*—From three to six ounces daily, or *ad libitum.*

In India considerable quantities of gum are yielded by **Acacia Arabica**, Willd.; but, for the most part, it is of very inferior quality, and often mixed with impurities. The gum of *Feronia Elephantum*, Corr. is preferable to it as a substitute for the officinal Gum Acacia.

## *ACACIA CATECHU, *Willd.* THE CATECHU ACACIA.

(*Roxb., Corom. Plants*, t. 175.)

*Habitat.*—Forests throughout India.

*Officinal Part.*—An extract of the heart-wood (*Catechu nigrum, Black Catechu*). It occurs in masses, consisting of layers occasionally enveloped in rough leaves (of *Nauclea Brunonis*), blackish brown, shining, heavy, bitter, and very astringent. *Active principles.*—A peculiar form of *Tannin* (*Mimotannic Acid*) and *Catechin.* Other varieties of Catechu are met with in the bazaars of India.

*Properties.*—Powerful astringent.

*Therapeutic Uses.*—In diarrhœa depending on a relaxed state of the intestinal mucous membrane, it is of much value. It has likewise been employed with alleged benefit in intermittent fevers, scurvy, &c. (30) Locally it is used with advantage in ptyalism, ulceration and sponginess of the gums, relaxation of the uvula, hypertrophy of the tonsils, &c., and in the form of injection in leucorrhœa and atonic menorrhagia.

*Dose.*—From ten to twenty grains in powder. It is, however, rarely administered in this form.

*Preparations.*—**Infusion of Catechu** (*Infusum Catechu*). Take of Catechu, in coarse powder, one hundred and sixty grains; Cinnamon Bark, bruised, thirty grains; Boiling Water, ten fluid ounces. Infuse in a covered vessel for half an hour, and strain.

*Dose.*—From one to two fluid ounces.

**Tincture of Catechu** (*Tinctura Catechu*). Take of Catechu, in coarse powder, two ounces and a half; Cinnamon Bark bruised, one ounce; Proof Spirit, one pint. Macerate for seven days in a closed vessel with occasional agitation; press, strain, filter, and add sufficient proof spirit to make one pint.

*Dose.*—From one half to two fluid drachms. A valuable adjunct to Mistura Cretæ and other astringent mixtures.

**Compound Powder of Catechu** (*Pulvis Catechu compositus*). Take of Catechu in powder, four ounces; Kino in powder, Rhatany Root in powder, of each, two ounces; Cinnamon Bark in powder, Nutmeg in powder, of each, one ounce. Mix them thoroughly, pass the powder through a fine sieve, and finally rub it lightly in a mortar. Keep it in a stoppered bottle.

*Dose.*—From fifteen to thirty grains. A valuable aromatic astringent.

## COPAIFERA MULTIJUGA, *Hayne*, AND OTHER SPECIES OF COPAIFERA YIELDING COPAIVA.

(*Woodville, Med. Bot.*, t. 216.)

*Habitat.*—Tropical America, especially Brazil; one species in the West Indian Islands.

*Officinal Part.*—An Oleo-resin (*Copaiba, Copaiva*) obtained from the trunk of the tree by incision; transparent, lighter than water, about the consistence of olive oil, light-yellow, transparent, with a peculiar odour and an acrid aromatic nauseous taste. Perfectly soluble in an equal volume of benzol. Does not become gelatinous after having been heated to 270°. Is scarcely fluorescent.

*Properties.*—Terebinthinate stimulant, acting principally on the mucous membrane of the genito-urinary organs.

*Therapeutic Uses.*—In gonorrhœa it is a remedy of great value. It has likewise been used with advantage in gonorrhœal rheumatism, leucorrhœa, hæmorrhoids, chronic cystitis, and in bronchorrhœa, chronic bronchitis, and other lung affections attended with excessive secretion.

*Dose.*—From twenty minims to one fluid drachm, twice or thrice daily, in emulsion or floating on water.

*Preparations.*—**Oil of Copaiva** (*Oleum Copaibæ*) obtained from the Oleo-resin by distillation. It is colourless, or of a pale-yellow colour, with the odour and taste of Copaiba.

*Dose.*—From five to twenty minims twice or thrice daily. It is applicable to all cases in which the Oleo-resin is generally employed.

## TAMARINDUS INDICA, *Linn.* THE TAMARIND TREE.

(*Rheede, Hort. Mal.*, vol. i. t. 23; *Woodville, Med. Bot.*, t. 161.)

*Habitat.*—A native of Africa, cultivated throughout the tropics of both hemispheres.

*Officinal Part.*—The pulp of the fruit (*Tamarindi Pulpa*). In the raw state, it is of a reddish-brown colour, and strongly acid, saccharine taste. Preserved in sugar for medicinal purposes, it is of a more or less brownish or blackish colour, a sweetish sub-acid taste, and contains strong fibres, and brown shining seeds, each enclosed in a membranous coat. Its acidity depends upon the presence of citric, malic, and tartaric acids; the last existing also in combination with potash, in the form of the Bitartrate. When prepared in copper vessels, it is apt to contain a portion of that metal, to detect which a piece of bright iron should be left in contact with the pulp for an hour, when copper, if present, will be deposited on it.

*Properties and Uses.*—Laxative and refrigerant; employed in the preparation of refrigerant drinks in febrile and inflammatory affections, in which it proves generally agreeable and useful. (29)

*Preparation.*—Tamarind pulp enters into the composition of Confectio Sennæ.

## CASSIA FISTULA, *Linn.* PURGING CASSIA.

(*Rheede, Hort. Mal.*, vol. i. t. 22.)

*Habitat.*—Forests of tropical India, cultivated in the tropics of both hemispheres.

*Officinal Part.*—The pulp of the pods (*Cassiæ Pulpa, Cassia Pulp*). It is of a blackish-brown colour, viscid, sweet to the taste, and somewhat sickly in odour. The pods or legumes are from one to two feet in length, about the thickness of the thumb, cylindrical, slightly curved, dark brown and shining, or nearly black and dull, and marked with two longitudinal streaks at the sutures of the valves. The pericarp is thin, hard, and brittle; its cavity divided by numerous thin transverse partitions; each cell contains a single hard, flattened, ovoid seed, surrounded by the pulp.

*Preparation.*—**Prepared Cassia** (*Cassia preparata*). Take of Cassia Pods, crushed in a mortar, one pound; Water, sufficient to cover the Cassia. Macerate for six hours, occasionally stirring; strain the softened pulp through a hair sieve, and evaporate to the consistence of a confection.

*Properties.*—Laxative in small, purgative in large doses. Given alone, it causes flatulence and griping; hence it should be combined with carminatives. Under its use, the urine occasionally assumes a dark brown colour.

*Therapeutic Uses.*—In constipation and other cases requiring aperients, it has been successfully employed.

*Dose.*—As a mild laxative, from one to two drachms; as a purgative, from one to two ounces.

Cassia pulp enters also into Confectio Sennæ.

[Dr. Irvine (*Med. Topog. of Ajmeer*, p. 124) states that he has found the root of this tree act as a very strong purgative.]

## 1. CASSIA OBOVATA, *Colladon.* } ALEXANDRIAN
## 2. CASSIA ACUTIFOLIA, *Delile,* } SENNA PLANT.
## 3. CASSIA LANCEOLATA, *Forsk.* { INDIAN OR TINNIVELLY SENNA PLANT.

(1. *Colladon, Hist. des Cass.*, t. 15, *Wight, Icones,* vol. iii. t. 757.
2. *Delile, Egypt,* t. 27.
3. *Royle, Illust.*, t. 37.)

*Habitat.*—*C. obovata* and *C. lanceolata* are indigenous in Eastern tropical Africa and Arabia; and in India, from Scinde and the Punjaub to the Carnatic. *C. acutifolia,* which is perhaps only a variety of *C. lanceolata*, is confined to Egypt and Nubia. All the species are cultivated.

*Officinal Part.*—The dried leaves or leaflets (*Senna*). Alexandrian Senna (*Senna Alexandrina*) possesses the following characters; lanceolate or obovate leaflets about an inch long, unequally oblique at the base, brittle, greyish green, of a faint peculiar odour, and mucilaginous sweetish taste. It is often adulterated with the leaves, flowers, and fruit of *Solenostemma Argel*, Hayne. The unequally oblique base, and freedom from bitterness, serve, however, to distinguish the Senna from the Argel leaves, which are also thicker and stiffer. Of Tinnivelly Senna (*Senna Indica*) the following are the usual characters; about two inches long, lanceolate, acute, unequally oblique at the base, flexible, entire, green, without any admixture; odour and taste those of Alexandrian Senna.

*Properties.*—Safe and efficient purgative, well adapted for childhood, old age, and delicate females.

*Therapeutic Uses.*—In constipation and other cases requiring aperients, it has long been held in deservedly high repute.

*Preparations.*—**Infusion of Senna** (*Infusum Sennæ*). Take of Senna, one ounce; Ginger, sliced, thirty grains; Boiling Water, ten fluid ounces. Infuse in a covered vessel for one hour, and strain.

*Dose.*—From one to two fluid ounces. The infusion, if taken hot, with the addition of milk and sugar, can hardly be distinguished from ordinary tea. It is in this manner easily administered to children.

**Compound Mixture of Senna** (*Mistura Sennæ composita*). Take of Sulphate of Magnesia four ounces; Extract of Liquorice, half an ounce; Tincture of Senna, two fluid ounces and a half; Compound Tincture of Cardamoms, ten fluid drachms; Infusion of Senna, a sufficiency. Dissolve the sulphate of magnesia and extract of liquorice in fourteen fluid ounces of the infusion of senna, with the aid of a gentle heat, then add the tinctures, and sufficient infusion of senna to make one pint.

*Dose.*—From one to one and a half fluid ounces.

**Tincture of Senna** (*Tinctura Sennæ*). Take of Senna, broken small, two ounces and a half; Raisins, freed from seeds, two ounces; Caraway Fruit, bruised, half an ounce; Coriander Fruit, bruised, half an ounce; Proof Spirit, one pint. Macerate the senna and the other ingredients for forty-eight hours, with fifteen ounces of the spirit, in a closed vessel, agitating occasionally; then transfer to a percolator, and when the fluid ceases to pass, pour into the percolator the remaining five ounces of the spirit. Afterwards subject the contents of the percolator to pressure, filter the product, mix the two liquids, and add sufficient proof spirit to make one pint.

*Dose.*—From one to three fluid drachms. A valuable adjunct to saline and other purgative mixtures.

**Confection of Senna** (*Confectio Sennæ*). Take of Senna, in fine powder, seven ounces; Coriander Fruit, in fine powder, three ounces; Figs, twelve ounces; Tamarind Pulp, nine ounces; Cassia Pulp, nine ounces; Prunes, six ounces; Extract of Liquorice, three quarters of an ounce; Refined Sugar, thirty ounces; Water, a sufficiency. Boil the figs and prunes gently with twenty-four ounces of water in a covered vessel for four hours; then, having added more water to make up the quantity to its original volume, mix the tamarind and cassia pulp, digest for two hours, and rub the softened pulp of the fruits through a hair sieve, rejecting the seeds and other hard parts. To the pulped product add the sugar and extract of liquorice, and dissolve them with a gentle heat. While the mixture is still warm, add to it gradually the mixed senna and coriander powders, and mix the whole thoroughly, making the weight of the resulting confection seventy-five ounces either by evaporation or by the addition of more water.

*Dose.*—From one to two drachms. A mild and useful purgative, long in popular use as "Lenitive Electuary." Often used as a vehicle for the exhibition of other medicines, as sulphur, acid tartrate of potash, &c.

## HÆMATOXYLON CAMPECHIANUM, *Linn.*
### LOGWOOD TREE.

(*Woodville, Med. Bot.*, t. 163.)

*Habitat.*—Central America and West Indies: introduced into India.

*Officinal Part.*—The heart-wood (*Hæmatoxyli Lignum, Logwood*). It occurs in logs, or in the form of chips, externally of a dark colour, internally of reddish brown; of a feeble agreeable odour and sweetish taste. A small portion chewed, imparts to the saliva a dark pink colour. It contains tannic acid, a resin, and a peculiar azotized crystalline colouring substance named *Hæmatoxyline*.

*Properties*.—Astringent, tonic.

*Therapeutic Uses*.—In chronic or atonic diarrhœa, especially in young subjects, it has been administered with advantage. Locally, in the form of injection, it has been used in leucorrhœa. In cancer, the Extract, in the form of ointment, has been found to destroy the fœtor and diminish the amount of the discharge.

*Preparations*.—**Decoction of Logwood** (*Decoctum Hæmatoxyli*). Take of Logwood, in chips, one ounce; Cinnamon Bark, in coarse powder, sixty grains; Water, one pint. Boil the logwood in the water for ten minutes, adding the cinnamon towards the end. Strain the decoction, and pour as much water over the contents of the strainer as will make the strained product measure a pint.

*Dose*.—From one to two fluid ounces.

**Extract of Logwood** (*Extractum Hæmatoxyli*). Take of Logwood, in fine chips, one pound; Boiling Water, one gallon. Macerate the logwood in water for twenty-four hours, then boil down to one half; strain, and evaporate to dryness by a water bath, stirring with a wooden spatula. Iron vessels should not be used.

*Dose*.—From ten to thirty grains.

## *CÆSALPINIA (GUILANDINA) BONDUCELLA, *Linn.* Bonduc.

(*Lam. Illust.*, t. 36.)

*Habitat*.—Tropical portions of both hemispheres.

*Officinal Part*.—The seeds (*Bonducellæ Semina, Bonduc seeds*); of a somewhat irregular sub-spherical or ovoid form, usually $\frac{4}{8}$ to $\frac{6}{8}$ of an inch in diameter, smooth, hard, and lead-coloured, and contain an amylaceous white nucleus, having a bitter taste. They contain a fixed oil, resin, and a bitter (crystallizable ?) principle. ([31])

*Properties*.—Tonic and antiperiodic.

*Therapeutic Uses*.—In intermittent fevers, especially in those of the natives, they have been employed with much success. They have also been advantageously prescribed in debility, and other cases requiring tonics. ([32])

*Dose*.—From ten to fifteen grains twice daily.

*Preparations*.—**Compound Powder of Bonduc** (*Pulvis Bonducellæ compositus*). Take of Bonduc seeds, deprived of their shells and powdered, one ounce; Black Pepper, powdered, one ounce. Mix thoroughly, and keep in a well-stoppered bottle.

*Dose.*—From fifteen to thirty grains, three times a day.

## MYROXYLON PEREIRÆ, *Klotzsch.* BALSAM OF PERU TREE.

(*Pharm. Journ.*, vol. x. p. 282.)

*Habitat.*—Western Coast of Central America, the so-called "Balsam coast," extending from the port of Acajutla to that of Libertad.

*Officinal Part.*—An oleo-resin (*Balsamum Peruvianum, Balsam of Peru*) which exudes from the trunk of the tree after the removal of the bark, which has been previously scorched by fire. It occurs in the form of a reddish-brown or nearly black liquid, translucent in thin films, having the consistence of syrup, a balsamic odour, and an acrid slightly bitter taste; soluble in five parts of rectified spirit; undergoes no diminution in volume when mixed with water.

*Properties.*—Mild stimulant and expectorant.

*Therapeutic Uses.*—It is applicable in the same cases as Balsam of Tolu (*infra*), but is less frequently employed. Inhalation of its vapour, generated by heat, has been found useful in chronic bronchitis and other pulmonary affections. Locally it is used as a stimulant to freshly incised wounds, indolent or phagædenic ulcerations, sore nipples, &c.; also in otorrhœa and in alopecia.

*Dose.*—From ten to fifteen minims in emulsion.

## MYROXYLON TOLUIFERUM, *H.B.K.* BALSAM OF TOLU TREE.

(*Nees, Düsseldorf.*, t. 321.)

*Habitat.*—New Granada.

*Officinal Part.*—A Balsam (*Balsamum Tolutanum, Balsam of Tolu*) obtained from the stem by incision. It is a soft tenacious solid, of a golden-brown colour, with a fragrant balsamic odour, less powerful than that of the Balsam of Peru, and a pleasant sweetish taste. By age, it becomes hard and brittle, with a granular, somewhat crystalline appearance. It is wholly soluble in rectified spirit.

*Properties.*—Mild stimulant and expectorant.

*Therapeutic Uses.*—In chronic bronchial affections unattended by inflammatory action, it is administered internally with benefit. In the same class of cases, inhalation of the vapour proves serviceable.

*Dose.*—From ten to twenty grains.

*Preparations.* — **Tincture of Tolu** (*Tinctura Tolutana*). Take of Balsam of Tolu, two ounces and a half; Rectified Spirit, a sufficiency. Macerate the balsam of tolu in fifteen fluid ounces of the spirit, in a closed vessel, with occasional agitation, for six hours, or until the balsam is dissolved; then filter, and add sufficient rectified spirit to make one pint.

*Dose.*—From twenty to forty minims. An excellent adjunct to other expectorant remedies. Each fluid ounce contains 54½ grains of the balsam.

**Syrup of Tolu** (*Syrupus Tolutanus*). Take of Balsam of Tolu, one ounce and a quarter; Refined Sugar, two pounds; Water, one pint, or a sufficiency. Boil the balsam in the water for half an hour in a lightly covered vessel, stirring occasionally. Then remove from the fire, and add water, if necessary, so that the liquid shall measure sixteen ounces. Filter the solution when cold, add the sugar, and dissolve with the aid of a steam or water bath. The product should weigh three pounds, and should have the specific gravity 1·330.

*Dose.*—From one to two fluid drachms, This is one of the few syrups which do not easily ferment under the action of tropical heat.

Balsam of Tolu enters also into Tinctura Benzoini composita, Trochisci Opii, Trochisci Morphiæ et Ipecacuanhæ, Trochisci Morphiæ, and Trochisci Acidi Tannici.

## PTEROCARPUS MARSUPIUM, *D.C.* THE INDIAN KINO TREE.

(*Roxb., Corom. Plants*, t. 116.)

*Habitat.*—Forests of Ceylon and all parts of the Madras Peninsula, extending north to the Rajmahl Hills, in Behar.

*Officinal Part.*—The inspissated juice obtained from incisions in the trunk (*Kino*). It occurs in the form of small angular, brittle, glistening, reddish black fragments, translucent and ruby-red on the edges, inodorous, very astringent. When chewed, it tinges the saliva blood-red. Active principles, a peculiar form of *Tannin* (*Mimotannic Acid*) and *Catechin*.

*Properties.*—Valuable astringent.

*Therapeutic Uses.*—Similar to those of Catechu, but being milder in its operation it is better adapted for children and delicate females.

*Dose.*—Of powdered Kino from ten to thirty grains or more.

*Preparations.*—**Tincture of Kino** (*Tinctura Kino*). Take of Kino, in coarse powder, two ounces; Rectified Spirit, one pint. Macerate for seven days in a closed vessel with occasional agitation, filter, and add sufficient rectified spirit to make one pint.

*Dose.*—From thirty minims to two fluid drachms. A useful adjunct to astringent mixtures.

**Compound Powder of Kino** (*Pulvis Kino compositus*). Take of Kino, in powder, three ounces and three quarters; Opium, in powder, a quarter of an ounce; Cinnamon Bark, in powder, one ounce. Mix them thoroughly, and pass the powder through a fine sieve, and finally rub it lightly in a mortar. Keep it in a stoppered bottle.

*Dose.*—From five to twenty grains. Twenty grains contain one grain of opium. A very useful preparation in pyrosis, and in dyspepsia attended with increased secretion.

Kino also forms an ingredient in Pulvis Catechu compositus.

[Botany Bay Kino, the Red Gum of Western Australia (*Gummi Rubrum*), is the produce of several species of **Eucalyptus** (especially of **E. resinifera**, Smith), which are widely distributed throughout the Australian continent. In physical characters and medical properties it is nearly allied to Kino. It has been introduced into British practice by Sir Ranald Martin, who has found it very effectual in the treatment of the chronic bowel complaints of invalids from India, but more especially in the chronic dysentery of Europeans. He regards it as less directly astringent and more demulcent than Catechu or Kino. It has been highly reported of by several medical officers who have served in Western Australia, where the tree yielding it is abundant. The dose is from five to ten grains in the form of powder or syrup. (See *Squire's Comp. to British Ph.*, p. 64.) This drug possesses additional interest to the practitioner in India from the fact that several species of Eucalyptus have become naturalized on the Neilgherries and other high lands of India.]

## PTEROCARPUS SANTALINUS, *Linn.* RED SANDAL-WOOD TREE.

(*Woodville, Med. Bot.*, t. 156.)

*Habitat.*—Mountains of the Coromandel Coast.

*Officinal Part.*—The wood (*Pterocarpi Lignum, Lignum Santalinum rubrum, Red Sandal-wood*); occurs in the form of dense heavy billets, or in chips; externally dark brown; internally variegated with dark and lighter red rings. Powder blood-red, of a faint peculiar odour, and obscurely astringent taste. It contains a peculiar colouring principle, *Santalin.*

*Properties and Uses.*—It is officinal only as a colouring agent, Tinctura Lavandulæ composita; but its use in this character may be extended in India as a substitute for cochineal in the preparation of Tinctura Cardamomi composita, Tinctura Cinchonæ composita, &c.

It is much in use amongst the natives of India as an astringent; but though it may possess some power in this character, as it contains a portion of tannin and gallic acid, it does not appear to possess any claims worthy of attention as an internal remedy.

## PHYSOSTIGMA VENENOSUM, *Balfour.* CALABAR BEAN PLANT.

(*Trans. Roy. Soc. Edinburgh,* vol. xxii. t. 16, 17.)

*Habitat.*—Old Calabar and other parts of Western Africa.

*Officinal Part.*—The seeds (*Physostigmatis semina*) about the size of a very large horse bean, with a very firm, hard, brittle, shining integument of a brownish-red, pale-chocolate, or ash-grey colour. Irregularly kidney-shaped, with two flat sides, and a furrow running longitudinally along its convex margin, and ending in an aperture near one end of the seed. Within the shell is a kernel, consisting of two cotyledons, weighing on an average about 46 grains; hard, white, and pulverisable; of a taste like that of the ordinary edible leguminous seeds, without bitterness, acrimony, or aromatic flavour. It yields its virtues to alcohol, and imperfectly to water.

*Properties.*—Powerful sedative of the spinal nervous system, producing in over-doses paralysis of the lower extremities and death by asphyxia, and in still larger doses by paralysis of the heart. Highly poisonous. Applied locally to the eye, it possesses the peculiar property of rapidly inducing contraction of the pupil.

*Therapeutic Uses.*—It has been prescribed internally in tetanus, chorea, and other nervous affections characterised by exalted sensibility of the spinal nervous system. Its chief use, however, is as a local application in diseases and injuries of the eye, and here it is especially valuable.

*Dose.*—One grain of the powdered seed gradually increased to four grains according to effect.

*Preparations.*—**Extract of Calabar Bean** (*Extractum Physostigmatis*). Take of Calabar Bean, in coarse powder, one pound; Rectified spirit, four pints, Macerate the bean for forty-eight hours, with one pint of spirit, in a closed vessel, agitating occasionally; then transfer to a percolator; and, when the fluid ceases to pass, add the remainder of the spirit, so that it may slowly percolate through the powder. Subject the residue of the bean to pressure, adding the pressed liquid to the product of the percolation; filter, distil off most of the spirit, and evaporate what is left in the retort by a water bath, to the consistence of a soft extract.

*Dose.*—From one-sixteenth to one-fourth of a grain. For the purpose of causing contraction of the pupil, a minute portion of the extract, in substance, or dissolved in glycerine, may be applied to the eye by means of a fine camel-hair pencil. Gelatine and bibulous paper impregnated with the tincture, are sold in the shops, and are convenient modes of application in ophthalmic diseases requiring this remedy.

## *MUCUNA PRURIENS, *D.C.* COWHAGE.

(*Hooker, Bot. Misc.*, vol. ii. Suppl. t. 13.)

*Habitat.*—West Indies. *Mucuna prurita,* Hooker, now regarded as identical with *M. pruriens,* D.C., is common throughout India.

*Officinal Part.*—The hairs of the pod (*Mucuna, Cowhage*). The pod or legume is of a brownish colour, oblong, compressed, slightly curved like the letter *f,* from two to three inches or more in length, densely clothed with strong, brown, bristly, stinging hairs, which under the microscope resemble porcupine quills, but are slightly notched or serrated towards the point.

*Properties.*—Mechanical anthelmintic.

*Therapeutic Uses.*—For the expulsion of Ascarides lumbricoides, cowhage has been chiefly employed; it has been used, though with less effect, in cases of A. vermiculares.

*Dose.*—Cowhage is best administered in the form of electuary with treacle, syrup, or honey. The pods, first dipped in the vehicle, should be scraped until the mass has the consistence of an electuary; of this the dose is a tablespoonful for an adult, and a teaspoonful for a child, for three or four successive mornings. This should be followed by a brisk purgative, when the worms are generally expelled.

## *BUTEA FRONDOSA, *Roxb.* BENGAL KINO TREE.

(*Roxb., Corom. Plants,* t. 21.)

*Habitat.*—Common all over India.

*Officinal Part.*—The inspissated juice obtained from the stem by incision (*Buteæ Gummi, Kino Bengalensis,*

*Bengal Kino*). It occurs in the form of irregular shining fragments, seldom as large as a pea; more or less mixed with adherent pieces of greyish bark; of an intense ruby colour and astringent taste; soluble, but not freely so, in water and in alcohol. Its astringency is due to the presence of tannic and gallic acids.

*Properties and Uses.*—Similar to those of Kino, for which it has been found an efficient substitute. (33)

*Preparations.*—The same as those of Kino.

An exudation, similar to the above, is yielded by **Butea superba,** *Roxb.*, (*Corom. Pl.*, t. 22), and **Butea parviflora,** *Roxb.*, (*Wight, Icones*, vol. i. t. 210). Both are employed medicinally by the natives, and doubtless are possessed of some efficiency as astringents.

## *ABRUS PRECATORIUS, *Linn.* INDIAN LIQUORICE PLANT.

(*Lam. Illust.*, t. 608.)

*Habitat.*—Tropical portions of both hemispheres.

*Officinal Part.*—The root (*Abri Radix, Indian Liquorice*). Occurs in pieces of various lengths, from ½ to 1 inch in diameter; pale brown externally, yellowish internally; inodorous; taste sweetish and mucilaginous, much resembling officinal liquorice root. (34)

*Properties and Uses.*—Similar to those of Liquorice, for which it forms an excellent substitute.

*Preparations.*—**Extract of Abrus** (*Extractum Abri*). Prepared as Extractum Glycyrrhizæ.

## *ARACHIS HYPOGÆA, *Linn.* GROUND NUT PLANT.

(*Lam. Illust.*, t. 615.)

*Habitat.*—Cultivated throughout the tropics of the Old and New World.

*Officinal Part.*—The oil of the seeds (*Oleum Arachis, Ground Nut Oil*). Obtained by expression. Limpid, clear, light yellow, almost inodorous or with a faint smell, and bland taste. Sp. gr. ·916.

*Properties and Uses.*—This oil affords a cheap and excellent substitute for Olive Oil for pharmaceutical and other purposes. (35)

## GLYCYRRHIZA GLABRA, *Linn.* THE LIQUORICE PLANT.

(*Woodville, Med. Bot.*, t. 152.)

*Habitat.*—Southern Europe; cultivated in England.

*Officinal Part.*—The root or underground stem (*Glycyrrhizæ Radix, Liquorice Root*). It occurs in long cylindrical branched pieces, an inch or less in diameter, tough and pliable; of a greyish-brown colour externally, yellow internally; with a somewhat disagreeable, earthy odour, and of a sweet mucilaginous and slightly acrid taste. Digested with water, it yields a solution which gives a precipitate with diluted sulphuric acid. Its sweetness resides in a peculiar principle named *Glycion*, and *Glycyrrhizin* or *Liquorice Sugar*.

*Properties.*—Demulcent and emollient.

*Therapeutic Uses.*—In coughs and catarrhal affections of the throat and pulmonary mucous membrane, also in dysuria, ardor urinæ, &c., it proves serviceable.

*Preparations.*—**Extract of Liquorice** (*Extractum Glycyrrhizæ*). Take of Liquorice Root, in coarse powder, one pound; Water, four pints. Macerate the liquorice with two pints of the water for twelve hours, strain and press; again macerate the pressed marc with the remainder of the water for six hours; strain and press. Mix the strained liquors, heat them to 212°, and strain through flannel; then evaporate by a water bath until the extract is of a suitable consistence for forming pills.

*Dose.*—*Ad libitum.* Much used for disguising the unpleasant taste of aloes, senna, hydrochlorate of ammonia, &c.

Liquorice root enters into the composition of Infusum Lini and Decoctum Sarsæ compositum; the Extract, into that of Decoctum Aloes compositum, Confectio Sennæ, Confectio Terebinthinæ, Tinctura Aloes, Trochisci Opii, and Mistura Sennæ composita.

## ASTRAGALUS VERUS, *Olivier*, AND POSSIBLY OTHER SPECIES OF ASTRAGALUS YIELDING TRAGACANTH.

(*Hayne*, vol. x. t. 7.)

*Habitat.*—Anatolia, Armenia, and Northern Persia.

*Officinal Part.*—A gummy exudation from the stem (*Tragacantha, Tragacanth*). It usually occurs in broad shell-like slightly curved plates, of a white or yellowish colour tough and elastic, but rendered more pulverizable by a heat of 120° Fahr.; very sparingly soluble in cold water, but swelling into a gelatinous mass, which is tinged violet by tincture of iodine. After maceration in cold water, the fluid portion is not precipitated by the addition of rectified spirit.

*Properties.*—Emollient and demulcent.

*Therapeutic Uses.*—In irritation of mucous membranes, especially the pulmonary and genito-urinary organs, it proves useful; its chief use, however, is as a vehicle for more active medicines.

*Preparations.*—**Mucilage of Tragacanth** (*Mucilago Tragacanthæ*). Take of Tragacanth, sixty grains; Water, ten fluid ounces. To the water contained in a pint bottle add the tragacanth; agitate briskly for a few minutes, and again at short intervals, until the tragacanth is perfectly diffused, and finally has formed a mucilage.

*Dose.*—From one to three fluid ounces. Occasionally used as a vehicle for suspending heavy powders in mixtures, &c.

**Compound Powder of Tragacanth** (*Pulvis Tragacantha compositus*). Take of Tragacanth in powder, Gum Acacia in powder, Starch in powder, of each, one ounce; Refined Sugar, in powder, three ounces. Rub them well together.

*Dose.*—A very convenient powder for the immediate preparation of a mucilage which is a good vehicle for other medicines, especially for heavy powders. Fifteen or twenty grains to an ounce of water make a mucilage of sufficient thickness.

Tragacanth also enters into Confectio Opii and Pulvis Opii compositus.

## CYTISUS SCOPARIUS, *Link.* COMMON BROOM.

(*Spartium Scoparium, Linn.*)

(*Engl. Bot.*, t. 1339; *ed. Syme*, t. 329.)

*Habitat.*—Great Britain and other parts of Europe.

*Officinal Part.*—The fresh and dried tops (*Scoparii Cacumina, Broom Tops*); straight, angular, dark-green, smooth, tough twigs, of a bitter nauseous taste, and of a peculiar odour when bruised. They contain a neutral principle, *Scoparin*, and a volatile liquid alkaloid, *Spartia*, in which their activity apparently resides.

*Properties.*—Diuretic and mildly laxative; in large doses purgative and emetic.

*Therapeutic Uses.*—In dropical affections it has been employed with manifest advantage. It also proves serviceable in other cases requiring the use of diuretics.

*Dose of the dried Tops.*—From twenty to thirty grains in decoction.

*Preparations.*—**Juice of Broom** (*Succus Scoparii*). Take of fresh Broom Tops, seven pounds; Rectified Spirit, a sufficiency. Bruise the broom tops in a stone mortar; press out the juice, and to every three measures of juice add one of the spirit. Set aside for seven days, and filter. Keep it in a cool place.

*Dose.*—From one to two fluid drachms.

**Decoction of Broom** (*Decoctum Scoparii*). Take of Broom Tops dried, one ounce; Water, one pint. Boil for ten minutes in a covered vessel, then strain and pour as much water over the contents of the strainer as will make the strained product measure a pint.

*Dose.*—From two to four fluid ounces.

(*Non-officinal.*)

**Acacia Arabica**, *Willd.* (*Roxb., Corom. Pl.*, t. 149.)—A common Indian tree. Its bark (*Babul Bark*) occurs in large thick pieces, coarsely fibrous, of a deep mahogany colour. It is a powerful astringent, and as such may be employed as a substitute for oak bark. In this character it is favourably noticed by Dr. M'Gregor (*Dis. of N.W. Provinces*, p. 175), who found the decoction a valuable application in prolapsus ani. Dr. S. Delpratt reports favourably of a decoction of Babul Bark as a local astringent, especially in leucorrhœa; and Sub-Assistant Surgeon Rama Churn Bose recommends poultices of the bruised tender leaves as an excellent astringent and stimulant application to ulcers attended with sanious discharge. Mr. L. Da Costa has published (*Journ. Asiat. Soc. of Bengal*, May 1837) an interesting paper on the properties and uses of this tree and its products according to Native ideas. The gum yielded by this tree has already been mentioned in Art. *Acacia vera*. The bark of several other indigenous species of Acacia, especially **A. Farnesiana**, *Willd.* (*Wight, Icones*, vol. i. t. 300), **A. ferruginea**, *D. C.*, **A. leucophlœa**, *Willd.* (*Roxb., Corom. Pl.*, t. 150), **A. amara**, *Willd.* (*Roxb., Corom. Pl.*, t. 122), and **A. Lebbek**, *Willd.* (*Siris*, Hind.), partake more or less of the astringent properties of *A. Arabica*. The gum yielded by *A. Farnesiana* and *A. Lebbek* is said to be of a superior quality.

**Cassia alata**, *Linn.* (*Wight, Icones*, vol. i. t. 253.)—A handsome shrub with large conspicuous erect racemes of yellow flowers, introduced from the West Indies, now naturalized in all parts of India. It is often cultivated by the natives for the sake of its leaves, which are held in high esteem as a local application in skin diseases. A belief in their powers in this character prevails also in the West Indies, Brazil, Mauritius, Java, and other tropical countries. Their efficiency, especially in *Herpes circinatus*, is confirmed by Dr. McKenna (*Madras Med. Journ.* vol. i. p. 431), Dr. Arthur (*Indian Ann. of*

*Med. Science*, 1856, vol. iii. p. 632), and others. Favourable statements as to their efficiency in this class of cases are contained in the reports of Dr. G. Bidie, Dr. W. J. Van Someren, Dr. L. Stewart, and Dr. Rean. As a general rule they appear to be more effectual in recent cases than in those of long standing. The Bengal Ph. contains the following formula for an ointment of the leaves, which is described as being almost a specific in ringworm :—Take of the fresh leaves of Cassia alata, a sufficiency, bruise into a paste, and incorporate with an equal weight of simple ointment. A more effectual mode of application, however, is thoroughly to rub in, over the affected part, the bruised leaves rubbed into a paste with a small portion of lime juice. In many cases it is productive of excellent effects. The leaves taken internally act as an aperient. Mr. J. Wood reports that a tincture of the dried leaves has been found to operate in the same manner as senna; and Dr. Pulney Andy states that an extract prepared from the fresh leaves is a good substitute for Extract of Colocynth. It is desirable that further trials should be made with them. Similar virtues are assigned to the leaves of **Cassia Sophora**, *Linn.* (*Bot. Reg.*, t. 856), **Cassia occidentalis**, *Linn.* (*Bot. Reg.*, t. 83), and **Cassia Tora**, *Linn.* (*Rheede, Hort. Mal.*, vol. ii. t. 53). Indeed, Ainslie states (*Mat. Ind.*, vol. ii. p. 405) that the leaves of *C. Tora*, rubbed up with lime juice, are regarded by the Hindú doctors as one of their best remedies in ringworm. Dr. H. E. Busteed reports having used an infusion of the leaves of *C. Sophora*, and found it a useful cathartic. He mentions also having found an infusion of the leaves of **Agati grandiflora**, *Desv.*, act in a similar manner. Dr. E. Bonavia confirms this statements, and he further speaks of the bark as a bitter tonic.

**Cassia Absus**, *Linn.* (*Nees, Düsseld*, t. 348).—The seeds of this plant, common alike in Northern Africa and in India, constitute the *Chaksú* (Hind.) of the Indian, and the *Chichm* of the Egyptian Materia Medica, and enjoy high repute as a local application in purulent ophthalmia. For this purpose the seeds are reduced to a fine powder, and a small portion, a grain or more, is introduced beneath the eyelids. In an epidemic of purulent ophthalmia which visited Brussels in 1822, Dr. Harbauer gave a fair trial to this treatment, and the results were on the whole confirmatory of its alleged efficacy (*Graëfe and Walther's Journal*, 1825, vol. vi. p. 1.) Dr. G. Smith, Superintendent of the Eye Infirmary at Madras, in his report, characterises it as a dangerous application in catarrhal ophthalmia and granular lids, adding that its application causes great pain. As met with in the bazaars, these seeds are of a black shining colour, somewhat flat, of an oval or oblong form, pointed at one extremity, about one-sixth of an inch long, having a bitter taste.

**Cassia auriculata**, *Linn.*—The seeds of this common Indian plant, like the preceding, are a valued local application in that form of purulent ophthalmia known in India by the name of "country sore eye." Dr. Kirkpatrick (*Cat. of Mysore Drugs*, No. 258) expresses his opinion that they constitute an undoubtedly useful application in these cases, when not severe. They are smooth flattish seeds, of an oval, oblong, or obscurely triangular form, obtusely pointed at one extremity, and varying in colour from brown to dull olive green: they are tasteless and inodorous. The bark is highly astringent; and Dr. Kirkpatrick states (*Op. cit.* No. 475) that he has employed it in the place of oak bark for gargles, enemas, &c., and found it a perfect substitute for the imported article. Both the seeds and bark appear worthy of further trials. A spirituous liquor is prepared in some parts of India by adding the bruised bark to a solution of molasses, and allowing the mixture to ferment.

**Cæsalpinia Sappan,** *Linn.* (*Roxb.*, *Corom. Pl.*, t. 16.)—A tree of the forests of the Madras and Malayan Peninsulas. The wood (*Sappan wood*), though chiefly used as a dye, is described (*Bengal Ph.*, p. 295) as a useful astringent, containing much tannic and gallic acids, and as a good substitute for logwood. The dose of the Extract, which may be prepared as Extract of Hæmatoxylon (*q.v.*), is from ten to fifteen grains twice or thrice daily.

**Cæsalpinia coriaria,** *Willd.* (*Divi-divi*).—The legumes of this tree, introduced from the western hemisphere, and now naturalized in some parts of India, contain a very large proportion of tannin. According to Dr. Cornish (*Indian Ann. of Med. Science*, 1856, vol. iv. p. 120), from 60 to 65 per cent. of the whole pod, exclusive of the seeds, consists of impure tannin, the remaining portion consisting of woody fibre, starch, and gum. The powder of the dried pods is of a light yellow colour, and purely astringent taste, strongly resembling tannin as met with in commerce. This powder has been brought forward as an antiperiodic by Dr. Cornish, who administered it in ninety-four cases of intermittent fever, many of them severe, with excellent results, the dose ranging from forty to sixty grains. Dr. Oswald reports that a decoction of the legumes forms a good injection in bleeding piles. Both as an astringent and as an antiperiodic, this drug appears to be well worthy of further attention.

**Pongamia glabra,** *Vent.* (*Wight, Icones*, vol. i. t. 59.)—From the seeds of this tree, met with in most parts of India, an oil is obtained by expression, which holds a high place in native Materia Medica, as an application in scabies, herpes, and other cutaneous diseases. Dr. Gibson states that he knows no article of the vegetable kingdom possessed of more marked properties in such cases than the above. The oil is also much used as an embrocation in rheumatism. Some remarks on the physical characters and properties of this oil are given by Dr. Crosse (*Journ. Agri.-Hort. Soc. of India*, 1858, vol. x. P. ii. p. 223).

**Butea frondosa,** *Roxb.*—The seeds of this tree enjoy a high repute as a vermifuge, especially amongst the Mahomedan doctors. As met with in the bazaars, they occur in the form of thin, flat, oval or reniform seeds, of a mahogany-brown colour, 1¼ to 1¾ inches in length, almost devoid of taste and smell. The late Dr. Butler (*Madras Med. Reports*, 1855, p. 425,) reported very favourably of their efficacy in this character; and his views are confirmed by other reports received from India from medical officers who have given them a trial. Dr. Oswald, who has had considerable experience in their use, directs the seeds to be first soaked in water, the testa to be carefully removed, and the kernel to be dried and reduced to powder. Of this, the dose is twenty grains three times a day for three successive days, and a dose of Castor oil on the fourth day. Thus administered, Dr. Oswald states that he has seen it cause the expulsion of 125 lumbrici in one instance, and from 70 to 80 in another. The remedy has the disadvantage of occasionally purging when its anthelmintic properties are not apparent. Dr. Kees further mentions that in large doses it is apt to induce vomiting; and Dr. G. Smith adds that it is apt to irritate the kidneys. These ill effects justify a caution given by Dr. Pulney Andy as to its indiscriminate use.

Of their powers as an anthelmintic there can be little doubt: further remarks as to their general safety are desirable. The pounded seeds, made into a paste, have in some instances, according to Dr. Oswald, been found useful in ringworm.

**Clitorea ternatea,** *Linn.* (*Bot. Mag.*, t. 1542.)—The seeds of this elegant climbing plant have purgative properties assigned to them. Dr. J. Shortt reports having employed the roasted seeds powdered, in drachm doses, with success in this character. Dr. W. Dymock bears similar testimony. Both these gentlemen advise their administration in combination with twice their bulk of Acid Tartrate of Potash. Their action appears to be mild and safe; and as they are to be procured in almost every locality throughout India for the cost of collecting, they are deserving of further attention. Mr. Moodeen Sheriff speaks highly from personal experience of the root bark, in doses of from one to two drachms in infusion as a demulcent in irritation of the bladder and urethra. It acts at the same time as a diuretic, and in some cases as a laxative. Dr. R. Haines recommends a syrup of the flowers as a colouring agent.

**Lathyrus sativus,** *Linn.*—Attention is here only called to this plant, from the fact that the continued use of its seeds (*Kisari dál*, Hind.) as an article of diet is apt, under certain circumstances, to induce paralysis of the lower extremities. In one district in Bengal, nearly four per cent. of the population were sufferers from it. Interesting papers on this subject are furnished by Dr. J. Irving (*Indian Ann. of Med. Sci.*, 1860, vol. vii. p. 127), and Dr. Kinloch Kirk (*Ibid.*, p. 145).

**Cicer arietinum,** *Linn.* (*Wight, Icones*, vol. i. t. 20)—*Chick Pea, Bengal Gram. Chaná*, Hind.—Much cultivated throughout India for the sake of its seeds, which are largely used as food for cattle, &c. The hairs of the stem, leaves, and other parts of the plant exude an acid liquid, containing oxalic, acetic, and perhaps malic acid, and, according to Dispan, another acid peculiar to the plant (Watts *Dict. of Chem.* vol. i. p. 962). Notices of this acid, its uses by the natives and mode of collection, are given by Dr. Christie (*Madras Lit. Sci. Journ.*, vol. iv. p. 476), Dr. Heyne (*Tracts*, p. 28), Ainslie (*Mat. Ind.*, vol. ii. p. 56), and Drury (*Useful Plants of India*, p. 135). It is employed by the natives as a refrigerant in fevers, &c., and it is probable that it is of some use in this character. In the Deccan, it is used by the Portuguese in the treatment of dysmenorrhœa; the fresh plant is put into hot water, and the patient sits over the steam. This, observes Dr. Walker (*Bombay Med. Phys. Trans.* 1840, p. 67), is only another way of steaming with vinegar.

**Alhagi Maurorum,** *Tourn.*—A shrub of the deserts of Africa and Western Asia; common in Northern India and the Deccan. A saccharine exudation from the stem constitutes a sort of Manna (*Túranjbin*, Arab.), which is said (*Bengal Disp.*, p. 296) to possess the medicinal properties of Ash Manna. It occurs in the form of small, brown granular tears, mixed with leaflets, stalks, and other impurities. Some interesting remarks on its production and collection have been published by M. Soubeiran (*Pharm Journ.*, 1861, p. 434), but they throw little additional light on its value as a medicinal agent. As far as our present knowledge extends, it is an article of minor importance.

## ROSACEÆ.

### ROSA GALLICA, *Linn.* French or Red Rose.

(*Woodville, Med. Bot.*, t. 179.)

*Habitat.*—South of Europe; cultivated in gardens everywhere.

*Officinal Part.*—The dried petals of the unexpanded flowers (*Rosæ Gallicæ Flores*) Colour fine purplish-red, retained after drying; taste bitterish, feebly acid and astringent; odour roseate, developed by drying.

*Properties and Uses.*—Slightly tonic and astringent. Chiefly employed in one of the forms mentioned below, as a vehicle for medicines.

*Preparations.*—**Acid Infusion of Roses** (*Infusum Rosæ Acidum*). Take of Red Rose Petals, broken up a quarter of an ounce; dilute Sulphuric Acid, one fluid drachm; Boiling Water, ten fluid ounces. Add the acid to the water, infuse the petals in the mixture in a covered vessel for half an hour, and strain.

*Dose.*—From one to two fluid ounces. An excellent vehicle for saline purgatives, quinine, &c.

**Confection of Roses** (*Confectio Rosæ Gallicæ*). Take of fresh Red Rose Petals, one pound; Refined Sugar, three pounds. Beat the petals to a pulp in a stone mortar, add the sugar, and rub them well together.

*Dose.*—From one to two drachms acts as a mild astringent, but it is rarely employed excepting as a vehicle in the preparation of pills, electuaries, &c. It enters into Pilula Hydrargyri, and other officinal pill masses.

### ROSA CANINA, *Linn.* Dog Rose.

(*Steph. et Church., Med. Bot.*, t. 100.)

*Habitat.*—Common in hedgerows throughout Europe and other portions of the globe.

*Officinal Part.*—The ripe fruit (*Rosæ caninæ Fructus, Hips*); an inch or more in length, ovate, scarlet, smooth, shining; taste sweet, subacid, pleasant.

*Properties and Uses.*—Officinal only as an ingredient in the following Confection, which is frequently used as the basis of electuaries, and also for the formation of pill masses.

*Preparation.*—**Confection of Hips** (*Confectio Rosæ caninæ*). Take of Hips, deprived of their seeds, one pound; Refined Sugar, two pounds. Beat the hips to a pulp in a stone mortar, and rub the pulp through a sieve, then add the sugar and rub them well together.

## ROSA CENTIFOLIA, *Linn.* The Hundred-leaved or Cabbage Rose.

*Habitat.*—Cultivated in gardens in all parts of the world.

*Officinal Part.*—The fresh fully expanded petals (*Rosæ centifoliæ Petala*). They possess a sweetish, bitter, and faintly astringent taste, and a roseate odour, both readily imparted to water.

*Properties and Uses.*—Mildly laxative; officinal only on account of their Distilled Water.

*Preparations.*—**Rose Water** (*Aqua Rosæ*). Take of the fresh petals of the Hundred-leaved Rose, ten pounds, or an equivalent quantity of the petals preserved, while fresh, with common salt; Water, two gallons. Distil one gallon.

Much employed, on account of its fragrant odour, as a vehicle for lotions, collyriums, &c.

**The Volatile Oil, Attar** or **Utr of Roses**, is manufactured chiefly in Turkey, but a small quantity is produced at Ghazipore, from the petals of *R. damascena*, or Damask Rose. A full description of its manufacture, as well as that of Rose Water, prepared at the latter locality, is given by Dr. Jackson (*Journ. of Asiatic Society*, 1839, *and Bengal Disp.*, p. 327). From its powerful aroma, Attar of Roses is well adapted for disguising the unpleasant odour of certain ointments, and other external applications.

## BRAYERA ANTHELMINTICA, *D.C.* Cusso, Kousso.

(*Hooker, Kew Journ.*, vol. ii. 1850, t. 10.)

*Habitat.*—Abyssinia.

*Officinal Part.*—The dried flowers and tops (*Cusso, Kousso*). Flowers small, reddish-brown, on hairy stalks; outer limb of calyx five-parted, the segments ovate, reticulated; odour balsamic; taste nauseous and slightly acrid, resembling senna. It contains a volatile oil, a bitter acrid resin and tannin, and a crystalline principle named *Kwoseine.*

*Properties.*—Anthelmintic.

*Therapeutic Uses.*—For the destruction of tænia, Kousso acts with tolerable certainty; to expel the entozoon, a subsequent aperient is necessary.

*Dose.*—For adults, half an ounce; for children of seven to twelve years, two drachms and a half; for those of three to seven years, two drachms; and for those not exceeding three years, one drachm to one drachm and a half. It may be administered in infusion (*infra*), or in the form of electuary, with honey.

*Preparations.*—**Infusion of Kousso** (*Infusum Cusso*). Take of Kousso, in coarse powder, a quarter of an ounce; Boiling Water, four fluid ounces. Infuse in a covered vessel for fifteen minutes.

This forms a dose for an adult, and should be taken, flowers and water together, on an empty stomach, followed in a few hours by an aperient.

## AMYGDALUS COMMUNIS, VAR. DULCIS, *D.C.*
### SWEET ALMOND TREE.

## AMYGDALUS COMMUNIS, VAR. AMARA, *D.C.*
### BITTER ALMOND TREE.

(*Woodville, Med. Bot.*, t. 182.)

*Habitat.*—Barbary and Syria; cultivated in Europe and temperate Asia.

*Officinal Part.*—1. The seeds (*Amygdalæ dulces, Sweet Almonds*). Usually about an inch in length, lanceolate, acute, with a clear cinnamon-brown seed-coat, and of a bland, sweetish nutty flavour. They do not evolve the odour of bitter almonds when bruised with water. 2. The seeds (*Amygdalæ amaræ, Bitter Almonds*): resemble sweet almonds in appearance, but are rather broader and shorter; have a bitter taste, and when rubbed with a little water emit a characteristic odour.

*Properties and Uses.*—Sweet almonds are emollient and nutritive. Bitter almonds (*Amygdalæ amaræ*) are officinal only for the sake of their expressed oil (*infra*).

*Preparations.*—**Compound Powder of Almonds** (*Pulvis Amygdalæ compositus; Confectio Amygdalæ, Lond. Ph.*) Take of Sweet Almonds, eight ounces; Refined Sugar, in powder, four ounces; Gum Acacia, in powder, one ounce. Steep the almonds in warm water until their skins can be easily removed; and when blanched, dry them thoroughly with a soft cloth, and rub them lightly in a mortar to a smooth consistence. Mix the gum and the sugar; and, adding them to the pulp gradually, rub the whole to a coarse powder. Keep it in a lightly-covered jar.

**Almond Mixture** (*Mistura Amygdalæ*).—Take of Compound Powder of Almonds, two ounces and a half; Distilled Water, one pint. Rub the powder with a little of the water into a thin paste; then add the remainder of the water, and strain through muslin.

*Dose.*—From one to two fluid ounces.

An excellent vehicle for expectorants, saline refrigerants, &c.

**Almond Oil** (*Oleum Amygdalæ*). Obtained by expression from sweet or bitter almonds. It is of a pale-yellow colour, nearly inodorous or of a slight nutty odour, and bland oleaginous taste.

Emollient, laxative; forms an ingredient in several officinal ointments.

## PRUNUS LAUROCERASUS, *Linn.* THE COMMON OR CHERRY LAUREL.

(*Woodville, Med. Bot.*, t. 185.)

*Habitat.*—Asia Minor; common in gardens all over temperate Europe.

*Officinal Part.*—The leaves (*Laurocerasi Folia*); ovate-lanceolate or elliptical, distantly toothed, furnished with glands at the base, smooth and shining, deep green, on strong foot stalks, inodorous until bruised, when they emit a ratafia odour, which is peculiarly observable in the leaf-buds; taste bitter, aromatic, and slightly astringent. Their activity depends upon a volatile oil, having hydrocyanic acid as one of its constituents. [This oil does not exist in the leaves in their natural state, but is developed, probably, by the reaction of different principles on each other when they are bruised and submitted to the action of moisture.]

*Properties.*—Powerful but uncertain sedative; in large doses, a violent poison. The leaf-buds are much more powerful than the full grown leaves.

*Therapeutic Uses.*—In nervous and spasmodic affections it has been employed, but every effect which can be expected from them may be procured with greater safety and certainty from dilute hydrocyanic acid. The bruised leaves have been used as an external anodyne application in certain painful affections; but they are not devoid of danger when applied to an abraded or ulcerated surface.

*Dose.*—From four to eight grains of the powdered leaves; rarely employed.

*Preparations.*—**Laurel Water** (*Aqua Laurocerasi*). Take of Fresh Leaves of Common Laurel, one pound; Water, two pints and a half. Chop the leaves, crush them in a mortar, and macerate them in the water for twenty-four hours. Then distil one pint of liquid, shake the product, filter through paper, and preserve in a stoppered bottle.

*Dose.*—From five to thirty minims. A dangerous remedy, on account of the variable quantity of hydrocyanic acid which it contains.

**Diluted Hydrocyanic Acid** (*Acidum Hydrocyanicum dilutum*). Hydrocyanic Acid, $HC_2N$ or **HCN**, dissolved in water, and constituting two per cent. by weight of the solution.

Hydrocyanic Acid may be obtained from the volatile oil and distilled water of the leaves of Prunus Laurocerasus, from the oil of Bitter Almonds, the seeds of other Amygdaleæ, and from the seeds of the Pomeæ; but for medicinal purposes it is prepared by the distillation of Sulphuric Acid with Yellow Prussiate of Potassium and water. *Characters and Tests.* — A colourless liquid with a peculiar odour; specific gravity 0·997. It only slightly and transiently reddens litmus paper. A fluid drachm evaporated in a platinum dish leaves no fixed residue. Treated with a minute quantity of a mixed solution of sulphate and persulphate of iron, afterwards with potash, and finally acidulated with hydrochloric acid, it forms Prussian blue. It gives no precipitate with chloride of barium, but with nitrate of silver it gives a white precipitate entirely soluble in boiling concentrated nitric acid. 270 grains of it, rendered alkaline by the addition of solution of soda, requires 1000 grain-measures of the volumetric solution of nitrate of silver to be added before a permanent precipitate begins to form, which corresponds to two per cent. of the real acid.

This acid contains rather more than half as much real acid as the *Acidum Hydrocyanicum* of the Edinburgh Pharmacopœia. It corresponds in strength with the *Acidum Hydrocyanicum Dilutum*, London and Dublin Ph.

*Properties.*—Powerfully sedative and anodyne. In large doses a rapid and energetic poison.

*Therapeutic Uses.*—In catarrhal and irritable states of the bronchial mucous membrane, and in some pulmonary spasmodic affections, as hooping cough, asthma, and angina pectoris, it has been often used with advantage. In dyspepsia attended with vomiting, in gastritis, gastrodynia, cardialgia, and pyrosis, it is a remedy of great value. In hypertrophy of the heart, especially when characterised by violent palpitation, it has been found serviceable. It has likewise been employed in gout, rheumatism, active hœmorrhage, chorea, tetanus, &c., with alleged benefit. Externally it has been employed, diluted in the form of lotion, for allaying pain and irritation in skin diseases; but if applied to a large or abraded surface, the practice is not devoid of danger.

*Dose.*—From two to eight minims diluted. As an external application the strength may vary from one to two drachms of the dilute acid to eight ounces of water.

*Preparation.*—**Inhalation of Hydrocyanic Acid** (*Vapor Acidi Hydrocyanici*). Take of Diluted Hydrocyanic Acid, ten to fifteen minims; Water (cold), one fluid drachm. Mix in a suitable apparatus, and let the vapour that arises be inhaled.

## PRUNUS DOMESTICA, *Linn.* THE PLUM TREE.

(*Engl. Bot.*, t. 1783; *ed. Syme*, t. 111.)

*Habitat.*—Cultivated in gardens throughout the temperate zone.

*Officinal Part.*—The dried drupe (*Prunum, Prune*); about an inch in length, ovate, wrinkled, black, and sweet to the taste.

*Properties and Uses.*—Demulcent and laxative; rarely employed alone for medicinal purposes. An agreeable and useful adjunct to electuaries; an ingredient in Confectio Sennæ.

(*Non-officinal.*)

**Pyrus Cydonia,** *Linn.* (*Hayne,* vol. iv. t. 47.)—This small tree (*Common Quince*) extends from Southern Europe, through Persia, to the Himalaya, Nepaul, and other parts of Northern India. Quince seeds (*Bhí-dana* or *Bhí-ka-bíj*, Hind.) are commonly met with in the bazaars. They are about ¼ inch in length, ovate or obconical, flattened, pointed at the extremities, of a reddish-brown colour. Ten or fifteen seeds, the contents of one cell of the fruit, are frequently found adhering together. The seed coat imparts to boiling water a peculiar kind of mucilage (*Cydonin*). They are highly valued as a demulcent tonic and restorative by the Mahomedans all over the East. According to the report of Dr. J. Newton, a decoction of these seeds proves particularly useful in dysentery where inflammatory action is present; it seems to line the mucous membrane, and protect it from the irritating fæcal matter. It has also been found a useful demulcent in gonorrhœa.

# LYTHRARIEÆ.

*(Non-officinal.)*

**Lawsonia alba,** *Lam.* (*Wight, Illust.* vol. i. t. 87)—*Henna.*—A shrub, common in dry jungles in tropical India, and cultivated throughout the East for the sake of its leaves, which are in common use amongst all classes of natives for staining the nails, &c. They are likewise esteemed for their medicinal properties, and are probably of some value as an astringent, Berthollet (*Journ. de Pharm.* vol. x. p. 405) having found them to contain gallic acid. In that obscure affection termed "Burning of the Feet," often met with in India, they are esteemed by the natives one of their most valued local applications. Dr. Grierson (*Calcutta Med. Phys. Trans.*, vol. ii. p. 279) mentions an obstinate case benefited by their use; and the Editor, when in Burmah, witnessed, in some cases, a great amount of temporary relief to the distressing sensation of burning from this remedy, when numerous other means had previously failed. The fresh leaves beaten up into a paste with vinegar, and applied as a poultice to the soles of the feet, was the common mode of application; but some patients obtained greater relief from using strong frictions with the bruised leaves over the part. Like all other remedies, however, they not unfrequently fail to afford more than temporary relief. (*See Madras Quarterly Journ. of Med.*, vol. i. p. 300, 1860.) Cataplasms of the bruised leaves, or fomentations with an infusion of the leaves, are much employed as a local application to bruises, sprains and other diseases. An extract prepared from the leaves and flowers is given in leprosy. (*Dr. J. Newton.*)

**Ammannia vesicatoria,** *Roxb.*—The leaves of this plant, common in India, are highly acrid, and are much employed by the natives as a vesicant; but from the trials made with them by Sir W. O'Shaughnessy, it is evident that, both from the length of time required to raise a blister, and the great pain caused by them, we are not justified in recommending their employment. They cause more pain than cantharides, and are far inferior to *Plumbago rosea* in celerity and certainty of action. (*Bengal Disp.*, p. 331.) Dr. Bholanauth Bose describes a mode of treatment of obstinate spleen disease, by the juice of the leaves administered internally; but the pain it causes is stated to be agonizing, and the results uncertain. It does not appear to be an eligible remedy.

# HAMAMELIDEÆ.

## LIQUIDAMBAR ORIENTALE, *Miller*. LIQUID STORAX TREE.

(*Hooker, Icon. Plant,* vol. xi.)

*Habitat.*—Asia Minor.

*Officinal Part.*—A balsam obtained from the bark, purified by rectified spirit and straining (*Styrax præparatus.*

*Prepared Storax*). It occurs in the form of a semi-transparent, brownish-yellow, semi-fluid resin, of the consistence of thick honey, with a strong agreeable fragrance and aromatic taste. Heated in a test tube on the vapour bath, it becomes more liquid, but gives off no moisture. Boiled with solution of bichromate of potash and sulphuric acid it evolves the odour of hydride of benzoyle. It contains a volatile oil (*Styrol*), a crystallizable principle (*Styracine*), and Cinnamic acid.

*Properties.*—Stimulant, expectorant.

*Therapeutic Uses.*—In chronic bronchitis, chronic coughs of the aged, and asthma, it proves beneficial. In gonorrhœa, leucorrhœa, and allied affections, it has been used as a substitute for copaiba. Applied to indolent and ill-conditioned ulcers it is a useful stimulant.

*Dose.*—From five to twenty grains in pill or emulsion.

*Preparations.*—Prepared Storax forms an ingredient in Tinctura Benzoini composita.

(*Non-officinal.*)

**Liquidambar Altingia,** *Blume* (*Nees, Düsseldorf, Suppl.*, t. 36.)—A large forest tree of Java, common also in some parts of the Tenasserim Provinces, especially at Panlow, about thirty miles from Mergui. It is the *Nan-ta-youk* of the Burmese. It yields a fragrant balsamic fluid, of which two varieties are met with in Burmah; one, pellucid, fragrant, and of a light yellowish colour, obtained by simple incision in the bark; the other, thick, dark, opaque, of a highly terebinthinate odour, obtained by boring holes in the stem, and the application of fire around the trunk of the tree. Of both these varieties the Editor forwarded specimens to the Madras Drug Committee in 1851. Analysed by Marquart (cited by Pereira) it was found to contain a volatile oil somewhat like styrol, and a substance similar to styracine, but their composition he found to be different. The Editor instituted some trials with it as an expectorant, but with no satisfactory results. As a medicinal agent it appears of little value.

## COMBRETACEÆ.

(*Non-officinal.*)

**Terminalia Bellerica,** *Roxb.* (*Wight, Illust.*, vol. i. t. 91), and **T. Chebula,** *Retz.* (*Roxb., Corom. Plants*, t. 197), two common forest trees of India, the ripe fruit of which constitute respectively the *Belleric* and *Chebulic Myrobalans.* Though obsolete in European practice, they retain a high place in the native Materia Medica. From some trials made with Chebulic Myrobalans, the Editor found that six of these fruits, bruised and given in decoction, acted efficiently and safely as a purgative, producing four or five copious stools, unattended by griping, nausea, or other ill effects. The addition of a little cinnamon rendered the medicine more palatable These fruits are procurable at a nominal cost throughout India, and when other aperients are not available, they may be resorted to with safety. (*Madras Journ. of Med.*, April 1861, p. 252.) Notwithstanding their aperient properties, they contain a large amount of astringent principles, which render them valuable in the arts, and as a substitute for galls in lotions, injections, &c. Dr. Oswald reports that a decoction of them proves serviceable in bleeding piles and in some vaginal discharges. They are of an ovoid shape, from 1 to 1½ inch long, sometimes tapering towards the lower extremity, obscurely five or six sided, more or less furrowed longitudinally, covered with a smooth yellowish-brown epidermis, within which is an astringent pulp, enclosing a large, rough, bony, one-celled endocarp. The unripe fruits constitute the *Indian* or *Black Myrobalans* of old writers. As found in commerce, they are shrivelled, black, ovoid bodies, from ⅓ to ¾ of an inch in length, having a shining fracture, and an extremely astringent taste. Their virtues are highly extolled by Rajah Kalikissen (*Calcutta Med. Phys. Trans.*, vol. v. p. 432), who regards them as combining mild purgative with carminative and tonic properties. Twining (*Diseases of Bengal*, vol. i. p 407) speaks very favourably of them in the same character, and expresses his surprise that a medicine with such useful properties should be so little employed in various forms of cachexia in Europe. He gives a case of enlargement of the spleen, in which it was productive of good effects. Curious gall-like excrescences, found on the leaves of *T. Chebula* (*Kadú-kai-pú*, *Tam.*), caused by the deposited ova of an undetermined insect, are held in high esteem as an astringent by the natives. The Rev. J. Kearns, of Tinnevelly, some years since, called the attention of the Editor to them. As the result of his own personal observation, he speaks in the highest terms of their efficacy in the dysentery and diarrhœa of the natives, especially in infantile diarrhœa; the dose for a child under a year old being one grain every three hours. He adds that in the last-named cases he has seen it administered in dozens of instances with signal benefit. Of the Belleric Myrobalans comparatively little is known. In the Bengal Dispensatory (p. 341) it is stated that the kernels, which are generally eaten by the natives, are intoxicating. That they will produce symptoms of narcotic poisoning, when taken in any quantity, is proved by four cases which fell under the care of Mr. C. E. Raddock (*Indian Ann. of Med. Sci.* 1855, vol. ii. p. 709). The symptoms in each were alarming, though the result in none of the cases was fatal. The dried fruit is much used in the arts as an astringent, &c.

**Terminalia Catappa,** *Linn.* (*Wight, Icones*, vol. i. t. 172.)—The kernels of this handsome Moluccan tree, cultivated throughout India, yield upwards of fifty per cent. of a pure bland oil, very similar to almond oil, for which it may be used as a substitute. Attention was called to it in 1843 by Mr. A. Smith (*Journ. Agri.-Hort. Soc. of India*, vol. ii. p. 539), and it was favourably reported on by Dr. F. J. Mouat (*loc cit.*), who observed that, by keeping, it deposited a large proportion of stearine. As prepared by the native process, however, it is apt to become turbid by long keeping. The kernels themselves, called in India *Country Almonds*, might probably be used as a substitute for the officinal almond. The bark possesses considerable astringency. This astringency is also well marked in the bark of **T. tomentosa,** *W. et A.*, which is favourably reported of by Dr. Æ. Ross, in the form of decoction, internally in atonic diarrhœa, &c., and locally as an application to weak indolent ulcers.

The dose of the decoction (two ounces of the bruised bark, water a pint) is two ounces thrice daily.

**Quisqualis Indica,** *Linn.* (*Wight, Illust.*, vol. i. t. 92.)—A scandent shrub of Burmah, the Malayan Peninsula and Archipelago, cultivated in gardens in India under the name of *Rangoon creeper*. The fruits are about an inch in length, oval or oblong, pointed at either extremity, and sharply pentagonal. The woody pericarp is thin, fragile, and of a deep mahogany colour, and encloses an oily seed. In the Moluccas the seeds have long enjoyed repute as an anthelmintic, and in 1833 they were brought forward in this character by Dr. Oxley and Mr. Gordon, of Singapore (*Calcutta Med. Phys. Trans.*, vol. vii. p. 488). The testimony adduced in their favour by these authorities is strong, and is to the effect that in cases of lumbrici, four or five of these seeds, bruised and given in electuary, with honey or jam, suffices for the expulsion of the entozoa in children. Bouton (*Med. Plants of Mauritius*, p. 58), who gives *Liane Vermifuge* as the name of the shrub in the Mauritius, states that if the seeds be given beyond four or five in number, they are apt, in some constitutions, to cause spasms and other ill effects. They seem worthy of further trials. (See *Indian Annals of Med. Science*, vol. vi. 1859.)

# MYRTACEÆ.

## MELALEUCA MINOR, *D.C.* THE LESSER MELALEUCA.

(*Melaleuca leucodendron, Linn.*)

(*Woodville, Med. Bot*, t. 195.)

*Habitat.*—Malayan Peninsula and Archipelago, and Northern Australia.

*Officinal Part.*—The oil distilled from the leaves (*Cajuputi Oleum, Oil of Cajuput*). A very mobile transparent fluid, of a fine pale bluish-green colour. It has a strong agreeable odour and aromatic camphoraceous taste, leaving a sensation of coldness in the mouth.

*Properties.*—Diffusible stimulant, antispasmodic, and diaphoretic; externally applied, rubefacient.

*Therapeutic Uses.*—In the advanced stages and adynamic forms of fever, in paralytic and rheumatic affections, and other cases marked by depression of the vital powers, it has been used with advantage. In cholera it has been lauded, but on insufficient grounds. It proves useful also in flatulent colic, painful spasmodic affections of the stomach, hysteria, &c. Externally it forms a valuable embrocation in rheumatic, neuralgic, and other painful affections, in paralysis, &c.

*Dose.*—From one to five drops.

It forms an ingredient in Linimentum Crotonis.

*Preparations.*—**Spirit of Cajuput** (*Spiritus Cajuputi*). Take of Oil of Cajuput, one fluid ounce; Rectified Spirit, forty-nine fluid ounces. Dissolve.

*Dose.*—From thirty minims to a fluid drachm. This is one fifth the strength of the preparation of the same name in the British Ph. 1864.

## CARYOPHYLLUS AROMATICUS, *Linn.* THE CLOVE TREE.

(*Bot. Mag.*, t. 2749, 2750; *Woodville, Med. Bot.*, t. 193.)

*Habitat.*—Moluccas; cultivated in the East and West Indies, Mauritius, Bourbon, and Zanzibar.

*Officinal Part.* — The dried unexpanded flower-bud (*Caryophyllum, Cloves*). About six lines in length, darkish-brown, plump, and heavy, consisting of a nearly cylindrical body, surmounted by four teeth and a globular head, with a strong fragrant odour, and a bitter, spicy, pungent taste. It emits oil when indented with the nail. Active principles, a volatile oil and a resinous crystalline principle, *Caryophyllin.*

*Properties.*—Aromatic stimulant and carminative.

*Therapeutic Uses.*—In atonic dyspepsia, and in gastric irritability, especially in the vomiting of pregnancy, the infusion or volatile oil (*infra*) proves serviceable, but its chief use is as an aromatic adjunct to other medicines.

*Preparations.*—**Infusion of Cloves** (*Infusum Caryophylli*). Take of Cloves, bruised, a quarter of an ounce; Boiling Water, ten fluid ounces. Infuse in a covered vessel for half an hour, and strain.

*Dose.*—From one to four fluid ounces.

**Oil of Cloves** (*Oleum Caryophylli*). Obtained by distillation from cloves. It is colourless when recent, but gradually assumes a red-brown colour, having the odour of cloves, and a pungent, spicy taste. Sinks in water.

*Dose.*—From two to six minims, on sugar or in emulsion. A small piece of cotton wool saturated with it, locally applied, not unfrequently relieves toothache.

Cloves form an ingredient in Pulvis Cretæ Aromaticus, Infusum Aurantii compositum, Mistura Ferri Aromatica, and Vinum Opii. The Oil enters into Pilula Colocynthidis composita, Pilula Colocynthidis et Hyoscyami, and Confectio Scammonii.

## EUGENIA PIMENTA, *D.C.* Pimento, Allspice Tree.

(*Steph. et Church., Med. Bot.*, t. 124.)

*Habitat.*—West Indies and tropical South America.

*Officinal Part.*—The dried unripe berries (*Pimenta, Pimento, Allspice*), of the size of a small pea, brown, rough, crowned with the teeth of the calyx, yellowish within, and containing two dark-brown seeds; odour and taste aromatic, hot, and peculiar. Its virtues reside in a volatile oil.

*Properties and Uses.*—Similar to those of the Clove.

*Preparations.* — **Oil of Pimento** (*Oleum Pimentæ*), obtained by distillation from pimento. It is colourless or slightly reddish when recent, but becomes brown by age, having the odour and taste of pimento; sinks in water.

*Dose.*—From one to five minims.

**Pimento Water** (*Aqua Pimentæ*). Take of Pimento, bruised, fourteen ounces; Water, two gallons. Distil one gallon.

*Dose.*—From one to two fluid ounces. A good vehicle for other medicines.

Pimento also forms an ingredient in Syrupus Rhamni.

(*Non-officinal.*)

**Psidium pyriferum**, *Linn.* (*White Guava tree*).—The bark, especially that of the root, of this tree, which is much valued for the sake of its delicious fruit, deserves notice as an astringent. Dr. Waitz (*Dis. of Children in Hot Climates*, p. 225) employed it with much success in chronic infantile diarrhœa. He administered it in the form of decoction (½ oz. of the root-bark; water, six oz. boiled to three oz.), in doses of one or more teaspoonfuls three or four times a day. This decoction he also found serviceable, as a local application, in the prolapsus ani of children (p. 233). The astringent properties of the bark have been noticed by Barham (*Hort. Amer.*, p. 70), Lunan (*Hort. Jamaic.*, vol. i. p. 351), Dr. Wright (*Med. Plants of Jamaica*, in his *Memoirs*, p. 279), Aublet (*Plant. Guian*, vol. i. p. 287), Horsfield (*Med. Plants of Java*), and others. The bark of **Psidium pomiferum**, *Linn.*, (*Red Guava tree*,) appears to possess similar properties, though it is not so much employed. In the cholera epidemic at the Mauritius, a decoction of the leaves of *P. pomiferum* is stated by M. Bouton (*Med. Plants of Mauritius*, p. 61), to have been frequently used for arresting the vomiting and diarrhœa.

**Syzigium Jambolanum**, *D.C.* (*Wight, Icones*, vol. ii. t. 535)—*Jám*, Hind.—Common in many parts of India. Its bark possesses astringent properties, and, in the form of decoction, is much used in Bengal in chronic dysentery. This statement of Mr. Rama Churn Bose is confirmed by Dr. Bhohanauth Bose, who adds that a syrup prepared with the juice of the ripe fruit is a pleasant stomachic, and acts as an efficient astringent in chronic diarrhœa.

# GRANATEÆ.

## PUNICA GRANATUM, *Linn.* THE POMEGRANATE TREE.

(*Wight, Illust.*, vol. ii. t. 97.)

*Habitat.*—Northern Africa, and Western Asia as far as the Western Himalaya.

*Officinal Parts.*—1. The root-bark (*Granati Radicis Cortex, Pomegranate Root Bark*). It occurs in quills or fragments of a greyish-yellow colour externally, yellow internally; having a short fracture, little odour, and an astringent slightly bitter taste. 2. *The dried rind or pericarp of the fruit (*Granati Cortex*) is met with in irregular-arched fragments, hard, smooth, about a line in thickness, of an olive or reddish-brown colour externally, yellowish within, inodorous, of a bitter astringent taste. Both the root-bark and the rind of the fruit contain a large proportion of tannin.

*Properties.*—Root-bark, anthelmintic. Rind of the fruit, astringent.

*Therapeutic Uses.*—For the destruction of tape worm the root-bark is very effectual; but as it possesses no purgative property, an aperient is required to ensure the expulsion of the entozoon. In diarrhœa (especially in that of the natives of India), in the advanced stages of dysentery, and in other cases requiring the use of astringents, the rind of the fruit has been used with advantage.

*Preparations.*—**Decoction of Pomegranate Root** (*Decoctum Granati Radicis*). Take of fresh Pomegranate Root-bark sliced, two ounces; Water, two pints. Boil down to a pint, and strain, making the strained product up to a pint, if necessary, by pouring water over the contents of the strainer.

*Dose.*—As an anthelmintic, two fluid ounces taken fasting, and the same quantity repeated every half hour until six doses have been taken; to be followed by an aperient.

* **Decoction of Pomegranate Rind** (*Decoctum Granati Corticis*). Take of dried Pomegranate Rind, bruised, two ounces; Water, one pint. Boil for fifteen minutes in a covered vessel, then strain, and pour as much water over the contents of the strainer as will make the strained product measure a pint.

*Dose.*—From one to one and a half fluid ounces. A good astringent for gargles, injections, &c. For internal use it is rendered more palatable by the addition of cloves or other aromatics. Combined with opium it proves most useful in the diarrhœa of the natives of India. ([36])

## CUCURBITACEÆ.

### CITRULLUS COLOCYNTHIS, *Schrad.* Bitter Cucumber or Colocynth Plant.

(*Wight, Icones,* vol. ii. t. 498.)

*Habitat.*—Southern Europe; also deserts of Northern Africa, Arabia, and India.

*Officinal Part.*—The dried decorticated fruit, freed from seeds (*Colocynthidis Pulpa, Colocynth Pulp.*) It is light, spongy, white, or yellowish white, intensely bitter. Active principle, a bitter resinoid substance, *Colocynthin.*

*Properties.*—Hydragogue cathartic.

*Therapeutic Uses.*—In constipation, hepatic and visceral congestions, dropsical affections, and other cases requiring purgatives, it is an eligible remedy. It is, however, rarely employed alone, one of the subjoined compounds being preferable.

*Dose.*—From two to eight grains.

*Preparations.*—**Compound Extract of Colocynth** (*Extractum Colocynthidis Compositum*). Take of Colocynth Pulp, six ounces; Extract of Socotrine Aloes, twelve ounces; Resin of Scammony, four ounces; Hard soap, in powder, three ounces; Cardamom seeds, in fine powder, one ounce; Proof Spirit, one gallon. Macerate the colocynth in the spirit for four days; press out the tincture; distil off the spirit; then add the extract of aloes, soap, and scammony, and evaporate by a water bath to a suitable consistence for forming pills, adding the cardamoms towards the end of the process. ([37])

*Dose.*—From three to ten grains.

**Compound Pill of Colocynth** (*Pilula Colocynthidis Composita*). Take of Colocynth Pulp, in powder, one ounce; Barbadoes Aloes, in powder, two ounces; Scammony, in powder, two ounces; Sulphate of Potash, in powder, a quarter of an ounce; Oil of Cloves, two fluid drachms; Water, a sufficiency. Mix the powders, add the oil of cloves, and beat into a mass with the aid of the water.

*Dose.*—From five to ten grains. A safe and active purgative.

**Pill of Colocynth and Hyoscyamus** (*Pilula Colocynthidis et Hyoscyami.*). Take of Compound Pill of Colocynth, two ounces; Extract of Hyoscyamus, one ounce. Beat them into a uniform mass.

*Dose.*—The same as that of compound colocynth pill; the addition of the hyoscyamus renders its operation milder and less irritant.

## ECBALIUM OFFICINARUM, *Rich.* THE SQUIRTING CUCUMBER.

(*Woodville, Med. Bot.* t. 72; *Bot. Mag.* t. 1914.)

*Habitat.*—Mediterranean region.

*Officinal Part.*—The sediment from the expressed juice of the fruit (*Elaterium, Extractum Elaterii,* Lond. Ph.); it occurs in light, friable, slightly incurved cakes, about a line in thickness, greenish-grey, acrid and bitter; fracture finely granular. Does not effervesce with acids; yields half its weight to boiling rectified spirit. This solution, concentrated and added to a warm solution of potash, yields on cooling not less than twenty per cent. of elaterin in colourless crystals. Active principle, *Elaterin,* which is obtained in delicate, striated, satiny, prismatic crystals, with rhombic bases, permanent in the air, inodorous, of a bitter acrid taste. It contains also a resin and a bitter principle.

*Properties.*—Powerful hydragogue cathartic.

*Therapeutic Uses.*—In dropsical affections, especially in that arising in connection with disease of the heart, it is a remedy of great value. In apoplexy and other cerebral affections it proves serviceable, not only by unloading the intestines, but by its derivative action.

*Dose.*—From one sixteenth to one half of a grain, repeated every four hours until it begins to operate. To obviate the griping and nausea which it is apt to create, it may be combined with a small portion of Pulvis Capsici or Extractum Hyoscyami. The dose of *Elaterin* is about one sixteenth of a grain in solution in rectified spirit.

(*Non-officinal.*)

**Cucumis trigonus,** *Roxb.*, (**C. Pseudo-Colocynthis,** *Royle, Illust.,* t. 47. f. 2,) and **C. Hardwickii,** *Royle* (*Illust.* t. 47. f. 3.) The former of these, called *Indrayan* and *Bislúmbhi,* inhabits the upper Gangetic plain; the latter, *Puhari Indrayan* or *Hill Colocynth,* is found on the lower range of the western Himalaya. Its native name on the Kumaon mountains, where it was observed by Madden, is *Airalú;* that of *Indrain* (or *Indrayan*) being applied to *Trichosanthes palmata,* Roxb. They are supposed to possess the purgative properties of officinal colocynth. Dr. Gibson, however, expresses a doubt as to the correctness of this opinion. Experiments are required to determine the point. According to the report of Dr. J. Newton, a decoction of the roots of these plants is used as a purgative; it is stated to be milder in its operation than the pulp of the fruit, and to cause less irritation.

**Trichosanthes nervifolia**, *Linn.*—**T. dioica**, Roxb. (*Rheede, Hort. Mal.*, vol. viii. t. 17.) A common weed, cultivated in many parts of India as an article of food. An alcoholic extract of the unripe fruit is described as a powerful and safe cathartic, in doses of from three to five grains, repeated every third hour till the desired effect is produced. (*Bengal Disp.*, p. 351.) According to Mr. Kanny Loll Dey the bulbous portion of the root is a hydragogue cathartic operating in a similar way to elaterium, for which he proposes it as a substitute. He describes the plant itself as a wholesome bitter, which imparts tone to the system after protracted illness. Dr. H. C. Bowser, from personal trials with it, describes it as a febrifuge and tonic. The old Hindú physicians placed much confidence in it in the treatment of leprosy. (Prof. Wilson, *Calcutta Med. Phys. Trans.*, vol. i. p. 42.)

**Trichosanthes cordata**, *Roxb.*, and **T. palmata**, *Roxb.* (*Wight, Illust.*, vol. ii. tt. 104, 105.) The large tuberous root of the former is regarded by the natives of Eastern Bengal as a valuable tonic, and is used by them as a substitute for Calumba (*Roxburgh*). The singularly bitter taste of the rind of the fruit of *T. palmata* induced Sir W. O'Shaughnessy to institute some trials with it, with the view of ascertaining whether it possessed tonic or purgative properties; but in doses of three grains, thrice daily, it failed to produce any sensible effect. (*Bengal Disp.*, p. 350.) According to Roxburgh (*op. cit.* p. 705), the fruit is regarded as poisonous, and is employed for destroying crows.

**Bryonia epigœa**, *Rottl.* (*Wight, Icones*, vol. ii. t. 503.) The large roots of this plant, common in many parts of India, in their fresh state much resemble a turnip, but are more pointed, and are marked externally with whitish, raised, circular rings; taste bitterish, mucilaginous, and sub-acid. As an alterative tonic it is highly valued by the natives, who prescribe it in syphilitic cases, and the advanced stages of dysentery. The people of the Deccan regard it as a powerful internal and local remedy in snake bites (Dr. Walker, *Bombay Med. Phys. Trans.* 1848, p. 60); and in 1861, Dr. George Bidie called the attention of the Editor to its use for a similar purpose by the people of Mysore. No cases, however, illustrative of its efficacy in this character appear to be on record. M. Jules Lepine, of Pondicherry, (*Exposition, &c.*, p. 118,) detected in it a bitter, yellow, uncrystallizable matter. Ainslie (*Mat. Ind.*, vol. ii. p. 158) justly remarks, that the root possesses virtues worthy of more definite investigation.

**Curcubita Pepo**, *Linn.*, (*Pumpkin*). This well-known vegetable is only mentioned here with the view of noticing the alleged anthelmintic properties of the seeds in cases of Tænia. Several American physicians have recorded evidence in their favour; the average dose being about two ounces of the fresh decorticated seeds, given in the form of emulsion, in the morning, fasting, and followed in an hour or two by a dose of castor oil. The expressed oil of the seeds, in doses of half an ounce, repeated once or twice at an interval of two hours, and followed by an aperient, is said to be equally effectual. (*See Dunglison's New Remedies*, p. 717.) Trials with this remedy might be advantageously made in India, where the fruit is so common, especially as the seeds obtained from plants grown in hot countries, have been found more effectual than those obtained from plants raised in cold latitudes. Dr. Rean reports favourably of the anthelmintic powers of the seeds of **Cucurbita maxima**, *Duch.* (cultivated in Burmah, as well as in many parts of India). He places the dose at from four to eight drachms, incorporated with sugar or honey. They were found principally effectual against tænia, which are usually expelled after ten or twelve hours.

**Luffa amara,** *Roxb.* (*Kerula, Bindál,* Hind.) Every part of this plant is extremely bitter; and, according to the report of Dr. J. A. Green, it is not only a grateful bitter tonic, but a powerful diuretic when given in infusion (two drachms of the fresh stalks; boiling water, one pint), in doses of from one to two fluid ounces, three or four times daily. Combined with nitro-hydrochloric acid, he has found it useful in dropsy supervening on enlargement of the spleen and liver from malarious poison. He makes no mention of the violent purgative and emetic properties which are assigned to the fruit by Roxburgh. Under the name *Bindaãl*, it is extolled by Mr. J. C. Dickenson as a remedy in spleen affections, especially in malarious enlargements of that organ. He relates cases successfully treated with it (*Indian Med. Gaz.*, Nov. 1, 1866, p. 322). He prescribes for young children the above infusion, in doses of a fluid drachm, three or four times daily.

## PAPAYACEÆ.

(*Non-officinal.*)

**Carica Papaya,** *Linn.* (*Wight, Illust.*, vol. ii. t. 106, 107.)—*Papaw tree.*—A native of the Western hemisphere, now domesticated in India and other tropical countries. The anthelmintic properties of the milky juice of the unripe fruit were first noticed in the 17th century by Hernandez; and the attention of the profession in India was called to it in 1810 by Dr. Fleming (*Asiatic Researches*, vol. xi.), who cites an interesting passage from the writings of M. Charpentier Cossigni in support of its alleged virtues. Further confirmatory evidence has more recently been adduced by M. Bouton (*Med. Plants of Mauritius*, 1857, p. 65), and it may justly be concluded that the statements as to its efficacy as an anthelmintic are founded on fact. The following mode of administration, employed by the late Dr. Lemarchand, of the Mauritius, (cited by Bouton,) it would be desirable to adopt in all future trials with this remedy: Take of fresh Papaw milk and honey, of each a tablespoonful; mix thoroughly, gradually add three or four tablespoonfuls of boiling water; and when sufficiently cool take the whole at a draught, following its administration two hours subsequently by a dose of castor oil, to which a portion of lime juice or vinegar may be added. This may be repeated two days successively if required. The above is a dose for an adult; half the quantity may be given to children between 7 and 10 years of age; and a third, or a teaspoonful, to children under three years. If it cause griping, as it occasionally does, enemas containing sugar have been found effectual in relieving it. Taking the dose above named as correct, the statement of Sir W. O'Shaughnessy (*Bengal*

*Disp.*, p. 352,) that he had administered the milky juice as an anthelmintic, in doses of from 20 to 60 drops, without obvious effect, is fully explained. It is principally effectual in the expulsion of lumbrici. On tænia it is reported to have little effect. Anthelmintic virtues have also been assigned to the seeds, which have a pungent taste, not unlike that of mustard and cress, but the evidence of their efficacy is very inconclusive. A belief in their powerfully emmenagogue properties prevails amongst all classes of women in Southern India; so much so, that they assert that if a pregnant woman partake of them, even in moderate quantities, abortion will be the probable result. This popular belief is noticed in many of the reports received from India. In them it is also stated that the milky juice of the plant is applied locally to the os uteri with the view of inducing abortion. Facts in support of the alleged emmenagogue properties of the papaw are still wanting. It is not within the scope of this work to consider the alleged power of the juice of the papaw to lessen the cohesion of the muscular fibre, or, in homely language, to render tough meat tender. The subject, which is discussed *in extenso* by Sir W. J. Hooker (*Bot. Mag.* Nos. 2998 and 2999), Dr. Wight (*Illust.*, vol. ii. p. 34 *et seq.*), and Dr. John Davy (*Edin. Med. Phil. Mag.*, Oct. 1855), must still be regarded as *sub judice*.

## UMBELLIFERÆ.

### CARUM CARUI, *Linn.* CARAWAY PLANT.

(*Engl. Bot.*, t. 1503; *ed. Syme*, t. 582.)

*Habitat.*—Meadows and pastures throughout Europe and Temperate Asia; abundant at high elevations in the Himalaya.

*Officinal Part.*—The dried fruit (*Carui Fructus, Caraway Fruit.*) It has the following characters:—Fruit usually separating into two parts, which are about two lines long, curved, tapering at each end, brown, with five paler longitudinal ridges; having an agreeable aromatic odour and a spicy taste. Active principle, a volatile oil.

*Properties.*—Stomachic and carminative.

*Therapeutic Uses.*—In flatulence, flatulent colic, atonic dyspepsia, and spasmodic affections of the bowels, it proves serviceable.

Caraway fruit is an ingredient in Confectio Opii, Confectio Piperis, Pulvis Opii compositus, Tinctura Cardamomi composita, and Tincura Sennæ.

*Preparations.*—**Oil of Caraway** (*Oleum Carui*). The oil obtained by distillation from the fruit. It is colourless or pale yellow, with an aromatic odour and spicy taste.

*Dose.*—From two to six drops on sugar or in emulsion. It enters into Confectio Scammoniæ, and Pilula Aloes Barbadensis.

**Caraway Water** (*Aqua Carui*). Take of Caraway Fruit, bruised, one pound; Water, two gallons. Distil one gallon.

*Dose.*—From one to two fluid ounces. A useful carminative, especially for children. A good vehicle for saline purgatives, &c.

[**Carum nigrum,** the fruit of which, under the name of *Zira siah*, Hind., is brought into India from Kunawur, and used as a carminative (*Royle*), does not appear to differ from the common Caraway.]

## *CARUM (PTYCHOTIS) AJOWAN, *D.C.* AJWAIN OR OMUM PLANT.

(*Ptychotis Coptica*, D.C.)

(*Wight. Icones*, vol. ii. t. 566.)

*Habitat.*—Tropical Africa? Much cultivated in India.

*Officinal Part.*—The fruit (*Fructus Ptychotis, Ajwain Fruit*). Occurs in the form of minute umbelliferous fruits, which, examined with a lens, are seen to be covered with prominent tubercles, extremely aromatic, evolving, when rubbed, a strong odour resembling that of common Thyme (*Thymus vulgaris*). Taste somewhat bitter and very pungent. Its virtues reside in a Volatile Oil.

*Properties.* — Valuable stimulant, carminative, and antispasmodic.[38]

*Therapeutic Uses.*—In flatulence, flatulent colic, atonic dyspepsia, and diarrhœa, it is a remedy of much value. It has obtained considerable repute, not only in the above affections, but in cholera; in the latter disease, however, its powers appear to be very limited.

*Preparations.*—**Oil of Ajwain** or **Omum** (*Oleum Ptychotis*). The Oil obtained by distillation from the fruit. Recently prepared, colourless, but soon acquiring a slightly yellow tinge. It has the odour of the fruit, and an acrid burning taste. Sp. gr. about 0·880.

*Dose.*—From one to three drops on sugar or in emulsion.

**Ajwain** or **Omum Water** (*Aqua Ptychotis*). Take of Ajwain Fruit, bruised, twenty ounces; Water, two gallons. Distil a gallon.

*Dose.*—From one to two fluid ounces. A valuable carminative, useful in disguising the taste of disagreeable drugs, especially Castor Oil, and obviating their tendency to cause nausea and griping.

[Under the name of *Ajwain-ka-phul* there is sold in the bazaars of the Deccan, Scinde, &c., a crystalline substance, first brought to notice by the late Dr. Stocks, who states that it is prepared from the fruits of *Carum Ajowan*, at Oojein and elsewhere in Central India, during the cold season, and also that it forms spontaneously on the surface of the distilled water of Ajwain. Examined by Dr. Stenhouse, it was found to be a stearopten ($C_{44}H_{31}O_{10}$), of a peculiar pungent odour, somewhat resembling the oils of thyme and marjoram, heavier than water, and melting at 127° F. (*Pharm. Journ.*, 1855, vol. xiv. p. 272.)

## PIMPINELLA ANISUM, *Linn.* COMMON ANISE.

(*Woodville, Med. Bot.*, t. 52.)

This plant, a native of Southern Europe, the Levant, &c is officinal only on account of the volatile oil obtained, by distillation from its fruit (*Oleum Anisi, Oil of Anise*), which, in characters, properties, and uses, agrees closely with the corresponding product of Illicium anisatum, *q.v.*

*Preparation.*—**Essence of Anise** (*Essentia Anisi*). Take of Oil of Anise, one fluid ounce; Rectified Spirit, four fluid ounces. Mix.

*Dose.*—From ten to twenty minims. A useful carminative. It is double the strength of the preparation of the same name in Dubl. Ph.

## FŒNICULUM VULGARE, *Gærtn.* COMMON FENNEL.

(*Wight, Icones*, vol. ii. t. 515.)

*Habitat.*—Southern Europe; commonly cultivated.

*Officinal Part.*—The fruit (*Fœniculi Fructus, Fennel Fruit*). About three lines long and one line broad, elliptical, slightly curved, beaked, having eight pale-brown longitudinal ribs, the two lateral being double; taste and odour aromatic. Its virtues reside in a volatile oil.

*Properties and Uses.*—Similar to those of Carum Carui.

*Preparations.*—**Fennel Water** (*Aqua Fœniculi*). Take of Fennel Fruit, bruised, one pound; Water, two gallons. Distil one gallon.

*Dose.*—From one to three fluid ounces. A useful carminative and stomachic. Chiefly used as a vehicle for other medicines.

[**Fœniculum Panmorium**, *D.C.*, the fruit of which constitutes the *Panmuhuri*, Hind., of the Indian bazaars, differs in no respect from *F. vulgare*. The Indian possesses all the characters and properties of the European article.]

## ANETHUM GRAVEOLENS, *Linn.* COMMON DILL.

(*Wight, Icones*, vol. ii. t. 572.)

*Habitat.*—Southern Europe; cultivated in England and India.

*Officinal Part.*—The dried fruit (*Anethi Fructus, Dill Fruit*). Oval, flat, about a line and a half in length, with a pale membranous margin; odour aromatic; taste warm, somewhat bitter. Active principle, a volatile oil.

*Properties and Uses.*—Similar to those of Carum Carui; but more grateful to the taste, and more effectual in operation.

*Preparations.*—**Oil of Dill** (*Oleum Anethi*). The oil obtained from distillation of the fruit. It is of a pale yellow colour, and acrid sweetish taste.

*Dose.*—From two to five drops on sugar or in emulsion.

**Dill Water** (*Aqua Anethi*). Take of Dill Fruit, bruised, one pound; Water, two gallons. Distil one gallon.

*Dose.*—From two fluid drachms to a fluid ounce or more. An excellent carminative for young infants, for relieving flatulence, &c.

[**Anethum Sowa,** *Roxb.*, cultivated in many parts of India for the sake of its aromatic fruit, sold in the bazaars under the Hindustani name *Sowa*, has no specific characters to distinguish it from *Anethum graveolens*, Linn. The fruit of the Indian-grown plant possesses the medicinal properties of the European, and may be substituted for it.]

## CORIANDRUM SATIVUM, *Linn.* THE COMMON CORIANDER.

(*Wight, Icones*, vol. ii. t. 516.)

*Habitat.*—Europe; cultivated in India.

*Officinal Part.*—The ripe fruit dried (*Coriandri Fructus, Coriander Fruit*). It is globular, nearly as large as white pepper, beaked, finely ribbed, yellowish-brown, with an agreeable aromatic odour and flavour. Its virtues reside in a volatile oil.

*Properties and Uses.*—Similar to those of Carum Carui. It forms an ingredient in Confectio Sennæ, Mistura Gentianæ, Syrupus Rhei, Tinctura Rhei, and Tinctura Sennæ.

*Preparations.*—**Oil of Coriander** (*Oleum Coriandri*). Obtained by distillation from the fruit. It is of a yellowish colour, and has a strong odour of Coriander.

*Dose.*—From two to five drops on sugar, or in emulsion.

It is an ingredient in Syrupus Sennæ.

## FERULA ASAFŒTIDA, *Linn.* ASSAFŒTIDA PLANT.

(*Bot. Mag.*, t. 5168. *Balfour, Trans. Roy. Soc. Edin.*, vol. xxii. t. 20, 21.)

*Habitat.*—Eastern Persia, Turkistan, Affghanistan and the extreme western Himalaya.

*Officinal Part.*—Gum-resin obtained by incision from the living root (*Assafœtida*). It occurs in irregular masses, partly composed of tears, moist or dry. The colour of a freshly cut or broken piece is opaque white, but it gradually becomes purplish-pink, and ultimately dull yellowish or pinkish-brown. Taste, bitter, acrid; odour fetid, alliaceous, and persistent. It dissolves almost entirely in rectified spirit. Its peculiar odour resides in a volatile oil.

*Properties.* — Powerful antispasmodic, stimulant, and anthelmintic.

*Therapeutic Uses.*—In hysteria and hysterical affections generally it is a remedy of great value, as it proves also in certain spasmodic affections, as asthma, hooping cough, angina pectoris, flatulent colic, &c. In the advanced stages of pneumonia and bronchitis in children, it produces excellent effects. As a vermifuge in cases of lumbrici, it is especially indicated, when the presence of these entozoa gives rise to sympathetic nervous affections.

*Dose.*—From five to twenty grains in the form of pill or emulsion.

*Preparations.*—**Tincture of Assafœtida** (*Tinctura Assafœtidæ*). Take of Assafœtida, in small fragments, two ounces and a half; Rectified Spirit, a sufficiency. Macerate the assafœtida in fifteen fluid ounces of the spirit for seven days in a closed vessel, with occasional agitation; then filter, and add sufficient rectified spirit to make one pint.

*Dose.*—From half a fluid drachm to one drachm.

**Compound Pill of Assafœtida** (*Pilula Assafœtidæ composita, Pilula Galbani composita,* Lond. Ph.) Take of Assafœtida, Galbanum, and Myrrh, of each two ounces; Treacle, by weight, one ounce. Heat all together by means of a water bath, and stir the mass until it assumes a uniform consistence.

*Dose.*—From five to ten grains. A valuable preparation, especially in the dyspepsia of hysterical women.

**Enema of Assafœtida** (*Enema Assafœtidæ, Enema Fœtidum, Edin. and Dubl. Ph.*) Take of Assafœtida thirty grains; Water, four fluid ounces. Rub the assafœtida in a mortar with the water added gradually, so as to form an emulsion.

A valuable stimulant and antispasmodic in hysteria, flatulent colic, infantile convulsions, &c., or when, from any cause, assafœtida cannot be administered by mouth. For children, a quarter or half the above quantity may be used, the dose being regulated by the age of the patient.

Assafœtida enters also into Pilula Aloes et Assafœtidæ, and Spiritus Ammoniæ Fœtidus.

[In addition to the gum-resin, the fruit of *Ferula Asafœtida* is imported into India from Persia and Affghanistan under the name of *Anjúdan*, and is extensively employed by the native physicians in India (*Royle*). Dr. Irvine includes the seeds and leaves of the Assafœtida plant under the name *Kashim*, and states that they are employed as a sudorific and carminative. [*Mat. Med. of Patna*, p. 53.]

## DOREMA AMMONIACUM, *Don*. AMMONIACUM PLANT.

(*Jaubert et Spach, Illust. Plant. Orient.*, vol. i. t. 40.)

*Habitat.*—Persia.

*Officinal Part.*—The gum-resinous exudation from the stem (*Ammoniacum*). It occurs in tears or masses; the tears, from two to eight lines in diameter, pale cinnamon-brown, breaking with a smooth, shining, opaque, white surface. The masses, composed of agglutinated tears; hard and brittle when cold, but readily softening with heat. Has a faint odour, and a bitter, acrid, nauseous taste. Rubbed with water it forms a milky emulsion. Its activity resides in a volatile oil and a resin.

*Properties.*—Stimulant and expectorant.

*Therapeutic Uses.*—In chronic catarrhs of old age, in spasmodic asthma, especially when occurring in hysterical women, and other pulmonary affections of an asthenic type, it is a remedy of established value.

*Dose.*—From ten to twenty grains n the form of pill or emulsion.

*Preparations.*—**Ammoniacum Mixture** (*Mistura Ammoniaci*). Take of Ammoniacum, in coarse powder, a quarter of an ounce; Water, eight fluid ounces. Triturate the ammoniacum with the water, gradually added, until the mixture assumes a milky appearance, then strain through muslin.

*Dose.*—From four fluid drachms to a fluid ounce. A valuable expectorant, especially when given in combination with squill and other remedies of the same class.

**Plaster of Ammoniacum with Mercury** (*Emplastrum Ammoniaci cum Hydrargyro*). Take of Ammoniacum, twelve ounces; Mercury, three ounces, Olive Oil, one fluid drachm; Sublimed Sulphur, eight grains. Heat the oil, and add the sulphur to it gradually, stirring till they unite. With this mixture triturate the mercury until globules are no longer visible; and, lastly, add the ammoniacum, previously liquified, mixing the whole carefully.

A useful application in hydarthrosis, chronic buboes, tumours, and syphilitic rheumatism.

Ammoniacum enters also into Emplastrum Galbani, Pilula Scillæ composita, and Pilula Ipecacuanhæ cum Scilla.

## FERULA GALBANIFLUA, *Buhse.* GALBANUM PLANT.

*Habitat.*—Persia.

*Officinal Part.*—Gum-resin (*Galbanum*). Imported into England from India and the Levant. It occurs in irregular tears about the size of a pea, usually agglutinated with masses of a greenish-yellow colour, translucent, having a strong disagreeable odour, and an acrid bitter taste. The two latter properties are due to the presence of a volatile oil.

*Properties.*—Stimulant, antispasmodic, and expectorant.

*Therapeutic Uses.*—Similar to those of Assafœtida, but milder in operation. Externally applied in the form of plaster (*infra*) as a stimulant to indolent tumours, and to the chest in chronic pulmonary affections.

*Dose.*—From ten to twenty grains in the form of pill or emulsion.

*Preparations.* — **Galbanum Plaster** (*Emplastrum Galbani*). Take of Galbanum, one ounce; Ammoniacum, one ounce; Yellow Wax, one ounce; Lead Plaster, eight ounces. Melt the galbanum and ammoniacum together, and strain. Then add them to the lead plaster and wax, also previously melted together, and mix the whole thoroughly.

Galbanum enters also into Pilula Assafœtidæ composita.

## CONIUM MACULATUM, *Linn.* SPOTTED HEMLOCK.

(*Engl. Bot.*, t. 1191; *ed. Syme*, t. 629.)

*Habitat.*—Europe and Temperate Asia; common in England.

*Officinal Part.*—1. The leaves (*Conii Folia*) and young branches, gathered from wild plants when the fruits begin to form, and carefully dried. The fresh leaves are decompound, smooth, arising from a smooth stem with dark purple spots; dried leaves of a full green colour and characteristic odour. The leaf, rubbed with caustic potash, gives out strongly the odour of conia. 2. The ripe fruit dried (*Conii Fructus*). They have the following characters:—broadly ovate, compressed laterally; half fruit with five waived or crenated ridges. Reduced to powder and rubbed with solution of potash, they give out strongly the odour of conia. The activity both of the fruit and leaves resides in a peculiar volatile oleaginous alkaloid, *Conia* or *Conein*.

*Properties.*—Narcotic, anodyne, antispasmodic; in over doses poisonous.

*Therapeutic Uses.*—In coughs and in irritable states of the bronchial mucous membrane, in rheumatic and neuralgic affections, in ulceration of the stomach, &c., it has been found of service. In cancer, both as a local application and as an internal remedy, it has been extensively employed, but with doubtful results. In scrofula it was once held in high repute. Cataplasms of the leaves are serviceable in allaying pain in scrofulous, syphilitic, and phagedenic ulcerations.

*Dose.*—From two to eight grains of the powdered leaves.

*Preparations of the Leaves.*—**Extract of Hemlock** (*Extractum Conii*). Take of the fresh Leaves and young Branches of Hemlock, one hundred and twelve pounds. Bruise in a stone mortar, and press out the juice; heat it gradually to 130°, and separate the green colouring matter by a calico filter. Heat the strained liquor to 200° to coagulate the albumen, and again filter. Evaporate the filtrate by a water-bath to the consistence of a thin syrup; then add to it the green colouring matter previously separated, and, stirring the whole together assiduously, continue the evaporation at a temperature not exceeding 140°, until the extract is of a suitable consistence for forming pills.

*Dose.*—From two to six grains or more. It loses much of its virtues by long keeping, especially in a hot climate.

**Compound Pill of Hemlock** (*Pilula Conii composita*). Take of Extract of Hemlock, two ounces and a half; Ipecacuanha, in powder, half an ounce; Treacle, a sufficiency. Mix the extract of hemlock and ipecacuanha, and add sufficient treacle to form a pill mass.

*Dose.*—From five to ten grains.

**Vapor Coniæ** (*Inhalation of Conia*). Take of Extract of Hemlock, sixty grains; Solution of Potash, one fluid drachm; Water, ten fluid drachms. Mix. Put twenty minims of the mixture on a sponge, in a suitable apparatus, so that the vapour of hot water passing over it may be inhaled.

A useful sedative in irritable states of the air passages, coughs, &c.

**Juice of Hemlock** (*Succus Conii*). Take of Fresh Leaves of Hemlock, seven pounds; Rectified Spirit, a sufficiency. Bruise the hemlock in a stone mortar; press out the juice; and to every three measures of juice add one of the spirit. Set aside for seven days, and filter. Keep it in a cool place.

*Dose.*—From one half to one fluid drachm. The most efficient form for internal use.

**Hemlock Poultice** (*Cataplasma Conii*). Take of Hemlock Leaf, in powder, one ounce; Linseed Meal, three ounces; Boiling Water, ten fluid ounces. Mix the hemlock and linseed meal, and add them to the water gradually, constantly stirring.

A useful application to painful swellings, and ulcerations.

*Preparation of the Fruit.*—**Tincture of Hemlock** (*Tinctura Conii*). Take of Hemlock Fruit, bruised, two ounces and a half; Proof Spirit, one pint. Macerate the hemlock fruit for forty-eight hours in fifteen ounces of the spirit, in a closed vessel, agitating occasionally; then transfer to a percolator, and, when the fluid ceases to pass, continue the percolation in the remaining five ounces of spirit. Afterwards subject the contents of the percolator to pressure, filter the product, mix the liquids, and add sufficient proof spirit to make one pint.

*Dose.*—From twenty to sixty minims.

## The Sumbul Plant.

*Officinal Part.*—The dried root (*Sumbul Radix, Sumbul Root*). Imported from Russia and also from India. It occurs in the form of transverse sections, nearly round, from 2½ to 5 inches in diameter, and from ¾ to 1½ inch in thickness. Bark, rough dusky brown, frequently beset with short bristly fibres. The interior is porous, and consists of irregular, easily separated fibres. It has a strong odour, resembling that of musk. The taste is at first sweetish, becoming, after a time, bitterish and balsamic. That brought from India differs from the Russian, being closer in texture, more dense and firm, and of a reddish tint.

*Properties.*—Nervine stimulant and antispasmodic.

*Therapeutic Uses.*—In hysteria, epilepsy, paralytic and other nervous affections attended with debility, it has been used with advantage; also in low typhoid fevers, asthenic dysentery and diarrhœa, chronic pulmonary affections, chlorosis, dysmenorrhœa, and hypochondriasis.

*Dose.*—From ten to twenty grains in powder.

*Preparation.*—**Tincture of Sumbul** (*Tinctura Sumbul*). Take of Sumbul Root, in coarse powder, two ounces and a half; Proof Spirit, one pint. Macerate the sumbul for forty-eight hours in fifteen fluid ounces of the spirit, in a closed vessel, agitating occasionally; then transfer to a percolator, and, when the fluid ceases to pass, continue the percolation with the remaining five ounces of spirit. Afterwards subject the contents of the percolator to pressure, filter the product, mix the liquids, and add sufficient proof spirit to make one pint.

*Dose.*—From ten to thirty minims.

[This root is distinct from that of *Nardostachys Jatamansi, D.C.*, one of the Persian and Hindústani names of which is *Sumbul Hindi.*]

## *HYDROCOTYLE ASIATICA, *Linn.* INDIAN HYDROCOTYLE OR PENNY-WORT.

(*Wight, Icones*, vol. ii. t. 565.)

*Habitat.*—Common throughout India.

*Officinal Part.*—The leaves (*Hydrocotyles Folia*); long petioled, reniform, crenate, half an inch or more in their longest diameter. In the fresh state they have little or no smell, but when bruised they exhale a peculiar aromatic odour; taste pungent, bitter, and disagreeable. *Active principle*, a pale-coloured, pungent, bitter volatile oil, named *Vellarine.* The dried leaves are not distinguished by any remarkable odour or taste.

*Properties.*—Alterative tonic; locally applied, stimulant.

*Therapeutic Uses.*—In anæsthetic leprosy good results have followed its use, but it possesses no claim to the character of a specific attributed to it by some. (39) It has been found more useful in secondary or constitutional syphilis, especially in those cases where the skin and subjacent cellular tissue are principally affected. In non-specific ulcerations, and in skin diseases, it is of value both as an internal and as a local remedy.

*Preparations.*—**Powder of Hydrocotyle** (*Pulvis Hydrocotyles*). Take of freshly gathered Hydrocotyle Leaves a sufficiency; remove the stalks, and dry thoroughly by exposure to the open air in the shade at a moderate temperature; when thoroughly dry, reduce to fine powder, and transfer to well stoppered bottles. [Thirty pounds of the fresh leaves prepared in this manner, yield between three and four pounds of the powder, which is of a pale green colour, and slight but pleasant aroma. Solar and a high artificial heat are objectionable, as they cause the dissipation of the volatile oil, on which the activity of the leaves depends.]

*Dose.*—From five to eight grains thrice daily. Sprinkled on ulcerated surfaces, it stimulates them to healthy action.

**Hydrocotyle Poultice** (*Cataplasma Hydrocotyles*). Take of the fresh Leaves of Hydrocotyle a sufficiency; bruise, and moisten with cold water.

A valuable stimulant application to syphilitic and other forms of ulceration.

(*Non-officinal.*)

**Dorema aureum,** *Stocks*. A shrub of Doobund and other parts of Upper Beloochistan, which yields a bitter, white gum, much resembling officinal Ammoniacum. The shrub often stands six feet high, very conspicuous from the golden hue of the loose and much branched panicles (*Stocks in Hooker's Journ. of Bot.* 1852, vol. xv. p. 149). Further information regarding the above exudation is very desirable.

**Carum (Ptychotis) Roxburghianum,** *Benth.—Apium involucratum, Roxb.* (*Wight, Icones*, t. 335, 567.) The small plump umbelliferous fruits of this plant (*Ajmud*, Hind.) are valued by the natives as a stomachic and carminative. They doubtless partake of the properties of *P. Ajowan;* but, unlike it, they do not appear to have been as yet subjected to trial in the hands of European medical officers. In aroma, however, they are inferior to Ajwain.

**Cuminum Cyminum,** *Linn.* (*Woodville, Med. Bot.*, t. 56.) The fruits (*Cumin seeds*), officinal in the Lond. Ph., are met with in bazaars throughout India, being much in use as a condiment. Their warm bitterish taste and aromatic odour reside in a volatile oil. Both fruit and oil possess carminative properties analogous to Coriander and Dill, but are comparatively rarely employed in medicine by Europeans, though much valued by the natives. In the absence of other remedies of the same class they may be had recourse to.

## ARALIACEÆ.

(*Non-officinal.*)

**Panax Pseudo-ginseng,** *Wallich*. This plant, first described and figured by Dr. Wallich (*Calcutta Med. Phys. Trans.* iv. p. 117, and *Plant. Asiat. Rar.* t. 137), is a native of Nepal, and is closely allied to *P. Ginseng*, Meyer, which yields the famed *Ginseng* of the Chinese. Nothing certain is known of its medicinal properties and uses, but, judging from the close resemblance it bears to the Chinese plant, it may be desirable to institute some trials with its root as to its value as an alterative tonic.

## LORANTHACEÆ.

(*Non-officinal.*)

**Viscum monoicum,** *Roxb.* The leaves of a Viscum, doubtfully referred to this species (*Kuchila ke molung*), growing on Nux Vomica trees (*Strychnos Nux Vomica*, Linn.) in the neighbourhood of Cuttack, have been found to possess poisonous properties similar to those of the tree on which it grows. The subject was investigated in 1837 by Sir W. O'Shaughnessy, who detected in the powdered leaves the presence of strychnine and brucine, Sir W. O'Shaughnessy, in a communication to the Editor, states that he saw an athletic European sailor killed in less than an hour by half a drachm of the powdered leaves taken by mistake for cubebs. It has been proposed as a substitute for strychnia.

and has indeed been used as such by Dr. Duncan Stewart and others (*Bengal Disp.* p. 376); but in cases requiring this powerful alkaloid it is far safer to employ a preparation of a known and uniform strength, as Liquor Strychniæ, than to have recourse to this plant, the composition of which is imperfectly known, and the active constituents of which are liable to variation according to the season of collection, mode of preparation, &c. M. Leon Souberain (*Pharm. Journ.* 1861, vol. i. N.S. p. 568) has published an account of a poisonous species of *Loranthus* found on the Neilgherries, growing on the Nux Vomica trees there. He gives *Poulourivi* as its Tamul name.

## CAPRIFOLIACEÆ.

### SAMBUCUS NIGRA, *Linn.* COMMON ELDER.

(*Engl. Bot.*, t. 476; *ed. Syme*, t. 637.)

*Habitat.*—Europe and Western Asia.

*Officinal Part.* — The flowers (*Sambuci Flores, Elder Flowers*). Small, white, fragrant, crowded in large cymes.

*Properties and Uses.*—Employed only in the preparation of a distilled water.

*Preparation.*—**Elder Flower Water** (*Aqua Sambuci*). Take of fresh Elder flowers ten pounds; Water, two gallons. Distil one gallon.

Used as a vehicle for other medicines, especially in lotions. It is mildly stimulant.

## RUBIACEÆ.

### CINCHONA CALISAYA, *Weddell.* CALISAYA OR YELLOW CINCHONA.

(*Weddell, Hist. Nat. des Quinquinas,* t. 3, 3 bis, and 28.)

*Habitat.*—Mountain Forests of Bolivia and Southern Peru, between 13° and 16° 30′ South lat., and from 68° to 72° West long. Under cultivation in India.(40)

*Officinal Part.*—The bark (*Cinchonæ flavæ Cortex, Cinchona flava, Yellow Cinchona Bark*). It occurs in flat pieces, uncoated or deprived of the periderm, rarely in coated quills, from six to eighteen inches long, one to three inches wide, and two to four lines thick, compact and heavy; outer surface brown, marked by broad, shallow, irregular longitudinal depressions; inner surface tawny-yellow, fibrous; transverse fracture, shortly and finely fibrous. Powder, cinnamon-brown, somewhat aromatic, persistently bitter. *Test.*—Boil 100 grains of the bark, reduced to very fine powder, for a quarter of an hour, in a fluid ounce of distilled water, acidulated with ten minims of hydrochloric acid; and allow it to macerate for twenty-four hours. Transfer the whole to a small percolator; and after the fluid has ceased to drop, add at intervals about an ounce and a half of similarly acidulated water, or until the fluid which passes through is free from colour. Add to the percolated fluid, solution of subacetate of lead, until the whole of the colouring matter has been removed, taking care that the fluid remains acid in reaction. Filter and wash with a little distilled water. To the filtrate add about thirty-five grains of caustic potash, or as much as will cause the precipitate which is at first formed to be nearly redissolved, and afterwards six fluid drachms of pure ether. Then shake briskly, and, having removed the ether, repeat the process twice with three fluid drachms of ether, or until a drop of the ether employed leaves on evaporation scarcely any perceptible residue. Lastly, evaporate the mixed ethereal solutions in a capsule. The residue, which consists of nearly pure Quinia, when dry, should weigh not less than two grains, and should be readily soluble in dilute sulphuric acid.

*Properties.*—Powerful antiperiodic, tonic, and astringent. The two former properties are due to the presence of Quinia; the last-named to Cincho-tannic and red Cinchonic acids.

*Therapeutic Uses.*—These are noticed in art. Quiniæ Sulphas, and under the various other preparations given below.

*Dose.*—From ten to sixty grains or more of the powdered bark; rarely administered in this form.

[The leaves of this and other species of Cinchona have been found to possess tonic and mildly antiperiodic properties. (41)]

*Preparations.*—**Sulphate of Quinia** (*Quiniæ Sulphas, Quinæ Disulphas, L. Ph.*) The Sulphate of an Alkaloid, $C_{40}H_{24}N_2O_4,HO,SO_3+7HO$, or $(\mathbf{C_{20}H_{24}N_2O_2})_2\mathbf{H_2SO_4.7H_2O}$, prepared from Yellow Cinchona Bark, and from the bark of Cinchona lancifolia *Mutis.* It possesses the following characters: filiform silky snow-white crystals, of a pure intensely bitter taste, sparingly soluble in water, yet imparting to it a peculiar bluish tint. The solution gives with chloride of barium a white precipitate insoluble in nitric acid, and when treated first with solution of chlorine, and afterwards with ammonia, it becomes of a splendid emerald green colour. *Tests.*—Dissolves in pure sulphuric acid with a feeble yellowish tint, and undergoes no further change of colour when gently warmed. Ten grains with ten minims of diluted sulphuric acid and half a fluid ounce of water form a perfect solution, from which ammonia throws down a white precipitate. This redissolves on agitating the whole with half a fluid ounce of ether, without the production of any crystalline matter floating on the lower of the two strata into which the agitated fluid separates on rest. 25 grains of the salt should lose 3·6 grains of water by drying at 212°.

*Properties.*—Similar to those of Cinchona flava (*ante*), more powerful, rapid, and certain in operation as a tonic and antiperiodic, less so as an astringent.

*Therapeutic Uses.*—In paroxysmal or periodical fevers, of whatever type, it holds a foremost place; it proves most effectual in intermittents, and least so in bilious remittent or yellow fever, though even here its effects are sometimes remarkable when given in large doses at the commencement of the attack. In continued fevers it is less beneficial. It has, however, proved serviceable in typhoid (enteric) fever in small doses in combination with mineral acids. In the advanced stages of exanthemata it is of great service in re-establishing the strength and restoring tone to the system. In splenic enlargement, particularly when of malarious origin, no remedy, especially when conjoined with the use of active purgatives, produces more certain effects. In rheumatic and neuralgic affections, particularly when they assume a periodical character, it is often productive of excellent results. Amongst other diseases in which it has been found serviceable are croup, laryngismus stridulus, hooping cough, the advanced stages of pneumonia and pleurisy, asthenic pneumonia, gangrene of the lungs, ophthalmia, iritis, and other affections of the eye connected with a scrofulous diathesis, erysipelas, urticaria, dysentery, and diarrhœa, especially when of malarious origin, gangrene, cancrum oris, tetanus, and phthisis. With the exception of opium, no single remedy perhaps has wider range of therapeutic uses than quinine.

*Dose.*—As a tonic, from one to three grains twice or thrice daily; as an antiperiodic, from three to ten grains in repeated doses during intermissions, or twenty grains or more in a single dose, either at the commencement of the attack, or at the conclusion of the sweating stage. It is best given in solution with sulphuric acid, and where the taste is objectionable, or irritability of the stomach exists, in the form of pill. Good results, though neither so uniform nor so speedy as when given by mouth, follow its use when administered in the form of enema, or when introduced into the system hypodermically or endermically. Its good effects are more speedily and certainly manifested if taken on an empty stomach.

*Preparations of Quinia.*—**Tincture of Quinia** (*Tinctura Quiniæ*). Take of Sulphate of Quinia, one hundred and sixty grains; Tincture of Orange Peel, one pint. Dissolve the sulphate of quinia in the tincture with the aid of a gentle heat; then allow the solution to remain for three days in a closed vessel, shaking it occasionally; and afterwards filter.

*Dose.*—From one half to two fluid drachms. Each fluid drachm contains one grain of the sulphate of quinia.

**Wine of Quinia** (*Vinum Quiniæ, Quinine Wine*). Take of Sulphate of Quinia, twenty grains; Citric Acid, thirty grains; Orange Wine, one pint. Dissolve, first the citric acid, and then the sulphate of quinia in the wine; allow the solution to remain for three days in a closed vessel, shaking it occasionally; and afterwards filter.

*Dose.*—From one half to one fluid ounce. Each fluid ounce contains one grain of quinia.

**Pill of Quinia** (*Pilula Quiniæ*). Take of Sulphate of Quinia, sixty grains; Confection of Hips, twenty grains. Mix them to a uniform mass.

*Dose.*—From two to ten grains. Every four grains contain three grains of quinia.

Quinia also forms an ingredient in Ferri et Quiniæ Citras.

*Preparations of Yellow Cinchona Bark.*—**Decoction of Yellow Bark** (*Decoctum Cinchonæ flavæ*). Take of Yellow Cinchona Bark, in coarse powder, one ounce and a quarter; Water, one pint. Boil for ten minutes in a covered vessel. Strain the decoction when cold, and pour as much water over the contents of the strainer as will make the strained product measure one pint.

*Dose.*—From one to two fluid ounces.

**Infusion of Yellow Cinchona** (*Infusum Cinchonæ flavæ*). Take of Yellow Cinchona Bark, in coarse powder, half an ounce; Boiling Water, ten fluid ounces. Infuse in a covered vessel for two hours, and strain.

*Dose.*—From one to two fluid ounces. This and the preceding preparation are good tonics; their efficacy is increased by the addition of a few drops of sulphuric acid. They are serviceable also as gargles in ulceration of the throat, and in scorbutic or idiopathic ulceration or sponginess of the gums, &c.

**Tincture of Yellow Cinchona** (*Tinctura Cinchonæ flavæ*). Take of Yellow Cinchona Bark, in moderately fine powder, four ounces; Proof Spirit, one pint. Macerate the cinchona bark for forty-eight hours in fifteen ounces of the spirit, in a closed vessel, agitating occasionally; then transfer to a percolator; and, when the fluid ceases to pass, continue the percolation with the remaining five ounces of spirit. Afterwards subject the contents of the percolator to pressure, filter the product, mix the liquids, and add sufficient proof spirit to make one pint.

*Dose.*—From one half to two fluid drachms. A valuable adjunct to other tonic remedies.

**Liquid Extract of Yellow Cinchona** (*Extractum Cinchonæ flavæ liquidum*). Take of Yellow Cinchona Bark, in coarse powder, one pound; Distilled Water, a sufficiency; Rectified Spirit, one fluid ounce. Macerate the cinchona bark in two pints of the water, for twenty-four hours, stirring frequently; then pack in a percolator, and add more water until twelve pints have been collected, or until the water ceases to dissolve anything more. Evaporate the liquor, at a temperature not exceeding 160°, to a pint; then filter through paper, and continue the evaporation to three fluid ounces, or until the specific gravity of the liquid is 1·200. When cold, add the spirit gradually, constantly stirring. The specific gravity should be about 1·100.

*Dose.*—From ten to thirty minims twice or thrice daily.

## CINCHONA CONDAMINEA, *D. C., vars.* C. CHAHUARGUERA, *Pavon,* and C. CRISPA, *Tafalla.* PALE CINCHONA.

(*Howard, Illustrations,* t. 1, 2.)

*Habitat.*—Mountain forests of Loxa, in the south-western angle of Columbia, at elevations of from 5,700 to 7,700 feet above the sea, having a mean temperature of from 64° to 68° F. Cultivated in India and Ceylon.

*Officinal Part.*—The bark (*Cinchonæ pallidæ Cortex, Cinchona pallida, Pale Cinchona Bark,* called also *Crown* or *Loxa Bark*). It has the following characters:—From half a line to a line thick, in single or double quills, which are from six to fifteen inches long, two to eight lines in diameter, brittle, easily splitting longitudinally, and breaking with a short transverse fracture; outer surface brown and wrinkled, or grey and speckled with adherent lichens, with or without numerous transverse cracks; inner surface, bright orange or cinnamon brown; powder, pale brown, slightly bitter, very astringent. *Test.*—200 grains of the bark, treated in the manner directed in the test for yellow cinchona bark, with the substitution of chloroform for ether, should yield not less than one grain of alkaloids.

*Properties, Therapeutic Uses, and Dose.*—The same as those of the Yellow-Cinchona Bark.

*Preparations.*—**Compound Tincture of Cinchona** (*Tinctura Cinchonæ Composita*). Take of Pale Cinchona Bark, in moderately fine powder, two ounces; Bitter Orange Peel, cut small and bruised, one ounce; Serpentary Root, bruised, half an ounce; Saffron, sixty grains; Cochineal, in powder, thirty grains; Proof Spirit, one pint. Macerate the cinchona bark, and the other solid ingredients, for forty-eight hours, in fifteen fluid ounces of the spirit, in a closed vessel, agitating occasionally; then transfer to a percolator; and when the fluid ceases to pass, continue the percolation with the remaining five ounces of spirit. Afterwards subject the contents of the percolator to pressure, filter the product, mix the liquids, and add sufficient proof spirit to make one pint.

*Dose.*—From one half to two fluid drachms as a tonic and stomachic.

Pale Cinchona Bark is also an ingredient in Mistura Ferri composita.

## CINCHONA SUCCIRUBRA, *Pavon.* RED CINCHONA.

(*Howard, Illustrations*, t. 9.)

*Habitat.*—Western slopes of Chimborazo, in the Republic of Ecuador; usually imported into England from Guayaquil. Cultivated in India and Ceylon.

*Officinal Part.*—The bark (*Cinchonæ rubræ Cortex, Cinchona rubra, Red Cinchona Bark*). It occurs in flat or incurved pieces, less frequently in quills, coated with the periderm, varying in length from a few inches to two feet, from one to three inches wide, and two to six lines thick, compact and heavy; outer surface, brown or reddish brown, rarely white from adherent lichens, rugged or wrinkled longitudinally, frequently warty, and crossed by deep transverse cracks; inner surface redder; fractured surface often approaching to brick red; transverse fracture finely fibrous; powder, red brown; taste, bitter and astringent. *Test.*—100 grains of the bark, treated in the manner directed in the test for yellow cinchona bark, with the substitution of chloroform for ether, should yield not less than 1·5 grains of alkaloids.

*Properties, Therapeutic Uses, and Dose.*—The same as those of Yellow Cinchona Bark.

All the above Cinchonas, as well as several other species, yield, in addition to Quinine, three other alkaloids, viz., Cinchonine, Cinchonidine, and Quinidine, in varying proportions. *C. micrantha* appears to be peculiarly rich in Cinchonine. The antiperiodic powers of these alkaloids have been examined by a Commission in India, appointed for the purpose, and the results are such as to justify a high opinion of their value in this character. The average dose of each as an antiperiodic is from grs. viii. to grs. x.; as a tonic, from grs. ii. to grs. v. [41a].

## CEPHAELIS IPECACUANHA, *D.C.* IPECACUANHA.

(*Woodville, Med. Bot.*, t. 274; *Bot. Mag.*, t. 4063.)

*Habitat.*—Brazil, in moist shady localities from 8° to 20° S. lat.

*Officinal Part.*—The root (*Ipecacuanhæ Radix, Ipecacuanha*). It occurs in pieces three or four inches long, about the size of a small quill, contorted and irregularly annulated. Colour, brown of various shades. It consists of two parts, the cortical or active portion, which is brittle, and a slender tough white woody centre. Powder, pale brown, with a faint, nauseous odour, and a somewhat acrid and bitter taste. Active principle, *Emetine*, which in its pure state is white, pulverulent, inodorous, of a slightly bitter taste, and alkaline in its properties.

*Properties.*—Emetic, diaphoretic, expectorant; in small doses, alterative. Powdered Ipecacuanha, in the form of ointment, rubbed into the skin, acts as a counter-irritant, producing a pustular eruption, resembling that produced by tartar emetic when similarly applied.

*Therapeutic Uses.*—In dysentery it is a remedy of established value. The treatment of this disease by large doses of Ipecacuanha (grs. xxx. to grs. lx.), of late years re-introduced, has been found most effectual.[42] In diarrhœa, and in some forms of dyspepsia, especially when connected with functional derangement or torpidity of the liver, it acts beneficially. As an expectorant it is in common use in catarrhs, chronic bronchitis, asthma, phthisis, the early stages of hooping cough, &c. In hœmorrhages, especially in uterine hœmorrhages, and in menorrhagia, it has proved an effectual remedy. For removing crude and indigestible matter from the stomach, ipecacuanha acts with certainty and safety as an emetic, without inducing nearly the same amount of subsequent depression that follows tartar emetic; it is especially adapted for childhood and for persons of a delicate constitution. As a counter-irritant (2 drs. of powdered ipecacuanha incorporated with 2 drs. of olive oil and 4 drs. of lard, rubbed into the skin for a few minutes once or twice daily) it has been advantageously used in hydrocephalus, chronic chest affections, &c. The powder, moistened and made into a paste, applied locally to the stings of venomous insects, is said often to allay the pain and irritation in a remarkable manner.

*Dose of the Powdered Root.*—As an emetic from fifteen to thirty grains, its action being promoted by warm diluents. As a nauseant and expectorant, from one to three grains. As an alterative, from a quarter to half a grain.

*Preparations.*—**Wine of Ipecacuanha** (*Vinum Ipecacuanhæ*). Take of Ipecacuanha, bruised, one ounce; Sherry, one pint. Macerate for seven days, in a closed vessel, with occasional agitation; strain, press, filter, and then add sufficient sherry to make one pint.

*Dose.*—As an emetic, from three to six fluid drachms; as an expectorant and diaphoretic, from five to forty minims. A safe and effectual emetic for young children, in doses of a fluid drachm repeated every half hour till it operates. Each fluid ounce contains the soluble portion of 22 grains of Ipecacuanha root.

**Compound Powder of Ipecacuanha** (*Pulvis Ipecacuanhæ compositus, Pulvis Ipecacuanhæ cum Opio,* Brit. Ph. 1864). Take of Ipecacuanha, in powder, half an ounce; Opium, in powder, half an ounce; Sulphate of Potash, in powder, four ounces. Mix them thoroughly, pass the powder through a fine sieve, and finally rub it lightly in a mortar. Keep it in a stoppered bottle.

*Dose.*—From five to fifteen grains, a valuable sedative and diaphoretic in rheumatic and neuralgic affections, dysentery, diarrhœa, calculous affections, &c. Ten grains contain one grain of opium.

**Pill of Ipecacuanha with Squill** (*Pilula Ipecacuanhæ cum Scillâ*). Take of compound powder of Ipecacuanha, three ounces; Squill in powder, Ammoniacum, in powder, of each one ounce; Treacle, a sufficiency. Mix the powders, and beat into a mass with the treacle.

*Dose.*—From five to ten grains, a serviceable expectorant in chronic coughs, &c.

**Ipecacuanha Lozenges** (*Trochisci Ipecacuanhæ*). Take of Ipecacuanha, in powder, one hundred and eighty grains; Refined Sugar, in powder, twenty-five ounces; Gum Acacia, in powder, one ounce; Mucilage of Gum Acacia, two fluid ounces; Distilled Water, one fluid ounce, or a sufficiency. Mix the powders, and add the mucilage and water to form a proper mass. Divide into 720 lozenges, and dry these in a hot-air chamber with a moderate heat.

*Dose.*—One to three lozenges. Each lozenge contains a quarter of a grain of ipecacuanha.

Ipecacuanha likewise enters into Pilula Conii composita, and Trochisci Morphiæ et Ipecacuanhæ.

## UNCARIA GAMBIR, *Roxb.* THE GAMBIR PLANT.

(*Hunter, Linnæan Trans.*, vol. ix. t. 22.)

*Habitat.*—Malayan Peninsula and Archipelago.

*Officinal Part.*—An Extract obtained from the leaves and young shoots (*Catechu pallidum, Pale Catechu*). It occurs in cubes, or masses formed of coherent cubes; the former about an inch in diameter, externally brown, internally ochrey-yellow or pale brick-red, breaking easily with a dull earthy fracture. Taste bitter, very astringent, and mucilaginous, succeeded by slight sweetness. *Tests.*—Entirely soluble in boiling water. The decoction, when cool, is not rendered blue by iodine.

*Properties, Uses, and Preparations.*—Similar to those of *Catechu nigrum* obtained from **Acacia Catechu**, over which it possesses the advantage of being more readily soluble.

*Preparations.*—**Catechu Lozenges** (*Trochisci Catechu*). Take of Pale Catechu, in powder, seven hundred and twenty grains; Refined Sugar, in powder, twenty-five ounces; Gum Acacia, in powder, one ounce; Mucilage of Gum Acacia, two fluid ounces; Distilled Water, a sufficiency. Mix the catechu, sugar and gum, and add the mucilage and water to form a proper mass. Divide into 720 lozenges, and dry these in a hot-air chamber with a moderate heat.

*Dose.*—One lozenge or more, several times daily. Each lozenge contains one grain of catechu. Allowed to dissolve slowly in the mouth, they prove useful in hoarseness, relaxation of the throat, uvula, and tonsils, in sponginess and ulceration of the gums, ptyalism, &c. In diarrhœa, pyrosis, and other cases in which astringents are indicated, they may be employed.

(*Non-officinal.*)

**Hymenodictyon excelsum,** *Wallich, Cinchona excelsa,* Roxb.—(*Wight, Icones,* vol. i. t. 79). A large tree inhabiting the forests of the Northern Circars and other parts of the Madras Peninsula. The inner coat of the bark, according to Roxburgh (*Flor. Ind.*, vol. i. p. 530), possesses the bitterness and astringency of Cinchona. The bitterness, however, is not so quickly perceived by the taste on chewing, but it is much more persistent, especially about the upper part of the fauces. The outer light spongy layer of the bark is comparatively tasteless. Considering the Natural Order to which the tree belongs, and the sensible properties of its bark, it is not improbable that it may prove a valuable remedy. In all future inquiries into the subject of Indian antiperiodics, this bark should be one of the first to which attention should be directed.

**Nauclea ovalifolia,** *Roxb.*—A forest tree of Cachar and Silhet, where it is known by the name of *Shal.* The bark, which is said to possess a bitterness equal to that of Cinchona, is in common use among the border tribes of Cachar in the treatment of endemic fevers and bowel complaints. (*Journ. of Agri.-Hort. Soc. of India*, 1857, vol. ix. App. p. 246.) It may prove worthy of further notice.

**Randia dumetorum,** *Lam.* (*Wight, Icones*, vol. ii. t. 580.)—A common shrub in most parts of India. The fruit is held in esteem by the natives for its emetic properties. The following note on its use has been communicated to the Committee by Dr. George Bidie:—"The fruit is about the size of a crab apple, round, two-"celled, many-seeded, and crowned with the rim of the calyx. It "has a peculiar sweetish sickly smell, which increases after the "fruit has been kept for a few days. It is very commonly used "as an emetic by the poorer classes in Mysore, and is said to "be safe and speedy in its action. I have myself seen it used "several times, when it produced emesis in about fifteen minutes. "The dose is one ripe fruit, well bruised, which may be repeated "if necessary. It is apparently an irritant emetic." The trials formerly made with this fruit in Calcutta led Sir W. O'Shaughnessy to conclude that little or no dependence was to be placed upon it as an emetic (*Bengal Disp.*, p. 399). According to Ainslie (*Mat. Ind.*, vol. ii. p. 185), an infusion of the bark of the root is employed by the natives to nauseate in bowel complaints. Roxburgh (*Flor. Ind.* vol. i. p. 714) mentions that the bruised fruit thrown into the water intoxicates and even kills fish, which, however, are not considered less wholesome in consequence.

**Gardenia lucida,** *Roxb.* (*Wight, Icones*, vol. ii. t. 575), and **G. gummifera,** *Linn.* (*Wight, Icones*, vol. ii. t. 576).—Both these trees, common in many parts of India, yield a resinous exudation (*Dikamali*, Hind.) It occurs in the form of irregular earthy-looking masses, of a dull olive-green colour, consisting of the resin, more or less mixed with bark, sticks, and other impurities. The twigs of the tree, coated and agglutinated with the exuding resin, are also sold in the bazaars. The odour is peculiar and offensive. It has been found useful in hospital practice in preventing the access of flies to ulcerated surfaces (*Cleghorn*). It is also extensively used by the natives as an anti-spasmodic. (See Dr. Walker, *Bombay Med. Phys. Trans.*, 1840, p. 70, and Rev. J. Long, *Journ. Agri.-Hort. Soc. of India*, 1858, vol. x. p. 10.) Nothing trustworthy, however, is known of its use as an internal remedy. According to Sprengel, the resin of *G. gummifera* constituted the *Cancamum* of the ancients, but this is doubtful, The people of Chittagong, according to Roxburgh (*Flor. Indica*, vol. i. p. 710), employ the fruit of **G. campanulata** as a cathartic and anthelmintic.

**Rubia cordifolia,** *Linn.* (*Wight, Illust.*, vol. ii. t. 128 bis, f. 1).—The root of this plant constitutes the Munjeth or Indian Madder, much used for dyeing purposes. Dr. George Playfair, in a note appended to his translation of the Taleef Shereef (p. 150), states that if taken to the extent of about three drachms several times daily, it powerfully affects the nervous system, inducing temporary delirium, &c., with evident determination to the uterine system. According to Ainslie (*Mat. Ind.*, vol. ii. p. 182), an infusion of the root is used as a grateful drink by Mahommedan women during the puerperal state, when the lochial discharge is deficient.

**Ophiorhiza Mungbos,** *Linn.*—A small perennial plant, common in many parts of India. The root, according to Dr. Wight and others, is intensely bitter, and may deserve notice as a tonic. Though held in high repute by the natives as a remedy against the bites of venomous snakes, mad dogs, &c., nothing trustworthy is known with regard to it. (See *Madras Quart. Med. Journ.*, Oct. 1861, p. 348.)

## VALERIANEÆ.

### VALERIANA OFFICINALIS, *Linn.* COMMON VALERIAN.

(*Engl. Bot.*, t. 698; *ed. Syme*, t. 666.)

*Habitat.*—Humid localities throughout Europe.

*Officinal Part.*—The root (*Valerianæ Radix, Valerian Root*). It occurs in the form of a short yellowish-white rhizome, with numerous fibrous roots about two or three inches long; of a bitter taste and penetrating odour, agreeable in the recent root, becoming fetid by keeping. *Active principle*, a volatile oil (*Oleum Valerianæ*). It likewise contains an oleaginous principle, *Valerole*, which, by oxidation in the air, becomes converted into *Valerianic Acid.*

*Properties.*—Stimulant and antispasmodic.

*Therapeutic Uses.*—In hysteria and hysterical affections it is of much value, especially when conjoined with other remedies of the same class. In epilepsy, chorea, and allied affections it has been used as an antispasmodic, but with doubtful results. As a stimulant it has been found useful in the advanced stages of fevers, low asthenic inflammations, &c.

*Dose.*—Of the powdered root, from twenty to forty grains. It is, however, rarely employed in this form. Of the volatile oil, an excellent form of administration, from three to five drops.

*Preparations.* — **Infusion of Valerian** (*Infusum Valerianæ*). Take of Valerian, bruised, one hundred and twenty grains; Boiling Water, ten fluid ounces. Infuse in a covered vessel for one hour, and strain.

*Dose.*—From one to two fluid ounces. A good ingredient in antispasmodic mixtures.

**Tincture of Valerian** (*Tinctura Valerianæ*). Take of Valerian Root, in coarse powder, two ounces and a half; Proof Spirit, one pint. Macerate the valerian root for forty-eight hours in fifteen fluid ounces of the spirit, in a closed vessel, agitating occasionally; then transfer to a percolator; and when the fluid ceases to pass, continue the percolation with the remaining five ounces of spirit. Afterwards subject the contents of the percolator to pressure, filter the product, mix the liquids, and add sufficient proof spirit to make one pint.

*Dose.*—From one to two fluid drachms.

**Ammoniated Tincture of Valerian** (*Tinctura Valerianæ ammoniata*). Take of Valerian Root, in coarse powder, two and a half ounces; Aromatic Spirit of Ammonia, one pint. Macerate for seven days in a well-closed vessel, with occasional agitation; then strain, press, filter, and add sufficient aromatic spirit of ammonia to make one pint.

*Dose.*—From thirty minims to one fluid drachm. A valuable antispasmodic in various forms of hysteria.

(*Non-officinal.*)

**Valeriana Hardwickii,** *Wall.* (*Plant. Asiat. Rar.*, t. 263.)—A plant of the temperate Himalaya. Its strong-scented roots are used for medicinal purposes in Nepal and Northern India (Royle, *Antiquity of Hindoo Med.*, p. 82). According to Dr. Adams (*Transl. of Paulus Ægineta*, vol. iii. p. 264) the *Syrian Nard* of the ancients was probably the root of this plant. It may deserve attention as an anti-spasmodic.

**Nardostachys Jatamansi**, *D.C.* (*Royle, Illust.*, t. 54.)—A plant of the Alpine Himalaya, from Kumaon to Sikkim. Its roots occur in the form of short pieces of an underground stem, about the thickness of a goose-quill, covered towards one extremity or almost entirely with coarse, dark, hair-like fibres. It has an aromatic odour resembling patchouli, with an aromatic bitterish taste. These roots have been identified by Sir W. Jones (*Asiat. Res.*, vol. ii. p. 405, vol. iv. p. 109), and Professor Royle (*Illust.*, vol. i. pp. 241, *seq.*), with the *Nardus Indicus* (*Spikenard*) of the ancients. Its sensible properties would lead to the supposition that it is possessed of the antispasmodic virtues of valerian; and Sir W. O'Shaughnessy states, as the result of his experience with it, that it is a perfect representative for that article (*Bengal Disp.*, p. 404). According to Virey, cited by Ainslie (*Mat. Ind.*, vol. ii. p. 368), it is employed by the people of India in the treatment of epilepsy, hysteria, and convulsive affections; and in this class of cases there is good reason for regarding it as a remedy of a considerable power. In the Susruta, the most ancient Hindu treatise on medicine, it enters into a nostrum highly recommended in the treatment of epilepsy. A Tincture of Jatamansi is officinal in the Bengal Ph. (Jatamansi root five ounces, Proof Spirit two pints); dose from one to two fluid drachms. It is very desirable that further trials should be instituted with this promising drug, which can be procured, at a small cost, in almost all the bazaars throughout India. Care should be taken to select good specimens for trial, as much of the drug sold in the bazaars is worm-eaten and worthless.

# COMPOSITÆ.

## ANTHEMIS NOBILIS, *Linn.* Common Chamomile.

(*Engl. Bot.*, t. 980; *ed. Syme*, t. 724.)

*Habitat.*—Open, gravelly pastures and commons throughout Europe. Cultivated in some parts of India.

*Officinal Part.*—The dried flower-heads, single or double (*Anthemidis Flores, Chamomile Flowers*). The single variety consists of both yellow tubular and white strap-shaped florets; the double, of white strap-shaped florets only; all arising from a conical scaly receptacle. Both varieties, especially the single, are bitter and very aromatic. *Active principles*, a volatile oil (*infra*), and a bitter extractive.

*Properties.*—Simulant tonic and carminative.

*Therapeutic Uses.*—In constitutional debility, hysteria, dyspepsia, and in all cases where the tone of the digestive organs or the system generally is depressed it proves serviceable. It was formerly employed in intermittent fevers, but has been superseded by cinchona and other more powerful antiperiodics.

*Preparations.*—**Infusion of Chamomile** (*Infusum Anthemidis*). Take of Chamomile Flowers, half an ounce; Boiling Water, ten fluid ounces. Infuse in a covered vessel for fifteen minutes, and strain.

*Dose.*—From a fluid ounce to an ounce and a half, twice or thrice daily, as a tonic. The warm infusion is often employed to promote the action of emetics. It is also used as a fomentation in sprains, &c.

**Oil of Chamomile** (*Oleum Anthemidis.*)—The oil distilled from Chamomile flowers. Recently prepared it is of a pale-blue or greenish-blue colour, but gradually becomes yellow. It has the peculiar odour and aromatic taste of the flowers.

*Dose.*—From one to five drops on sugar or in emulsion. In dyspeptic flatulence and flatulent colic few remedies are more effectual.

**Extract of Chamomile** (*Extractum Anthemidis*).—Take of Chamomile Flowers, one pound; Oil of Chamomile, fifteen minims; Water, a gallon. Boil the chamomile with the water until the volume is reduced to one half; then strain, press, and filter. Evaporate the liquor by a water-bath until the extract is of a suitable consistence for forming pills, adding the oil of chamomile at the end of the process.

*Dose.*—From five to ten grains. A good serviceable adjunct to other tonics in dyspepsia, &c.

[Chamomile flowers (*Bábúna ka phul*, Hind.) are met with in most Indian bazaars. They form a perfect substitute for the European article.]

## ARTEMISIA, Sp. of. Santonica.

*Habitat.*—Russia ?

*Officinal Part.*—The unexpanded flower-heads (*Santonica, Semen Santonicum, Wormseed*). They are rather more than a line in length, and nearly half a line in breadth, fusiform, blunt at each end, pale-greenish brown, smooth ; resembling seeds in appearance, but consisting of imbricated involucral scales, with a greenish mid-rib, enclosing four or five tubular flowers ; odour strong ; taste bitter and camphoraceous. *Test.*—Flower-heads not round or hairy. This serves to distinguish them from the flower-heads of *Artemisia vulgaris*, Linn. (*Mugwort*), and *A. Absinthium*, Linn. (*Wormwood*). Their activity resides in a crystalline neutral principle, *Santonin* (*infra*).

*Properties.*—Anthelmintic.

*Dose.*—From one to two drachms, repeated night and morning, followed by a purgative.

*Preparation.*—**Santonin** (*Santoninum*). $C_{30}H_{18}O_6$ or $C_{15}H_{18}O_3$. A crystalline neutral principle obtained from Santonica. It occurs in colourless flat rhombic prisms, feebly bitter, fusible and sublimable by a moderate heat ; scarcely soluble in cold water, sparingly in boiling water, but abundantly in chloroform and in boiling rectified spirit. Sunlight renders it yellow. Not dissolved by diluted mineral acids. Entirely destructible by a red heat with free access of air.

*Properties.*—Valuable anthelmintic.

*Therapeutic Uses.*—For the destruction of ascarides lumbricoides its action is speedy and certain. In chorea, hysteria, and other anomalous convulsive affections connected with the presence of these entozoa in the intestines, it proves valuable. The peculiar yellow discolouration of the vision (chromatopsy) which occasionally follows its use, led to its being employed in amaurosis and other diseases of the eye, but without any marked benefit. It has likewise been used in intermittents as a substitute for quinine, but with doubtful results.

*Dose.*—For children under four years of age, from two to four grains ; above twelve years, from six to eight grains ; with an equal quantity of white sugar or syrup. A dose at night, repeated in the morning, and followed in a few hours by a dose of castor oil, is the best form of administration.

## ARNICA MONTANA, *Linn.* MOUNTAIN ARNICA.

(*Bot. Mag.*, t. 1749.)

*Habitat.*—Mountains of Central and Southern Europe.

*Officinal Part.*—The root (*Arnicæ Radix, Arnica Root*). It occurs in the form of a rhizome, from one to three inches in length, and about two or three lines in thickness, cylindrical, contorted, rough from the scars of coriaceous leaves, and furnished with numerous long slender fibres; odour peculiar, taste pungent. *Active Principles,* an alkaloid, *Arnicine,* and a bitter acrid extractive matter analogous to Cytisin.

*Properties.*—Stimulant; in large doses, an acro-narcotic poison. Externally applied, sedative and resolvent.

*Therapeutic Uses.*—In paralytic affections, low types of fever, asthenic dysentery, amaurosis, and other affections, it has been employed with alleged benefit, but in British practice its use is limited to the application of the tincture to bruises, sprains, and local painful affections.

*Dose.*—Of the powdered root from five to ten grains.

*Preparations.*—**Tincture of Arnica** (*Tinctura Arnicæ*). Take of Arnica Root, in coarse powder, one ounce; Rectified Spirit, one pint. Macerate the arnica for forty-eight hours in fifteen fluid ounces of the spirit, in a closed vessel, agitating occasionally; then transfer to a percolator; and when the fluid ceases to pass, continue the percolation with the remaining five ounces of spirit. Afterwards subject the contents of the percolator to pressure, filter the product, mix the liquids, and add sufficient rectified spirit to make one pint.

*Dose.*—From one to two fluid drachms. Its principal use is as an external application.

## TARAXACUM DENS LEONIS, *D.C.* TARAXACUM OF DANDELION.

(*Engl. Bot.*, t. 510; *ed. Syme*, t. 802.)

*Habitat.*—Throughout Europe and temperate Asia; abundant throughout the Himalaya; cultivated in India.

*Officinal Part.*—The root (*Taraxaci Radix, Taraxacum*). Collected between the months of September and February: tap-shaped, smooth, dark brown externally, white within, easily broken, and giving out an inodorous bitter milky juice, which becomes pale-brown by exposure. Not wrinkled or pale-coloured externally; juice not watery; any adherent leaves runcinate and quite smooth.

*Properties.*—Alterative tonic and cholagogue.

*Therapeutic Uses.*—In dyspepsia, in chronic hepatic affections, especially in torpor and congestion of the liver, and in jaundice, it has been employed with advantage. In chronic cutaneous diseases connected with visceral and hepatic derangement it has likewise been found useful.

*Preparations.*—**Decoction of Taraxacum** (*Decoctum Taraxaci*). Take of Dried Taraxacum Root, sliced and bruised, one ounce; Water, one pint. Boil for ten minutes in a covered vessel; then strain, and pour as much distilled water over the contents of the strainer as will make the strained product measure a pint.

*Dose.*—From two to four fluid ounces.

**Extract of Taraxacum** (*Extractum Taraxaci*). Take of Fresh Taraxacum Root, four pounds. Crush the root; press out the juice, and allow it to deposit; heat the clear liquor to 212°, and maintain the temperature for ten minutes; then strain, and evaporate by a water bath at a temperature not exceeding 160° until the extract has acquired a suitable consistence for forming pills.(43)

*Dose.*—From ten to thirty grains, or more, three or four times a day.

**Juice of Taraxacum** (*Succus Taraxaci*). Take of Taraxacum Root, seven pounds; Rectified Spirit, a sufficiency. Bruise the Taraxacum root in a stone mortar; press out the juice; and to every three measures of juice add one of the spirit. Set aside for seven days, and filter. Keep it in a cool place.

*Dose.*—From one to three fluid drachms.

### LACTUCA VIROSA, *Linn.* STRONG-SCENTED LETTUCE.

(*Engl. Bot.*, t. 1957; *ed. Syme*, t. 805.)

*Habitat.*—Europe.

*Officinal Part.*—The flowering herb (*Lactuca, Lettuce*), which is officinal only as the source of the following preparation.

*Preparation.*—**Extract of Lettuce** (*Extractum Lactucæ*). Take of the flowering herb of Lettuce, one hundred and twelve pounds. Bruise in a stone mortar, and press out the juice; heat it gradually to 130°, and separate the green colouring matter by a calico filter. Heat the strained liquor to 200° to coagulate the albumen, and again filter. Evaporate the filtrate by a water bath to the consistence of a thin syrup; then add to it the green colouring matter previously separated; and stirring the whole together assiduously, continue the evaporation at a temperature not exceeding 140° until the extract is of a suitable consistence for forming pills.

*Properties.*—Mild sedative, anodyne, and antispasmodic.

*Therapeutic Uses.*—As a means of allaying cough in phthisis, bronchitis, asthma, and pertussis, it has been used with doubtful results; it has likewise been prescribed in rheumatism, insanity, spermatorrhœa, dropsy, &c.

*Dose.*—From five to twenty grains.

[Sir W. O'Shaughnessy (*Bengal Disp.*, p. 407) mentions that he gave a trial to an Extract of Lettuce prepared in Calcutta, and found it distinctly sedative in six-grain doses. Dr. Graham (*Calcutta Med.. Phys. Trans.*, vol. iv. p. 1) furnishes some interesting remarks on the use of this drug in India.]

## ANACYCLUS PYRETHRUM, *D.C.* PELLITORY OF SPAIN.

(*Steph. and Church, Med. Bot.*, vol. ii. t. 97.)

*Habitat.*—Northern Africa, whence it has been introduced into Southern Europe.

*Officinal Part.*—The root (*Pyrethri Radix, Pellitory Root*). Occurs in pieces about the length and thickness of the little finger, covered with a thick brown bark, studded with black shining points; breaks with a resinous fracture, internal structure radiated. When chewed, it excites a prickling sensation in the lips and tongue, and a glowing heat. Its activity resides in an acrid resinous principle, *Pyrethrin*.

*Properties.*—Stimulant; locally applied, irritant and rubefacient; sialagogue.

*Therapeutic Uses.*—In toothache, relaxation of the uvula and tonsils, in some forms of aphonia, and in paralysis of the tongue, it has been used as a local application with advantage.

*Preparation.* — **Tincture of Pellitory** (*Tinctura Pyrethri*). Take of Pellitory Root, in coarse powder, four ounces; Rectified Spirit, one pint. Macerate the pellitory for forty-eight hours in fifteen fluid ounces of the spirit, in a closed vessel, agitating occasionally; then transfer to a percolator; and when the fluid ceases to pass, continue the percolation with the remaining five ounces of spirit. Afterwards subject the contents of the percolator to pressure, filter the product, mix the liquids, and add sufficient proof spirit to make one pint.

Chiefly used as a local application in toothache, &c.

[Pyrethrum root is met with in most of the larger bazaars of India. It is an imported article, and is probably introduced viâ Bombay, from Arabia. See Ainslie, *Mat. Ind.*, vol. i. p. 300.]

### (*Non-officinal.*)

**Vernonia anthelmintica,** *Willd.* (*Rheede, Hort. Mal.*, vol. ii. t. 24). — Common in waste places near villages throughout India. The seeds, commonly met with in all bazaars, are about an eighth of an inch in length, of a dark-brown colour, covered with whitish scattered hairs, cylindrical, tapering toward the base, marked with about ten paler longitudinal ridges, and crowned with a circle of short brown scales; taste nauseous and bitter. These seeds enjoy a high repute amongst the natives as an anthelmintic, in cases of ascarides lumbricoides, which, under their use, are stated to be expelled in a lifeless state, thus showing that they exercise a specific influence on the entozoa. The ordinary dose of the bruised seed, administered in electuary with honey, is about one and a half drachm, given in two equal doses at the interval of a few hours, and followed by an aperient. Dr. Æ. Ross speaks favourably of an infusion of the powdered seeds (in doses of from ten to thirty grains) as a good and certain anthelmintic in ascarides. In this character they seem well worthy of further trials. In Travancore, the bruised seeds, ground up in a paste with lime juice, are largely employed as a means of destroying pediculi. Dr. Gibson, as the result of personal experience, regards them as a valuable tonic and stomachic, in doses of twenty to twenty-five grains. Diuretic properties are also assigned to them.

**Artemisia Indica,** *Willd.* (*Wight, Icones*, vol. iii. t. 1112.) — A common plant on the mountains of India. The strong aromatic odour and bitter taste of this plant, scarcely distinct from *A. vulgaris*, indicate stomachic and tonic properties; and, according to Ainslie (*Mat. Ind.*, vol. ii. p. 194), it is regarded as such by the people of Southern India. Dr. Wight (*Illust.*, vol. ii. p. 92) states that the leaves and tops are administered in nervous and spasmodic affections connected with debility, and also that an infusion of them is used as a fomentation in phagedenic ulceration. Dr. L. Stewart describes an infusion of the tops and leaves as a good mild stomachic tonic.

**Berthelotia lanceolata,** *var.* **Indica,** *D.C.*—A native of Scinde, the Punjaub, and the drier parts of Central India. The leaves (*Rae-Suna*, Hind.) possess aperient properties, and are stated by the late Dr. Falconer to be an excellent substitute for senna. They much resemble the leaves of *Salvadora Indica*. (See Royle, *Illust.*, vol. i. p. 319.)

**Notonia grandiflora,** *D.C.*, of which **N. corymbosa,** *D.C.* (*Wight, Icones*, vol. ii. t. 484,) is only a many flowered variety, inhabits dry rocky localities in the Madras Peninsula. It was brought forward in 1860, by Dr. A. Gibson, as a preventive of hydrophobia. The mode of administration is as follows: About four ounces of the freshly gathered stems, infused in a pint of cold water for a night, yield in the morning, when subjected to pressure, a quantity of viscid greenish juice, which, being mixed with the water, is taken at a draught. In the evening, a further quantity of the juice, made up into boluses with flour, is taken. These medicines are directed to be repeated for three successive days. From official documents placed at the disposal of the Editor by Dr. Gibson, it appears that the remedy has been tried in numerous cases; but as, at the time of the infliction of the wound, caustic was applied locally in the majority of cases, it is difficult to determine how far the *Notonia* operated, if at all, as a prophylactic. Further trials may solve the question.

**Cacalia Kleinia,** *Linn.* —Ainslie [*Mat. Ind.*, vol. ii. p. 118,] and other subsequent writers on Indian Materia Medica, regard this plant as the source of the drug sold in the bazaars under the name of *Gouzabán.* There is probably a double error here: 1, *C. Kleinia* of Linnæus (*Kleinia neriifolia, Haw.*) is a plant of the Canaries, and not of India; and, 2, specimens of the leaves and imperfect flowers of *Gouzabán*, forwarded to the Committee by Mr. Moodeen Sheriff, are pronounced by Drs. Wight and Thomson to be those of a species of *Echium,* Nat. Ord. Boragineæ, *q.v.*

**Eupatorium Ayapana,** *Vent.* (*Malm.*, t. 3.)—A South American plant, naturalized in various parts of India, Java, Ceylon, &c., and generally known, with very slight variations, by its Brazilian name, *Aya-pana.* The whole plant is aromatic, with a slightly bitter, sub-astringent taste. The exaggerated ideas of its virtues formerly entertained are now exploded; but there is reason to believe that it is a good stimulant, tonic, and diaphoretic. According to the statements of Bouton (*Med. Plants of Mauritius*, p. 96), it appears to hold a high place amongst the medicinal plants of the Mauritius, being there in daily use, in the form of infusion, in dyspepsia and other affections of the bowels and of the lungs. In the cholera epidemics in that island, in 1854 and 1856, it was extensively used for restoring the warmth of the surface, the languid circulation, &c. As an antidote in snake bites, it has been used, both internally and externally, with alleged success. (*Madras Quart. Med. Journ.*, vol. iv. p. 7.) The bruised leaves are stated by Ainslie (*Mat. Ind.*, vol. ii. p. 35) to be one of the best applications with which he is acquainted to foul and ill-conditioned ulcers. They are also favourably spoken of by Bouton. A decoction of the leaves proves useful also as a fomentation. It appears probable that this plant has fallen into unmerited neglect.

**Aplotaxis auriculata,** *D.C.*—(*Aucklandia Costus, Falconer.*)—Inhabiting N.W. Himalaya. It was first shown by the late Dr. Hugh Falconer (*Linnæan Trans.*, vol. xix.) to be the source of the *Costus Arabicus* of the ancients, which Dr. Royle (*Illust.*, vol. i. p. 360) had previously identified with the *Putchuk* or *Koot* root, met with in Indian bazaars. Dr. Irvine (*Med. Topog. of Ajmeer*, p. 107) states that formerly, when opium was not produced in Rajwarra, this root was extensively smoked as a stimulant. He adds (p. 142) that it is said to be narcotic when thus used, and that formerly great quantities went to China for smoking purposes. It is chiefly used as a perfume, as a protection of bales of cloth from insects.

**Chrysanthemum Roxburghii,** *Desv.*—Is common in gardens throughout India. The flowers, which impress a peculiar pricking sensation on the tongue when dried, are stated by Dalzell and Gibson (*Bombay Flora*, P. ii. p. 48) to form a tolerable substitute for chamomile for medicinal purposes. The root, chewed, communicates the same tingling sensation to the tongue as pellitory, and might doubtless be used as a substitute for it. The people of the Deccan administer the plant, in conjunction with black pepper, in gonorrhœa (Dr. Walker, *Bombay Med. Phys. Trans.*, 1840, p. 71).

**Blumea grandis**, *D.C.*—One of the commonest weeds in waste places in the Tenasserim Provinces, where it is known by the Burmese name of *Pung-ma-theing*. Some years since, Mr. E. O'Riley prepared from it upwards of a hundredweight of camphor, which the authorities of Calcutta pronounced identical, in all its properties, with the camphor imported from China. (*Mason's Nat. Productions of Burmah*, p. 151.) Dr. Rean, from experiments instituted with this plant in Burmah, expresses a doubt of its yielding as much camphor as has been reported.

**Blumea balsamifera**, *D.C.*—This plant, which inhabits the Moluccas, Ceylon, and many parts of India, possesses a strong camphoraceous odour and pungent taste. According to Horsfield (*Asiat. Journ.*, vol. viii. p. 272), a warm infusion of the plant acts as a powerful sudorific; and is in very general use, amongst the Javanese and Chinese, as an expectorant. Several European medical men, practising at Samarang, assured Horsfield that they had repeatedly employed it in catarrhal affections. Loureiro (*Flor. Coch.*, p. 603) mentions its use in Cochin China as a stomachic, antispasmodic, and emmenagogue.

**Eclipta prostrata**, *Linn.* (*Rheede, Hort. Mal.*, vol. x. t. 41.)—A common plant in wet places throughout India. The root has purgative and emetic properties assigned to it; and its use in affections of the liver and spleen, and in dropsy, is noticed in the reports of Dr. G. Smith, Mr. J. Wood, and native surgeons Moodeen Sheriff and Iyaswammy. Mr. Wood, indeed, states that, from what he has learnt of its properties, he considers that it will be found eventually of greater service than Taraxacum in hepatic derangements. The expressed juice appears to be the best form of administration.

## LOBELIACEÆ.

---

### LOBELIA INFLATA, *Linn.* LOBELIA.

(*Nees, Düsseldorf*, t. 205.)

*Habitat.*—North America, from Canada to Carolina.

*Officinal Part.*—The flowering herb (*Lobelia*), usually imported into England in compressed rectangular parcels. It has the following characters:—Stem, angular; leaves, alternate, ovate, toothed, somewhat hairy beneath; capsule ovoid, inflated, ten-ribbed; smell, nauseous and disagreeable; taste, burning and acrid. *Active principles*, a volatile oil, and a peculiar acrid, alkaline principle, *Lobelin*. In addition to these, it contains an acrid resin and a peculiar acid, *Lobelic Acid*.

*Properties.*—Emetic, sedative, diaphoretic, expectorant, and antispasmodic; in large doses, a powerful acro-narcotic poison.

*Therapeutic Uses.*—In spasmodic asthma, angina pectoris, the chronic stage of hooping cough, chronic bronchitis, and pneumonia it is of great value, allaying cough and dyspnœa, and promoting expectoration.

*Dose.*—Of the powdered leaves, from one to five grains, as a sedative, diaphoretic, and expectorant; from fifteen to twenty grains as an emetic. In the latter character it is inferior to ipecacuanha in safety and certainty of operation.

*Preparations.*—**Tincture of Lobelia** (*Tinctura Lobeliæ*). Take of Lobelia, in coarse powder, two ounces and a half; Proof Spirit, one pint. Macerate the lobelia for forty-eight hours in fifteen fluid ounces of the spirit, in a closed vessel, agitating occasionally. Then transfer to a percolator; and when the fluid ceases to pass, continue the percolation with the remaining five ounces of spirit. Afterwards subject the contents of the percolator to pressure, filter the product, mix the liquids, and add sufficient proof spirit to make one pint.

*Dose.*—From ten to thirty minims as an expectorant and sedative; from a drachm to two fluid drachms, repeated every two or three hours according to circumstances, as an antispasmodic and emetic.

**Ethereal Tincture of Lobelia** (*Tinctura Lobeliæ Ætherea*). Take of Lobelia, in coarse powder, two ounces and a half; Spirit of Ether, one pint. Macerate for seven days in a closed vessel, with occasional agitation; then strain, press, filter, and add sufficient spirit of ether to make one pint.

*Dose.*—From ten to thirty minims; especially useful in spasmodic asthma.

(*Non-officinal.*)

**Lobelia nicotianæfolia**, *Heyne* (*Wight, Icones*, vol. iv. t. 1172.)—This plant, inhabiting the mountain ranges of Ceylon and the Madras Peninsula, is known by the Mahratti names *Dawul, Deonul*, and *Boke-Nul*. The last of these names signifies *Tubular-poison-plant*, *Boke* being the native name of a poisonous species of Euphorbia. Its seeds are extremely acrid (Dalzell and Gibson, *Bombay Flora*, p. 133). Sub-assistant Surgeon Odoy Chund Newgee reports that an infusion of the leaves is used by the natives as an anti-spasmodic. Further information with regard to this plant and its properties is desirable.

## ERICACEÆ.

### ARCTOSTAPHYLOS UVA URSI, *Sprengel.* UVA URSI, BEAR-BERRY.

(*Engl. Bot.*, t. 714; *ed. Syme*, t. 881.)

*Habitat.* — Stony alpine peaks of Europe, Asia, and North America.

*Officinal Part.* — The dried leaves (*Uvæ Ursi Folia*, *Bear-berry Leaves*). They are obovate, entire, coriaceous, shining, about three fourths of an inch in length, reticulated beneath; with a strong astringent taste, and a feeble hay-like odour when powdered; the infusion giving a bluish-black precipitate with the perchloride of iron. Leaves not dotted beneath, nor toothed on the margin. In addition to tannic and gallic acids and a volatile oil, they contain a peculiar crystallizable principle, *Arbutine*.

*Properties.*—Astringent and diuretic.

*Therapeutic Uses.*—In irritable states of the genito-urinary system, in chronic cystitis and cystirrhœa, in obstinate gonorrhœa, gleet, also in leucorrhœa and menorrhagia, they have been used with advantage.

*Dose.*—From ten to thirty grains of the powdered leaves.

*Preparation.*—**Infusion of Bear-berry** (*Infusum Uvæ Ursi*). Take of Bear-berry Leaves, bruised, half an ounce; Boiling Water, ten fluid ounces. Infuse in a covered vessel for two hours, and strain.

*Dose.*—From one to two fluid ounces twice or thrice daily.

## SAPOTACEÆ.

(*Non-officinal.*)

**Bassia longifolia,** *Linn.*, (*Wight, Illust.*, vol. ii. t. 147,) and **Bassia latifolia,** *Roxb.* (*Corom. Pl.*, t. 19.)—These two trees, common in most parts of India, deserve notice as yielding two important products, a fixed concrete oil and a spirit; the former obtained by expression from the seeds, the latter by distillation from the flowers. The oil is generally coarse and thick, and soon becomes rancid on exposure to the air; hence it is of little service as a pharmaceutical agent, except in the manufacture of soap, for which it is said to be well adapted. It retains its solid form under 95° F. The spirit distilled from the flowers of *B. latifolia* (*Baia* or *Mahwa Spirit*) has a strong smoky odour, somewhat resembling Irish whiskey, and rather a pungent fetid flavour, which, however, disappears with age. The freshly distilled spirit proves very deleterious, exciting gastric irritation, and other unpleasant effects. (See

Dr. Gibson in *Hooker's Journ. Botany*, vol. v. p. 90.) Sub-assistant Surgeon Odoy Chund Dutt reports having used the weaker (diluted?) spirit extensively; and in his opinion it is less injurious to the digestive system than rum, more resembling beer in its effects on the constitution, and nutrition of the body. This view is coincident with that of Dr. W. Wright. It is evidently a powerful diffusible stimulant, and when matured by age may be used as such, when brandy and other agents of the same class are not available. The residuum or cake left after the expression of the oil (*Ilúpai púnak, Tam*), is employed as an emetic. Some cases of poisoning by Stramonium, in which it was so employed, are given by Dr. J. Shortt (*Madras Quart. Med. Journ.*, vol. vi. p. 286). It appears to act efficiently in this character.

**Bassia butyracea,** *Roxb.*—A tree of the sub-tropical Himalaya, known by the Hindústani name of *Fulwa* or *Phulwara*. The seeds by expression yield a concrete oil known by the name of *Fulwa Butter;* it has the consistence of lard, is almost inodorous, of a delicate white colour, is a soft solid at 95°, and melts completely at 120° F. Unlike the oil of *B. longifolia* and *B. latifolia*, it does not become rancid by keeping. For a full account of its properties and uses, see *Trans. of Agri.-Hort. Soc. of India*, vol. i. p. 19. It is held in high esteem as an external application in rheumatic and other painful affections, and is well worthy of further attention.

**Mimusops Elengi,** *Linn.* (*Wight, Icones*, vol. iv. t. 1586.)—The bark of this tree, much cultivated for the sake of its fragrant flowers, possesses, according to Horsfield (*Asiat. Journ.*, vol. vii. p. 262), astringent tonic properties. It is much esteemed by the Javanese, and is stated by the same authority to have proved useful in fevers and as a general tonic. According to Dr. Bholanauth Bose, a decoction of the bark forms a good gargle in salivation. A water distilled from the flowers is in use amongst the natives of Southern India, both as a stimulant medicine and as a perfume.

## EBENACEÆ.

### *DIOSPYROS EMBRYOPTERIS, *Persoon.* GAB. (Hind.)

(*Embryopteris glutinifera, Roxb.*)

(*Wight, Icones*, vol. iii. t. 843, 844.)

*Habitat.*—Common in forests throughout India.

*Officinal Part.*—The fruit (*Diospyri Fructus*), about the size of a small apple, of a yellowish rusty colour, covered with a rubiginous farina, eight-seeded, abounding with a viscid very astringent juice.

*Properties.*—Powerfully astringent.

*Therapeutic Uses.*—See Extract of Diospyros (*infra*).

*Preparation.*—**Extract of Diospyros** (*Extractum Dyospyri*). Take of Diospyros fruit a sufficiency; bruise and subject the mass to pressure; evaporate the expressed juice on a water bath to dryness. Preserve in stoppered bottles.

This extract is of a reddish brown colour, in flexible plates, and readily soluble in water. It is an excellent astringent, and very useful in diarrhœa and chronic dysentery. A solution of two drachms in a pint of water is a valuable vaginal injection in leucorrhœa.(44)

*Dose.*—From one to five grains thrice daily.

(*Non-officinal.*)

**Diospyros melanoxylon,** *Roxb.* (*Corom. Pl.*, t. 46). The bark of this tree, known as *the Ebony Tree* of Malabar and Coromandel, according to the report of Dr. Æ. Ross, possesses tonic and astringent properties, and in decoction proves very useful in atonic diarrhœa, dyspepsia, and diseases of debility.

## STYRACACEÆ.

### STYRAX BENZOIN, *D.C.* BENZOIN TREE.

(*Steph. et Church, Med. Bot.*, vol. ii. t. 112.)

*Habitat.*—Borneo, Java, Sumatra, Siam.

*Officinal Part.*—A balsamic resin (*Benzoinum, Benzoin*), procured by making incisions into the bark of the tree, and allowing the liquid which exudes to concrete by exposure to the air. Imported into Great Britain from Siam and Sumatra. It occurs in lumps, consisting of agglutinated tears, or of a brownish mottled mass, with or without white tears embedded in it; has little taste, but an agreeable odour; gives off, when heated, fumes of benzoic acid; is soluble in rectified spirit and in solution of potash. It contains a resin (76 to 80 per cent.), a volatile oil, and a peculiar acid, *Benzoic Acid.*

*Properties.*—Stimulant expectorant; locally applied, stimulant.

*Therapeutic Uses.*—In chronic coughs and other chronic affections of the lungs, it has been used both internally and in the form of fumigation. It has likewise been employed in pyrosis, irritable states of the bladder, &c. It has in a great measure been superseded by more effectual remedies of the same class.

*Dose.*—From ten to twenty grains; rarely given alone.

*Preparations.*—**Compound Tincture of Benzoin** (*Tinctura Benzoini composita*). Take of Benzoin, in coarse powder, two ounces; Prepared Storax, one ounce and a half; Balsam of Tolu, half an ounce; Socotrine Aloes, one hundred and sixty grains; Rectified Spirit, one pint. Macerate for seven days in a closed vessel, with occasional agitation, then filter, and add sufficient rectified spirit, if required, to make one pint.

*Dose.*—From half a fluid drachm to one fluid drachm. Under the name of *Friars Balsam* it has long enjoyed great popular repute as a stimulant application to wounds, ulcers, &c.

**Benzoated Lard** (*Adeps Benzoatus*). Take of Prepared Lard, one pound; Benzoin, reduced to coarse powder, one hundred and sixty grains. Melt the lard by the heat of a water-bath, add the benzoin, and, frequently stirring them together, continue the application of heat for two hours; finally remove the residual benzoin by straining.

Benzoated Lard is said to become rancid less speedily than lard which has not been so treated. It is used for the same purposes as prepared lard.

**Benzoic Acid** (*Acidum Benzoicum*). An acid, HO, $C_{14}H_5O_3$ or $\mathbf{HC_7H_5O_2}$. obtained from Benzoin by sublimation. It occurs in the form of light feathery crystalline plates and needles, which are flexible, nearly colourless, and have an agreeable aromatic odour, resembling that of benzoin. It is sparingly soluble in water, but is readily dissolved by rectified spirit; soluble also in solutions of the caustic alkalies and of lime, and it is precipitated from these on the addition of hydrochloric acid, unless the solution be very dilute. It melts at 248°, and boils at 462.° When heated to the last-named temperature, it passes off in vapour, leaving only a slight residue.

*Properties.*—Stimulant, particularly of mucous surfaces. Is eliminated by the urine in the form of hippuric acid.

*Therapeutic Uses.*—Proposed on theoretical grounds as a remedy in the uric or lithic acid diathesis, but failed; has been found more useful in removing phosphatic deposits in the urine. In jaundice it has been found useful; also in incontinence of urine in children.

*Dose.*—From ten to fifteen grains.

Benzoic acid is an ingredient in Tinctura Camphoræ composita, Tinctura Opii Ammoniata, and Ammoniæ Benzoas.

## OLEACEÆ.

### OLEA EUROPÆA, *Linn.* EUROPEAN OLIVE.

(*Woodville, Med. Bot.*, t. 98.)

*Habitat.*—Asia Minor, South of Europe, islands of the Mediterranean, and Northern Africa.

*Officinal Part.*—The oil expressed from the fruit (*Olivæ Oleum, Olive Oil*). It is of a pale-yellow colour, almost inodorous, with a bland oleaginous taste. Congeals partially at about 36° F At 20° F. it separates into portions; one fluid, *Elaine* or *Oleine*, and the other a pearly solid, *Margarine*. The proportion of the former is about 72, to 28 of the latter.

*Properties.*—Mild laxative; principally used as an emollient ingredient in enemas, in bowel affections, and also as a mechanical antidote in cases of poisoning, enveloping the poisonous particles, and protecting the surface of the stomach from their action. Much employed as an emollient vehicle for liniments and other external applications. Applied also to relieve pruritus in skin diseases, and to protect the surface from the action of the air in burns and scalds. Inunction with it has been thought to be a preventative of the plague.

*Dose.*—From one to two fluid ounces as a laxative; rarely, however, used in this character.

Olive Oil enters into the following preparations:—Charta Epispastica, Cataplasma Lini, Emplastrum Ammoniaci cum Hydrargyro, Emp. Cerati Saponis, Emp. Hydrargyri, Emp. Picis, Emp. Plumbi, Enema Magnesiæ Sulphatis, Linimentum Ammoniæ, Lin. Calcis, Lin. Camphoræ, Unguentum Cantharidis, Ung. Hydrargyri compositum, Ung. Hydrargyri Nitratis, Ung. Veratriæ, Ung. Aconitiæ.

*Preparations.*—**Hard Soap** (*Sapo Durus*), called also *Castile* or *Spanish Soap*, prepared with Olive Oil and Soda. It is of a greyish white colour, dry, inodorous; horny and pulverisable when kept in dry warm air; easily moulded when heated; soluble in rectified spirit; does not impart an oily stain to paper. Incinerated it yields an ash which does not deliquesce.

*Preparations of Hard Soap.*—**Soap Liniment** (*Linimentum Saponis*). Take of Hard Soap, cut small, two ounces and a half; Camphor, one ounce and a quarter; Oil of Rosemary, three fluid drachms; Rectified Spirit, eighteen fluid ounces; Water, two fluid ounces. Mix the water with the spirit, and add the oil of rosemary, the soap and the camphor. Macerate for seven days at a temperature not exceeding 70° with occasional agitation, and filter.

An excellent vehicle for embrocations in rheumatic and other painful affections. It forms an ingredient in Linimentum Opii.

**Soap Plaster** (*Emplastrum Saponis*). Take of Hard Soap, six ounces; Lead Plaster, two pounds and a quarter; Resin, one ounce. To the lead plaster, melted by a gentle heat, add the soap and the resin, first liquified; then, constantly stirring, evaporate to a proper consistence.

Chiefly employed as a support in affections of the joints, sprains, &c.

**Soap Cerate Plaster** (*Emplastrum Cerati Saponis*). Take of Hard Soap, in powder, ten ounces; Yellow Wax, twelve ounces and a half; Olive Oil, one pint; Oxide of Lead, fifteen ounces; Vinegar, one gallon. Boil the vinegar and oxide of lead together by the heat of a steam-bath, constantly stirring them until the oxide has combined with the acid; then add the soap, and boil again until most of the moisture is evaporated; finally, add the wax and oil melted together, and stir the whole continuously, maintaining the heat until, by the evaporation of the remaining moisture, the product has acquired the proper consistence for a plaster.

Hard soap enters into the composition of the following preparations:—Emplastrum Resinæ, Emp. Saponis, Extractum Colocynthidis compositum, Linimentum Potassii Iodidi cum Sapone, Lin. Saponis, Pilula Aloës Barbadensis, Pil. Aloës et Assafœtidæ, Pil. Aloës Socotrinæ, Pil. Cambogiæ composita, Pil. Rhei composita, Pil. Saponis composita, Pil. Scillæ composita.

**Soft Soap** (*Sapo mollis*), prepared with Olive Oil and Potash. It is yellowish-green, inodorous, of a gelatinous consistence. Soluble in rectified spirit; not imparting an oily stain to paper. Incinerated it yields an ash which is very deliquescent.

*Properties and Uses.*—Emollient, detergent, employed externally in tinea capitis and other skin diseases, especially in the form of baths in syphylitic eruptions. It forms an ingredient in Linimentum Terebinthinæ.

**Glycerine** (*Glycerinum*). A sweet principle, $C_6H_8O_6$ or $C_3H_8O_3$, obtained from fixed oils and fats. A clear colourless fluid, oily to the touch, without odour, of a sweet taste, freely soluble in water and in alcohol. When decomposed by heat it evolves intensely irritating vapours. Sp. gr. 1·25.

*Properties and Uses.*—A valuable emollient. Being a ready solvent of Morphia, Iodine, &c., it forms an excellent vehicle for embrocations and other external applications. Introduced into the external meatus auditorius, it has been thought useful in some forms of deafness; its effects are only temporary. It has been proposed, on insufficient grounds, as a substitute for cod liver oil in phthisis.

*Dose.*—From one to two fluid drachms.

Glycerine enters into the following preparations:—Glyycerinum Acidi Carbolici, Glyc. Acidi Gallici, Glyc. Acidi Tannici, Glyc. Amyli, Glyc. Boracis, and Linimentum Potassii Iodidi cum Sapone.

## FRAXINUS ORNUS, *Linn.* FLOWERING ASH.

(*Woodville, Med. Bot.*, t. 36.)

## FRAXINUS ROTUNDIFOLIA, *D.C.* ROUND-LEAVED ASH.

(*Hayne*, vol. xiii. t. 12.)

*Habitat.*—Mountains of the South of Europe, especially Calabria and Sicily.

*Officinal Part.*—A concrete saccharine exudation from the stem, obtained by incisions (*Manna*). It occurs in stalactiform pieces from one to six inches in length, and one or two inches in width, uneven, porous, and friable, curved on one side, of a yellowish-white colour, with a faintly nauseous odour, and a sweetish taste. It consists principally of mannite, $C_6H_7O_6$ or $\mathbf{C_3H_7O_3}$, together with common sugar and extractive matter. The mannite, which forms from 60 to 80 per cent. of the manna, may be extracted by means of boiling rectified spirit, from which it will afterwards separate on cooling in colourless, shining crystals. It requires five parts of cold water for its solution, and this does not undergo vinous fermentation in contact with yeast.

*Properties and Uses.*—Laxative. Well adapted for childhood, on account of its sweet taste and generally mild action. It is a good adjunct to senna, and the saline purgatives, for the purpose of disguising their nauseous taste, and assisting their operation. Applicable in the same cases as Senna.

*Dose.*—For children, from one to three drachms; for adults, from one to two ounces.

# JASMINEÆ.

(*Non-officinal.*)

**Jasminum Sambac,** *Aiton* (*Wight, Icones*, vol. ii. t. 704). — Cultivated throughout India for the sake of its fragrant flowers, which are used as votive offerings. The flowers, according to the report of Mr. J. Wood, possess considerable power as a lactifuge; he speaks of them as effectual in arresting the secretion of milk in the puerperal state, in cases of threatened abscess. For this purpose about two or three handfuls of the flowers are bruised, and unmoistened are applied to each breast, and renewed once or twice a day. The secretion is sometimes arrested in twenty-four hours, though this generally requires two or even three days. Mr. Wood speaks of this fact as being well known at Madras.

# APOCYNEÆ.

## *ALSTONIA SCHOLARIS, *R. Br.*

(*Wight, Icones*, vol. ii. t. 442.)

*Habitat.*—Common in forests throughout India.

*Officinal Part.*—The bark (*Alstoniæ Cortex*). It occurs in thick, irregular, more or less contorted pieces, easily broken. It consists of a rough greyish epidermis, investing a buff or pale cinnamon coloured bark; internally still lighter in colour, and of a spongy texture, having a very bitter taste, but devoid of odour.

*Properties.*—Astringent tonic, anthelmintic; antiperiodic.

*Therapeutic Uses.*—In chronic diarrhœa and the advanced stages of dysentery, it has proved valuable.(45) It has also been found effectual in restoring the tone of the stomach, and of the system generally, in debility after fevers and other exhausting diseases.

*Dose.*—From three to five grains, either alone or combined, in bowel affections, with small doses of Ipecacuanha and Extract of Gentian.

*Preparations.* — **Tincture of Alstonia** (*Tinctura Alstoniæ*). Take of Alstonia Bark, bruised, two ounces and a half; Proof Spirit, one pint. Macerate for seven days in a closed vessel, with occasional agitation; filter, and add sufficient proof spirit to make one pint. Or prepare by percolation, as Tincture of Calumba.

*Dose.*—From one to two fluid drachms.

**Infusion of Alstonia** (*Infusum Alstoniæ*). Take of Alstonia Bark, bruised, half an ounce; Boiling Water, ten fluid ounces. Infuse in a covered vessel for an hour, and strain.

*Dose.*—From one to two fluid ounces twice or thrice daily. A good serviceable tonic.

(*Non-officinal.*)

**Holarrhena antidysenterica,** *R. Br.* (*Wight, Icones*, vol. ii. t. 439.) —A shrub or small tree, common throughout India, the bark of which has long enjoyed considerable repute, and was formerly imported into Europe under the names of *Conessi bark*, *Codaga pala*, *Corte de Pala*, and *Tellicherry bark*. It is a spongy bark, of a dull rusty colour, and bitter taste. Though held in esteem as a tonic and febrifuge, it has obtained most repute as a remedy in dysenteric affections: hence its specific name. Its efficacy in this character is testified to by Dr. Alexander Munro (*Edin. Med. Essays*, vol. iii. p. 32), and Dr. Ives (*Voyage to India*, p. 464). A strong opinion of its efficacy, based on its employment in numerous cases, is expressed by Sub-assistant Surgeon Odoy Chund Dutt. And it is favourably noticed in the reports of Dr. H. C. Bowser, Dr. Bholanauth Doss, and others. Sub-assistant Surgeon A. C. Kastagree (*Indian Med. Gaz.* 1866, vol. i. p. 352) publishes the case of a child at 15 months suffering from dysentery, in which this remedy succeeded after ipecacuanha and all ordinary means had failed. He employed a decoction (Bark two ounces, Water O ii. boiled to O i.) Doses of four drachms, four times a day, with the addition of one drop of Tr. Opii to each dose. Dr. Gibson states that he has employed it extensively as an antiperiodic. It has, however, fallen into disrepute, principally, according to Sir Walter Elliot, who regards it as one of the most valuable medicinal products of India, from the comparatively or wholly inert bark of *Wrightia tinctoria*, R. Br., a tree very similar in general appearance to *H. antidysenterica*, and known by very similar native names, having been often confounded with it. (46) This bark and its properties are well deserving of the notice of future investigators. It may be prescribed in decoction (eight ounces, water two pints boiled to one pint) in doses of one ounce and a half or two ounces twice or thrice daily; but Mr. Odoy Chund Dutt prefers a watery extract of the root-bark, of which the average dose is about three grains in combination with half a grain or more of opium. The oat-like seeds (*Anderjow* of the Taleef Shereef, No. 75,) are also highly valued by the natives of India in dysenteric cases. They are narrow, elongated, about half an inch in length, of a cinnamon brown colour, convex on one side, concave and marked with a longitudinal pale line on the other, easily broken, of a bitter taste, and heavy unpleasant odour. They are often confounded with the seeds of *Wrightia tinctoria, Roxb.*, to which they bear a general resemblance. According to Ainslie (*Mat. Ind.*, vol. ii. p. 483), an infusion of the toasted seeds is a gentle and safe astringent in bowel complaints, and is given to allay the vomiting of cholera. In the Taleef Shereef, the infusion is said to be effectual in arresting hæmorrhage from piles. Anthelmintic virtues are also assigned to them. During the last cattle plague epidemic at Backergunge (Bengal) they were extensively employed, being regarded as possessing certain specific virtues (*Indian Med. Gaz.* 1866, vol. i. p. 352.) The results are not stated.

**Holarrhena pubescens,** *Wall.*—The seeds of this shrub, common in many parts of India, apparently only a variety of the above, are an esteemed remedy in native practice in dysentery and other bowel affections. They are known by the names of *Indurjuo tulk* (bitter), to distinguish them from *Indurjuo sherin* (mild), those of *Wrightia tinctoria*, R. Br., to which they bear a resemblance (Royle, *Illust.*, vol. i. p. 271). The bark possesses astringent tonic properties, and is employed in fevers (*Wight*). Our knowledge of their virtues at present rests on native testimony.

**Ichnocarpus frutescens,** *R. Br.* (*Wight, Icones*, vol. ii. t. 430.)—A native of Bengal, Sylhet, Assam, Kumaon, and other parts of India. The root is considered to possess alterative tonic properties, and has been employed as a substitute for sarsaparilla (Royle, *Illust.*, vol. i. p. 271, and Wight, *Illust.*, vol. ii. p. 162).

**Thevetia neriifolia,** *Juss.* (*Hooker, Bot. Mag.*, t. 2309.)—A West Indian shrub, domesticated in India, and cultivated under the name of *The Exile* or *Yellow Oleander*. The antiperiodic properties of the bark, first noticed by M. Descourtilz (*Flor. Med. des Antilles*, vol. iii. p. 40), have been confirmed by Dr. G. Bidie (*Madras Quart. Med. Journ.*, 1862, vol. v. p. 178), and Dr. J. Shortt

(*Ibid.*, 1865, vol. viii. p. 294). Their trials with it in various forms of intermittent fever proved highly satisfactory, and leave little doubt that it is a remedy of considerable power. It was employed in the form of Tincture (one ounce of the freshly dried bark macerated for eight days in five ounces of Rectified Spirit) in doses of from ten to fifteen drops thrice daily. In larger doses, from thirty to sixty drops, it acts as an acrid purgative and emetic, and carried to a greater extent is evidently powerfully poisonous. The kernels are extremely bitter, and when chewed produce a slight feeling of numbness and heat in the tongue; by expression they yield a clear pale-amber coloured, slightly viscid, acrid oil, which is sometimes recommended as a cathartic by the natives, but it produces violent vomiting and hypercatharsis (Dr. Shortt). An interesting case of poisoning by one of these kernels is recorded by Dr. J. Balfour (*Madras Journ. of Lit. and Science*, 1857, vol. iii. N.S. p. 140). Recovery ensued; but, from the symptoms detailed, they belong evidently to the class of acro-narcotic poisons. In all trials with this remedy, much caution is necessary.

**Nerium odorum**, *Aiton* (*Bot. Mag.*, t. 2032.)—*The Sweet-scented Oleander*. Much cultivated in India for the sake of its flowers, which are used in certain religious ceremonies by the Hindús. All parts of the plant, especially the root, are recognized by the natives as poisonous, and as such are used for criminal and suicidal purposes; yet we find, in the Taleef Shereef (p. 129), and other works on Indian Materia Medica, it is prescribed in leprosy and other diseases. It is mentioned here chiefly with the view of enforcing caution in any trials which may be made with it, as in over-doses it is productive of serious and even fatal effects. Two interesting cases of poisoning with it are recorded, one by Dr. J. Broughton (*Bombay Med. Phys. Trans.*, vol. iv. N.S. p. 4, in Appendix), and the other by Dr. A. Greig (*Indian Annals of Med. Science*, vol. ii. p. 295). In the latter, which proved fatal, death, according to Dr. Greig, was due to the directly depressing influence which the drug exercised on the nervous system. A case in which tetanic symptoms followed the exhibition of the root-bark is recorded by Mr. Kamikhyá Nath Acherjee (*Indian Med. Gaz.*, 1866, vol. i. p. 218).

**Cerbera Odollam** (*Gaertn*), or **C. Manghas**, *Linn.* (*Wight, Icones*, vol. ii. t. 441.) Common in low swampy sites on the seacoasts of India. Emetic and purgative properties are assigned to the milky juice and to the leaves; but their use is to be condemned, as the number of safe and efficient medicines of both classes is quite large enough, and there is reason for believing that these trees, even in moderate quantities, are possessed of poisonous properties.

**Ophioxylon serpentinum**, *Linn.* (*Wight, Icones*, vol. iii. t. 849.) —An erect or twining shrub, common throughout India. It is held in high esteem by the natives as an antidote to snake bites, but reliable evidence of its utility is wanting. It is also valued as a tonic and febrifuge. Horsfield (*Asiat. Journ.*, vol. viii. p. 148) states that the root yields a strong bitter infusion, and that its sensible properties indicate considerable activity. According to the same authority, it is employed by the Javanese as an anthelmintic. Dr. Pulney Andy reports that a decoction of the root is employed in labours to increase uterine contractions.

**Rhazya stricta,** *Dec.* (*Jacquemont, Voy. Bot.*, t. 111.)—A native of Scinde, the Punjaub, and Affghanistan, where it is known by the names of *Sewur, Sihar,* and *Ishwurg*. The dried leaves and stalks are sold in the Scinde bazaars. Dr. Stocks describes it as a good and peculiar bitter tonic, and recommends it for future trial. (Letter to Dr. J. Forbes Watson, June 13th, 1852.)

## ASCLEPIADEÆ.

### HEMIDESMUS INDICUS, *R. Brown.* HEMIDESMUS.

(*Wight, Icones*, t. 594.)

*Habitat.*—Common throughout India.

*Officinal Part.*—The root (*Hemidesmi Radix, Hemidesmus Root*). It occurs in pieces of various lengths, of a yellowish-brown colour, cylindrical, tortuous, furrowed longitudinally; the cortex divided by annular cracks; odour, peculiar and aromatic; taste, feebly bitter and agreeable. Its virtues reside in a volatile oil, and a crystallizable principle, *Hemidesmine.*[47]

*Properties.*—Valuable alterative tonic, diuretic, and diaphoretic.
*Therapeutic Uses.*—In constitutional debility, cachexia, especially of children, constitutional syphilis, chronic rheumatism, and skin diseases, it has been employed with signal benefit.

*Preparations.*—***Infusion of Hemidesmus** (*Infusum Hemidesmi*). Take of the roots of Hemidesmus, bruised, one ounce; Boiling Water, ten fluid ounces. Infuse in a covered vessel for an hour, and strain.

*Dose.*—From two to three fluid ounces, thrice daily.

[This is the best form for administration. Its efficacy is increased if taken while the infusion is still warm. The addition of milk and sugar renders it so like ordinary tea that children will take it readily. It forms an excellent vehicle for Iodide of Potassium and other medicines. The fresher the root the greater is its efficacy.]

**Syrup of Hemidesmus** (*Syrupus Hemidesmi*).—Take of the Roots of Hemidesmus, four ounces; Refined Sugar, twenty-eight ounces; Boiling Water, one pint. Infuse the hemidesmus in the water, in a covered vessel, for four hours, and strain. Set it by till the sediment subsides; then decant the clear liquor, add the sugar, and dissolve by means of a gentle heat. The product should weigh two pounds ten ounces, and should have the specific gravity 1·335.

*Dose.*—From one to two fluid drachms, or more. As it readily ferments, it is ill adapted for use in the tropics.

## *CALOTROPIS PROCERA, *R. Br.* CALOTROPIS GIGANTEA, *R. Br.* } MUDAR.(48)

(*Wight, Illust.*, vol. ii. t. 155; *Icones*, vol. iv. t. 1278)

*Habitat.*—One or other of these species is found everywhere in India. *C. procera*, the smaller of the two, prefers the drier climate of the Deccan, the Upper Provinces of Bengal, the Punjaub and Scinde; *C. gigantea*, Lower Bengal, the Madras and Malayan Peninsulas, and Ceylon.

*Officinal Part.*—The root-bark dried (*Calotropis Cortex*). It occurs in small flat or arched pieces, brownish externally, of a yellow-greyish colour internally, with a peculiar smell, and mucilaginous, nauseous, acrid taste. Its activity appears to reside in a peculiar extractive matter named *Mudarine.* (49)

*Properties.*—Alterative tonic; diaphoretic, and in large doses emetic.

*Therapeutic Uses.*—In leprosy, constitutional syphilis, mercurial cachexia, syphilitic and idiopathic ulcerations, in dysentery, diarrhœa, and chronic rheumatism, it has been used with alleged benefit. (50)

*Preparations.*—**Powder of Mudar** (*Pulvis Calotropis*). Take of the Roots of Mudar, collected in the months of April and May from sandy soils, a sufficiency; carefully remove, by washing, all particles of sand and dirt, and dry in the open air, without exposure to the sun, until the milky juice contained in it becomes so far inspissated that it ceases to flow on incisions being made in it. The bark is then to be carefully removed, dried, and reduced to powder. Preserve in well corked bottles.

*Dose.*—As an alterative tonic, three grains, gradually increased to ten grains or more, thrice daily. As an emetic, from half a drachm to a drachm.

[The emetic properties of Mudar, first pointed out by Dr. Duncan in 1829 (*Edin. Med. Surg. Journ.*, vol. xxxii. p. 65), have been fully confirmed by the subsequent observations of Sir W. O'Shaughnessy (*Bengal Disp.*, p. 453), Dr. Bonavia (*Indian Lancet*, Sept. 1st, 1859, p. 42), Dr. J. Hutchinson (*Ibid.*, Oct. 1st, 1859), Mr. J. J. Durant (*Indian Med. Gaz.*, May 1st, 1866, p. 112), and others (*Indian Lancet*, Dec. 1st, 1859). Further testimony in its favour is to be found in the reports of Dr. L. Stewart, Dr. J. Newton, Dr. Æ. Ross, Mr. Odoy Chund Dutt, &c. The root dug up at the proper season, carefully prepared in accordance with the above directions, and preserved from contact with the air, is doubtless possessed of valuable emetic properties; but in this character, as well as in that of an alterative tonic, it is apt to prove almost inert, should the above cautions be neglected. Ainslie (*Mat. Ind.*, vol. i. p. 488) regards the inspissated milky juice of the plant as infinitely more efficacious than the root-bark; evidence, however, is wanting to confirm this opinion. He places the dose at about twelve grains daily, in divided doses.]

## *TYLOPHORA ASTHMATICA, *W. et A.*

(*Wight, Icones*, vol. iv. t. 1277.)

*Habitat.*—Common in sandy localities in Bengal, the Madras Peninsula, and other parts of India; Ceylon.

*Officinal Part.* — The dried leaves (*Tylophoræ Folia*). From two to three inches in length, entire, ovate-roundish, acuminated, cordate at the base, glabrous above, downy beneath. They have a heavy disagreeable smell when bruised, and a nauseous taste.

*Properties.*—Emetic, diaphoretic, and expectorant.

*Therapeutic Uses.* — In over-loaded states of the stomach, and other cases requiring the use of emetics, it acts efficiently. It has been found useful also in dysentery, catarrh, and other affections in which ipecacuanha is generally employed.

*Dose.*—As an emetic, from five and twenty to thirty grains of the powder of the dried leaves, conjoined with half a grain or a grain of Tartar Emetic. As a diaphoretic and expectorant, from three to five grains thrice daily, or oftener, combined with opium, and other remedies of the same class.

[The root of this plant, which is met with in the bazaars in the form of thick contorted pieces of a pale colour, and a bitterish, somewhat nauseous taste, has long been known to possess diaphoretic and emetic properties, and its efficacy in dysentery is asserted by Dr. J. Anderson. (Roxburgh, *Flor. Ind.*, vol. ii. p. 34.) Its value has also been confirmed by Sir W. O'Shaughnessy. It has, however, been superseded by the dried leaves, the operation of which has been found more uniform and certain. It may be regarded as one of the best indigenous (Indian) substitutes for Ipecacuanha. ([51])]

(*Non-officinal.*)

**Secamone emetica,** *R. Br.* (*Wight, Icones*, vol. iv. t. 1283.)—A climbing shrub, common in low jungles in many parts of India. Regarded by the natives as possessing powerfully emetic properties (Dr. Wight in *Madras Journ. of Lit. and Sci.*, vol. ii. p. 80). Dr. G. Bidie, however, gave it a trial in several instances, and found it almost inert. The propriety of its specific name is therefore doubtful.

**Asclepias curassavica,** *Linn.*—A West Indian plant naturalized in India. It has been named *Bastard* or *Wild Ipecacuanha* by the West Indian colonists, from the emetic properties of its root; but as its operation is said to be attended by powerful action on the bowels, it is little applicable in the generality of cases, or where simple emesis is required. The dose of the powder of the dried root is from 20 to 40 grains. The expressed juice of the leaves is stated to act efficiently as an anthelmintic. Lunan (*Hort. Jamaicensis*, vol. i. p. 63) and Hamilton (*Pharm. Journ.*, 1847, vol. vi. p. 214).

**Dœmia extensa,** *R. Br.* (*Wight, Icones*, vol. ii. t. 596) has emetic and expectorant virtues ascribed to it by the natives, and is much employed by them in the diseases of children. Dr. Oswald reports that it is used as an expectorant in the treatment of catarrhal affections, in ten-grain doses, at the Pettah Hospital, Mysore. It attracted some attention in Madras, in 1858, as a remedy in snake bites; but the identification of this plant with the one employed in a case which recovered under very hopeless circumstances is incomplete, and no other evidence of its value in this character is on record. The leaves of **Hoya viridiflora**, *R. Br.* (*Wight, Icones*, vol. ii. t. 586), are much employed by the natives as an application to boils and abscesses. It has, according to native testimony, the same emetic and expectorant virtues as *Dæmia extensa.*

**Gymnema sylvestre**, *R. Br.* (*Wight, Icones*, vol. ii. t. 349), has properties similar to those of *Dæmia extensa* ascribed to it by the natives, who hold the root in esteem as a local and internal remedy in snake bites (Ainslie, *Mat. Ind.*, vol. ii. p. 390). A curious circumstance connected with this plant was first noticed by Mr. Edgeworth; namely, that if chewed it destroys the power of the tongue to appreciate the taste of sugar and all saccharine substances. In his own person he found that powdered sugar, taken immediately after masticating some of the leaves, appeared like so much sand in his mouth, and this effect lasted nearly twenty-four hours, when he recovered the power of distinguishing the taste of sugar (*Pharm. Journ.*, vol. vii. p. 551).

## LOGANIACEÆ.

### STRYCHNOS NUX VOMICA, *Linn.* NUX VOMICA TREE.

(*Roxb., Corom. Plants*, t. 4.)

*Habitat.*—Most parts of India.

*Officinal Part.*—The seed (*Nux Vomica*): nearly circular and flat, about an inch in diameter, umbilicated, and slightly convex on one side; externally of an ash-grey colour, thickly covered with short satiny hairs, internally translucent, tough and horny; taste intensely bitter, inodorous. It contains two crystallizable principles, *Strychnia* and *Brucia*, which exist in combination with *Igasuric acid.*

*Properties.*—Valuable nervine tonic and stimulant, in over-doses a virulent poison.

*Therapeutic Uses.*—In paralytic and neuralgic affections, in atonic diarrhœa and chronic dysentery, also in habitual constipation dependent on torpor of the colon, in prolapsus of the rectum, in incontinence of urine, in spermatorrhœa, and in other cases referrible to debility or inactivity of the spinal system of nerves, it is a remedy of great value. It has also been employed with alleged benefit in intermittent fevers, epiplepsy, diabetes, anæmia, chlorosis, and other affections.

*Dose.*—Of the powdered seeds from two to three grains, gradually increased to ten grains or more, twice or thrice daily.

*Preparations.*—***Infusion of Nux Vomica** (*Infusum Nucis Vomicæ*). Take of Nux Vomica Seeds, bruised, two drachms; Boiling Water, twelve fluid ounces. Infuse in a covered vessel for an hour and strain.

*Dose.*—Four fluid drachms gradually increased to eight and ten fluid drachms thrice daily. A valuable bitter tonic, especially adapted to debilitated states of the system and dropsical affections of the natives of India. Its effects require careful watching.

**Tincture of Nux Vomica** (*Tinctura Nucis Vomicæ*). Take of Nux Vomica, two ounces; Rectified Spirit, one pint. Apply steam to the nux vomica until it is thoroughly softened, then dry rapidly, and reduce it to fine powder. Macerate the powder for forty-eight hours in fifteen fluid ounces of the spirit in a closed vessel, agitating occasionally; then transfer to a percolator; and when the fluid ceases to pass, continue the percolation with the remaining five ounces of spirit. Afterwards subject the contents of the percolator to pressure, filter the product, mix the liquids, and add sufficient rectified spirit to make one pint.

*Dose.*—From ten to twenty drops as a nervine stimulant; from five to ten drops as a tonic.

**Extract of Nux Vomica** (*Extractum Nucis Vomicæ*). Take of Nux Vomica, one pound; rectified Spirit, a sufficiency. Apply steam to the Nux Vomica until it is thoroughly softened, then dry rapidly, and reduce to fine powder. Exhaust the powder by boiling it with successive portions of the spirit until the latter comes off nearly free from bitterness. Strain, distil off the spirit, and evaporate by a water bath to the consistence of a soft extract.

*Dose.*—From a quarter of a grain to two grains. A valuable preparation, especially in intestinal affections characterised by a want of nervous energy.

**Strychnia** (*Strychnia*). An alkaloid, $C_{42}H_{22}N_2O_4$ or $C_{21}H_{22}N_2O_2$. obtained from Nux Vomica. It occurs in the form of right square octahedrons or prisms, colourless and inodorous; is sparingly soluble in water, but communicating to it, its intensely bitter taste; soluble in boiling rectified spirit and in chloroform, but not in absolute alcohol or in ether. Pure sulphuric acid forms with it a colourless solution, which on the addition of bichromate of potash acquires an intensely violet hue, speedily passing through red to yellow. *Tests.*—Not coloured by nitric acid; leaves no ash when burned with free access of air.

*Properties and Uses.* — The same as those of Nux Vomica. Being powerfully poisonous, even in small doses, its administration requires much caution and careful watching. It is especially adapted for paralytic affections of an asthenic type. In nervous exhaustion, from whatever cause arising, it is a remedy of great value. In amaurosis, nyctalopia, chorea, intermittent fevers, and other affections, it has been used with alleged benefit.

*Dose.*—One fiftieth part of a grain thrice daily as a tonic. From one thirtieth to one twelfth of a grain, gradually increased, as a nervine stimulant. It should in all cases be immediately discontinued on the occurrence of slight convulsive twitchings in the muscles of the extremities.

*Preparations.*—**Solution of Strychnia** (*Liquor Strychniæ*). Take of Strychnia, in crystals, four grains; Dilute Hydrochloric Acid, six minims; Rectified Spirit, two fluid drachms; Distilled Water, six fluid drachms. Mix the hydrochloric acid with four drachms of the water, and dissolve the strychnia in the mixture by the aid of heat; then add the spirit, and the remainder of the water.

*Dose.*—From three to ten minims. Each minim contains one ninetieth of a grain of strychnia. Nine minims, therefore, contain one tenth of a grain. In this, as in all preparations of strychnia, small doses at the commencement, gradually increased, are the best and safest form of administration.

[The bark of Strychnos Nux Vomica found its way, some years since, into European commerce, under the name of "False Angustura bark;" the distinctions between the true and the false barks were pointed out by Sir W. O'Shaughnessy in 1837. (*Calcutta Quart. Journ. of Med.*, Jan. 1st, 1837, p. 9.) It contains strychnine and brucine, and hence is powerfully poisonous. It is commonly sold in Calcutta under the name of *Rohun*, and is sometimes substituted for the comparatively harmless bark of *Soymida febrifuga*, which is known by the same native name. The latter may readily be distinguished by the application of nitric acid to the inner surface of the bark; in the Nux Vomica bark a bright red stain is caused, which is not observed in the Soymida bark under the same circumstances. Professor Christison considers it probable that Nux Vomica bark might be advantageously substituted for the seed in the preparation of strychnia. It forms the principal ingredient in the chief of the medicated oils commonly in use by the natives as local applications to leprous, syphilitic, and other obstinate eruptions. Mr. Moodeen Sheriff reports that these oils in some instances prove very effectual.]

(*Non-officinal.*)

**Strychnos colubrina,** *Linn.* (*Rheede, Hort. Mal.*, vol. viii. t. 24.)—A climbing shrub of Malabar, Coromandel, and other parts of the Madras Peninsula, also of Ceylon, the Moluccas, &c. Its wood is supposed to constitute the *Lignum Colubrinum* of old writers, the *Pao de Cobra* of the Portuguese, from its efficacy, imaginary or real, in the treatment of the most venomous snake bites, even of the Cobra de Capello. In these cases it was employed both locally and internally. No trustworthy evidence, however, of its efficacy in this character is on record. According to Horsfield (*Asiat. Journ.*, vol. vii. p. 147) it has long been employed by the Javanese as a remedy in intermittent fevers. Its claims as an antiperiodic have been examined by Dr. Berdenis Van Berkelow (*Schmidt's Jahrbucher,* May 24th, 1866, and *Brit.*

*and For. Med. Chir. Rev.*, April 1867, p. 527); and after a trial with it in twenty-two cases, quartan and tertian, he reports favorably of its action, and considers that from its cheapness it may advantageously be used as a febrifuge in pauper practice. The fact of its containing strychnia in considerable quantities indicates the necessity for great caution in its use. Whatever efficacy it possesses in this character is doubtless due to this alkaloid; and as the proportion in which it exists in this wood is undetermined, and is likely to vary according to the season of collection, it is far safer to employ in its stead the alkaloid itself, a preparation of uniform strength, and which can be regulated with comparative ease. In the present state of our information, Lignum Colubrinum must be looked upon as a dangerous remedy. These remarks apply with equal force to the seeds of **Ignatia amara,** *Linn.* (*St. Ignatius's Bean,*) which are met with commonly in Indian bazaars, and are largely used in native practice. The Taleef Shereef (p. 29) contains a long account of their uses. It appears, as far as we at present know, that every good effect expected from them may be more certainly and safely obtained by employing strychnia or one of the officinal preparations of Nux Vomica. These seeds are about the size of olives, rounded and convex on one side, and somewhat angular on the other. Externally they are brownish, with a bluish-grey tint. Within the envelopes of the seed is a very hard horny or cartilaginous albumen, in whose cavity is contained the embryo.

**Strychnos Potatorum,** *Linn.* (*Wight, Illust.*, vol. ii. t. 156.)—The seeds of this tree are devoid of poisonous properties, and are used in native practice as an emetic (*Ainslie*), as a remedy in diabetes (*Kirkpatrick*), gonorrhœa (*Taleef Shereef*), &c. Their chief use, however, is as a means of clearing muddy water, and rendering it fit for drinking purposes; hence their Anglo-Indian name, *Clearing Nut*. Looked at in this point of view, they may be regarded as a valuable aid to medical officers and others during the marches of troops in India in the rainy season, when little but muddy water can be procured. Dr. Pereira (*Pharm. Journ.*, 1850, vol. ix. p. 478) suggests that this property depends upon the albumen and casein which they contain. If the seeds be sliced and digested in water, they yield a thick mucilaginous liquid, which, when boiled, yields a coagulum (albumen), and by subsequent addition of acetic acid, it furnishes a further coagulum (casein). The mode of employing them is simple, consisting only of rubbing the inside of the vessel with the sliced or bruised seeds, previous to the water being poured into it. The muddiest water is stated, under these circumstances, to be speedily rendered clear and wholesome. Carefully conducted experiments, in illustration of the properties of these seeds in the above character, are desirable. The seeds are of a flattened spherical form, and yellowish grey colour, having the testa coated with short close hairs; albumen horny and tasteless.

**Fagræa fragrans,** *Roxb.*—A tree of China and Malayan Peninsula, the bark of which has been found effectual in the treatment of the malarious fevers of Malacca. Dr. A. C. Maingay called the attention of the medical authorities of Bengal to it, and, examined chemically by Mr. Kanny Loll Dey (*Ind. Drugs*, p. 54), it was found to contain strychnia. The remedy appears worthy of further investigation.

# GENTIANACEÆ.

## GENTIANA LUTEA, *Linn.* COMMON OR YELLOW GENTIAN.

(*Woodville, Med. Bot.*, t. 95.)

*Habitat.*—Sub-alpine regions of Central and Southern Europe.

*Officinal Part.*—The dried root (*Gentianæ Radix, Gentian Root*); occurs in pieces from half an inch to an inch in thickness, several inches in length, often twisted, much wrinkled or marked with close transverse rings, brown externally, yellow within, tough and spongy; taste at first sweetish, afterwards very bitter. Its activity resides in a bitter extractive, *Gentianite;* it also contains a crystallizable principle, *Gentianin*, and a volatile oil.

*Properties.*—Valuable bitter tonic.

*Therapeutic Uses.*—In debility, in convalescence after exhausting diseases, and in some forms of dyspepsia, especially in that of gouty subjects, it is a remedy of proved value. In intermittents, it formerly was held in repute.

*Preparations.*—**Compound Infusion of Gentian** (*Infusum Gentianæ compositum*). Take of Gentian Root, sliced, Bitter Orange Peel, cut small, of each sixty grains; Fresh Lemon Peel, cut small, a quarter of an ounce; Boiling Water, ten fluid ounces. Infuse in a covered vessel for one hour, and strain.

*Dose.*—From one to two fluid ounces, twice or thrice daily.

**Gentian Mixture** (*Mistura Gentianæ; Infusum Gentianæ compositum, Brit. Ph.*, 1864). Take of Gentian Root, sliced, a quarter of an ounce; Bitter Orange Peel, cut small, Coriander Fruit, bruised, each thirty grains; Proof Spirit, two fluid ounces; Water, eight fluid ounces. Macerate the gentian, orange peel, and coriander in the proof spirit for two hours; then add the water; macerate again for two hours, and strain through calico.

*Dose.*—From one half to two fluid ounces, twice or thrice daily.

**Extract of Gentian** (*Extractum Gentianæ*). Take of Gentian Root, sliced, one pound; Boiling Water, one gallon. Infuse the gentian in the water for two hours; boil for fifteen minutes; pour off, press, and strain. Then evaporate the liquor by a water-bath until the extract is of a suitable consistence for forming pills.

*Dose.*—From two to ten grains. A useful adjunct, in the form of pill, to other tonics.

**Compound Tincture of Gentian** (*Tinctura Gentianæ composita*). Take of Gentian Root, bruised, one ounce and a half; Bitter Orange Peel, cut small and bruised, three quarters of an ounce; Cardamom seeds, freed from the pericarps and bruised, a quarter of an ounce; Proof Spirit, one pint. Macerate the solid ingredients for forty-eight hours in fifteen fluid ounces of the spirit, in a closed vessel, agitating occasionally; then transfer to a percolator; and when the fluid ceases to pass, continue the percolation with the remaining five ounces of spirit. Afterwards subject the contents of the percolator to pressure, filter the product, mix the liquids, and add sufficient proof spirit to make one pint.

*Dose.*—From one half to two fluid drachms.

## OPHELIA CHIRATA, *D.C.* CHIRETTA. (52)

(*Wallich, Plant. Asiat. Rar.*, t. 252.)

*Habitat.*—Temperate Himalaya, east of Kumaon.

*Officinal Part.*—The entire plant (*Chirata, Chiretta*), collected when the fruit begins to form. It usually presents the following characters:—Stems about three feet long, of the thickness of a goose quill, round, smooth, pale brown, branched, branches opposite; flowers small, numerous, panicled; the whole plant intensely bitter. It contains a very bitter extractive, and a resinous matter, in which its virtues reside.

*Properties.*—Powerful pure bitter tonic.

*Therapeutic Uses.*—Similar to those of Gentian.

*Preparations.*—**Infusion of Chiretta** (*Infusum Chiratæ*). Take of Chiretta, cut small, a quarter of an ounce; Water at 120° F., ten fluid ounces. Infuse in a covered vessel for half an hour, and strain.

*Dose.*—From one to two fluid ounces, twice or thrice daily.

*__Compound Tincture of Chiretta__ (*Tinctura Chiratæ*). Take of Chiretta, bruised, one ounce and a half; Orange Peel, bruised, three quarters of an ounce; Cardamom seeds, freed from the pericarps and bruised, a quarter of an ounce; Proof Spirit, one pint. Macerate for seven days in a closed vessel, with occasional agitation; strain, press, filter, and add sufficient proof spirit to make one pint.

*Dose.*—From one to two fluid drachms. A valuable adjunct to other tonics.

[In Southern India some confusion occasionally arises from confounding Chiretta, our present article, with Kariyát, *Andrographis paniculata*, Nat. Ord. Acanthaceæ, *q.v.*]

(*Non-officinal.*)

**Gentiana Kurroo**, *Royle* (*Illustr.*, t. 68.)—The root of this plant, indigenous at Mussoorie, Simla, and other portions of Himalaya, possesses the bitterness of, and is applicable to the same uses as the Gentian of Europe, for which it affords a good substitute. It may be given in the form of Compound Infusion, in the same doses as the corresponding preparation of officinal Gentian.

**Ophelia angustifolia**, *D. Don* (*Wallich, Plant. Asiat. Rar.*, t. 204), **Ophelia elegans**, *Wight* (*Icones*, vol. iv. t. 1331), and **Ophelia densifolia**, *Gris.* (**O. multiflora**, *Dalzell.*) These and other species of Ophelia are common throughout the Himalaya, and several others occur in the mountains of the Madras Peninsula. They all possess strong bitter properties, and may, therefore, where they are indigenous, be substituted for the officinal Chiretta, which is rare to the west of Nepal, and is not found in Central or Southern India. In the North Western Provinces of Bengal, O. angustifolia, *D. Don*, a common Himalayan species, is much used instead of O. Chirata, and is called *Pahari* or *Hill Chiretta*, while the officinal plant, imported from the plains, is called *Dukhani* or *Southern Chiretta* (Royle). According to Dr. Cleghorn (*Indian Annals of Med. Sci.*, vol. iii. p. 271), **O. elegans**, *Wight*, which inhabits the mountains of the Madras Peninsula, possesses powerful and persistent bitterness. He states that frequent trials with it confirm the belief that it exercises a tonic influence on the digestive organs, thereby improving the general health; it appears also to possess some power as an antiperiodic. It is best given in the form of infusion in the proportion of two drachms to a pint of cold water. It appears equal, if not superior, to the officinal Chiretta. **O. multiflora**, *Dalz.*, a native of the mountains of the Concans, forms, in like manner, an excellent substitute for Chiretta, and is so used in Bombay (Dalzell and Gibson, *Bombay Flora*, p. 156). Particular attention has been called to it by Dr. Broughton (*Bombay Med. Phys. Trans.* vol. vi., N.S., App. p. 58). The dried root, he states, occurs in pieces about two inches in length, of the diameter of a quill, giving off two or three rootlets, covered with a whitish brown epidermis, wrinkled longitudinally, white internally; brittle. He considers that its medicinal action and uses are similar to those of Gentian and Chiretta, for which it may be advantageously substituted. The dried plant appears also to be used for the same purposes.

**Exacum tetragonum**, *Roxb.* (*Wallich, Plant. Asiat. Rar.*, t. 276), and **E. bicolor**, *Roxb.* (*Wight, Icones*, vol. iv. t. 1321.)—The former of these is common in the Himalaya and the mountains and plains of Bengal and Central India, as far south as Bombay. The whole plant possesses a powerfully bitter taste; and, according to Royle (*Illust.* vol. i. p. 277), it is called by the natives *Ooda* (*purple*) *Chiretta.* As a tonic it appears to possess considerable power. The second species (*E. bicolor*) is common from the Concan and Cuttack throughout the Madras Peninsula. Its dried stalks are sold at Mangalore and elsewhere in Southern India under the name of *Country Kariyát*, It possesses the tonic stomachic properties of Gentian, and may, in localities where it is procurable, be advantageously substituted for it (Dr. Cleghorn, *op. cit.* p. 270). In addition to these, Dr. G. Bidie (*Madras Quart. Med. Journ.* 1862, vol. v. p. 283) enumerates another species, **E. pendunculatum**, *Linn.* (*Wight, Icones,* vol. ii. t. 336), common in the western districts of Mysore, which possesses all the virtues of its congeners. He states that its bitterness is not so strong and harsh as that of Chiretta, and approaches more nearly to Gentian, for which, he adds, it may always be substituted. He directs the plant to be gathered when the flowers begin to fade, and to be carefully dried in the shade. For administration it may be given in infusion and tincture of the same strength as those of Chiretta. Many other species occur in India, and they are all worthy of a trial where they are indigenous.

**Cicendia hyssopifolia**, *W. et A.* (*Wight, Icones,* vol. ii. t. 600.)—Common in moist localities in most parts of India. It is the *Chota* (*small*) *Chiretta* of the natives. Like many others of this family, it possesses marked bitterness, and according to Dr. Cleghorn (*op. cit.* p. 272) it is much used by the natives of Madras as a stomachic, as, in addition to its tonic property, it is also somewhat laxative.

**Erythræa Roxburghii**, *G. Don* (*Wight, Icones*, vol. iv. t. 1325.)—A native of Mysore, the Deccan, and Bengal. The whole plant is described as powerfully bitter, and is held in high esteem by the natives (*Bengal Disp.*, p. 461). It doubtless might prove a useful tonic.

## BIGNONIACEÆ.

(*Non-officinal.*)

**Bignonia xylocarpa**, *Roxb.* (*Wight, Icones*, vol. iv. t. 1335, 1336.)—A small tree inhabiting forests from Kandeish to Malabar and other parts of India, known by the native name *Kúrsing.* An oil obtained by distillation from the wood is a powerful remedy in cutaneous diseases (Gibson and Dalzell, *Bombay Flora*, p. 160). Dr. Gibson is of opinion that it is well worthy of attention as an external application in these cases.

## SESAMEÆ.

(*Non-officinal.*)

**Sesamum Indicum**, *Linn.* (*Wight, Illust.*, vol. ii t. 163.)—This plant is cultivated in all parts of India, as well as in the tropical and warmer portions of the globe, for the sake of the expressed oil of its seeds, *Til* or *Jinjili oil*, which is stated in the Bengal Dispensatory (p. 479) to be, when well prepared, quite equal to olive oil for medicinal and pharmaceutical purposes. Dr. A. Burn (*Bombay Med. Phys. Trans.*, 1838, vol. i.) warmly advocates "oil dressing" in the treatment of wounds, ulcers, &c. He states that in his hospital practice he is in the habit of employing only a pledget of common country cloth, dipped in pure sesamum oil, to any wound, and to almost all ulcers. As a simple dressing he regards it as superior to any other, during the hot season of the year particularly. The Editor for many years employed it as a substitute for olive oil in the preparation of Linimentum Calcis, and found it answer well. The poorer natives use it much for dietetical purposes. The seeds have powerfully emmenagogue properties assigned to them, and it is believed by the natives and Indo-Britons that, if taken largely, they are capable of producing abortion. In amenorrhœa, the employment of a warm sitz bath containing a handful of the seeds, bruised, has been reported to the Editor, on good authority, to be an efficient mode of treatment. The alleged emmenagogue properties of these seeds deserve further investigation. The leaves (*Sesami folia* or *Benne leaves*) are officinal in the secondary list of the U.S. Pharmacopœia; they abound with thick viscid mucilage, which is readily imparted to water, and an infusion of them is much used in the Southern States of North America in all affections requiring demulcents. One or two full-sized fresh leaves, infused or agitated in half a pint of cold water, will soon render it sufficiently viscid for this purpose. If the dried leaves be used hot water should be substituted for the cold. The leaves also serve for the preparation of emollient poultices (*U.S. Disp.*, p. 714). How far the leaves of the Indian grown plant may be used in this way remains to be determined.

**Pedalium Murex**, *Linn.* (*Wight, Icones*, vol. iv. t. 1617.)—A common plant in many parts of the Madras Peninsula, especially near the sea. The fresh leaves and stems, briskly agitated in cold water, speedily convert it into a thick mucilage, nearly of the consistence of the white of a raw egg, inodorous and tasteless. An infusion, thus prepared, is a highly prized remedy amongst the people of Southern India, in gonorrhœa and dysuria. Facts, communicated to the Editor, leave little doubt that in these cases it is a remedy of considerable value, and that as a diuretic its action is speedy and marked. Dr. Ives (*Voyage to India*, p. 466) speaks very favourably of the virtues of this plant, under the name of *Ghanti-gura* or *Gocrow* (*Gokeroo*, Hind.); and he adds to his own testimony that of Dr. Thomas, as to the power of the mucilage to cure gonorrhœa without the aid of any other medicine. Water thus rendered mucilaginous, soon returns to its original fluidity, and it therefore requires to be freshly prepared each time before its exhibition. Its virtues are well deserving of further investigation. The fruits, met with in all the bazaars of India, are quadrangular, spiny, about half an inch in length, inodorous, tasteless. Demulcent and diuretic properties are assigned to them, and they are extensively employed as such by the natives.

# CONVOLVULACEÆ.

## EXOGONIUM PURGA, *Bentham*. JALAP PLANT.

(*Bot. Mag.*, t. 4280.)

*Habitat.*—Mountain forests of Mexico.

*Officinal Part.*—The dried tubercles (*Jalapa, Jalap*): they vary from the size of a walnut to that of an orange, ovoid, the larger tubercles frequently incised, covered with a thin, brown, wrinkled cuticle, presenting, when cut, a yellowish gray colour, with dark brown concentric circles; odour faint and disagreeable; taste at first sweetish and nauseous, subsequently acrid. *Active Principle*, a resin, *Jalapæ Resina* (*infra*).

*Properties.*—Cathartic, anthelmintic.

*Therapeutic Uses.*—In constipation, dropsical affections, and other cases requiring active catharsis, it is a remedy of established value, especially when given in the form of Pulvis Jalapæ compositus (*infra*). As an anthelmintic it is chiefly adapted for the expulsion of lumbrici in children.

*Dose.*—From ten to thirty grains of the powdered root. For young children, from two to five grains.

*Preparations.*—**Compound Powder of Jalap** (*Pulvis Jalapæ compositus*). Take of Jalap, in powder, five ounces; Acid Tartrate of Potash, nine ounces; Ginger, in powder, one ounce. Mix them thoroughly, pass the powder through a fine sieve, and finally rub it lightly in a mortar.

*Dose.*—From twenty grains to a drachm. An excellent mode of administration.

**Tincture of Jalap** (*Tinctura Jalapæ*). Take of Jalap, in coarse powder, two ounces and a half; Proof Spirit, one pint. Macerate the jalap for forty-eight hours in fifteen fluid ounces of the spirit, in a closed vessel, agitating occasionally; then transfer to a percolator; and when the fluid ceases to pass, continue the percolation with the remaining five ounces of spirit. Afterwards subject the contents of the percolator to pressure, filter the product, mix the liquids, and add sufficient proof spirit to make one pint.

*Dose.*—From one half to two fluid drachms; chiefly used as an adjunct to purgative draughts.

**Extract of Jalap** (*Extractum Jalapæ*). Take of Jalap, in coarse powder, one pound; Rectified Spirit, four pints; Water, one gallon. Macerate the jalap in the spirit for seven days; press out the tincture, then filter, and distil off the spirit, leaving a soft extract. Again macerate the residual jalap in the water for four hours; express, strain through flannel, and evaporate by a water bath to a soft extract. Mix the two extracts, and evaporate at a temperature not exceeding 140° until it has acquired a suitable consistence for forming pills.

*Dose.*—From five to fifteen grains.

**Resin of Jalap** (*Jalapæ Resina*). Take of Jalap, in coarse powder, eight ounces; Rectified Spirit, a sufficiency; Water, a sufficiency. Digest the jalap with sixteen fluid ounces of the spirit in a covered vessel, at a gentle heat, for twenty-four hours; then transfer to a percolator; and, when the tincture ceases to pass, continue the percolation with successive portions of spirit until it ceases to dissolve anything more. Add to the tincture four fluid ounces of the water, and distil off the spirit by a water bath. Remove the residue while hot to an open dish, and allow it to become cold. Pour off the supernatant fluid from the resin, wash this two or three times with hot water, and dry it on a porcelain plate by the heat of a stove or water bath. *Characters.*—It occurs in the form of dark-brown opaque fragments, translucent at the edges, brittle, breaking with a resinous fracture, readily reduced to a pale-brown powder, sweetish in odour, acrid in the throat, easily soluble in rectified spirit, but only partially so in ether, and insoluble in oil of turpentine.

*Dose.*—From two to five grains or more; a safe and effectual cathartic.

[For the preparation of this resin, the root, when in a worm-eaten state, as it is often met with in India, answers as well, if not better than the fresher drug, as the insects, although they destroy the ligneous portion of the root, leave the resin untouched.]

## CONVOLVULUS SCAMMONIA, *Linn.* Scammony Plant.

(*Woodville, Med. Bot.*, t. 86.)

*Habitat.*—Greece, Asia Minor, and Syria.

*Officinal Parts.*—1. The dried root (*Scammoniæ Radix*).

2. Gum-resin (*Scammonium, Scammony*) obtained by incision from the living root: it occurs in amorphous pieces of an ash-grey colour, and rough externally; fresh fracture resinous, splintery, shining, black when dry; odour and flavour cheesy; causes, when chewed, a slight prickly sensation in the back of the throat; easily triturated into a dirty grey powder, and converted with water into a smooth emulsion. It does not effervesce with hydrochloric acid. Boiling water, agitated with the powder, cooled and filtered, does not strike a blue colour with tincture of iodine. Ether removes from 80 to 90 per cent. of resin; and what remains is chiefly soluble gum, with a little moisture. Its activity resides in a resin, *Resina Scammonii* (*infra*).

*Properties.*—Cathartic and anthelmintic.

*Therapeutic Uses.*—Similar to those of Jalap.

*Dose.*—From five to ten grains. The dose requires to be increased to fifteen grains or more, should the drug, as is often the case, be impure.

*Preparations.* — **Compound Powder of Scammony** (*Pulvis Scammonii compositus*). Take of Scammony, in powder, four ounces; Jalap, in powder, three ounces; Ginger, in powder, one ounce. Mix them thoroughly, pass the powder through a fine sieve, and finally rub it lightly in a mortar.

*Dose.*—From ten to twenty grains for adults. For children under ten years, from six to eight grains. For infants, from three to five grains.

**Confection of Scammony** (*Confectio Scammonii*). Take of Scammony, in fine powder, three ounces; Ginger, in fine powder, one ounce and a half; Oil of Caraway, one fluid drachm; Oil of Cloves, half a fluid drachm; Syrup, three fluid ounces; Clarified Honey, one ounce and a half. Rub the powders with the syrup and the honey into a uniform mass, then add the oils, and mix.

*Dose.*—From ten to thirty grains.

**Resin of Scammony** (*Scammonii Resina*). Take of Scammony Root, in coarse powder, eight ounces; Rectified Spirit, a sufficiency; Distilled Water, a sufficiency. Digest the scammony root with sixteen fluid ounces of the spirit in a covered vessel, at a gentle heat for twenty-four hours; then transfer to a percolator; and, when the tincture ceases to pass, add more spirit, and let it percolate slowly until the root is exhausted. Add to the tincture four fluid ounces of the water, and distil off the spirit by a water-bath. Remove the residue while hot to an open dish, and allow it to become cold. Pour off the supernatant fluid from the resin, wash this several times with hot water, and dry it on a porcelain plate with the heat of a stove or water-bath. It may also be prepared in a similar way from scammony. *Characters.*—It occurs in brownish translucent pieces, brittle, resinous in fracture, of a sweet fragrant odour if prepared from the root. It cannot form singly an emulsion with water. Its tincture does not render the fresh cut surface of a potato blue. Ether dissolves it entirely.

*Dose.*—From three to eight grains, best given in the form of mixture.

[As a purgative this resin is superior to the ordinary Scammony of commerce, on account of its greater purity, and its consequent greater certainty and uniformity of action.]

**Scammony Mixture** (*Mistura Scammonii*). Take of Resin of Scammony, four grains; Milk, two fluid ounces. Triturate the resin of scammony with a little of the milk, and continue the trituration, gradually adding the remainder of the milk, until a uniform emulsion is obtained.

*Dose.*—From one half to two fluid ounces for a child. It is well adapted for children, on account of its being devoid of disagreeable taste.

Scammony enters into Pilula Colocynthidis composita, Pilula Colocynthidis et Hyoscyami, and Extractum Colocynthidis compositum.

## *PHARBITIS NIL, *Choisy*. KALADANA.

(*Ker, Bot. Reg.*, vol. iv. t. 276.)

*Habitat.*—Common throughout India.

*Officinal Part.*—The Seeds (*Pharbitis Semina, Kaladana*). Black, angular, a quarter of an inch or more in length, weighing on an average about half a grain each, having the form of the segment of an orange; of a sweetish and subsequently rather acrid taste, and heavy smell. *Active principle*, a resin, *Pharbitisin* (*infra*).

*Properties and Uses.*—Safe and effectual cathartic, closely resembling in properties and uses officinal jalap, for which it forms an excellent substitute, though not quite so active in operation.

*Dose.*—From thirty to fifty grains of the powdered seeds.

*Preparations.* — **Extract of Kaladana** (*Extractum Kaladanæ*). — Take of Kaladana Seeds, in coarse powder, one pound; Rectified Spirit, four pints; Water, one gallon. Macerate the Kaladana in the spirit for seven days; press out the tincture, then filter, and distil off the spirit, leaving a soft extract. Again macerate the residual Kaladana in the water for four hours, express, strain through flannel, and evaporate by a water-bath to a soft extract. Mix the two extracts, and evaporate at a temperature not exceeding 140° until it has acquired a suitable consistence for forming pills.

*Dose.*—From five to ten grains, in the form of pill. Thus given, its action is speedy and certain, and seldom occasions either griping or vomiting.

**Tincture of Kaladana** (*Tinctura Kaladanæ*).—Take of Kaladana Seeds, two ounces and a half; Proof Spirit, one pint. Macerate for seven days in a closed vessel, with occasional agitation, filter, and add sufficient rectified spirit to make one pint. It may be prepared also by percolation in the same manner as Tincture of Jalap.

*Dose.*—From two to three drachms. A good adjunct to purgative draughts.

**Compound Powder of Kaladana** (*Pulvis Kaladanæ compositus*).—Take of Kaladana Seeds, in powder, five ounces; Acid Tartrate of Potash, nine ounces; Ginger, in powder, one ounce. Rub them well together, and pass the powder through a fine sieve.

*Dose.*—From fifty to sixty grains. An efficient substitute for the corresponding preparation of jalap.

**Resin of Kaladana** (*Kaladanæ Resina, Pharbitisin*).—Take of Kaladana Seeds, in coarse powder, eight ounces; Rectified Spirit, a sufficiency; Water, a sufficiency. Prepare as Resin of Jalap.

*Dose.*—From five to eight grains. A safe and efficient purgative.

[This resin, introduced into practice by Dr. G. Bidie, is of a brown colour in mass, but becomes grey when reduced to powder. It has a peculiar sweetish but rather disagreeable odour, and a taste at first sweetish but afterwards acrid, very nauseous and persistent, exciting salivation and irritation of the fauces.]

(*Non-officinal.*)

**Ipomœa Turpethum,** *R. Brown* (*Wight*, in *Hooker's Bot. Misc.*, vol. iii. t. 38.)—The root of this species, common throughout India, has been held in reputation in the East, as a purgative, from the time of Avicenna (lib. ii. 2. 701). It was the *Turbith Root* of old pharmacologists. Roxburgh (*Flor. Indica*, vol. i. p. 476) gives a full account of its properties and uses, in accordance with the views of Wallich, Glass, Gordon, and others; but it has entirely fallen into disuse in European practice; and Sir W. O'Shaughnessy (*Bengal Disp.*, p. 504) found it so uncertain in its operation that he pronounced it unworthy of a place in the Pharmacopœia. The dose of the powdered root is from half a drachm to a drachm; that of the extract, from ten to twenty grains. According to the analysis of M. Andouard (*Journ. de Pharm. et de Chim.*, 1866, vol. iii. p. 111) it contains 10.20 per cent. of resin, in which the purgative properties of the root appear to reside. If this were obtained in sufficient quantities (by the process advised for the resin of jalap), it might prove worthy of clinical experiment.

**Pharbitis Sp. of?** Mr. Kanny Loll Dey (*Ind. Drugs*, p. 86) calls attention to a seed, the produce of a species of *Pharbitis*, sold in the bazaars of Bengal and Upper Provinces by the name of *Shapussundo*. Each capsule contains three seeds of a brownish-red colour, and studded with minute hairs. When soaked in water they swell and yield a mucilage. In doses of from a scruple to half a drachm of the sun-dried and powdered seed, it acts as a gentle and safe aperient. It is at the same time considered to exercise a beneficial influence, as an alterative, in skin diseases. This is evidently the same seed described as a good purgative by Mr. Turruck Chunder Lahory under the name of *Lal-dana* (*Red Seed*) in contradistinction to *Kala-dana* (*Black Seed*). They are probably the seeds of **Ipomœa cymosa**, *Röm. et Schultes* (*Bot. Reg.* vol. xxix. t. 24) and **I. sepiaria**, *Kön* (*Wight, Icones*, t. 838), which have their seeds covered with short brown hairs. Both species are widely diffused throughout India.

**Argyreia speciosa**, *Choisy*.—A common Indian plant, the leaves of which are in use among the natives as a local stimulant and rubefacient. In a case which came under the observation of Dr. Wight (*Illust.*, vol. ii. p. 201) they acted as a powerful vesicant.

# BORAGINACEÆ.

(*Non-officinal.*)

**Cordia Myxa**, *Linn.* (*Wight, Illust.*, vol. ii. t. 169) and **Cordia latifolia**, *Roxb.* (which differs only by its larger fruit), two trees common in many parts of India, yield the *Large and Small Sebestens*, which formerly held a place in European Materia Medica. These fruits, the larger of the size of a small plum, the smaller that of a cherry, are black, ovoid, inodorous, of a sweetish mucilaginous taste, and were in considerable repute as an emollient and demulcent, especially in affections of the lungs and genito-urinary organs, but have now fallen into disuse in European practice. They still, however, are employed in the East, and are met with in the bazaars under the names of *Lasora* (Hind.) and *Bahúrai* (Beng.) In doses of from ten to twelve drachms the pulp acts as a laxative. The bark, according to Horsfield (*Asiat. Journ.*, 1819), is one of the chief remedies of the Javanese, who employ it in fevers, &c. It is, apparently, a mild tonic. In the Bengal Dispensatory (p. 499) it is stated that the seeds of Cordia Myxa are called *Chakoon ke benje*, and are deemed an infallible remedy in ringworm. This is erroneous, this being the Hindústani name of the seeds of the *Cassia Tora*, Linn. The bark of **C. angustifolia**, another Indian species, is much used for making astringent gargles (*Bengal Disp.*, p. 499).

**Trichodesma Indicum,** *R. Br.* (*Wight, Illust.*, vol. ii. t. 172.)—An Indian plant, which is held in repute in snake bites. A case of recovery under its use, in the practice of Dr. Maxwell, is on record (*Spry's Modern India*, vol. i.); but there is no other evidence of its utility in this character, and its virtues may be justly doubted. (See Col. Munro, in *Trans. of Agri.-Hort. Soc. of India*, vol. vi. p. 15.) The people of the Deccan employ the mucilaginous leaves of this plant, and of **T. Zeylanica,** *R. Br.*, for making emollient poultices (Dr. Walker, *Bombay Med. Phys. Trans.*, 1840, p. 72.)

**Ehretia buxifolia,** *Roxb.* (*Corom. Pl.*, t. 57), a shrub or small tree common on the barren tracts of the Coromandel coast and other parts of India. The root, which in a fresh state has a sweetish and somewhat warm taste, is employed by the Hindú doctors as an alterative (Ainslie, *Mat. Ind.*, vol. ii. p. 80.) Dr. Æ. Ross reports having employed it in the form of decoction, in proportion of two ounces of the root to a pint of water, and that this in doses of two ounces appeared to be decidedly beneficial in secondary and constitutional syphilitic affections.

**Tiaridium Indicum,** *Lehm.* (*Wight, Illust.*, vol. ii. t. 171.)—The leaves of this widely-distributed plant are held in esteem in various parts of the world as an external application to ulcers, wounds, and local inflammations. (See Barham, *Hort. Amer.*, p. 42; Martius, *Mat. Med. Bras.*, p. 6; Ainslie, *Mat. Ind.*, vol. ii. p. 414; Bouton, *Med. Pl. of Mauritius*, p. 115; Loureiro, *Flor. Cochin.* vol. i. p. 126.) Their action is probably only that of an emollient. Diuretic properties are also assigned to the plant by Lunan (*Hort. Jamaic.*, vol. ii. p. 248).

**Echium, Sp. of.** Under the name of *Gouzabán*, (*Hind.*) are sold in most bazaars of India the broken leaves, stems, and flowers of a plant which in most works on Indian Materia Medica have been erroneously referred to *Cacalia Kleinia*, *L.* This drug has long held a high place in native practice as an alterative tonic in syphilitic, leprous, and rheumatic cases, and has been favourably noticed in this character by Sir W. O'Shaughnessy (*Bengal. Disp.*, p. 420.), and others (*Indian. Journ. of Med. Phys. Sci.*, Jan. 1st, 1838, p. 9.) Not only as an alterative tonic, but as a demulcent and diuretic, it is extolled by Mr. Moodeen Sheriff, who states in his report that he has employed it extensively, and that he regards it as an efficient substitute for Pareira Brava and Sarsaparilla, in all cases in which those agents are indicated. He advises its administration in decoction. (Bruised leaves, one ounce; Boiling Water, one pint. Macerate for two hours, and strain.) The dose is from two to four ounces, twice or thrice daily, or oftener. It appears well worthy of further trials. The leaves are readily distinguished by numerous well marked white spots on their surface; taste, mucilaginous; odour, in the dry state, faint, but in the fresh state they are said be strong smelling, approaching to Conium.

# SCROPHULARIACEÆ.

## DIGITALIS PURPUREA, *Linn.* PURPLE FOXGLOVE.
(*Engl. Bot.*, t. 1297; *ed. Syme*, t. 1952.)

*Habitat.*—Great Britain and other parts of Europe, chiefly on a sandy or gravelly soil. Thrives well on the mountain ranges of India.

*Officinal Part.*—The Leaves (*Digitalis Folia*), gathered when about two-thirds of the flowers are expanded.† They are ovate-lanceolate, shortly petiolate, rugose, downy, of a dull-green colour, paler on the under surface, crenate, with a faint odour and bitter nauseous taste. Their activity resides in a peculiar bitter principle, *Digitalin.*

*Properties.*—Sedative, especially of the heart's action, and diuretic. Given in small and long-continued doses, it is apt to accumulate in the system, and suddenly to evidence its presence by poisonous or even fatal effects. Hence, though the dangers resulting from its cumulative action may have been over-rated, much caution is necessary in its use. In large doses it is an acro-narcotic poison.

*Therapeutic Uses.*—In dropsical affections, especially when connected with cardiac complications, it is a remedy of established value. In diseases of the heart it has been used too indiscriminately; but in proper cases, those mainly characterised by too forcible action, it is a powerful remedy. Amongst other diseases in which it has been employed with alleged benefit are hydrocephalus, asthma, bronchitis, phthisis, hæmoptysis, insanity, delirium tremens, epilepsy, croup, menorrhagia, and other forms of uterine hæmorrhage.

*Dose.*—Of the powdered leaves from half a grain to two grains every six or eight hours as a sedative. When its diuretic action is desired the infusion is a better form. In all cases the action of the remedy should be carefully watched.

*Preparations.*—**Infusion of Digitalis** (*Infusum Digitalis*). Take of Digitalis Leaves, dried, thirty grains; Boiling Water, ten fluid ounces. Infuse in a covered vessel for one hour, and strain.

*Dose.*—From two to four fluid drachms, repeated every six hours. This infusion has half the strength of Infusum Digitalis, *Edin. and Dub. Ph.*

---

† The leaves should be collected in the second year of the plant's growth; the full-grown and perfect leaves should be selected, and they should be dried at a moderate temperature. Both the dried leaves and powder should be protected from the action of air and light by being kept in well-stoppered bottles in a dark cupboard; and, as by long keeping their medicinal activity is diminished or lost, the supply should be renewed annually. The dried leaves have a dull-green colour, faint odour, and bitter, nauseous taste.

**Tincture of Digitalis** (*Tinctura Digitalis*). Take of Digitalis, in coarse powder, two ounces and a half; Proof Spirit, one pint. Macerate the digitalis for forty-eight hours, in fifteen ounces of the spirit, in a closed vessel, agitating occasionally; then transfer to a percolator; and when the fluid ceases to pass, continue the percolation with the remaining five ounces of the spirit. Afterwards subject the contents of the percolator to pressure, filter the product, mix the liquids, and add sufficient proof spirit to make one pint.

*Dose.*—From ten to thirty minims, gradually increased, as a sedative and diuretic. In epilepsy and delirium tremens much larger doses have been advised, but it is doubtful if the efficacy of the treatment is commensurate with the danger incurred by the practice.

**Digitalin** (*Digitalinum*). The active principle of Digitalis. It occurs in the form of porous mammillated masses or small scales, white, inodorous, and intensely bitter; readily soluble in spirit, but almost insoluble in water and in pure ether; dissolves in acids, but does not form with them neutral compounds; its solution in hydrochloric acid is of a faint yellow colour, but rapidly becomes green. It powerfully irritates the nostrils, and is an active poison. It leaves no residue when burned with free access of air.

*Dose.*—From one sixtieth to one thirtieth of a grain, in solution in alcohol or acetic acid, or in the form of pill. Its action and uses are similar to those of Digitalis. It is a powerful anaphrodisiac, and hence has been found useful in spermatorrhœa. From its powerfully poisonous action, its administration, even in the smallest doses, demands the greatest caution.

(*Non-officinal.*)

**Picrorrhiza kurroa,** *Royle* (*Illust.*, t. 71), a plant of Kumaon and other parts of Northern India. According to Royle (*Illust.*, vol. i. p. 291) its root possesses much bitterness, and is employed medicinally by the natives. Irvine (*Materia Medica of Patna*, p. 58) assigns *Kootki* as its Hindústani name, and mentions its use as a tonic. It occurs in short pieces of a brittle, dark-coloured rhizome, sometimes contorted, as thick as a goose quill at the upper extremity, tapering downwards, beset with rootlets below and the remains of leaves above. It has a very bitter taste. It would be desirable to have more information with regard to this root and its properties. The root sold in the bazaars under the name of *Kali Kútki* (*Hind.*) and *Kadagaroganie* (*Tam.*) approximates very closely in physical characters to the above, and is probably the produce of a species of *Picrorrhiza*. Its botanical origin, however, is undetermined. Mr. Moodeen Sheriff reports that the plant which yields it grows in the Madras Peninsula, but he had not himself seen it.

Ainslie (*Mat. Ind.*, vol. i. p. 165) and most subsequent writers regard this root as Black Hellebore; but from this, it differs materially in many respects. In large doses it is an acrid hydragogue cathartic. Antiperiodic virtues have been assigned to it by Dr. Tripe (*Madras Medical Reports*, 1855, p. 422).

**Herpestis Monniera,** *H. B. et K.* (*Bot. Mag.*, t. 2557), a small creeping plant of the tropical portions of both hemispheres. It is regarded by the Hindûs as a powerful diuretic and aperient (Ainslie, *Mat. Ind.*, vol. ii. p. 239), but there is no trustworthy evidence of its value in these respects. According to Roxburgh (*Flor. Ind.*, vol. i. p. 141), the juice of the leaves, conjoined with petroleum, is used in India as a local application in rheumatism. Whatever benefit is derived from this formula is doubtless due to the petroleum.

**Celsia Coromandeliana,** *Vahl.*, (*Wight, Icones*, vol. iv. t. 1406,) a common weed in gardens and cultivated grounds in various parts of India during the wet season. Under its Bengali name, *Kukshima*, it is brought to notice by Sub-Assistant Surgeon B. M. Chatterjee, who prescribed the inspissated juice of the leaves in several cases of acute and chronic dysentery with manifest advantage. Its action appears to be that of a sedative and astringent. Dose not mentioned.

## ACANTHACEÆ.

### *ANDROGRAPHIS PANICULATA, *Nees.* KARIYÁT.

(*Wight, Icones*, vol. ii. t. 518.)

*Habitat.*—Common in shady places all over India.

*Officinal Part.*—The dried stalks and root (*Andrographis Caules et Radix, Kariyát, Creyat*). The stem, which is usually met with, with the root attached, occurs in pieces of about a foot or more in length, quadrangular, of a lightish brown colour, and persistent bitter taste.

*Properties.*—Bitter tonic and stomachic, very analogous to Quassia in its action.(54)

*Therapeutic Uses.*—In general debility, in convalescence after fevers, and in the advanced stages of dysentery, it has been found serviceable.

*Preparations.*—**Compound Infusion of Kariyát** (*Infusum Andrographis compositum*). Take of Kariyát, bruised, half an ounce; Orange Peel and Coriander Fruit, bruised, of each, sixty grains; Boiling Water, ten fluid ounces. Infuse in a covered vessel for an hour, and strain.

*Dose.*—From one and a half fluid ounces to two ounces, twice or thrice daily.

**Compound Tincture of Kariyát** (*Tinctura Andrographis composita*). Take of Kariyát Root, cut small, six ounces; Myrrh and Aloes, in coarse powder, of each, one ounce; Brandy, two pints. Macerate for seven days in a closed vessel, with occasional agitation; strain, press, filter, and add sufficient brandy to make two pints.

*Dose.*—From one to four fluid drachms. This tincture is given in the Bengal Pharm. as equivalent to the celebrated nostrum "*Drogue amère.*" It is said to be tonic, stimulant, and gently aperient, and to prove valuable in the treatment of several forms of dyspepsia, and in torpidity of the alimentary canal.

[The expressed juice of the fresh leaves is a common native domestic remedy in the bowel complaints of children. Its bitterness being a strong objection to its use, Mr. Nil Madhub Mookerjee (*Indian Med. Gaz.*, 1866, vol. i. p. 220) substitutes a decoction, prepared by boiling two ounces of the fresh leaves in a pint and a half of water down to six ounces, of which the dose is one ounce every two or three hours. He mentions cases treated with it, but as morphia, sinapisms, and other remedies were employed at the same time, it is doubtful how far the recoveries can be said to be due to the Andrographis.]

(*Non-officinal.*)

**Hygrophila spinosa,** *T. And.*—*Asteracantha longifolia, Nees.*—(*Wight, Icones,* vol. ii. t. 449.)—Common in moist sites in most parts of India; has valuable diuretic properties assigned to it by the natives. Dr. Kirkpatrick (*Cat. of Mysore Drugs,* No. 451) states that he frequently employed it in dropsical cases, and that it undoubtedly possesses considerable power as a diuretic. Dr. Gibson also bears testimony to its powers as a diuretic; and it is favourably reported on by Dr. Æ. Ross and Native Surgeon Iyaswamy. Mr. Kanny Loll Dey (*Ind. Drugs,* p. 18) furnishes the two following formulæ. *Decoction.*—Take of Asteracantha Root, one ounce; Water, one pint; boil to fourteen ounces; strain. Dose, from one to one and a half ounce daily. *Acetum.*—Take of Asteracantha leaves, freshly dried, two ounces; Distilled vinegar, sixteen ounces. Macerate for three days, press and strain. Dose, four drachms to one ounce. The ashes of the burnt dried plant, in dose of about half a teaspoonful twice or thrice daily, is a form of administration followed by the natives (Dr. J. Shortt).

**Justicia Gendarussa,** *Linn.*,—*Gendarussa vulgaris, Nees.*—(*Wight, Icones,* vol. ii. t. 468.)—The *Ganda-rusa* of the Malays, who employ it as a febrifuge (Motley, in *Hooker's Journ. of Bot.,* 1855, vol. vii. p. 166). According to Horsfield (*Asiat. Journ.,* vol. vii. p. 266) emetic qualities are ascribed to it in Java. The leaves and tender shoots, which, when bruised, emit a strong but not unpleasant odour, are, according to Ainslie (*Mat. Ind.,* vol. ii. p. 68), prescribed in decoction in chronic rheumatism. Its action is apparently that of a diaphoretic. Our knowledge of its virtues rests principally on native testimony.

**Justicia Adhatoda,** *Linn.*,—*Adhatoda vasica, Nees.*—(*Bot. Mag.,* t. 861.) *Bakas, Hind.*—A shrub, common in most parts of India; has antispasmodic and expectorant virtues ascribed to it by the natives, who employ it in coughs, asthma, ague, &c.

(*See* Royle, *Illust.*, vol. i. p. 289; Ainslie, *Mat. Ind.*, vol. ii. p. 3; and Long, *Journ. Agri.-Hort. Soc. of India*, 1858, vol. x. p. 28). Strong testimony in favour of its remedial properties, drawn from personal experience, is furnished Dr. N. Jackson and Sub-Assistant Surgeon Odoy Chund Dutt, who have employed it with marked success in chronic bronchitis, asthma, and other pulmonary and catarrhal affections when not attended with febrile action. In phthisis even it is reported to prove serviceable by its expectorant operation. The dose of the aqueous extract, prepared by evaporating the juice, is from four to ten grains; but this preparation is objectionable on account of the readiness with which it spoils. A tincture prepared by dissolving the extract in alcohol is preferable, the dose being from one half to one fluid drachm. An alcoholic extract also keeps well; dose about three grains. The addition of Long Pepper seems to increase its efficacy. It is very desirable that further trials should be made to test the value of this remedy. Cases illustrative of its effects in catarrh, bronchitis, and phthisis, together with much information on this drug, have been published by Mr. Odoy Chund Dutt (*Indian Annals of Med. Sci.*, 1865, vol. x. p. 156 *seq.*)

**Rhinacanthus communis,** *Nees.* (*Wight, Icones*, vol. ii. t. 464.) —The seeds of this plant are held in high esteem as a local application in ringworm. Royle, (*Illust.*, vol. i. p. 298) speaks of them as very efficacious; and Ainslie (*op. cit.* p. 216) states that the fresh root, bruised and mixed with lime juice, is, in the native opinion, a sovereign remedy for cutaneous affections. It is desirable to know how far these statements are correct.

## VERBENACEÆ.

(*Non-officinal.*)

**Vitex Negundo,** *Linn.* (*Wight, Icones*, vol. ii. t. 519), and **V. trifolia,** *Linn.* (*Rheede, Hort. Mal.*, vol. ii. t. 11.)—These two shrubs, widely distributed throughout India, have long enjoyed high repute in native practice. They appear to be possessed of similar properties, and to be used indiscriminately, though *V. trifolia* is regarded as the more powerful of the two. The latter is highly extolled by Bontius (*Diseases of India*, p. 226), under its Malayan name *Lagondi;* he speaks of it as anodyne, diuretic, and emmenagogue, and testifies to the value of fomentations and baths prepared with "this noble herb," as he terms it, in the treatment of Beri-beri, and in the allied and obscure affection Burning of the Feet (*Ignipedites*) in natives. *V. Negundo* is no less prized by the natives of India. Its leaves, Dr. Fleming remarks (*Asiat. Researches*, vol. xi.), have a better claim to the title of discutient than any other vegetable remedy with which he is acquainted; and he adds that their efficacy in dispelling inflammatory swellings of the joints from acute rheumatism, and of the testes from suppressed gonorhœa, has often excited his surprise. The mode of application followed by the natives, and adopted, according to Dr. Fleming, by some European practitioners in India, is simple: the fresh leaves, put into an earthen pot, are heated over a fire till they are as hot as can be borne without pain; they are then applied to the affected part, and kept *in situ* by

L 2

a bandage; the application is repeated three or four times daily until the swelling subsides. A very interesting account of the treatment of febrile, catarrhal, and rheumatic affections, as practised by the people of Mysore, by means of a sort of rude vapour bath prepared with this plant, is furnished by Dr. W. Ingledew (*Edin. Med. Surg. Journ.*, Oct. 1817, p. 530). Roxburgh (*Flor. Ind.*, vol. iii. p. 70) mentions the use of baths prepared with the aromatic leaves of this plant, in the puerperal state of women in India; and according to Ainslie (*Mat. Ind.*, vol. ii. p. 252), the Mahomedans are in the habit of smoking the dried leaves in cases of headache and catarrh. The dried fruit (*Filfil burrí*, Hind.) is deemed vermifuge. Amongst the natives few plants appear to have a much wider range of uses than *V. Negundo.*

**Gmelina parvifolia,** *Roxb.* (*Corom. Pl.*, t. 162.)—The leaves and young shoots of this shrub abound with a thick viscid mucilage, which is imparted readily to cold water, which, when thus impregnated, is employed by the natives in the treatment of gonorrhœa to allay ardor urinæ. Water stirred with the leaves and stem of *Pedalium Murex* (*ante*) rapidly becomes mucilaginous in the same manner as when this article is used, but it soon loses this character and resumes its original fluidity, whereas the leaves of *G. parviflora* cause the water to remain mucilaginous until decomposition ensues (Roxburgh, *Flor. Ind.*, vol. iii. p. 88). The root of **Gmelina Asiatica,** *Linn.*, according to Horsfield (*Asiat. Journ.*, vol. vii. p. 263), was formerly held in high esteem by the Portuguese under the name of *Rais Madre de Deos;* but its virtues, if any, are forgotten; Ainslie merely mentions that the Hindú doctors regard it as a demulcent and alterative.

**Clerodendron serratum,** *Blume.* (*Wight, Icones*, vol. iv. t. 1472.) —A shrubby plant common in hill districts in most parts of India, the roots of which constitute the *Gantu-Bharangi, Tel* (*Gunti Paringaie* of Ainslie, vol. ii. p. 112), which, according to Sir Walter Elliot (*Flor. Andhrica*, p. 57), is exported largely from Vizagapatam for medicinal purposes. It is used by the natives in febrile and catarrhal affections. It occurs in the form of a brittle, wiry, woody root, in short pieces, of a thickness varying from that of large packthread to that of a small quill, frequently swollen into hard, woody, globular excrescences. It has scarcely any odour or taste. As a medicinal agent it is probably of little value. Dr. Bholanauth Bose calls attention to the leaves of **Clerodendron infortunatum,** *Linn.* (*Wight, Icones*, vol. iv. t. 1471), as a cheap and efficient substitute for chiretta as a tonic and antiperiodic. He refers to a special report on the drug, forwarded by him, but it has not been received by the Committee. The fresh juice of the leaves is stated by Mr. Kanny Loll Dey (*Ind. Drugs*, p. 35) to be employed by the natives as a vermifuge, and also as a bitter tonic and febrifuge in malarious fevers, especially in those of children.

**Tectona grandis,** *Linn.* (*Roxb., Corom. Pl.*, t. 6.)—*Teak tree.*—The statements made with reference to the medicinal virtues of this tree by Rumphius, Horsfield, and others, are very doubtful; but the property of the wood, rubbed down on a stone with a little water to the consistence of a thin paste, to allay the pain and inflammation caused by handling the Burmese black varnish *Thit-tsi* (*Melanorrhœa usitatissima*), is worthy of note. Colonel Burney (*Journ. of Asiat. Soc. of Bengal*, vol. i. p. 170) has published some interesting remarks on its use. It is deserving of a trial as a local application in inflammations arising from the action of the Marking nut (*Semecarpus Anacardium*) and Cashew nut (*Anacardium occi-*

*dentale*). Dr. Gibson states that in two cases he observed marked diuresis follow the application of an epithem of the bruised fruit to the pubes. He considers it worthy of the notice of future inquirers.

## LABIATÆ.

---

### LAVANDULA VERA, *D.C.* COMMON LAVENDER.

(*Hayne*, vol. viii. t. 37. *Steph. et Church. Med. Bot.*, vol. i. t. 40.)

*Habitat.*—A native of the South of Europe. Cultivated in gardens in all parts of Europe.

*Officinal Part.*—The Oil (*Oleum Lavandulæ*) obtained by distillation from the flowers; it is colourless or pale yellow, with the peculiar fragrant odour of lavender, and a hot bitter aromatic taste.

*Properties and Uses.*—Carminative and antispasmodic, rarely administered internally, except in the form of Tinctura Lavandulæ composita. Employed for disguising the unpleasant odour of ointments and other preparations. It is an ingredient in Linimentum Camphoræ compositum.

*Dose.*—From two to five drops.

*Preparations.*—**Spirit of Lavender** (*Spiritus Lavandulæ*). Take of Oil of Lavender one fluid ounce; Rectified Spirit, forty-nine fluid ounces. Dissolve.

*Dose.*—From thirty minims to one fluid drachm. This is one fifth the strength of the preparation of the same name in the *Brit. Pharm.* 1864.

**Compound Tincture of Lavender** (*Tinctura Lavandulæ composita*). Take of Oil of Lavender, one fluid drachm and a half; Oil of Rosemary, ten minims; Cinnamon Bark, bruised, Nutmeg bruised, of each one hundred and fifty grains; Red Sandal Wood, three hundred grains; Rectified Spirit, two pints. Macerate the cinnamon, nutmeg, and red sandal wood in the spirit for seven days in a closed vessel, with occasional agitation; then strain and press, dissolve the oils in the strained tincture, filter, and add sufficient rectified spirit to make two pints.

*Dose.*—From half a fluid drachm to two drachms. A good stimulant. Much employed in nervous and hysterical cases, incipient syncope, flatulence, and flatulent colic.

## MENTHA PIPERITA, *Linn.* PEPPERMINT.

(*Engl. Bot.*, t. 687 ; *ed. Syme*, t. 1024.)

*Habitat.*—Moist localities in various parts of Europe, Asia, and America. Cultivated at Mitcham and elsewhere.

*Officinal Part.*—The oil (*Oleum Menthæ piperitæ*), obtained by distillation from the fresh herb when in flower. It is colourless, or pale-yellow, with the peculiar odour of peppermint; taste, warm aromatic, succeeded by a sensation of coldness in the mouth. It consists of two isomeric oils; one liquid, and the other solid and crystalline; the latter is termed *Peppermint Camphor*, or the Stearoptene of Oil of Peppermint.

*Properties.*—Valuable carminative, stomachic, and antispasmodic.

*Therapeutic Uses.*—In flatulence, flatulent colic, nausea, and spasmodic affections of the bowels, it is a remedy of established value. It has been proposed as a substitute for the nauseous oil of turpentine in the treatment of puerperal fever. ([55])

*Dose.*—From two to five drops on sugar, or suspended in mucilage.

*Preparations.*—**Peppermint Water** (*Aqua Menthæ piperitæ*). Take of Oil of Peppermint, one fluid drachm and a half; Water, one gallon and a half. Distil one gallon.

*Dose.*—From one to three fluid ounces. An excellent vehicle for other carminatives, in flatulence and spasmodic affections of the bowels. It is an ingredient in Mistura Ferri Aromatica.

**Spirit of Peppermint** (*Spiritus Menthæ piperitæ*). Take of Oil of Peppermint, one fluid ounce; Rectified Spirit, forty-nine fluid ounces. Dissolve.

*Dose.*—From thirty to sixty minims. This is one fifth the strength of the preparation of the same name in *Brit. Pharm.* 1864.

## MENTHA VIRIDIS, *Linn.* SPEARMINT.

(*Engl. Bot.*, t. 2424 ; *ed. Syme*, t. 1023.)

*Habitat.*—Marshy localities in Europe, Asia, and America.

*Officinal Part.*—The oil (*Oleum Menthæ viridis*) obtained by distillation from the fresh herb when in flower. It is colourless, or of a pale-yellow colour, with the peculiar odour of spearmint, and hot, pungent, aromatic taste.

*Properties and Uses.*—Similar to those of Peppermint, but less powerful in operation.

*Dose.*—From two to five drops on sugar, or in emulsion.

*Preparations.*—**Spearmint Water** (*Aqua Menthæ viridis*). Take of Oil of Spearmint, one fluid drachm and a half; Water, a gallon and a half. Distil one gallon.

*Dose.*—From one to three ounces, chiefly used as a vehicle for other carminative medicines.

## ROSMARINUS OFFICINALIS, *Linn.* COMMON ROSEMARY.

(*Hayne*, vol. vii. t. 25. *Steph. et Church. Med. Bot.*, vol. i. t. 24.)

*Habitat.*—South Europe, North Africa, and Asia Minor. Cultivated in gardens in England.

*Officinal Part.*—The oil (*Oleum Rosmarini*) obtained by distillation from the flowering tops. It is colourless, with the peculiar odour of rosemary, and a warm aromatic taste.

*Properties and Uses.*—Carminative, but rarely exhibited internally. Used externally as an ingredient in stimulating liniments for alopecia.

*Dose.*—From two to five drops. It is an ingredient in Tinctura Lavandulæ composita and Linimentum Saponis.

*Preparations.*—**Spirit of Rosemary** (*Spiritus Rosmarini*). Take of Oil of Rosemary, one fluid ounce; Rectified Spirit, forty-nine fluid ounces. Dissolve.

Chiefly employed, for the sake of its odour, in lotions and other external applications. It is one-fifth the strength of the preparation of the same name in the *Brit. Pharm.*, 1864.

(*Non-officinal.*)

**Ocimum sanctum,** *Linn.* (*Rheede, Hort. Mal.*, vol. x. t. 92.) and **O. Basilicum,** *Linn.* (*Wight, Icones*, vol. iii. t. 868), and other species of Ocimum distributed throughout India, possess in common a fragrant camphoraceous odour, and pungent aromatic taste. Stimulant, diaphoretic, and expectorant virtues are assigned to them by the natives, who employ them in these characters, but they appear to be worthy of little or no attention on the part of the European practitioner. The leaves of *O. sanctum,* dried and pulverised, are used by the Bengali natives as snuff in the endemic affection of the nasal cavities termed Peenash; it is said to be an effectual means of dislodging the maggots (*Dr. J. Newton*). Dr. Fleming (*Asiatic Researches*, vol. xi.) mentions a peculiar quality of the seeds of **O. pilosum,** which, when, infused in cold water, form a mucilage much used by the natives as a demulcent in catarrhs, and as a means of relieving the after-pains of parturition. Martius (*Mat. Med. Bras.*, p. 105) mentions that in Brasil a decoction of the mucilaginous seeds of

**O. gratissimum,** *Linn.* (cultivated in India) is an esteemed remedy in gonorrhœa. Dr. Waitz (*Dis. of Children in Hot Climates,* p. 196) speaks of the last-named species under the Malay name of *Daun selasse,* and states that in the aphthæ of children he found a strong decoction of the plant effectual when ordinary European remedies had failed. He also advises (*Ibid.*, p. 230) the use of aromatic baths prepared with it, in cases of atrophy. In the Mauritius, baths or fumigations prepared with this plant are employed in the treatment of rheumatism and paralysis (Bouton, *Med. Plants of Mauritius,* p. 120).

**Micromeria capitellata,** *Bentham,* a small plant inhabiting the Neilgherries and the Mahableshwur mountains. According to Mr. Dalzell, who first brought it to notice, under the name of **Marrubium Malcolmianum,** "it is entitled to be called East Indian Peppermint, being possessed of all the aromatic and carminative qualities of Mentha piperita." (*Hooker's Journ. of Bot.,* 1852, vol. iv. p. 109.)

**Anisomeles Malabarica,** *R. Br.* (*Wight, Icones,* vol. iii. t. 864).—In Southern India few plants are held in higher esteem, or are more frequently employed in native practice, than this. An infusion of the aromatic bitter leaves is in common use in affections of the stomach and bowels, catarrhal affections, and intermittent fevers. According to Dr. Wight (*Illust.*, vol. ii. p. 221), in addition to its internal use in the cure of fevers, patients are made to inhale the vapour of a hot infusion so as to induce copious diaphoresis. An infusion of the leaves is reported by Dr. Æ. Ross to be powerfully diaphoretic, and very useful in the low continued fevers of the natives. An oil obtained by distillation of the leaves is likewise stated to prove an effectual external application in rheumatism. The virtues of this plant seem worthy of further investigation. **Anisomeles ovata,** *R. Br.* (*Wight, Icones,* vol. iii. t. 865), partakes of the physical characters of the preceding species, and, like it, appears worthy of notice. A distilled oil prepared from it in Ceylon, is said by Burmann (*Thes. Zeylan,* p. 153) to have been found useful in uterine affections.

**Coleus aromaticus,** *Bentham* (*Wight, Illust.,* vol. ii. t. 175).—A native of the Moluccas, cultivated in gardens in many parts of India; has a pleasant aromatic odour and pungent taste, and is employed in Cochin China, according to Loureiro (*Flor. Cochin.*, p. 452), in asthma, chronic coughs, epilepsy, and other convulsive affections. Dr. Wight (*Illust.* vol. ii.) speaks of it as a powerful aromatic carminative given in cases of colic in children, in the treatment of which the expressed juice is prescribed mixed with sugar or other suitable vehicle. In his own practice he observed it produce so decidedly an intoxicating effect that the patient, an European lady, who had taken it on native advice for dyspepsia, had to discontinue it, though otherwise benefitting under its use. Further information on this point is desirable. The Rev. J. Long (*Journ. of Agri.-Hort. Soc. of India,* 1858, vol. x. p. 23) also notices its intoxicating properties, and states that the people of Bengal employ it in colic and dyspepsia.

Amongst the plants of this Natural Order held, more or less, in repute in native practice, the following may be mentioned; they are all, as far as is known, of minor importance:—**Roylea elegans,** *Wallich,* (*Plant Asiat. Rar.*, t. 74), employed as a febrifuge. **Dracocephalum Royleanum,** *Wallich,* the seeds of which are used in forming mucilaginous drinks (Royle, *Illust.*, vol. i. p. 303). **Me-**

**riandra Bengalensis**, *Benth.*, (*Jacquemont Voy. Bot.*, t. 139), and **M. strobilifera**, *Benth.*, camphoraceous-smelling bitter-tasted plants, possessed of all the properties of sage (*Salvia officinalis*); the leaves named *Káfúr ka pattá*, i.e., *Camphor leaves*, are much used in native practice. An infusion of them is a serviceable application to aphthæ and sore throats, according to Mr. Rama Churn Bose, who likewise notices its alleged power of diminishing or arresting the secretion of milk. **Geniosporum prostratum**, *Benth.*, is regarded as febrifuge at Pondicherry, where it is known by the Tamul name of *Nazel-nagai:* **Anisochilus carnosum**, *Benth.*, a stimulant, diaphoretic, and expectorant, is used in cynanche (*Ainslie*), and by the native doctors of Travancore, in catarrhal affections; Dr. G. Bidie (*Madras Quart. Med. Journ.*, 1862, vol. v. p. 269) characterises it as a mild stimulant expectorant, and particularly useful in the coughs of childhood. Its properties depend upon a volatile oil. **Leucas aspera**, *Sprengel*, proposed on insufficient grounds by Mr. Oslen (*Calcutta Med. Phys. Trans.*, vol. ii. p. 403) as an antidote for snake bites. The juice of the leaves, according to Dr. J. Shortt, is applied successfully in psora and other chronic eruptions. **Pogostemon Patchouli**, *Pelletier* (*Hooker's Kew Journ.*, 1849, vol. i. t. 11), a native of Silhet and the Malayan Peninsula, the dried tops of which constitute the *Patchouli* of commerce, of little or no value as a medicine; much used as a perfume.

# PLUMBAGINEÆ.

(*Non-officinal.*)

**Plumbago rosea**, *Linn.* (*Bot. Mag.*, t. 230 and 5263), a common plant throughout India. The vesicant properties of the root were noticed by Burman, Rumphius, and other old writers; but Sir W. O'Shaughnessy was the first to institute a series of trials with it. As the result of clinical observation in between three and four hundred cases, he states that he found that the root-bark, rubbed into a paste with water and a little flour, and applied to the skin, occasioned pain in about five minutes, which increased in severity till in a quarter of an hour it was equal to that of an ordinary blister. The paste was removed in half an hour, and within twelve or eighteen hours afterwards a large uniform blister filled with serum followed. The blistered surfaces were found to heal readily without troublesome ulceration. On the whole, Sir W. O'Shaughnessy regards it as a cheap substitute for cantharides, possessing the additional advantage of not causing irritation of the genito-urinary organs (*Bengal Disp.*, p. 508). The results met with by the Editor in trials with this vesicant were far less satisfactory than those mentioned above. The pain occasioned was often much greater than that of an ordinary blister, whilst the resulting vesication was far from uniform in extent or rapidity of healing. It is, however, a powerful vesicant, and may be resorted to where cantharides is unavailable. Taken internally it is an acrid stimulant, and in large doses acts as an acro-narcotic poison, in which character it is not unfrequently employed by the people of Bengal (Dr. Norman Chevers, *Med. Juris. of Bengal*, p. 287). Its action is apparently directed chiefly to the uterine system; and, according to Dr. Allan Webb (*Pathologia Indica*, p. 281), it is one of the articles in use amongst the natives for procuring abortion. For this purpose, the scraped root-bark is introduced *per vaginam* into the os uteri. Death not unfrequently results from the introduction of this highly acrid agent, metritis and peritonitis rapidly following its use (*Dr. Chevers*). Its use as an abortive amongst the women of Southern India, both when given internally and when applied locally to the os uteri, is noticed in Dr. J. Shortt's Report. The dose of the fresh root beaten up into a paste for this purpose is from one to two drachms. An embrocation, formed by macerating the root in any bland oil, is used externally in rheumatic and paralytic cases (Ainslie, *Mat. Ind.*, vol. ii. p. 397). The Javanese apply the root topically for the cure of toothache; it doubtless acts in these cases as a powerful sialogogue. In Southern India the dried root, which is comparatively inert, is in high repute as a remedy in secondary syphilis and leprosy, but caution is necessary in its use. **P. Zeylanica**, *Linn.* (*Wight, Illust.*, vol. ii. t. 179), appears to possess the properties of the preceding species, but is regarded as milder in its operation. A tincture of the root-bark has been employed as an antiperiodic. Dr. Oswald states that he has employed it in the treatment of intermittents with good effect. It acts as a powerful sudorific. The activity of both species resides in a peculiar crystalline principle, *Plumbagin.* They are well worthy of further trials.

## SALVADORACEÆ.

(*Non-officinal.*)

**Salvadora Wightiana**, *Planch.* (**S. Persica**, *Roxb.*, *Corom. Pl.*, t. 26, and **S. Indica**, *Wight, Illust.*, vol. ii. t. 81), a tree widely diffused over India, but not very common; generally known by the Hindústani name *Pilú.* The leaves, bark, and fruit possess a peculiar, pungent smell and taste, resembling that of garden cress. The root-bark is very acrid, and, when powdered and applied to the skin, acts as a vesicant. Dr. Irvine (*Med. Topog. of Ajmeer*, p. 178) has employed it successfully in this character. The bark, according to Ainslie (*Mat. Ind.*, vol. ii. p. 266), is used by the Hindú doctors in adynamic fevers and in amenorrhœa. In Dr. Imlach's Report on Snake-bites in Scinde (*Bombay Med.-Phys. Trans.*, vol. iii. N.S., p. 80), several cases are mentioned in the tabular record, in which "Pilloo seeds" (the fruit of this tree) were administered internally, with good effect. They are likewise said to be a favourite purgative. There appears little doubt that all parts of this tree, especially the root-bark, are possessed of acrid stimulant properties. Roxburgh (*Flor. Ind.*, vol. i. p. 390) considers that it promises to prove valuable as a medicinal agent; an opinion fully endorsed by Dr. Gibson. Sir W. O'Shaughnessy (*Bengal Disp.*, p. 527) regards the properties of this tree, as well as those of **S. oleoides**, *Decaisne* in *Jacquemont, Voy. Bot.*, t. 144 (**S. Indica**, *Royle*), as highly deserving of further investigation. This latter species is said to partake, though in a minor degree, of the acrid properties of *S. Wightiana.* It is known by the name of *Miswak*, or *Tooth-brush tree*, from the fact of the young branches being in common use amongst the natives of Northern India, for the purpose of cleansing and strengthening the teeth and gums.

# SOLANACEÆ.

---

ATROPA BELLADONNA, *Linn.* DEADLY NIGHTSHADE.
(*Engl. Bot.* t. 592; *ed. Syme*, t. 934.)

*Habitat.*—Hedges, woods, and shady places in Europe and Western Asia.

*Officinal Parts.*—1. The Leaves (*Belladonnæ Folia*), gathered when the fruit has begun to form. They are alternate, from three to six inches in length, ovate, acute, entire, smooth, the uppermost in pairs and unequal. When fresh, they have a feeble bitterish sub-acid taste, and exhale a disagreeable odour when bruised. The expressed juice or an infusion, dropped into the eye, dilates the pupil. 2. The dried Root (*Belladonnæ Radix*). Occurs in pieces from one to two feet long, and from half an inch to two inches thick, branched and wrinkled, brownish-white. An infusion, dropped into the eye, dilates the pupil. The activity of both leaves and root resides in an alkaloid, *Atropia.*

*Properties.*—Powerfully sedative, anodyne, and antispasmodic; lactifuge; exercises, in common with some other plants of this Natural Order, the peculiar power of dilating the pupil, whether taken internally or applied locally to the eye. In over doses, powerfully poisonous.

*Therapeutic Uses.*—As an antispasmodic, it is a remedy of value in the advanced stages of hooping cough, spasmodic asthma, laryngismus stridulus, chorea, epilepsy, and spasmodic stricture of the urethra; as a sedative and anodyne, in various forms of neuralgia, rheumatism, tetanus, hydrophobia, delirium tremens, dysmenorrhœa and other painful uterine affections, cancerous and other painful ulcerations. In cataract and other eye affections in which it is desirable to dilate the pupil, or to keep the edge of the iris free, as in cases of deep ulceration of the cornea, it is invaluable in surgical practice. In rheumatic and scrofulous iritis it affords great relief. Its alleged powers as a prophylactic against scarlet fever must be regarded as still *sub judice.*

*Dose.*—Of the powdered leaves, one grain, gradually increased to two grains or more. It is, however, best administered in one of the following forms.

*Preparations of the Leaves.*—**Tincture of Belladonna** (*Tinctura Belladonnæ*). Take of Belladona Leaves, in coarse powder, one ounce; Proof Spirit, one pint. Macerate the leaves for forty-eight hours in fifteen fluid ounces of the spirit, in a closed vessel, agitating occasionally; then transfer to a percolator; and when the fluid ceases to pass, continue the percolation with the remaining five ounces of spirit. Afterwards subject the contents of the percolator to pressure, filter the product, mix the liquids, and add sufficient proof spirit to make one pint.

*Dose.*—From five to twenty minims. It is about one half the strength of Tinctura Belladonnæ, *Lond. and Dub. Ph.*

**Extract of Belladonna** (*Extractum Belladonnæ*). Take of the fresh Leaves and young Branches of Belladonna, one hundred and twelve pounds. Bruise the belladonna in a stone mortar, press out the juice, heat it gradually to 130°, and separate the green colouring matter by a calico filter. Heat the strained liquor to 200° to coagulate the albumen, and again filter. Evaporate the filtrate by a water-bath to the consistence of a thin syrup; then add to it the green colouring matter previously separated; and stirring the whole together assiduously, continue the evaporation at a temperature not exceeding 140°, until the extract is of a suitable consistence for forming pills.

*Dose.*—From a quarter of a grain to one grain twice or thrice daily, and gradually increased until its physiological effects manifest themselves. Much employed locally in affections of the eye.

**Ointment of Belladonna** (*Unguentum Belladonnæ*). Take of Extract of Belladonna, eighty grains; Prepared Lard, one ounce. Rub the extract smooth with a few drops of water; then add the lard, and mix thoroughly.

A very useful topical application for rheumatic, neuralgic, and other painful affections. Applied to the perinæum, in chordee, piles, and affections of the bladder.

**Belladonna Plaster** (*Emplastrum Belladonnæ*). Take of Extract of Belladonna, Resin Plaster, of each, three ounces; Rectified Spirit, six fluid ounces. Rub the extract and spirit together in a mortar, and when the insoluble matter has subsided decant the clear solution, remove the spirit by distillation or evaporation, and mix the alcoholic extract thus obtained with the resin plaster melted by the heat of a water-bath, continuing the heat until with constant stirring the plaster has required a suitable consistence.

Applied to the chest in asthma, angina pectoris, chronic bronchitis, and other pulmonary affections; also to the joints in rheumatic and other painful enlargements.

*Preparations of the Root.*—**Liniment of Belladonna** (*Linimentum Belladonnæ*). Take of Belladonna Root, in coarse powder, twenty ounces; Camphor, one ounce; Rectified Spirit, a sufficiency. Moisten the belladonna with some of the spirit, and macerate in a closed vessel for three days; then transfer to a percolator, and, adding more spirit, percolate slowly into a receiver containing the camphor, until the product measures one pint.

Applicable to the same class of cases as Belladonna Ointment.

**Atropia** (*Atropia*). — An alkaloid, $C_{34}H_{23}NO_6$ or $C_{17}H_{23}NO_3$, obtained from Belladonna Root. *Characters.* — Colourless acicular crystals, sparingly soluble in water, more readily in alcohol and in ether. Its solution in water has an alkaline reaction, gives a citron-yellow precipitate with terchloride of gold, has a bitter taste, and powerfully dilates the pupil. It leaves no ash when burned with free access of air. It is an active poison.

*Properties and Uses.*—Similar to belladonna, but much more powerful. The dose is from one fiftieth to one twentieth of a grain, but it is rarely given internally. As an internal remedy it is inferior, on account of its energetic action, to belladonna; but it is superior to it as a local application in eye affections.

*Preparations of Atropia.* — **Solution of Atropia** (*Liquor Atropiæ*). Take of Atropia, in crystals, four grains; Rectified Spirit, one fluid drachm; Distilled Water, seven fluid drachms. Dissolve the atropia in the spirit, and add this gradually to the water, shaking them together.

Each fluid ounce contains four grains of Atropia. The dose is from two to five drops. It has occasionally been used hypodermically. For the purpose of dilating the pupil, from two to five drops may be employed. Its use requires much caution.

**Ointment of Atropia** (*Unguentum Atropiæ*). — Take of Atropia, eight grains; Rectified Spirit, half a fluid drachm; Prepared Lard, one ounce. Dissolve the atropia in the spirit; add the lard, and mix thoroughly.

A powerful external application in neuralgia and other painful affections.

**Sulphate of Atropia** (*Atropiæ Sulphas*). Take of Atropia, one hundred and twenty grains; Distilled Water, four fluid drachms; Diluted Sulphuric Acid, a sufficiency. Mix the atropia with the water, and add the acid gradually, stirring them together until the alkaloid is dissolved and the solution is neutral. Evaporate it to dryness at a temperature not exceeding 100°. It occurs in the form of a colourless powder, soluble in water, forming a solution which is neutral to test paper, and when applied to the eye dilates the pupil as the solution of atropia does. It leaves no ash when burned with free access of air.

Intended for external application. It is a powerful poison.

**Solution of the Sulphate of Atropia** (*Liquor Atropiæ Sulphatis*). Take of the Sulphate of Atropia, four grains; Distilled Water, one fluid ounce. Dissolve.

Applicable to the same purposes as Liquor Atropiæ.

## DATURA STRAMONIUM, *Linn.* STRAMONIUM, THORN APPLE.

(*Engl. Bot.*, t. 1298; *ed. Syme*, t. 935.)

*Habitat.*—Waste places throughout Europe, extending to the Himalaya; also in North America.

*Officinal Part.*—The leaves (*Stramonii Folia*); large ovate, sinuous, deeply cut, of a heavy odour, most marked whilst they are drying, and of a mawkish, faintly bitter, nauseous taste. They should be collected when the plant is in flower. 2. The seed (*Stramonii Semina*); blackish brown, reniform, flat, rough; in taste feebly bitter and mawkish; inodorous, unless bruised, when they emit a peculiar heavy odour. The active principle of both leaves and seeds is an alkaloid, *Daturia.*

*Properties.*—Anodyne and antispasmodic; in over doses, a powerful poison.

*Therapeutic Uses.*—Analogous to those of belladonna, but its operation is neither so well tested nor so well ascertained. In spasmodic asthma, dyspnœa of phthisis, emphysema of the lungs, and in some forms of chronic catarrh, smoking the dried leaves and stems affords relief to urgent symptoms, and facilitates expectoration; but caution is necessary in its use. Locally applied to the eye, and also when taken internally in large doses, it causes marked dilatation of the pupil.

*Dose.*—Of the powdered leaves, from one to three grains. Of the dried leaves and stems, for smoking purposes, from ten to thirty grains. In both cases it is desirable to commence with the smaller doses, and gradually to increase them as required.

*Preparations.*—**Extract of Stramonium** (*Extractum Stramonii*). Take of Stramonium Seeds, in coarse powder, one pound; Ether, one pint, or a sufficiency; Distilled Water, Proof Spirit, of each, a sufficiency. Shake the ether in a bottle with half a pint of the water, and after separation decant the ether. Pack the stramonium in a percolator, and free it from its oil by passing the washed ether slowly through it. Having removed and rejected the ethereal solution, pour the spirit over the residue of the stramonium in the percolator, and allow it to pass through slowly until the powder is exhausted. Distil off most of the spirit from the tincture, and evaporate the residue by a water-bath, until the extract has acquired a suitable consistence for forming pills.

*Dose.*—A quarter of a grain, gradually increased to two grains. Incorporated with four times its weight of lard, it forms a useful local anodyne application in chronic rheumatism and other painful affections.

**Tincture of Stramonium** (*Tinctura Stramonii*). Take of Stramonium Seeds, bruised, two ounces and a half; Proof Spirit, one pint. Macerate the stramonium for forty-eight hours in fifteen fluid ounces of the spirit, in a closed vessel, agitating occasionally; then transfer to a percolator; and when the fluid ceases to pass, continue the percolation with the remaining five ounces of spirit. Afterwards subject the contents of the percolator to pressure, filter the product, mix the liquids, and add sufficient proof spirit to make one pint.

*Dose.*—From ten to thirty minims.

### *DATURA ALBA, *Linn.* DHATURA.

(*Wight, Icones,* vol. iii. t. 855.)

*Habitat.*—Waste places throughout India.

*Officinal Part.*—The leaves and seeds (*Daturæ Folia et Semina*). 1. The leaves are ovate, acuminate, repandly-toothed, unequal at the base, downy, emitting, especially when bruised, a peculiar heavy disagreeable odour. 2. The seeds are about three-eighths of an inch in length, reniform, flattened, of a darkish-brown colour, having a disagreeable, bitter, somewhat acrid taste. The activity both of leaves and seeds resides in an alkaloid, *Daturia.*

*Properties, Uses, and Dose.*—Similar to those of *Datura Stramonium, Linn.* Epithems of the bruised leaves, or embrocations formed by macerating the bruised seeds in any bland oil, are often very effectual in allaying the pain in rheumatic swellings, nodes, boils, and tumours. Its poisonous properties in large doses are well known to the natives, who employ it frequently for criminal purposes. (56)

*Preparations.*—**Tincture of Dhatura** (*Tinctura Daturæ*). Take of Dhatura seeds, bruised, two ounces and a half; Proof Spirit, one pint. Macerate for seven days in a closed vessel, with occasional agitation; then strain, press, filter, and add sufficient proof spirit to make one pint; or prepare by percolation in the same manner as Tincture of Stramonium.

*Dose.*—Ten minims, gradually increased to twenty or thirty minims or more.

[The Editor for some years employed a Tincture of Dhatura seed in hospital practice in India, and found it generally produce all the sedative and narcotic effects which could have been expected from opium. A great saving of expenditure was thus effected, as opium is expensive, and this tincture can be prepared at a comparatively small cost. The dose requires to be regulated in each individual case; and it was found better to commence with small doses, and increase them according to circumstances. Twenty drops were found usually to be equal in effect to a grain of opium.]

**Extract of Dhatura** (*Extractum Daturæ*). Take of Dhatura seeds, in coarse powder, one pound; Ether, one pint, or a sufficiency; Proof Spirit and Distilled Water, of each a sufficiency. Prepare as Extract of Stramonium.

*Dose.*—A quarter of a grain, gradually increased to a grain and a half, thrice daily. A substitute for Extract of Belladonna.

[Dr. George Bidie suggests the employment of an extract prepared from the leaves and young branches in the same manner as Extract of Henbane. He prepared various specimens of this extract at Húnsúr, one of which was sent for trial to the General Hospital at Madras. Dr. Blacklock reported that "in a case of phthisis, in which it was employed in two-grain doses, it acted favourably on the dyspnœa, and produced much the same effect as Extract of Belladonna in doses of a third of a grain." Dr. Bidie adds that his own experience fully confirms that of Dr. Blacklock as to the value of this preparation, and he considers that the larger dose in which it may be administered, compared with the officinal extract, is an advantage.]

**Dhatura Plaster** (*Emplastrum Daturæ*). Take of Extract of Dhatura, three ounces; Soap Plaster and Resin Plaster, of each, one ounce and a half. Melt the plasters by the heat of a steam or water bath; then add the extract of dhatura, and mix intimately.

A good local anodyne application in rheumatic and other chronic painful affections; also to the chest in asthma and chronic pulmonary affections.

**Dhatura Poultice** (*Cataplasma Daturæ*). Take of Dhatura Leaves, fresh and bruised, and of Flour, equal parts. Add sufficient water to render the mass of the consistence of a poultice.

An effectual anodyne application to nodes, rheumatic enlargements of the joints, painful tumours, and to external piles. It should not be applied to abraded or ulcerated surfaces, on account of the danger which would result from the absorption of the poisonous principle of the plant.

[**Datura fastuosa,** *Linn.* (*Wight, Icones*, vol. iv. t. 1396).—The large purple-flowered variety is closely allied to *D. alba*, not only in botanical characters, but in medicinal properties. It is generally thought to be the more powerful of the two, but there is no evidence of this being the case. The probability is that they possess equal powers as a narcotic and anodyne; but clinical observation is wanting to confirm this. Dr. Oswald reports having seen great and immediate relief follow smoking a small quantity of the leaves of this species in cases of asthma.

Under the Tamul name of *Maratia Mooghoo*, Ainslie (*Mat. Ind.*, vol. ii. p. 185) describes certain broken-down capsules and small seeds sold in the bazaars of Southern India, which have sedative and slightly intoxicating properties assigned to them. These have been carefully examined by Dr. Wight, who found them to consist of the calyx, ovary, and base of the corolla of the young unexpanded flowers of the Datura.]

## HYOSCYAMUS NIGER, *Linn.* HYOSCYAMUS, COMMON HENBANE.

(*Engl. Bot.*, t. 591; *ed. Syme*, t. 936.)

*Habitat.*—Waste places throughout Europe and Western Asia as far west as the Western Himalaya. Cultivated in India for medicinal purposes.(57)

*Officinal Part.*—The dried leaves (*Hyoscyami Folia*), collected when about two thirds of the flowers are expanded. The leaves are sinuated, clammy, and hairy, of a dull pale green colour. The fresh herb has a strong unpleasant odour, and slightly acrid taste, which nearly disappear on drying. The fresh juice dropped into the eye dilates the pupil. Its activity resides principally in an alkaloid, *Hyoscyamia*.

*Properties.*—Sedative, anodyne, and antispasmodic.

*Therapeutic Uses.*—In nervous irritability, mental excitement, sleeplessness, and palpitations connected with debility or hysteria, it exercises a favourable influence. As an external application, it has been employed in neuralgic and rheumatic affections, painful glandular enlargements, irritable and cancerous ulcerations, and hæmorrhoids. In diseases of the eye it proves valuable from the power it possesses of dilating the pupil when locally applied.

*Dose.*—From five to ten grains of the powdered leaves.

*Preparations.*—**Tincture of Hyoscyamus** (*Tinctura Hyoscyami*). Take of Hyoscyamus Leaves, in coarse powder, two ounces and a half; Proof Spirit, one pint. Macerate the hyoscyamus for forty-eight hours in fifteen fluid ounces of the spirit, in a closed vessel, agitating occasionally; then transfer to a percolator; and when the fluid ceases to pass, continue the percolation with the remaining five ounces of spirit. Afterwards subject the contents of the percolator to pressure, filter the product, mix the two liquids, and add sufficient proof spirit to make one pint.

*Dose.*—From twenty to sixty minims repeated as necessary.

**Extract of Hyoscyamus** (*Extractum Hyoscyami*). Take of the fresh Leaves and young Branches of Hyoscyamus, one hundred and twelve pounds. Bruise in a stone mortar, and press out the juice; heat it gradually to 130°, and separate the green colouring matter by a calico filter. Heat the strained liquor to 200° to coagulate the albumen, and again filter, Evaporate the filtrate by a water bath to the consistence of a thin syrup; then add to it the green colouring matter previously separated, and, stirring the whole assiduously, continue the evaporation at a temperature not exceeding 140°, until the extract is of a suitable consistence for forming pills.

*Dose.*—From five to ten grains. A useful local application in many painful affections. A solution dropped into the eye, or the extract rubbed on the temple, causes dilatation of the pupil.

[Henbane seeds (*Khórasání Ajwain*, Hind., *Kórasání ómum*, Tam.) are commonly met with in the Indian bazaars. They are stated to be imported from Turkey, and are prescribed by the Mahomedan doctors "to soothe the mind, procure sleep, and keep the bowels gently open in cases of melancholia and mania." (*Ainslie.*)]

## NICOTIANA TABACUM, *Linn.* TOBACCO.

(*Steph. et Church., Med. Bot.*, vol. i. t. 37.)

*Habitat.*—Tropical America. Cultivated throughout the warmer portions of the globe.

*Officinal Part.*—The dried Leaves (*Tabaci Folia, Tobacco Leaves*). They are large mottled-brown ovate or lanceolate-acuminate, bearing numerous short glandular hairs; having a peculiar heavy odour, and nauseous bitter acrid taste; yielding, when distilled with solution of potash, an alkaline fluid, which has the peculiar odour of nicotia, and precipitates with bichloride of platinum and tincture of galls. Their activity resides in a liquid alkaloid, *Nicotia*, and a volatile oil, *Nicotianin*.

*Properties.*—Powerful sedative and antispasmodic; in over doses an acro-narcotic poison.

*Therapeutic Uses.*—In tetanus (58), dropsical affections, spasmodic affections of the abdomen, retention of urine, and as a means of inducing muscular relaxation, and thus aiding in the reduction of strangulated hernia and dislocations, it has been employed; but, as a general rule, it is unfitted for internal administration, on account of the great nervous depression it produces. As a local application, it has been used for relieving pain and irritation in rheumatic swellings, syphilitic nodes, and skin diseases; but its ungrateful smell is an objection to its use, whilst there are other remedies of greater and more uniform efficacy. Tobacco smoking is sometimes effectually resorted to in asthma, spasmodic coughs, nervous irritability, and sleeplessness.

*Preparation.*—**Enema of Tobacco** (*Enema Tabaci*). Take of Tobacco Leaves, twenty grains; Boiling Water, eight fluid ounces. Infuse in a covered vessel for half an hour, and strain.

Only employed, and that rarely, in strangulated hernia, spasmodic affections of the abdomen, and retention of urine from spasmodic stricture. The greatest caution is necessary in its use. The above quantity (twenty grains) should not be exceeded at the commencement.

## SOLANUM DULCAMARA, *Linn.* DULCAMARA OR BITTER-SWEET.

(*Engl. Bot.*, t. 565; *ed. Syme*, t. 930.)

*Habitat.*—Europe, and temperate Asia.

*Officinal Part.*—The dried young branches (*Dulcamara*), collected after the plants have shed their leaves. They are about the thickness of a goose-quill, light, hollow, cylindrical, bitter, and subsequently sweetish to the taste.

*Properties.*—Alterative, diuretic, diaphoretic.

*Therapeutic Uses.*—In cachectic and constitutional syphilitic cases, in chronic rheumatism, but especially in psoriasis, lepra, eczema, and other obstinate skin diseases, it has been used with alleged benefit, but its efficacy is doubtful.

*Preparation.*—**Infusion of Dulcamara** (*Infusum Dulcamaræ*). Take of Dulcamara, bruised, one ounce; Boiling Water, ten fluid ounces. Infuse in a covered vessel for one hour, and strain.

*Dose.*—From one to two fluid ounces, thrice daily or oftener.

[With the fresh Hemidesmus root at hand the practitioner in India is independent of this article.]

## CAPSICUM FASTIGIATUM, *Blume.* CAPSICUM.
(*Capsicum annuum*, Linn.)
(*Wight, Icones*, vol. iv. t. 1617.)

*Habitat.*—Cultivated throughout the tropics of both hemispheres.

*Officinal Part.*—The ripe fruit dried (*Capsici Fructus, Capsicum Fruit*). Pod membraneous, from five to eight lines in length, about two lines in breadth, straight, conical, pointed, smooth, shining, but somewhat corrugated; of an orange red colour, and intensely hot taste. Its activity resides in a resinous principle, *Capsicine.*

*Properties.*—Acrid stimulant; locally applied, rubefacient.

*Therapeutic Uses.*—In atonic dyspepsia, and in diarrhœa arising from putrid or crude ingesta in the intestines, and in the vomiting of bilious remittent fever, it acts beneficially. In scarlatina it has been used with great repute in the West Indies. In various forms of cynanche, and in hoarseness or aphonia, depending upon a relaxed condition of the chordæ vocales, it has been found a useful adjunct to gargles. As a rubefacient and counter-irritant, the bruised fruit, in the form of poultice, acts energetically; added to sinapisms it greatly increases their activity.

*Dose.*—From one to four grains; rarely prescribed alone.

*Preparations.*—**Tincture of Capsicum** (*Tinctura Capsici*). Take of Capsicum Fruit, bruised, three quarters of an ounce; Rectified Spirit, one pint. Macerate the capsicum for forty-eight hours in fifteen fluid ounces of the spirit, in a closed vessel, agitating occasionally; then transfer to a percolator; and when the fluid ceases to pass, continue the percolation with the remaining five ounces of spirit. Afterwards subject the contents of the percolator to pressure, filter the product, mix the liquors, and add sufficient rectified spirit to make one pint.

*Dose.*—From ten to twenty minims. A good adjunct to stimulant and other gargles, *e.g.*, Tincture of Capsicum, one fluid drachm; Decoction of Cinchona, six fluid ounces.

(*Non-officinal.*)

**Hyoscyamus insanus**, *Stocks.*—A common plant of Belúchistan, where it is known by the name of *Kohí bung* or *Mountain Hemp.* Its powerfully poisonous properties are well known, and it is stated to be smoked in small quantities by debauched faquirs, and to be used also for criminal purposes. The chief symptoms produced by it are dryness and constriction of the throat, and furious delirium (Stocks in *Hooker's Journ. of Bot.*, 1852, vol. iv. p. 178). It would be desirable to know more of this plant and its properties.

**Scopolia lurida**, *Dunal*,—*Anisodus luridus*, *Link*. (*Icones*, t. 35; *Sweet*, *Brit. Fl. Gard.*, vol. iii. t. 125.)—A herbaceous plant of the Himalaya, introduced into Europe in 1824, and now cultivated there in gardens. The leaves, which are of a pale-green colour, emit, especially when bruised, a peculiar tobacco-like odour. A tincture prepared from them, in the proportion of one ounce to eight ounces of alcohol, administered to different patients, was found to produce extreme dilatation of the pupil; and in two instances it induced blindness, which only disappeared when the medicine was discontinued. The largest dose given was twenty drops of the above tincture during the twenty-four hours (*Gaz. Med.*, Nov. 4th, 1843, and *Braithwaite's Retrospect of Med.*, vol. ix. p. 119.) The subject demands further investigation.

**Solanum Jacquini**, *Willd.* (*Wight*, *Icones*, vol. iv. t. 1401.)—This is one of the most popular medical plants of the people of India, having expectorant, diuretic, and other properties assigned to it, and being largely employed in catarrhal and febrile affections, asthma, consumption, &c. The stems, flowers, and fruit, according to Dr. Wilson (*Calcutta Med. Phys. Trans.*, vol. ii. p. 406), are bitter and carminative, and are prescribed in those forms of burning of the feet (*Ignipeditis*) which are attended with a vesicular, watery eruption (Dr. Grierson, *ibid.*, vol. ii. p. 278). Fumigations with the vapour of the burning seeds of this plant are in high repute in the cure of toothache. The mode of application followed by the natives is given in detail by Dr. Morehead (*ibid.*, vol. vii. P. ii. p. 489). It acts as a powerful sialogogue, and by this means probably relief is obtained.

**Solanum nigrum**, *Linn.* (*Engl. Bot.*, t. 566; *ed. Syme*, t. 931, 932.) —Mr. Moodeen Sheriff reports having used with advantage a decoction of the leaves of this plant, and also an aqueous extract prepared from it, the latter in drachm doses thrice daily, in the treatment of dropsical affections. Its action is diuretic and laxative. The juice of the leaves of **S. incertum**, *Dunal*, is stated by Dr. Shortt to be an excellent remedy in the aphthæ of childhood. Several other species of Solanum, *e.g.* **S. indicum**, *Linn.*, **S. trilobatum**, *Linn.*, **S. verbascifolium**, *Linn.*, and **S. ferox**, *Linn.*, are mentioned by Ainslie, Drury, and other writers, as being employed medicinally by the natives; but their virtues, if any, are very unimportant, and rest solely on native testimony.

**Withania (Puneeria) coagulans**, *Dunal* (*Wight*, *Icones*, vol. iv. t. 1616.)—A small shrub, common on hilly ground throughout Belúchistan and Scinde, where it is known by the name of *Punír* or *Punírbad*. It is densely covered with minute stellate hairs arranged in tufts, which form a short ash-grey covering to the whole plant. It may be recognized at a considerable distance by its dusky ash-grey hue, which in the young leafy shoots has a blueish tinge. There is not a shade of green in the whole plant. The ripe fruits are brown and shining on the surface, and when fresh are used as an emetic; when dried they are sold in the Scinde bazaars under the name of *Punír ja fota* (*Puneer cardamoms*), and are regarded by Dr. Stocks as constituting the *Kakinj* or *Hub-ul-Kakinj* of Arabian and Persian writers on Materia Medica (*Punír ka bíj*, *Hind.*) They are employed in dyspepsia and flatulent colic, and other intestinal affections, and enjoy an immense reputation in Scinde, Belúchistan, and Affghanistan. They are prescribed in infusion, either alone or conjoined with the leaves and twigs of

*Rhazya stricta*, Dec., an excellent bitter tonic, known in Scinde by the name of *Sihar* or *Sewur*. The dried fruit is in almost universal use throughout Belúchistan and Affghanistan for coagulating milk in the process of cheese manufacture. (See Dr. Stocks, *Journ. of Bombay Asiat. Soc.*, January 1849, p. 55.)

**Withania (Physalis) somnifera,** *Dunal* (*Wight, Icones*, vol. iii. t. 853.)—A common plant in many parts of India. It has narcotic, diuretic, and other properties assigned to it, but nothing trustworthy is known regarding it. The root, sold in the bazaars of Southern India under the Tamul name *Amúlang kalung*, resembles Gentian root in external appearance, but has little taste or smell (Ainslie, *Mat. Ind.*, vol. ii. p. 14). This root, ground up with water, and also the bruised leaves, are much employed as a local application to carbuncles, ulcers, and painful swellings. The Rajpoots regard the root as useful in rheumatic affections, and in dyspepsia, especially when accompanied by flatulence. Dr. Irvine (*Med. Topog. of Ajmeer*, p. 123), on whose authority this is stated, adds that the root is of a warm nature, and calculated to promote all the secretions. It has been thought especially to stimulate the kidneys, but Dr. Oswald reports that its diuretic properties, according to his experience, are not very marked.

# PLANTAGINEÆ.

## *PLANTAGO ISPAGHULA, *Roxb.* ISPAGHÚL.

*Habitat.*—Persia ; cultivated in India.

*Officinal Part.*—The seeds (*Ispaghulæ Semina, Ispaghúl Seeds*): ovate-elliptical, concave, about an eighth of an inch in length, of a greyish colour; they yield to water an abundance of tasteless mucilage.

*Properties.*—Demulcent, mildly astringent.

*Therapeutic Uses.*—In febrile, catarrhal, and renal affections, they have been found serviceable, but their chief use is in diarrhœa and dysentery. The bruised seeds, moistened with water, form a good emollient poultice.

*Dose.*—From two to three drachms.

*Preparations.*—**Decoction of Ispaghúl** (*Decoctum Ispaghúlæ*). Take of Ispaghúl Seeds, bruised, two drachms ; Water, a pint. Boil for ten minutes in a covered vessel, and strain.

*Dose.*—From two to four ounces, repeated three or four times daily.

[This decoction is well adapted for catarrhal and renal affections; but for diarrhœa and dysentery the following mode of administration, advised by the late Mr. Twining, is preferable: "In the chronic diarrhœa of Europeans who have been long resident in India, benefit," he remarks, "often follows the use of demulcents followed by mild tonics. For this purpose the Ispaghúl seeds seem to answer better than any other remedy. The dose for an adult is two drachms and a half mixed with half a drachm of sugar-candy. The seeds are exhibited whole, and in their passage through the intestines they absorb as much fluid as makes them swell, and by the time they reach the central or lower portions of the canal, they give out a bland mucilage; and in general they continue to possess the same mucilaginous properties until they have passed through the intestines. If the frequency of the dejections be restrained by an anodyne enema, and by using only a small quantity of food, the mucilaginous properties of these seeds are most evident. It is said that a slight degree of astringency and some tonic property may be imparted to the seeds by exposing them to a moderate degree of heat, so that they shall be dried and slightly browned. This remedy sometimes cures the protracted diarrhœa of European and Native children after many other remedies have failed." (*Diseases of Bengal*, vol. i. p. 212.)]

## PHYTOLACCACEÆ.

(*Non-officinal.*)

**Gisekia pharnaceoides,** *Linn.* (*Wight, Icones,* vol. iv. t. 1167), a common plant in the drier parts of India, from the Carnatic to the Punjaub and Oude. It has been brought to notice by Capt. W. H. Lowther (*Journ. of Agri.-Hort. Soc. of India*, 1857, vol. ix. p. 285) as a powerful anthelmintic in cases of tænia. The fresh plant, including the leaves, stalks, and capsules, is directed to be employed, in doses of about an ounce ground up in a mortar with sufficient water to make a draught. This is to be repeated three times at an interval of four days, the patient each time taking it after fasting for some hours. Capt. Lowther's estimate of it is very high, but as yet no medical evidence has been adduced in support of its alleged virtues.

## SALSOLACEÆ.

(*Non-officinal.*)

**Salicornia Indica,** *Willd.* (*Wight, Icones,* vol. iii. t. 737), **S. brachiata,** *Roxb.* (*Ibid.*, t. 738), and **Suaeda nudiflora,** *Willd.*, which abound on the sea coasts of India, yield on incineration considerable quantities of barilla, sufficient, in the opinion of Royle (*Illust.*, vol. i. p. 319), to make soap and glass for the whole world. Sir W. O'Shaughnessy, however, expresses a just doubt whether Indian prepared barilla could compete in point of cheapness with that manufactured in Europe (*Bengal Disp.*, p. 526). In Irvine's Materia Medica of Patna (p. 47) an impure soda is described under the name of *Khar-suji* or *Suji-Khar* (*Hind.*) imported from Scinde, employed in the manufacture of soap and glass, and applied locally to tumours with the view of causing their resolution. **Salsola (Suaeda) Indica** (*Wight, Icones,* vol. v. t. 1797) is the plant named as yielding this. The greater part, if not the whole of the impure soda sold in the bazaars under the Hindústani name of *Saji-mati* is a mineral product, obtained in large quantities from Monghyr and other parts of Bengal.

## AMARANTACEÆ.

(*Non-officinal.*)

**Amarantus spinosus,** *Linn.* (*Wight, Icones*, vol. ii. t. 513), and other indigenous species included under the generic name of *Nutí* or *Nutíya* (*Beng.*), possess mucilaginous properties. A poultice of the bruised leaves is officinal in the Bengal Ph.; but it is a simple emollient, inferior to many others, and may be safely omitted. In the Mauritius a decoction of the leaves and root is administered internally as a diuretic. (Bouton, *Med. Plant of Mauritius*, p. 128.)

**Achyranthes aspera,** *Linn.* (*Wight, Icones*, vol. v. t. 1777.)—A common weed in most parts of India. Astringent and diuretic properties are assigned to it. Of its value in the former character little is known, although it is said to be successfully used in native practice in menorrhagia and diarrhœa. As a diuretic it is favourably reported of by Dr. Cornish, who, in a communication to the Editor (dated November 14th, 1860), states that he has employed it largely in general dropsy with very satisfactory results. It is also favourably noticed in this class of cases in the Reports of Dr. G. Smith, Dr. J. Shortt, Mr. Kanny Loll Dey, and others. It is best administered in decoction, prepared by boiling two ounces of the fresh plant in a pint and a half of water till reduced to one pint, and straining. Of this the dose is two fluid ounces or more until its diuretic operation is established. The whole plant, when incinerated, yields a considerable quantity of potash; hence its Sanscrit name, *Apamarga*, i.e. *The Washerman*, from the circumstance of the ashes being used in washing clothes. (Rev. J. Long, *Journ. of Agri.-Hort. Soc. of India*, 1858, vol. x. p. 31.) These ashes, in conjunction with infusion of ginger, are likewise esteemed in dropsical affections. The flowering spike has the repute in Oude and other parts of India of being a safeguard against scorpions, which it is believed to paralyse. (*Ibid.*, May 1848, p. 340.) It is also believed to be a curative agent in the bites of these and other venomous insects and reptiles. Dr. Shortt reports having used it as a successful local application in scorpion stings. Dr. Turner has called attention to it as a remedy in snake bites. (See *Madras Quart. Journ. of Med.*, 1862, vol. iv. p. 10.)

## NYCTAGINACEÆ.

(*Non-officinal.*)

**Mirabilis Jalapa,** *Linn.* (*Rheede, Hort. Mal.*, vol. x. t. 75.)—This plant, cultivated in gardens throughout India under the name of *Four o'clock* (from the circumstance of its flowers opening at that hour), was formerly thought to be the source of the Jalap of commerce; an idea, however, now exploded. In the Taleef Shereef

(p. 110) the root is stated to be a mild and efficient purgative, equal, if not superior, to common jalap. Subjected to clinical trials by Drs. Shoolbred and Hunter (*Fleming's Cat. of Indian Drugs*, p. 29), Ainslie (*Mat. Ind.*, vol. ii. p. 285), and Sir W. O'Shaughnessy (*Bengal Disp.*, p.512), its powers as a purgative have been found to be feeble and uncertain, and unworthy of attention in this or any other character. The bruised leaves form a favourite application amongst the natives to abscesses and boils, to hasten the suppurative process. The Editor on one occasion witnessed a greatly increased amount of pain and local inflammation follow the use of this application, in the case of a lady who had been induced to apply it to a boil by her native attendant.

**Boerhaavia diffusa,** *Linn.* (*Wight, Icones*, vol. iii. t. 874.) — A troublesome weed throughout India. Sub-Assistant Surgeon B. M. Chatterjee reports having found it a very good expectorant, and that he has prescribed it in several cases of asthma with marked success. He employed it in the form of powder, decoction, and infusion, but the doses and proportions are not furnished. Taken largely it acts as an emetic.

## POLYGONACEÆ.

### RHEUM, ONE OR MORE UNDETERMINED SPECIES OF, YIELDING RHUBARB.

*Habitat.*—Thibet and Tartary.

*Officinal Part.*—The dried decorticated Root (*Rhei Radix, Rhubarb Root*). It is imported into Europe from Chinese Thibet and Tartary in trapezoidal roundish cylindrical or flattish pieces, frequently bored with one hole, yellow externally, internally marbled with fine waving greyish and reddish lines, finely gritty under the teeth; taste bitter, faintly astringent and aromatic; odour peculiar. Free from decay, not worm-eaten. Boracic Acid does not turn the yellow exterior brown. It contains a peculiar neutral principle, *Rheine* (supposed to be the active constituent), tannic and gallic acids, and a bitter extractive.

*Properties.*—Primarily, a mild and efficient cathartic; secondarily, astringent; in small doses, stomachic and astringent.

*Therapeutic Uses.*—In the constipation of children, anæmic females, gouty subjects, and in the puerperal state, it is especially recommended by the mildness of its operation. In diarrhœa depending upon the presence of crude or irritating ingesta, it proves highly useful. In some forms of dyspepsia it is a remedy of great value, either alone or combined with other agents.

*Dose.*—As a cathartic, from twenty to forty grains; as a stomachic, from three to eight grains.

*Preparations.*—**Infusion of Rhubarb** (*Infusum Rhei*). Take of Rhubarb Root, in thin slices, a quarter of an ounce; Boiling Water, ten fluid ounces. Infuse in a covered vessel for one hour, and strain.

*Dose.*—From one to two fluid ounces.

**Extract of Rhubarb** (*Extractum Rhei*). Take of Rhubarb Root, sliced or bruised, one pound; Rectified Spirit, ten fluid ounces; Distilled Water, five pints. Mix the spirit and the water, and macerate the rhubarb in the mixture for four days; then decant, press and set by, that the undissolved matter may subside; pour off the clear liquor, filter the remainder, mix the liquors, and evaporate by a water bath at a temperature not exceeding 160° until the extract has acquired a suitable consistence for forming pills.

*Dose.*—From three to eight grains as a stomachic; from ten to twenty grains as a carthartic.

**Tincture of Rhubarb** (*Tinctura Rhei*). Take of Rhubarb Root, in coarse powder, two ounces; Cardamom Seeds, freed from the pericarps, and bruised, Coriander Fruit bruised, Saffron, of each a quarter of an ounce; Proof Spirit, one pint. Macerate the solid ingredients for forty-eight hours in fifteen fluid ounces of the spirit, in a closed vessel, agitating occasionally; then transfer to a percolator; and when the fluid ceases to pass, continue the percolation with the remaining five ounces of spirit. Afterwards subject the contents of the percolator to pressure, filter the product, mix the liquids, and add sufficient proof spirit to make one pint.

*Dose.*—From one to two fluid drachms as a stomachic. A good adjunct to purgative draughts.

**Wine of Rhubarb** (*Vinum Rhei*). Take of Rhubarb Root, in coarse powder, one ounce and a half; Canella Alba Bark, in coarse powder, sixty grains; Sherry, one pint. Macerate for seven days in a closed vessel with occasional agitation, then strain, press, filter, and add sufficient sherry to make one pint.

*Dose.*—From one to two fluid drachms.

**Syrup of Rhubarb** (*Syrupus Rhei*). Take of Rhubarb Root in coarse powder, Coriander Fruit in coarse powder, of each two ounces; Refined Sugar, twenty-four ounces; Rectified Spirit, eight fluid ounces; Distilled Water, twenty-four fluid ounces.

Mix the rhubarb and coriander; pack them in a percolator; pass the spirit and water, previously mixed, slowly through them; evaporate the liquid that has thus passed until it is reduced to thirteen fluid ounces, and in this, after it has been filtered, dissolve the sugar with a gentle heat.

*Dose.*—From one to four fluid drachms.

**Compound Rhubarb Pill** (*Pilula Rhei Composita*). Take of Rhubarb Root, in powder, three ounces; Socotrine Aloes, in powder, two ounces and a quarter; Myrrh, in powder, Hard Soap, in powder, of each one ounce and a half; Oil of Peppermint, one fluid drachm and a half; Treacle by weight, four ounces. Mix the powders with the oil, then add the treacle, and beat the whole into a uniform mass.

*Dose.*—From five to ten grains.

**Compound Powder of Rhubarb** (*Pulvis Rhei Composita*). Take of Rhubarb, in powder, two ounces; Light Magnesia, six ounces; Ginger, in powder, one ounce. Mix them thoroughly, and pass the powder through a fine sieve.

*Dose.*—From twenty to sixty grains for adults; from five to ten grains for children. This preparation has long enjoyed repute in domestic practice under the name of "Gregory's Powder."

(*Non-officinal.*)

**Rheum Emodi**, *Wallich* (*Bot. Mag.* t. 3508); **R. Moorcroftianum**, *Royle*; **R. Webbianum**, *Royle*. (*Illust.*, t. 78 a.) The roots of these plants, inhabiting the elevated portions of Himalaya, constitute the principal portion of the Indian or Himalayan Rhubarb. There are two principal varieties. 1. *The large* (from *R. Emodi?*); occurs in twisted or cylindrical pieces of various sizes and shapes, furrowed; cut obliquely at the extremities, about four inches long and an inch and a half in diameter; of a dark brown colour, feeble rhubarb odour, and bitter astringent taste; texture radiated, rather spongy, not presenting on fracture the marbled texture characteristic of ordinary rhubarb; pulverized with difficulty; powder of a dull brownish yellow colour. 2. *The small* (from *R. Webbianum*); consists of short transverse segments of the root branches; of a dark-brownish colour, odourless, or nearly so, with a very bitter astringent taste. Both kinds are liable to considerable variation in physical characters. The trials made with Himalayan rhubarb by Prof. Royle (*Calcutta Med. Phys. Trans.*, vol. iii. p. 439), and Mr. Twining (*Diseases of Bengal*, vol. i. p. 220), were productive of satisfactory results; the latter authority, indeed, regarded it as superior to imported rhubarb as a stomachic tonic. Subsequent experience has not confirmed this view. The general tenor of all the reports received from India in which this drug is noticed is to the effect that the indigenous rhubarb procured in the bazaars is generally worthless, and unfitted to replace the imported article. Dr. Hugh Cleghorn (*Madras Quart. Med. Journ.* 1862, vol. v. p. 461), who furnishes some interesting remarks on Himalayan Rhubarb, states that it is only an inferior variety that reaches the plains of Hindústan. He tested the action of the fresh root, and found it resemble that of Russian rhubarb. Cultivated with due care, there is reason to believe that a good serviceable drug, equal to Chinese or Turkey Rhubarb, might be obtained from the Himalayan plants.

## THYMELACEÆ.

### DAPHNE MEZEREUM, *Linn.* MEZEREON.

(*Steph. et Church. Med. Bot.*, vol. ii. t. 65.)

### DAPHNE LAUREOLA, *Linn.* SPURGE LAUREL.

(*Engl. Bot.*, t. 119.)

*Habitat.*—Europe.

*Officinal Part.*—The dried Bark (*Mezerei Cortex, Mezereon Bark*). It occurs in strips or quilled pieces of various lengths, tough and pliable, olive-brown on the surface, white within, fibrous; odour faintly nauseous; taste hot and acrid. Its activity resides in an acrid resin and a volatile oil. In addition to these, it contains a neutral crystalline principle, *Daphnia*.

*Properties.*—Stimulant, diaphoretic, and diuretic. Externally applied, rubefacient and vesicant. To obtain the latter effect it should be first steeped in hot vinegar, and kept in contact with the skin by a bandage. It has been proposed as a substitute for Unguentum Sabinæ in dressing blisters.

*Therapeutic Uses.*—In syphilitic and rheumatic cases, and various skin affections, it has been used, but with doubtful results.

*Dose.*—From ten to twelve grains in infusion, twice or thrice daily. It is rarely, if ever, prescribed alone. It is an ingredient in Decoctum Sarsæ compositum.

*Preparations.*—**Ethereal Extract of Mezereon** (*Extractum Mezerei Æthereum*). Take of Mezereon Bark, cut small, one pound; Rectified Spirit, eight pints; Ether, one pint. Macerate the mezereon in six pints of the spirit for three days, with frequent agitation; strain and press. To the residue of the mezereon add the remainder of the spirit, and again macerate for three days, with frequent agitation; strain and press. Mix and filter the strained liquors; recover the greater part of the spirit by distillation, evaporate what remains to the consistence of a soft extract; put this into a stoppered bottle with the ether, and macerate for twenty-four hours, shaking them frequently. Decant the ethereal solution; recover part of the ether by distillation, and evaporate what remains to the consistence of a soft extract.

Externally applied, irritant. It is an ingredient in Linimentum Sinapis compositum.

## MYRISTICEÆ.

### MYRISTICA OFFICINALIS, *Linn. fil.* Officinal Nutmeg Tree.

(*Bot. Mag.*, t. 2756, 2757. *Steph. et Church. Med. Bot.*, vol. ii. t. 104.)

*Habitat.*—Moluccas; cultivated in the Malayan peninsula and archipelago, Ceylon, Malabar, and in some parts of tropical America.

*Officinal Part.*—The kernel of the fruit (*Myristica, Nutmeg*); oval or nearly round, about an inch in length, marked externally with reticulated furrows; internally greyish-red, with dark-brownish veins; odour strong and peculiar; taste bitter and aromatic. Its activity resides in a volatile oil (*Oleum Myristicæ*).

*Properties.*—Stimulant and carminative; in larger doses narcotic.

*Therapeutic Uses.*—In atonic diarrhœa, flatulence, flatulent colic, and some forms of dyspepsia, it has been used with advantage, but it is principally employed as an adjunct to other remedies. Used largely as a condiment.

*Dose.*—From ten to twenty grains.

Nutmegs enter into the composition of Pulvis Catechu compositus, Pulvis Cretæ aromaticus, Spiritus Armoraciæ compositus, and Tinctura Lavandulæ composita.

*Preparations.*—**Volatile Oil of Nutmeg** (*Oleum Myristicæ*). The oil obtained by distillation from Nutmegs. It is colourless or straw-coloured, having the odour and taste of nutmegs.

*Dose.*—From one to five minims. Used locally for the relief of toothache. The oil forms an ingredient in Spiritus Myristicæ, Spiritus Ammoniæ Aromaticus, and Pilula Aloes Socotrinæ.

**Spirit of Nutmeg** (*Spiritus Myristicæ*). Take of Volatile Oil of Nutmeg, one fluid ounce; Rectified Spirit, forty-nine fluid ounces. Dissolve.

*Dose.*—From thirty to sixty minims.

**Expressed Oil of Nutmeg** (*Oleum Myristicæ Expressum, Adeps Myristicæ, Brit. Pharm.* 1864). A concrete oil obtained by means of expression and heat from nutmegs. It is of an orange colour, firm consistence, and fragrant odour like that of nutmeg; soluble in four times its weight of boiling alcohol, or half that quantity of ether.

A useful application in rheumatism, paralysis, and sprains, for which purpose it should be diluted with a little bland oil or Soap Liniment. It forms an ingredient in Emplastrum Picis and Emplastrum Calefaciens.

[Mace, the false aril or arillode investing the shell of the kernel as met with in commerce, occurs in single or double blades, flat, irregularly slit, smooth, slightly flexible or brittle; of a pale cinnamon-yellow or golden-yellow colour, and an odour and taste analogous to those of nutmegs. It yields by distillation a volatile oil, which, in composition, effects, and uses, is similar to that of nutmegs. It is chiefly used as a condiment.]

(*Non-officinal.*)

**Myristica Malabarica,** *Lam.* (*Rheede, Hort. Mal.*, vol. iv. t. 5). A common forest tree of Malabar and Travancore. Yields a variety of nutmeg (Malabar Nutmeg?), larger and much longer than the officinal nutmeg, and possessing little of its fragrance or its warm aromatic taste. When bruised and subjected to boiling, it yields a considerable quantity of a yellowish concrete oil, analogous to expressed oil of nutmeg, which has been represented to the Editor as a most efficacious application to indolent and ill-conditioned ulcers, allaying pain, cleansing the surface, and establishing healthy action. For this purpose it requires to be melted down with a small quantity of any bland oil. It may be found serviceable as an embrocation in rheumatism.

## LAURACEÆ.

### CINNAMOMUM CAMPHORA, *Nees et Ebermaier.*

(CAMPHORA OFFICINARUM, *Nees, Brit. Pharm.*)

(*Wight, Icones*, vol. v. t. 1818.)

*Habitat.*—China, Japan, and Cochin China: introduced into Java.

*Officinal Part.*—The concrete volatile oil (*Camphora, Camphor*) obtained from the wood by sublimation. It occurs in white translucent masses, of a crystalline structure; powerful penetrating odour, and pungent taste, followed by a sensation of cold. Floats on water; volatilizes slowly at ordinary temperatures; is slightly soluble in water, but readily soluble in rectified spirit and in ether; tough, not easily pulverised. Burns with a bright flame. Sublimes entirely when heated. Crude camphor is imported into Great Britain from China and Japan.

*Properties.*—Its primary action is that of a diffusible stimulant and diaphoretic; its secondary, that of a sedative, anodyne, and antispasmodic. In large doses it is an acro-narcotic poison.

*Therapeutic Uses.*—Amongst the numerous diseases in which Camphor has been most extensively employed, and found most serviceable, are the advanced stages and adynamic forms, of fevers and inflammation, insanity, especially the puerperal form, asthma, angina pectoris, hooping cough, and palpitations connected with hypertrophy of the heart, affections of the genito-urinary system, comprising dysmenorrhœa, nymphomania, spermatorrhœa, cancer, and irritable states of the uterus, chordee, incontinence of urine, hysteria, rheumatism, gangrene, and gout. It has also been employed as an antidote to strychnia, but with doubtful results. As an external application, it is used in the form of embrocation, for rheumatism, sprains, and other painful affections, for preventing bed sores, and for allaying pruritus in skin diseases.

*Dose.*—From one to five grains; may be increased, in cases requiring it, to double these quantities.

*Preparations.*—**Camphor Water** (*Aqua Camphoræ, Mistura Camphoræ, Lond. Ph.*) Take of Camphor, broken into pieces, half an ounce; Water, one gallon. Enclose the camphor in a muslin bag, and attach this to the end of a glass rod, by means of which it may be kept at the bottom of the bottle containing the water, the other end of the rod terminating just below the stopper of the bottle. Having thus put the camphor into the water, close the mouth of the bottle, macerate for at least two days, and then pour off the solution when it is required.

*Dose.*—From one to two fluid ounces; used chiefly as a vehicle for other medicines.

**Spirit of Camphor** (*Spiritus Camphoræ*). Take of Camphor, one ounce; Rectified Spirit, nine fluid ounces. Dissolve.

*Dose.*—From ten to thirty minims suspended in water by means of mucilage. Chiefly used as an external application in sprains, bruises, chilblains, chronic rheumatism, and paralysis.

**Compound Tincture of Camphor** (*Tinctura Camphoræ composita; Tinctura Camphoræ cum Opio, Brit. Ph.* 1864; *Tinctura Opii Camphorata, Edin. et Dubl. Ph.*) Take of Opium, in coarse powder, forty grains; Benzoic Acid, forty grains; Oil of Anise, half a fluid drachm; Proof Spirit, one pint. Macerate for seven days in a closed vessel, with occasional agitation, then filter, and add sufficient proof spirit to make one pint.

*Dose.*—From fifteen minims to two fluid drachms or more. Each fluid drachm contains a quarter of a grain of opium. Under the name of *Paregoric*, or *Paregoric Elixir*, this preparation has long enjoyed popular repute as a sedative. It is a frequent ingredient in cough mixtures.

**Liniment of Camphor** (*Linimentum Camphoræ*). Take of Camphor, one ounce; Olive Oil, four fluid ounces. Dissolve the camphor in the oil.

**Compound Liniment of Camphor** (*Linimentum Camphoræ compositum*). Take of Camphor, two ounces and a half; Oil of Lavender, one fluid drachm; Strong Solution of Ammonia, five fluid ounces; Rectified Spirit, fifteen fluid ounces. Dissolve the camphor and oil of lavender in the spirit; then add the solution of ammonia gradually, shaking them together until a clear solution is formed.

This and the preceding preparation are useful applications in rheumatism and other painful affections.

Camphor is an ingredient also in many officinal Liniments; also in Unguentum Plumbi Subacetatis compositum and Ung. Hydrargyri compositum.

[Camphor exists in the form of white crystalline fragments, in the wood of **Dryobalanops Camphora,** *Colebr.*, a forest tree of Sumatra, Borneo, and Java, from 1° 10′ to 2° 10′ N. lat. A good account of its mode of collection, &c., is given by Dr. De Vriese (*Hooker's Journ. of Bot.*, vol. iv. p. 33). A notice of its medicinal properties and uses, by Mr. Motley, is published in the same Journal (vol. iv. p. 202). In these respects it appears to possess no advantage over officinal camphor, whilst its price is far greater. Camphor exists in small quantities in other plants, and has been prepared in the Tenasserim Provinces, in considerable quantities, from the leaves and stems of *Blumea grandis, D.C.* (q.v.)]

## SASSAFRAS OFFICINALE, *Nees*. OFFICINAL SASSAFRAS.

(*Hayne*, vol. xii. t. 19. *Steph. et Church, Med. Bot.* vol. iii. t. 126.)

*Habitat.*—Woods of North America from Canada to Florida.

*Officinal Part.*—The dried Root (*Sassafras Radix*). Occurs in branched pieces, sometimes eight inches in diameter at the crown. Bark externally greyish-brown, internally rusty-brown, of an agreeable odour, and a peculiar aromatic warm taste. Wood light, porous, greyish-yellow, more feeble in odour and taste than the bark. It is met with also in the form of chips. It contains a volatile oil (*Oleum Sassafras*), resin, and a peculiar principle, *Sassafrin.*

*Properties.*—Alterative tonic, and sudorific.

*Therapeutic Uses.*—In chronic rheumatism, secondary syphilis, scurvy, and skin diseases, it has been employed, but generally conjoined with sarsaparilla, guaiacum, and other remedies of the same class.

Sassafras forms an ingredient in Decoctum Sarsæ compositum.

[The volatile oil obtained by distillation of the wood is stimulant, carminative, and reputed to be diaphoretic, in doses of from two to ten drops. It, as well as the pith (*Sassafras Medulla*), is officinal in the United States Ph. The latter abounds in mucilaginous gummy matter; and, in infusion, is employed as a demulcent in cases requiring that class of remedies. (See Wood and Bache, *United States Disp.*, 11th ed., p. 692.)]

## NECTANDRA RODIÆI, *Schomburgk.* GREENHEART TREE.

*Habitat.*—British Guiana.

*Officinal Part.*—1. The bark (*Nectandræ Cortex, Beberu Bark*). It occurs in large flat heavy pieces, from one to two feet long, from two to six inches broad, and about a quarter of an inch thick. External colour greyish-brown; internal, dark cinnamon-brown. Taste strongly and persistently bitter, with considerable astringency.

*Properties and Uses.*—Astringent tonic. Officinal only for the sake of its alkaloid (*Beberia*).

*Preparation.*—**Sulphate of Beberia** (*Beberiæ Sulphas*), $C_{35}H_{20}NO_6$, HO, $SO_3$, or $\mathbf{C_{35}H_{40}N_2O_6.H_2SO_4}$. It occurs in the form of dark-brown thin translucent scales, yellow when in powder, with a strong bitter taste, soluble in water and in alcohol. Its watery solution gives a white precipitate with chloride of barium; and with caustic soda a yellowish-white precipitate, which is dissolved by agitating the mixture with twice its volume of ether. The ethereal solution, separated by a pipette and evaporated, leaves a yellow translucent residue, entirely soluble in dilute acids. Entirely destructible by heat. Water forms with it a clear brown solution.

*Properties.*—Tonic and antiperiodic.

*Therapeutic Uses.*—In intermittent and remittent fevers, neuralgia, tic douloureux, and other affections exhibiting periodicity, it has been used as a substitute for sulphate of quinine, to which, however, it is much inferior in power.

*Dose.*—From one to five grains as a tonic; from five to ten grains thrice daily as an antiperiodic. It is conveniently exhibited in solution with a few drops of dilute sulphuric acid.

## CINNAMOMUM ZEYLANICUM, *Nees*. CEYLON CINNAMON TREE.

(*Wight, Icones*, vol. i. t. 123.)

*Habitat.* — Ceylon. Cultivated in India, Java, Cayenne, &c.

*Officinal Part.*—The inner bark of shoots from the truncated stocks (*Cinnamomi Cortex, Cinnamon Bark*). It occurs in closely-rolled quills, which are about four lines in diameter, containing several smaller quills within them, of a light yellowish-brown colour, fragrant odour, and warm, sweet, aromatic taste. Breaks with a splintery fracture. Its virtues reside principally in a volatile oil (*Oleum Cinnamomi*), in addition to which it contains tannin and a peculiar acid, *Cinnamic Acid.*

*Properties.*—Aromatic, stimulant, and carminative.

*Therapeutic Uses.*—In flatulence, flatulent colic, spasmodic affections of the bowels, atonic diarrhœa, and gastric irritation, it often proves effectual. It has been supposed to act as a stimulant of the uterine muscular fibre, and hence has been employed in menorrhagia, and in tedious labours depending upon insufficiency of uterine contractions. Given also as a stimulant, with other medicines of the same class, in the advanced stages of fever.

*Dose.*—From five to twenty grains of the powdered bark. Rarely prescribed alone.

*Preparations.* — **Cinnamon Water** (*Aqua Cinnamomi*). Take of Cinnamon Bark, bruised, twenty ounces; Water, two gallons. Distil one gallon.

*Dose.*—From one to two ounces. Chiefly used as a vehicle for other medicines. It enters into Mistura Cretæ, Mistura Guaiaci, and Mistura Spiritus Vini Gallici.

**Oil of Cinnamon** (*Oleum Cinnamomi*). The oil obtained by distillation from Cinnamon Bark; of a yellowish colour when recently prepared; gradually becomes red; has the odour and taste of cinnamon. Sinks in water.

*Dose.*—From two to five minims. A good stimulant carminative, used as an adjunct to other stimulants in the advanced stages of fever. A drop or two, introduced into a carious tooth, occasionally relieves toothache. Applied to the temples it often relieves headache (Dr. Shortt).

**Tincture of Cinnamon** (*Tinctura Cinnamomi*).—Take of Cinnamon Bark, in coarse powder, two ounces and a half; Proof Spirit, one pint. Macerate the cinnamon for forty-eight hours in fifteen fluid ounces of the spirit, in a closed vessel, agitating occasionally; then transfer to a percolator, and, when the fluid ceases to pass, continue the percolation with the remaining five ounces of spirit. Afterwards subject the contents of the percolator to pressure, filter the product, mix the liquids, and add sufficient proof spirit to make one pint.

*Dose.*—From one to two fluid drachms. A good adjunct to stimulant and carminative mixtures.

**Compound Cinnamon Powder** (*Pulvis Cinnamomi compositus, Pulvis Aromaticus, Edin. Ph.*) Take of Cinnamon Bark, in powder, Cardamom Seeds, in powder, Ginger, in powder, of each one ounce. Mix them thoroughly, pass the powder through a fine sieve, and finally rub it lightly in a mortar. Keep it in a stoppered bottle.

*Dose.*—From three to ten grains.

Cinnamon also forms an ingredient in Infusum Catechu, Decoctum Hæmatoxyli, Acidum Sulphuricum aromaticum, Pulvis Catechu compositus, Pulv. Cretæ aromaticus, Pulv. Kino compositus, Tinctura Cardamomi composita, Tinct. Catechu, Tinct. Lavandulæ composita, and Vinum Opii.

[From the leaves of the Cinnamon tree there is prepared in Ceylon, by maceration in sea water and subsequent distillation, a volatile oil (*Oleum Cinnamomi foliorum*). It is of a dark-yellow or brownish colour, and taste and odour analogous to those of cloves. Sp. gr. 1·050. It has been examined by Dr. Stenhouse (*Pharm. Journ.*, Jan. 1855, vol. xiv. p. 320), who found it to be, like the oil of cloves, essentially a mixture of eugenic acid and a neutral hydrocarbon having the formula $C^{20}H^{16}$. It is remarkable, however, for containing a small quantity of benzoic acid. In its medicinal properties and uses it approximates closely to oil of cloves.]

(*Non-officinal.*)

**Cinnamomum aromaticum**, *Nees.*—*C. Cassia, Blume.*—(*Wight, Icones*, vol. i. t. 136.) A native of China, supposed to yield the Cassia bark (*Cortex Cassiæ, Cassia lignea*) of commerce, or at any rate that portion of the article imported into Europe and India from China viâ Singapore. It appears certain that Cassia bark is a produce also of the Malabar coast; but the tree which yields it is undetermined, though probably it is **Cinnamomum Zeylanicum**, *var.* **Cassia**, *Nees*, which is not uncommon in Travancore, Malabar, and other portions of the western coast of the Madras Peninsula. The inner bark of **C. iners**, *Reinw.* (*Wight, Icones*, vol. i. t. 130. (*C. Malabathrum, G. Don.*) possesses in the fresh state a powerful cinnamomic odour and taste, and by careful drying and preparation appears capable of affording cassia lignea of good quality.([58]) Cassia bark usually occurs in single quills, very seldom more than double, considerably thicker than cinnamon. The outer surface, as compared with cinnamon, is darker, reddish-brown, and duller; the fracture of the inner portion of the bark, sharper and less fibrous. The powder possesses a deeper reddish-brown tint; and the taste and odour, though strongly cinnamomic, are less purely so, the taste being not so sweet but more pungent, leaving an impression of bitterness in the mouth; odour far less agreeable. By distillation it yields a volatile oil (*Oleum Cassiæ*), which in properties and uses closely resembles Oil of Cinnamon. *Cassia Buds*, the immature flowers of an undetermined species of Cinnamomum, are chiefly brought from China. A variety of these, however, met with in the Travancore bazaars, was found by the Editor to be the produce of *C. iners*. They are employed by the natives of that part of India, variously combined, in diarrhœa, dysentery, and coughs. They partake of the carminative properties of Cinnamon and Cassia.

**Cinnamomum Tamala**, *Nees*, and **C. eucalyptoides**, *Nees* (*C. nitidum, Hooker*). The leaves of these two species, and probably of other allied species indigenous or naturalized in India, are supposed to have furnished the *Folia Malabathri* seu *Tamalpathri* or *Indian Leaf* of old pharmacologists. They were held in considerable repute by the ancients for their stomachic and sudorific properties (*Dr. Adams' Transl. of Paulus Ægineta*, vol. iii. p. 238), and they still constitute an article of the Indian Materia Medica under the name of *Tej* or *Tedj pat*, the *Tudje* of the Taleef Shereef (p. 55, No. 291). They partake of the aroma and pungency, and probably also of the carminative properties of Cinnamon. They are of minor importance.

**Cinnamomum parthenoxylon**, *Meissner* (*Wight, Icones*, vol. v. t. 1832). A forest tree of Penang, Sumatra, and Java, the *Kayogadis* of the Malays. The fruit has a strong balsamic smell, and yields an oil, which is regarded as highly serviceable in rheumatic affections. An infusion of the root is employed in the same class of cases in which sassafras is usually administered. Jack suggests that this may be the *Oriental Sassafras wood* mentioned in the article *Laurus* in Rees' Cyclopœdia; and if this surmise be correct, it is probably identical with that Lauraceous tree of the Tenasserim provinces, known to the Burmese by the name of *Hman-then;* the root, much used for carpentry and housebuilding, closely resembles in odour the officinal Sassafras, as a substitute for which it was used by the Editor, but with no very satisfactory results (*Indian Ann. of Med. Sci.*, 1858, vol. v. p. 600). The "Sassafras of Nepal," supposed to be an excellent substitute for the officinal article, is the produce of **Cinnamomum glanduliferum**, *Meissner*, a tree of the mountains of Nepal, Sikkim, Bhootan, and Khasia, an account of which is given by Dr. Wallich (*Calcutta Med. Phys. Trans.*, vol. i. p. 45, *cum tab.*) It seems worthy of more attention than has been awarded to it.

## SANTALACEÆ.

(*Non-officinal.*)

**Santalum album**, *Linn.—Sirium myrtifolium, Linn.*—(*Bot. Mag.*, t. 3235.) The wood of this tree, *Sandal wood* (*Saféd Chandan*, i.e. *White Sandal wood*, in contradistinction to *Lal Chandan, Red Sandal wood*, the product of *Pterocarpus santalinus*), has long held a place in Eastern Materia Medica (see *Adams' Transl. of Paulus Ægineta*, vol. iii. p. 448), and is employed in fevers, indigestion, palpitations, and many other affections. The wood, ground up with water to the consistence of paste, is one of the most common applications at the present day, amongst all classes of natives, to erysipelatous and local inflammations, or to the temples in fevers, and to skin diseases to allay heat and pruritus. Dr. Æ. Ross reports having subjected to trial the wood, both in a state of powder and in decoction; and whilst its effects as a stimulant were very slight, he observed as a secondary effect a sedative action on the circulation; in some cases it occasioned nausea. In remittent fevers in which it was administered, it acted as a diaphoretic, diminishing at the same time the rapidity rather than the violence of the heart's action. By distillation it yields between two and three per cent. of a pale yellow volatile oil, with the peculiar fragrant odour of the wood.[59] In India the chief use of this oil is as a perfume; but attention has recently been called to it by Dr. T. B. Henderson, of Glasgow, as a remedy in gonorrhœa. In a communication from that gentleman to the Editor, he states that he has employed it during the last five years in more than one hundred cases, and with the most satisfactory results. He prescribes from thirty to forty minims thrice daily, diluted with three parts of Rectified Spirit, and flavoured with Oil of Cassia or Cinnamon. In some cases beneficial effects were evident within forty-eight hours. He regards it as equal, and frequently superior, to Copaiba and Cubebs, having found it sometimes to succeed when both these remedies had previously failed. Its comparatively pleasant taste and smell also give it a great advantage over Copaiba. It has not been observed to communicate any strong odour to the urine. The success of Dr. Henderson with this remedy fully justifies extended trials with it in India, where it can be procured abundantly at a moderate cost.

## ARISTOLOCHIACEÆ.

### ARISTOLOCHIA SERPENTARIA, *Linn.* SERPENTARY OR VIRGINIAN SNAKE ROOT.

(*Woodville, Med. Bot.*, t. 59; *Steph. et Church, Med. Bot.*, vol. iii. t. 180.)

*Habitat.*—North America.

*Officinal Part.*—The dried Root (*Serpentariæ Radix, Serpentary Root*). A small roundish rhizome, with a tuft of numerous slender radicles about three inches long, yellowish, of an agreeable camphoraceous odour, and warm bitter camphoraceous taste. It contains a volatile oil and a bitter extractive principle.

*Properties.*—Stimulant, tonic, and diaphoretic.

*Therapeutic Uses.*—In the advanced stages and in the adynamic forms of fever, it has been found serviceable. In the bites of venomous snakes it formerly enjoyed high repute; it has also been employed in some forms of dyspepsia, gout and skin disease, and locally as a gargle in various affections of the throat.

*Dose.*—From ten to thirty grains of the dried root in infusion.

*Preparations.*—**Infusion of Serpentary** (*Infusum Serpentariæ*). Take of Serpentary Root a quarter of an ounce; Boiling Water, ten fluid ounces. Infuse in a covered vessel for two hours and strain.

*Dose.*—From one to two fluid ounces, three or four times daily.

**Tincture of Serpentary** (*Tinctura Serpentariæ*). Take of Serpentary Root, bruised, two ounces and a half; Proof Spirit, one pint. Macerate the serpentary for forty-eight hours in fifteen fluid ounces of the spirit, in a closed vessel, agitating occasionally; then transfer to a percolator, and, when the fluid ceases to pass, continue the percolation with the remaining five ounces of the spirit. Afterwards subject the contents of the percolator to pressure, filter the product, mix the liquids, and add sufficient proof spirit to make one pint.

*Dose.*—From one to two fluid drachms. A good adjunct to stimulant and diaphoretic mixtures.

Serpentaria is an ingredient in Tinctura Cinchonæ composita.

(*Non-officinal.*)

**Aristolochia Indica**, *Linn.* (*Rheede, Hort. Mal.*, vol. viii. t. 25.). This twining shrub is common throughout India. The root, which is very bitter, is held in much esteem by the natives as a stimulant, tonic, and emmenagogue, and is employed by them in intermittent fevers and other affections. Nothing certain is known of its virtues; but Dr. Kirkpatrick (*Cat. of Mysore Drugs*, No. 455) considers that its properties as a febrifuge are deserving of investigation; and Dr. Fleming, judging from the aromatic bitterness of the root, is of opinion that it will be found useful in dyspepsia (*Asiat. Researches*, vol. xi.) Dr. Gibson regards it as valuable n bowel affections. From its sensible properties, and the high esteem in which it is held by the natives, it may be worthy of further notice. It is as an antidote to snake bites, however, that it has obtained most repute, and by the early Portuguese settlers was termed *Raiz de Cobra*, from its supposed efficacy in those cases, even in the bite of the Cobra de Capello. The leaves, and the expressed juice of the leaves, have more recently been brought to notice in the same class of cases by Mr. Lowther (*Journ. of Agri.-Hort. Soc. of India*, 1846, vol. v. pp. 138, 742, and vol. vii. p. 42.) His testimony in its favour is very strong[60]; but so many elements of doubt surround the subject of snake bites and their antidotes, that further evidence is required to establish its character (*Madras Quart. Med. Journ.*, 1861, vol. iii. p. 336 *et seq.*).

**Aristolochia bracteata**, *Retz.* A common plant throughout India. Agrees with the preceding species as being nauseously bitter. It is well known by its Hindústani name, *Kirá-már*, from its supposed anthelmintic properties, and also probably from the fact of the expressed juice of the leaves being applied to foul and neglected ulcers, for the purpose of destroying the larvæ of insects. A belief in the anthelmintic virtues of the leaves is common amongst the natives, but facts based on European experience are wanting to substantiate its claims to this character. In Dalzell and Gibson's Flora of Bombay (p. 225) it is spoken of as possessing "a merited reputation as an antiperiodic in intermittent fevers." Emmenagogue properties are also assigned to it. Dr. J. Newton reports that in Scinde the dried root, in doses of about a drachm and a half, in the form of powder or in infusion, is administered during labours to increase uterine contractions.

**Bragantia Wallichii**, *R. Brown.* (*Wight, Icones*, vol. ii. t. 520.) A small shrub of the Malabar Coast, where it is known by the name of *Alpam.* The juice of the leaves, like that of many plants of this Natural Order, is valued as an antidote in venomous snake bites, especially in that of the Cobra. Fra Bartolomeo (Voyage, p. 416) quotes a Malabar proverb, to the effect "as soon as Alpam enters the body, poison leaves it." **B. tomentosa**, *Blume*, possesses intense bitterness, and, according to Horsfield, is employed by the Javanese as an emmenagogue.

# EUPHORBIACEÆ.

## CROTON ELUTERIA, *Bennett.* CASCARILLA.

(*Bennett, Pharm. Journ., 2nd Series*, vol. iv. p. 150. t. 1.)

*Habitat.*—The Bahamas.

*Officinal Part.*—The Bark (*Cascarillæ Cortex, Cascarilla Bark*). It occurs in quills, two or three inches in length, and from two to five lines in diameter, dull brown, but more or less coated with white crustaceous lichens; breaks with a short resinous fracture; is warm and bitter to the taste; and emits a fragrant odour when burned. It contains a volatile oil, tannin, and a bitter crystallizable principle, *Cascarilline.*

*Properties.*—Aromatic, bitter, and tonic.

*Therapeutic Uses.*—In general debility, in atonic dyspepsia, and in the advanced stages of diarrhœa and dysentery, it proves serviceable. It was formerly employed in intermittent fevers, though it has now fallen into disuse for this purpose; it is an excellent tonic in convalescence after febrile attacks.

*Dose.*—From ten to thirty grains of the powdered bark.

*Preparations.*—**Infusion of Cascarilla** (*Infusum Cascarillæ*). Take of Cascarilla, in coarse powder, one ounce; Boiling Water, ten fluid ounces. Infuse in a covered vessel for one hour, and strain.

*Dose.*—From one to two fluid ounces, twice or thrice daily.

**Tincture of Cascarilla** (*Tinctura Cascarillæ*). Take of Cascarilla, bruised, two ounces and a half: Proof Spirit, one pint. Macerate the cascarilla for forty-eight hours, in fifteen fluid ounces of the spirit, in a closed vessel, agitating occasionally; then transfer to a percolator, and, when the fluid ceases to pass, continue the percolation with the remaining five ounces of the spirit. Afterwards subject the contents of the percolator to pressure, filter the product, mix the liquids, and add sufficient proof spirit to make one pint.

*Dose.*—From one to two fluid drachms; a useful adjunct to tonic mixtures.

## CROTON TIGLIUM, *Linn.* THE PURGING CROTON.

(*Rheede, Hort. Mal.*, vol. ii. t. 332; *Steph. et Church, Med. Bot.*, vol. i. t. 4.)

*Habitat.*—Both Peninsulas of India, the Moluccas, Ceylon.

*Officinal Part.*—The Seeds (*Crotonis Semina, Croton seeds*). About the size of a grain of coffee, oval or oval-oblong, of a rounded or imperfectly quadrangular form; testa, dark brown or blackish, and marked with the ramifications of the raphé; endocarp, thin, brittle, and of a light odour; nucleus consists of yellowish albumen, inclosing a large dicotyledonous leafy embryo; inodorous; taste at first mild, subsequently acrid and pungent.

*Properties and Uses.*—Powerful drastic purgative; in over doses an acro-narcotic poison. Externally applied, stimulant and rubefacient (61).

*Preparations.*—**Croton Oil** (*Oleum Crotonis, Croton Oil*); the oil obtained by expression from Croton seeds; it is slightly viscid, of a brownish yellow colour, acrid taste, and faintly nauseous odour. *Test.*—Agitated with its own volume of alcohol, and gently heated, it forms a clear solution, from which about three fourths of the oil separate on cooling.

*Properties.*—Powerful hydragogue cathartic. Externally rubefacient and counter-irritant.

*Therapeutic Uses.*—In dropsical affections, in obstinate constipaion, especially in that met with in insanity and other affections of the brain, in apoplexy and other cases when it is desired to act speedily and powerfully on the bowels, it may be employed with advantage.

*Dose.*—From half a drop to two or even three drops, made into pills with bread crumb. In apoplexy, coma, and other cases where the patient is unable to swallow, it is sufficient to place the oil at the base of the tongue. Hypercatharsis may be controlled by copious draughts of diluted lemon or lime juice, or vinegar.

**Liniment of Croton Oil** (*Linimentum Crotonis*). Take of Croton Oil, half a fluid ounce; Olive Oil, three fluid ounces and a half. Mix.

A useful stimulant application in chronic rheumatism, paralytic affections, diseases of the joints, and to the chest in phthisis, chronic bronchitis, and other pulmonary affections. It gives rise to a vesicular eruption.

[The seeds of **Baliospermum montanum**, *Müll.*—*Croton Roxburghii, Wall.*—(*Wight, Icones*, vol. v. t. 1885)—**Croton Pavana**, *Ham.*, and **C. oblongifolius**, *Roxb.*, partake of the purgative properties of *C. Tiglium*. These species are more or less common throughout India.]

## RICINUS COMMUNIS, *Linn.* THE CASTOR OIL PLANT.

(*Rheede, Hort. Mal.*, vol. ii. t. 32; *Steph. et Church, Med. Bot.*, vol. i. t. 50.)

*Habitat.*—Cultivated in the temperate and tropical portions of both hemispheres.

*Officinal Part.*—The Seeds (62) (*Ricini Semina*). Oval, somewhat compressed, about four lines long and three lines broad, varying in weight from two to eight grains, and marked externally with grey, reddish-brown, or blackish-brown spots and stripes. The seed is covered with a thin, coriaceous, smooth seed-coat, composed of two layers, the external one thick and dark brown, the inner one thinner and paler. The nucleus consists of an oily albumen, enclosing a large dicotyledonous leafy embryo.

*Properties and Uses.*—Purgative; in large doses an acro-narcotic poison. The seeds are only officinal as the source of Castor Oil.

*Preparation.*—**Castor Oil** (*Oleum Ricini*). The oil obtained by expression from Castor Oil seeds. It is viscid, colourless, or of a pale straw colour, having a slightly nauseous odour, and somewhat acrid taste. Entirely soluble in one volume of alcohol and in two volumes of rectified spirit.

*Properties and Therapeutic Uses.*—A mild and efficient purgative, well adapted for childhood, the puerperal state, inflammatory conditions of the alimentary canal (when aperients are admissible), or of the genito-urinary organs. In some forms of dyspepsia and spasmodic affections of the bowels, it produces beneficial results.

*Dose.*—From six to ten fluid drachms for adults; from one to two fluid drachms for children.

Castor oil is an ingredient in Collodion Flexile, Linimentum Sinapis compositum, and Pilula Hydrargyri Subchloridi composita.

[The leaves of the Castor Oil plant possess considerable power as a lactagogue. For this purpose a decoction, or the expressed juice, is prescribed internally; and fomentations with the decoction, together with cataplasms of the boiled leaves, applied locally to the mammæ, are employed. Dr. J. Shortt reports having employed successfully for this purpose the leaves simply warmed and applied to the mammæ.]

## MALLOTUS PHILIPPIENSIS, *Müll.*

(*Rottlera tinctoria*, Roxb., *Brit. Pharm.*)

(*Roxb., Corom. Plants*, t. 168.)

*Habitat.*—Hilly districts throughout India.

*Officinal Part.*—A powder which consists of minute glands that cover the capsules (*Kamala*). It is a fine granular mobile powder, of a dark purplish-red colour: it is with difficulty mixed with water, but when boiled with alcohol the greater part is dissolved, forming a red solution. Ether dissolves most of it; the residue consisting principally of tufted hairs. It should be free from sand or earthy impurities.

*Properties and Therapeutic Uses.*—Anthelmintic, especially adapted for the expulsion of tænia ([63]); purgative.

*Dose.*—From two to three drachms. In these doses it acts freely on the bowels, causing in many cases considerable nausea and griping; the entozoa are generally expelled in a lifeless state in the third or fourth stool.

*Preparation.*—**Tincture of Kamala** (*Tinctura Kamalæ*). Take of Kamala, six ounces; Rectified Spirit, one pint. Macerate for seven days in a closed vessel with occasional agitation; then strain, press, and filter, and add sufficient rectified spirit to make one pint.

*Dose.*—Half a fluid ounce, in two equal doses, at an interval of three hours, in some aromatic water. This preparation has been found to act as a purgative more mildly than the powder in substance, and at the same time to be equally efficient as an anthelmintic.

(*Non-officinal.*)

**Aleurites triloba,** *Forst.* (*Belgaum* or *Indian Walnut*). The kernels of this Molluccan tree, cultivated in many parts of India, yield on expression a large proportion of a fixed oil, which has been pronounced by the Madras Drug Committee (*Madras Med. Reports*, 1855, p. 428) to be superior to linseed oil for purposes connected with the arts. Its medicinal properties have been examined by Dr. O'Rorke (*Ann. de Thérap.*, 1859, p. 117), who found that in doses varying from one to two ounces it acted as a mild and sure purgative, producing in from three to six hours after ingestion free bilious evacuations, its operation being unattended either by nausea, colic, or other ill effects. It was found to approach nearly to castor oil in the mildness and certainty of its operation, but superior to it as having neither taste nor smell, and as producing its cathartic action without causing any degree of nausea, whether administered in emulsion or in a pure state. It may be worthy of further attention.

**Jatropha Curcas,** *Linn.* Is common in the tropical portions of both hemispheres. Its seeds (*English Physic Nuts*) yield on expression about 30 per cent. of a colourless, or pale yellow, very mobile fixed oil, which, according to Guibourt (*Hist. des Drogues Simpl.*, vol. ii. p. 334), differs from castor oil by its very slight solubility in alcohol, not dissolving in 24 parts of alcohol. For a chemical history of this oil see *Chemical Gazette*, Dec. 15th, 1854, p. 496. Prof. Christison (*On Poisons*, p. 591) found by experiment that twelve or fifteen drops of the oil produced exactly the same effect as an ounce of castor oil, though not with such certainty. The want of uniformity observed in its action, mentioned more in detail in the Edinburgh Dispensatory, p. 794, is a serious drawback to its general employment as a purgative. In over doses the seeds act as an acro-narcotic poison. The diluted oil forms a useful embrocation in chronic rheumatism. The leaves are extensively employed in the Cape de Verd Islands, in the form of decoction and cataplasm to the mammæ, as a lactagogue, in the same manner as those of the castor oil plant (Dr. McWilliam, *Lancet*, 1850, vol. i. p. 294). The seeds of **Jatropha multifida,** *Linn.* (*French Physic Nuts*) are regarded as even more powerfully purgative than those of *C. purgans*. The Editor once saw a case of poisoning from three of these nuts. Violent vomiting and purging, intense pain and heat in the stomach, with great prostration of the vital powers, were the principal symptoms. The patient, a young man, recovered under the use of lime juice diluted with water, and stimulants. Under the name of *Coral Plant* (so called from the peculiar coral-like appearance of the flowering tops), it is often cultivated in the gardens of Europeans in India. The seeds of **Jatropha glandulifera**, *Roxb.*, a plant probably of African origin, now common near tanks throughout India, yield by expression a fixed oil, held in much esteem by the Hindús as a stimulant application in rheumatism and paralysis (Ainslie, *Mat. Ind.*, vol. ii. p. 6, and *Madras Med. Topog.*, *art. Ceded Districts*, p. 6).

**Euphorbia antiquorum**, *Linn.* (*Wight, Icones*, vol. iii. t. 897), **E. Tirucalli**, *Linn.* (*Rheede, Hort. Mal.*, vol. ii. t. 44), and **E. Nivulia**, *Ham.* (*Wight, Icones*, vol. v. t. 1862). These three Indian species abound in a milky juice, which in the fresh state is highly acrid. Cathartic, anthelmintic, and other virtues are ascribed to them by the natives, but little trustworthy is known concerning them. *E. antiquorum* was long supposed to yield the Euphorbium of the shops; but this has been disproved by Hamilton (*Linn. Trans.*, vol. xiv.), and Royle (*Illust.*, vol. i. p. 328). The fresh milky juice of *E. Tirucalli* is said to be an effectual application for the removal of warts, and, incorporated with any bland oil, is used in common with the milky juice of other species as a rubefacient embrocation in rheumatism. The inspissated milky juice formerly enjoyed great repute in India as an antisyphilitic (*Ives' Voyage to India*, p. 462, and *Sonnerat Voyage*, vol. i. p. 146); and Dr. J. Shortt reports having found it an excellent alterative in these cases in doses of five grains night and morning. Horsfield (*Asiat. Journ.*, vol. vii. p. 265) mentions a case of dropsy in which he prescribed the inspissated juice of *E. Nivulia* in doses of a few (?) grains as a diuretic, and states that it was productive of evident relief.

**Euphorbia nerlifolia**, *Linn.*—*E. ligularia*, *Roxb.* (*Munsa Sij*, *Beng.*), common in many parts of India, is sacred to Munsa, the goddess of serpents. The root enjoys almost universal repute as a remedy in snake bites, but there is no reliable evidence of its utility in these cases. The expressed juice of the leaves is reported to prove very effectual in relieving the paroxysms of spasmodic asthma. Six cases in which it afforded marked and uniform relief are recorded by Dr. S. C. Amesbury, of the Bengal Medical Service (*Indian Ann. of Med. Sci.* 1861, vol. vii. p. 516). Considering the acrid nature of the plants of this family, caution should be employed in its use.

**Phyllanthus Emblica**, *Linn.* (*Wight, Icones*, vol. v. t. 1896), a tree common throughout India, the fruit of which constitutes *Emblic Myrobalans* (*Amla*, Hind.) In the fresh state they are round, of the size of a gall nut, with six valves projecting externally; pulp, fleshy, acidulous, enveloping white angular seeds, and possessed of purgative properties. In the dry state they are roundish, sub-hexagonal, wrinkled, of a blackish grey colour, slightly aromatic odour and acidulous astringent taste. In the latter state they are employed in the process of tanning, and are highly valued as an astringent in bowel complaints. Bontius (*Diseases of India*, p. 200) testifies to their value in the treatment of diarrhœa and dysentery, in the hospitals of Batavia in his day. Antiscorbutic virtues have also been attributed to them by Dr. D. McNab (*Calcutta Med. Phys. Trans.*, vol. viii., and *Calcutta Quart. Med. Journ.* 1837, vol. i. p. 306); but Dr. Irvine (*Med. Topog. of Ajmeer*, p. 118) is of opinion that they do not possess any peculiar virtue in this respect, and that they are not superior to any other acid vegetable astringent. He mentions that they contain a large proportion of gallic acid. The flowers of this tree are employed by the Hindu doctors for their supposed refrigerent and aperient qualities (Ainslie, *Mat. Ind.*, vol. ii. p. 244). The bark partakes of the astringency of the ripe fruit. Dr. Æ. Ross reports having prepared from the root, by decoction and evaporation, an astringent extract equal to catechu, both for medicinal purposes and in the arts; he adds, that chips of the wood or small branches thrown into impure or muddy water, clear it effectually; hence the wood is much employed by the natives in making well rings. This point is worthy of further inquiry.

**Phyllanthus Niruri,** *Linn.* (*Wight, Icones*, vol. v. t. 1894), and **P. urinaria,** *Linn.* (*Rheede, Hort. Mal.*, vol. x. t. 16), two plants indigenous throughout India, are held in considerable repute by the natives as diuretics, and as such are much employed in dropsical affections, also in gonorrhœa, and other genito-urinary affections. They have been mentioned favourably by Horsfield and others, but they do not appear to possess any special claims to notice.

**Acalypha Indica,** *Linn.* (*Wight, Icones*, vol. iii. t. 877). With reference to this plant, which is widely distributed throughout India, Dr. George Bidie furnishes the following remarks:—"The "expressed juice of the leaves is in great repute, wherever the "plant grows, as an emetic for children, and is safe, certain, "and speedy in its action. Like Ipecacuanha, it seems to have "little tendency to act on the bowels or depress the vital powers, "and it decidedly increases the secretion of the pulmonary or-"gans. Probably an infusion of the dried leaves, or an extract "prepared from the green plant, would retain all its active "properties. The dose of the expressed juice, for an infant, is "a teaspoonful." Dr. Æ. Ross speaks highly of its use as an expectorant, ranking it in this respect with Senega; he found it especially useful in the bronchitis of children. He reports also favorably of a cataplasm of the leaves as a local application to syphilitic ulcers; and as a means of relieving the pain and irritation attendant on the bites of venomous insects. The alleged purgative action of the root noticed by Ainslie (*Mat. Ind.*, vol. ii. p. 161) is confirmed by Dr. H. E. Busteed, who reports having used the expressed juice of the root and leaves as a laxative for children.

## PIPERACEÆ.

### PIPER NIGRUM, *Linn.* BLACK PEPPER VINE.

(*Wight, Icones,* vol. vi. t. 1934.)

*Habitat.*—India; cultivated in the West Indies.

*Officinal Part.*—The dried unripe Berries (*Piper Nigrum, Black Pepper*); small, roundish, wrinkled; tegument brownish-black, containing a greyish-yellow globular seed; odour, aromatic; taste, pungent and bitterish. They contain a volatile oil, an acrid resin, and a crystalline principle, *Piperine.*

*Properties.*—Stimulant, carminative, antiperiodic; externally applied, rubefacient.

*Therapeutic Uses.*—Amongst other affections in which it has been employed are hæmorrhoidal affections, intermittent fevers, cholera, and gonorrhœa. Locally, in the form of gargle, it has been employed in various affections of the throat.

*Dose.*—From ten to fifteen grains or more; of Piperine, as an antiperiodic, from six to ten grains twice daily.

*Preparation.*—**Confection of Pepper** (*Confectio Piperis*). Take of Black Pepper, in fine powder, two ounces; Caraway Fruit, in fine powder, three ounces; Clarified Honey, fifteen ounces. Rub them well together in a mortar.

*Dose.*—From one to two drachms twice or thrice daily. It is especially adapted for the hæmorrhoidal affections of the aged, or in persons of debilitated constitution; it also proves useful in relaxed conditions of the rectum attended with prolapsus.

Black pepper is also an ingredient in Confectio Opii, and Pulvis Opii compositus.

## CUBEBA OFFICINALIS, *Miquel.* OFFICINAL CUBEB.

(*Hayne,* vol. xiv. t. 8.; *Steph. et Church, Med. Bot.,* vol. iii. t. 175.)

*Habitat.*—Java and the Moluccas.

*Officinal Part.*—The dried unripe Fruit (*Cubeba, Cubebs*), usually about the size of black pepper, globular, wrinkled, blackish, supported on a stalk of rather more than its own length; has an acrid camphoraceous taste, and a peculiar aromatic odour. Within the shell is a hard, spherical, whitish, oily seed. It contains a volatile oil, an acrid resin, and a crystalline principle (*Cubebin*) very similar to Piperine.

*Properties.*—Stimulant, its action being chiefly directed to mucous membranes, especially to that of the genito-urinary organs.

*Therapeutic Uses.*—In gonorrhœa it is a remedy of established value. It has likewise been employed with advantage in leucorrhœa, cystirrhœa, chronic inflammation of the prostate gland, hæmorrhoids, and in chronic bronchitic and other pulmonary affections.

*Dose.*—From thirty grains to two drachms, three or four times daily.

*Preparations.*—**Oil of Cubebs** (*Oleum Cubebæ*). Oil obtained by distillation from Cubebs; it is colourless, or of a pale greenish-yellow colour, having the peculiar odour and taste of cubebs.

*Dose.*—From five to twenty minims.

**Tincture of Cubebs** (*Tinctura Cubebæ.*) Take of Cubebs, in powder, two ounces and a half; Rectified Spirit, one pint. Macerate the cubebs for forty-eight hours in fifteen fluid ounces of the spirit, in a closed vessel, agitating occasionally; then transfer to a percolator, and, when the fluid ceases to pass, continue the percolation with the remaining five ounces of spirit. Afterwards subject the contents of the percolator to pressure, filter the product, mix the liquids, and add sufficient rectified spirit to make one pint.

*Dose.*—From thirty minims to two fluid drachms.

## ARTANTHE ELONGATA, *Miquel.* MATICO PLANT.

(*Piper angustifolium, Ruiz et Pavon.*)

(*Ruiz et Pavon, Flor. Peruv.*, t. 57.)

*Habitat.*—Peru.

*Officinal Part.*—The dried Leaves (*Maticæ Folia, Matico Leaves*); from two to eight inches in length; veined and tessellated on the upper surface, downy beneath, with an aromatic slighty astringent taste, and an agreeable aromatic odour.

*Properties.*—Astringent; locally applied a powerful styptic.

*Therapeutic Uses.*—In hæmatemesis, hæmaturia, hæmoptysis, menorrhagia, and other passive forms of hæmorrhage, also in leucorrhœa and atonic diarrhœa, it has been employed with alleged benefit. For the purpose of arresting hæmorrhage from superficial wounds, it proves very effectual; for this purpose the under surface of the leaf, or the powdered leaves, should be applied to the bleeding surface.

*Dose.*—From half a drachm to one drachm of the powdered leaves.

*Preparation.*—**Infusion of Matico** (*Infusum Maticæ*). Take of Matico Leaves, cut small, half an ounce; Boiling Water, ten fluid ounces. Infuse in a covered vessel for half an hour, and strain.

*Dose.*—From one to four fluid ounces.

*(Non-officinal.)*

**Chavica Roxburghii,** *Miquel — Piper longum,* Linn. — (*Wight, Icones,* vol. vi. t. 1928). A native of India, cultivated in Bengal and other parts of India for the sake of its fruit, the *Long Pepper* of commerce. It is an inch or more in length, cylindrical, of a greyish-brown colour, mild aromatic odour, and acrid very pungent taste. Like Black Pepper, it contains a volatile oil, an acrid resin and piperine; and, like it, it possesses stimulant carminative properties, but more powerful. Its chief use is as a condiment. Dr. Herklots reports favourably of the following Mahomedan nostrum in the treatment of beri-beri: Take of Long Pepper, bruised, four ounces; Black Pepper and Ginger, of each half an ounce; Arrack, twenty ounces. Macerate for seven days and strain. Dose, a drachm twice or thrice daily. A powerful stimulant, with probably no special claim to notice. The root is in great repute amongst the natives of India; it is the *Peepla-mool* of the Taleef Shereef (p. 55, No. 275), where it is described as bitter, stomachic, and useful in promoting digestion. In Travancore an infusion of the root is prescribed after parturition, with the view of causing the expulsion of the placenta. It appears to partake, in a minor degree, in the stimulant properties of the fruit. Ainslie (*Mat. Ind.*, vol. ii. p. 416) states that in Southern India the aromatic jointed root of **Piper dichotomum,** *Rottler,* is prescribed in dyspepsia.

**Chavica Betle,** *Miquel — Piper Betle,* Linn. — (*Wight, Icones,* vol. vi. t. 1926). Cultivated throughout India for the sake of its leaves, which, in conjunction with lime and the nut of *Areca Catechu,* are almost universally employed as a masticatory. The juice of the leaves is regarded as a valuable stomachic. Amongst the Indo-Britons of Southern India a use is made of the leaves, which merits notice. In catarrhal and pulmonary affections generally, especially of children, the leaves warmed and smeared with oil are applied in layers over the chest; and the Editor, from personal observation in many instances, can testify to the relief afforded to the cough and dyspnœa, far more than can be accounted for by the warmth and exclusion of air, or by any rubefacient effect it produces, which indeed is very slight in most cases. Dr. Gibson, who corroborates this statement, states that he has often seen the application afford marked relief in congestion and other affections of the liver. Mr. J. Wood reports that the leaves warmed by the fire and applied in layers over the mammæ are used effectually for arresting the secretion of milk. Their use in this manner is also noticed by Dr. J. Shortt, who adds that the leaves are similarly employed as a resolvent to glandular swellings.

**Chavica officinarum,** *Miquel—Piper Chaba,* Hunter. A native of the Moluccas, cultivated in India for the sake of its fruit, which constitutes the *Chaab* of the Indian Materia Medica. It partakes of the stimulant and carminative properties of Black and Long Pepper, but does not appear to possess any special claim to notice. Its use in hæmorrhoidal affections is noticed in the Taleef Shereef (p. 66, No. 340).

# CUPULIFERÆ.

## QUERCUS ROBUR, *Linn.* THE COMMON OAK.

(*Steph. et Church, Med. Bot.*, vol. iii. t. 151.)

*Habitat.*—Woods and hedge-rows of Europe.

*Officinal Part.*—The dried Bark of the small branches and young stems (*Quercûs Cortex, Oak Bark*), collected in the spring. It occurs in pieces from one to two feet in length, covered with a greyish shining epidermis, cinnamon-coloured on the inner surface, fibrous, brittle, almost inodorous, of a strongly astringent taste. Its active constituents are Tannic and Gallic acids.

*Properties.*—Powerful astringent.

*Therapeutic Uses.*—In chronic diarrhœa, the advanced stages of dysentery, and intermittent fevers, it has been thought useful. It is chiefly employed, however, as a local or external application, in decoction, as an injection in leucorrhœa, atonic menorrhagia, and prolapsus of the uterus, as an enema in prolapsus of the rectum, and hæmorrhoidal affections, and as a gargle in relaxation of the uvula or tonsils, and in sponginess and ulceration of the gums. Poultices of the powdered bark have been applied with advantage to gangrenous and ill-conditioned ulcers.

*Dose.*—From half a drachm to a drachm of the powdered bark.

*Preparation.*—**Decoction of Oak Bark** (*Decoctum Quercûs*). Take of Oak Bark, bruised, one ounce and a quarter; Water, one pint. Boil for ten minutes in a covered vessel, then strain and pour as much distilled water over the contents of the strainer as will make the strained product measure a pint.

*Dose.*—From one to two fluid ounces, principally used as an external or local application.

## QUERCUS INFECTORIA, *Olivier.* THE GALL OR DYERS' OAK.

(*Steph. et Church, Med. Bot.*, vol. iii. t. 152.)

*Habitat.*—Asia Minor, extending to the borders of Persia.

*Officinal Part.*—Excrescences (*Galla, Galls*) caused by the punctures and deposited ova of Diplolepis Gallæ tinctoriæ, *Latr.* They are hard, heavy, globular bodies, varying in size from half to three fourths of an inch in diameter, tuberculated on the surface, the tubercles and intervening spaces smooth; of a bluish-green colour on the surface; yellowish-white within, with a small central cavity; intensely astringent. Their active constituents are Tannic and Gallic acids.

*Properties.*—Astringent, tonic, antiperiodic? (64)

*Therapeutic Uses.*—Very similar to those of Oak Bark. In the form of decoction, they are used also as an antidote in poisoning by Emetine and the alkaloids generally, and those vegetable products whose activity resides in an alkaloid, as opium and aconite. They have also been advised in poisoning by Tartar Emetic, but their antidotal powers require further investigation.

*Dose.*—From ten to twenty grains of powdered galls, three or four times daily.

*Preparations.*—***Decoction of Galls** (*Decoctum Gallæ*). Take of Galls, bruised, one ounce and a quarter; Water, one pint. Boil for ten minutes in a covered vessel, then strain, and pour as much distilled water over the contents of the strainer as will make the strained product measure a pint.

*Dose.*—From one to two fluid ounces. Chiefly used as an astringent gargle, enema, injection, or wash. May be exhibited freely in the cases of poisoning mentioned above.

**Tincture of Galls** (*Tinctura Gallæ*). Take of Galls, bruised, two ounces and a half; Proof Spirit, one pint. Macerate the galls for forty-eight hours in fifteen fluid ounces of the spirit, in a closed vessel, agitating occasionally; then transfer to a percolator, and, when the fluid ceases to pass, continue the percolation with the remaining five ounces of the spirit. Afterwards subject the contents of the percolator to pressure, filter the product, mix the liquids, and add sufficient proof spirit to make one pint.

*Dose.*—From half a drachm to two fluid drachms. Diluted, it is sometimes used as an astringent lotion.

**Ointment of Galls** (*Unguentum Gallæ*). Take of Galls, in very fine powder, eighty grains; Benzoated Lard or Simple Ointment, one ounce. Mix thoroughly.

**Ointment of Galls with Opium** (*Unguentum Gallæ cum Opio*). Take of Ointment of Galls, one ounce; Opium, in powder, thirty-two grains. Mix thoroughly.

Both these last preparations, the latter especially, are efficient applications to hæmorrhoids.

**Tannic Acid** (*Acidum Tannicum*). An Acid, $C_{54}H_{22}O_{34}$ or $C_{27}H_{22}O_{17}$, extracted from Galls. It occurs in the form of pale yellow vesicular masses or thin glistening scales, with a strongly astringent taste, and an acid reaction; readily soluble in water and rectified spirit, very sparingly soluble in ether. The aqueous solution precipitates solution of gelatine yellowish-white, and the persalts of iron of a bluish-black colour. It leaves no residue when burned with free access of air.

*Properties.*—Powerful astringent.

*Therapeutic Uses.*—In passive hæmorrhage from the lungs, stomach, uterus, or kidneys, it is an internal remedy of considerable value. In superficial hæmorrhage from the gums, or hæmorrhoidal tumors, and in epistaxis, tannin applied locally in substance suffices in many cases to arrest the discharge. Amongst the other diseases in which it has been prescribed internally with advantage are atonic dyspepsia, diarrhœa, bronchorrhœa, and phthisis, (chiefly with the view of checking the profuse perspiration and diarrhœa,) the chronic stage of hooping cough, leucorrhœa, nervous exhaustion, and intermittent fevers. As a local application, it has been found serviceable in ophthalmic and other diseases of the eye, ulcers and skin diseases attended with much discharge, hæmorrhoids, prolapsus and fissures of the anus, gonorrhœa and gleet (in the form of injection), ptyalism, sponginess of the gums, toothache, and sore or fissured nipples.

*Dose.*—From two to ten grains, three or four times daily or oftener, in powder, pill, or solution.

*Preparations of Tannic Acid.*—**Tannic Acid Suppositories** (*Suppositoria Acidi Tannici*). Take of Tannic Acid, thirty-six grains; Benzoated Lard, forty-four grains; White Wax, ten grains; Oil of Theobroma, ninety grains. Melt the wax and oil of theobroma with a gentle heat, then add the tannic acid and benzoated lard previously rubbed together in a mortar, and mix all the ingredients thoroughly. Pour the mixture while it is fluid into suitable moulds of the capacity of fifteen grains; or the fluid mixture may be allowed to cool, and then be divided into twelve equal parts, each of which shall be made into a conical or other convenient form for a suppository.

A useful application in affections arising from a relaxed condition of the mucous coat of the rectum and adjacent parts. Each suppository contains two grains of Tannic Acid.

**Tannic Acid Lozenges** (*Trochisci Acidi Tannici*). Take of Tannic Acid, three hundred and sixty grains;

Tincture of Tolu, half a fluid ounce; Refined Sugar, in powder, twenty-five ounces; Gum Acacia, in powder, one ounce; Mucilage of Gum Acacia, two fluid ounces; Distilled Water, one fluid ounce. Dissolve the tannic acid in the water; add this solution to the tincture of tolu, previously mixed with mucilage, and with the gum and the sugar, also previously mixed. Form the whole into a proper mass, and divide into 720 lozenges, and dry these in a hot-air chamber with a moderate heat.

Each lozenge contains half a grain of Tannic Acid.

In various affections of the mouth and throat, requiring the application of an astringent, these lozenges, allowed to dissolve slowly in the mouth, prove serviceable. As an internal remedy, they may be taken to the extent of ten or twenty daily.

**Glycerine of Tannic Acid** (*Glycerinum Acidi Tannici*). Take of Tannic Acid, one ounce; Glycerine, four fluid ounces. Rub them together in a mortar; then transfer the mixture to a porcelain dish, and apply gentle heat until complete solution is effected.

A valuable external astringent application.

**Gallic Acid** (*Acidum Gallicum*). A crystalline acid, $3HO,C_{14}H_3O_7 + 2HO$ or $\mathbf{H_3C_7H_3O_5.H_2O}$, prepared from Galls. *Characters.*—Crystalline, in acicular prisms or silky needles, sometimes nearly white, but generally of a pale-fawn colour. It requires about a hundred parts of cold water for its solution, but dissolves in three parts of boiling water; soluble also in rectified spirit. The aqueous solution gives no precipitate with solution of isinglass. It gives a bluish-black precipitate with a persalt of iron. The crystalline acid, when dried at 212°, loses 9·5 per cent. of its weight. It leaves no residue when burned with free access of air.

*Properties and Therapeutic Uses.*—Similar to those of Tannic Acid. As a remote astringent it is regarded as more effectual than an equal quantity of Tannic Acid, as the latter becomes converted in the blood into gallic acid and grape sugar; hence a portion of it only s available for therapeutic action.

*Dose.*—From two to ten grains or more, three or four times daily.

*Preparations.*—**Glycerine of Gallic Acid** (*Glycerinum Acidi Gallici*). Take of Gallic Acid, one ounce; Glycerine, four fluid ounces. Rub them together in a mortar; then transfer the mixture to a porcelain dish, and apply a gentle heat until complete solution is effected.

(*Non-officinal.*)

**Salix tetrasperma**, *Roxb.*, (*Corom. Pl.*, t. 97, *Wight, Icones*, vol. vi. t. 1954.) a small ornamental tree of Northern and Central India, the bark of which is stated by Dalzell and Gibson (*Flora of Bombay*, p. ii. p. 82) to be of some account as a febrifuge. Mr. Long (*Journ. of Agri.-Hort. Soc. of India*, 1858, vol. x. p. 43) states that the bark yields "a tonic substance." If by this he means Salicine (the crystalline principle found in some European species of Salix), he is under a mistake, as Sir W. O'Shaughnessy carefully examined this bark, and failed to detect any trace of this principle (*Bengal Disp.*, p. 606). Under the Hindústani names *khilaf* and *Bed-i-músk* is included **Salix Caprea**, *Linn.* (*Eng. Bot.*, t. 1488.) the flowers of which yield, on distillation, an aromatic water (*Ma-ûl-khilaf*, Hind.) which has valuable stimulant properties assigned to it, and is held in high repute in a variety of diseases. The ashes of the wood of this tree are also prescribed in hæmoptysis (*Journ. Agri.-Hort. Soc. of the Punjaub*, Feb. 10th, 1852, p. 161).

## ULMACEÆ.

### ULMUS CAMPESTRIS, *Linn.* BROAD-LEAVED ELM.

(*Engl. Bot.*, t. 1886.)

*Habitat.*—Europe and temperate Asia.

*Officinal Part.*—The dried inner bark (*Ulmi Cortex, Elm bark*). Of a brownish-yellow colour, tough, about half a line in thickness, without smell; taste mucilaginous, slightly bitter and astringent. Its decoction is turned green by perchloride of iron, and precipitates with a solution of gelatine. In addition to the tannin, the presence of which is indicated by the above tests, it contains a peculiar gummy principle, *Ulmin.*

*Properties.*—Alterative tonic, and demulcent.

*Therapeutic Uses.*—In chronic skin diseases, especially in lepra, psoriasis, and herpes, it is thought to exercise considerable influence.

*Preparation.*—**Decoction of Elm Bark** (*Decoctum Ulmi*). Take of Elm Bark, cut in small pieces, two ounces and a half; Water, one pint. Boil for ten minutes in a covered vessel; then strain, and pour as much water over the contents of the strainer as will make the strained product measure a pint.

*Dose.*—From two to four fluid ounces.

# URTICEÆ.

## HUMULUS LUPULUS, *Linn.* THE HOP PLANT.

(*Engl. Bot.*, t. 427.)

*Habitat.*—Common in Europe and temperate Asia; extensively cultivated in temperate Europe and the United States.

*Officinal Part.*—The dried strobiles of the female plant (*Lupulus, Hop*). They consist of scales of a greenish-yellow colour, with an adherent golden-yellow powder (*Lupuline*) at their base; odour aromatic; taste bitter. They contain a volatile oil and a peculiar bitter principle, *Lupulite* or *Humulin.*

*Properties.*—Tonic, stomachic, and mildly narcotic. Lupuline possesses considerable power as an anaphrodisiac.

*Therapeutic Uses.*—Atonic dyspepsia, nervous affections attended with sleeplessness, hysteria, intermittent fevers, and rheumatism, are amongst the principal affections in which hops have been used with advantage. In certain irritable states of the genito-urinary system, as spermatorrhœa, chordee, and enuresis, Lupuline exercises a well-marked influence.

*Dose.*—Of Lupuline, from six to twelve grains in the form of pills.

*Preparations.*—**Infusion of Hop** (*Infusum Lupuli*). Take of Hops, half an ounce; Boiling Water, ten fluid ounces. Infuse in a covered vessel for two hours, and strain.

*Dose.*—From one to two fluid ounces.

**Extract of Hop** (*Extractum Lupuli*). Take of Hop, one pound; rectified Spirit, one pint and a half; Distilled Water, one gallon. Macerate the hop in the spirit for seven days; press out the tincture, filter, and distil off the spirit, leaving a soft extract. Boil the residual hop with the water for one hour; press out the liquor, strain, and evaporate by a water-bath to the consistence of a soft extract. Mix the two extracts, and evaporate at a temperature not exceeding 140° until it has acquired a suitable consistence for forming pills.

*Dose.*—From five to fifteen grains.

**Tincture of Hop** (*Tinctura Lupuli*). Take of Hop, two ounces and a half; Proof Spirit, one pint. Macerate the hop for forty-eight hours in fifteen fluid ounces of the spirit, in a closed vessel, agitating occasionally; then transfer to a percolator, and, when the fluid ceases to pass, continue the percolation with the remaining five ounces of spirit. Afterwards subject the contents of the percolator to pressure, filter the product, mix the liquids, and add sufficient proof spirit to make one pint.

*Dose.*—From half a fluid drachm to two fluid drachms.

## MORUS NIGRA, *Linn.* MULBERRY TREE.

(*Steph. et Church. Med. Bot.*, vol. i. t. 397.)

*Habitat.*—Western Asia; cultivated throughout the temperate zone.

*Officinal Part.*—The juice of the ripe fruit (*Mori Succus*); it is of a dark violet colour, with faint odour and acidulous sweet taste.

*Properties and Uses.*—Only employed as a colouring agent.

*Preparation.*—**Syrup of Mulberries** (*Syrupus Mori*). Take of Mulberry Juice, one pint; Refined Sugar, two pounds; Rectified Spirit, two and a half fluid ounces. Heat the mulberry juice to the boiling point, and when it has cooled, filter it. Dissolve the sugar in the filtered liquid with a gentle heat, and add the spirit. Sp. gr. 1·33.

*Dose.*—One fluid drachm. From the readiness with which it ferments it is little suited for tropical practice. A syrup prepared with the flower of *Clitorea ternatea* has been proposed as a substitute.

## FICUS CARICA, *Linn.* THE COMMON FIG.

(*Woodville, Med. Bot.*, t. 244.)

*Habitat.*—Asia and Southern Europe.

*Officinal Part.*—The dried fruit (*Ficus, Fig*); compressed, soft but tough, brown, covered with a saccharine efflorescence, containing a viscid sweet pulp, and numerous small hard seeds.

*Properties and Uses.*—Emollient, demulcent, laxative, nutritive. Rarely employed medicinally, except as an ingredient in Confectio Sennæ.

[A full account of the medicinal uses of this fruit, according to native writers, is given by Mr. L. Da Costa (*Corbyn's Ind. Med. Journ.*, Nov. 1, 1837, p. 733).]

## CANNABIS SATIVA, *Linn.* INDIAN HEMP.

(*Rheede, Hort. Mal.*, vol. x. t. 60, 61.)

*Habitat.*—Persia, extending to Western Himalaya; extensively cultivated.

*Officinal Part.*—The dried flowering tops of the female plant grown in India, from which the resin has not been removed (*Indian Hemp, Gunjah*, Hind.) *Characters:*—Tops consisting of one or more alternate branches, bearing the remains of the flowers and smaller leaves and a few ripe fruits, pressed together in masses which are about two inches long, harsh, of a dusky-green colour, and a characteristic odour. *Active principle*, a bitterish acrid resin (*Churrus*, Hind.)

*Properties.*—Primarily stimulant; secondarily anodyne, sedative, and antispasmodic. Narcotic, diuretic, and parturifacient properties have been assigned to it; but these require confirmation. (65)

*Therapeutic Uses.*—In tetanus, hydrophobia, delirium tremens, ebrietas, infantile convulsions, various forms of neuralgia and other nervous affections, its use has been attended with benefit. Amongst other diseases in which it has been employed are cholera, menorrhagia, and uterine hæmorrhage, rhuematism, hay fever, asthma, cardiac functional derangement, and skin diseases attended with much pain and pruritus. It has likewise been employed in lingering and protracted labours depending upon atony of the uterus, with the view of inducing uterine contractions.

*Preparations.*—**Extract of Indian Hemp** (*Extractum Cannabis Indicæ*). Take of Indian Hemp, in coarse powder, one pound; Rectified Spirit, four pints. Macerate the hemp in the spirit for seven days, and press out the tincture. Distil off the greater part of the spirit, and evaporate what remains by a water-bath to the consistence of a soft extract.

*Dose.*—From half a grain to two grains or more.

**Tincture of Indian Hemp** (*Tinctura Cannabis Indicæ*). Take of Extract of Indian Hemp, one ounce; Rectified Spirit, one pint. Dissolve the extract of hemp in the spirit.

*Dose.*—From five to twenty minims, repeated according to the effects produced.

[The three principal forms in which Indian Hemp is met with in India are,—1, *Gunjah*, the dried flowering plant from which the resin has not been removed; 2, *Churrus*, the resinous exudation from the leaves, stems, and flowers; and, 3, *Bang*, *Subjee*, or *Sidhee*, the larger leaves and capsules without the stalks. In addition to these is *Majoon*, a compound of bang, butter, sugar, flour, and milk. A careful chemical examination of Indian hemp and its preparations is a desideratum.]

(*Non-officinal.*)

**Ficus Bengalensis**, *Linn.*,—*Ficus Indica*, Roxb.—(*Hooker, Journ. Bot.*, 1841, vol. iii. t. 13, 14.) The white glutinous juice of this tree, the well known *Banyan Tree*, is a much used application to those troublesome cracks on the soles of the feet to which the natives of India are so liable. It is said to be very effectual, and may be worthy of a trial when, as is so often the case in this affection, European drugs fail. The natives, according to Ainslie (*Mat. Ind.*, vol. ii. p. 10), ascribe powerfully tonic properties to the bark. We have no other evidence of the fact.

**Ficus oppositifolia**, *Roxb.* (*Wight, Icones*, vol. ii. t. 638.) A small tree chiefly inhabiting the banks of rivers in Bengal, Coromandel, and other parts of India. According to the report of Mr. Moodeen Sheriff, the fruit, seeds, and bark are possessed of valuable emetic properties. The most eligible form of administration appears to be the seeds of the ripe fruit, dried and preserved from moisture in stoppered bottles. The dose is about one drachm, which in effect is equal to four or six of the ripe fruit. The emetic action of the bark is generally attended with more or less purging. The dose is placed at from forty to sixty grains. The bark, in doses of from fifteen to thirty grains three or four times daily, is stated to act effectually as an antiperiodic, and in half those quantities as a good tonic. **F. polycarpa**, *Roxb.*, (*Wight, Icones*, vol. ii. t. 632.) possesses, according to the experience of Mr. Moodeen Sheriff, all the medicinal properties of the preceding. It is desirable to know more of the properties of these trees.

**Antiaris saccidora**, *Nimmo.* (*Wight, Icones*, vol. vi. t. 1958.) A forest tree of Western India, where it is known by the names of *Juzoogry* and *Kurwut*. It is chiefly valued for the sake of its bark, composed of very strong tenacious fibres, which, with little manipulation, form sacks; hence its specific name. It is mentioned here only on account of its intensely bitter seeds, which, according to Mr. Nimmo, contain a peculiar principle, which may prove an active medicinal agent (*Graham, Cat. of Bombay Plants*, p. 193). It would be very desirable to obtain further information regarding the properties of these seeds.

## MYRICEÆ.

(*Non-officinal.*)

**Myrica sapida**, *Wall.* (*Tent. Nepal.*, t. 45.) A tree of the Himalaya from the Sutlej to Silhet. Its bark (*Káephul*, Hind.) forms an export to Patna and the low country, where it enjoys much repute as an aromatic stimulant, and is used as a rubefacient and sternutatory. Dr. Irvine (*Med. Topog. of Ajmeer*, p. 140) states that he has found Kaephul and ginger mixed the best substance with which to rub cholera patients to promote reaction. It is not prescribed internally.

**Casuarina muricata**, *Roxb.* (*Casuarina* or *Tinian Pine*); an Arracan and Malayan tree, much cultivated in India. Its bark, according to Dr. Gibson, is an excellent and often readily available astringent in the treatment of chronic diarrhœa and dysentery; in these affections he thinks highly of its powers. Its use in the same class of cases is noticed by Bouton (*Med. Plants of the Mauritius*, p. 148).

## CONIFERÆ.

---

### ABIES BALSAMEA, *Aiton*. BALM OF GILEAD FIR.

(*Lambert, Gen. Pinus*, t. 31. *Steph. et Church. Med. Bot.*, vol. ii. t. 74.)

*Habitat.*—North America, from Canada and Nova Scotia to Carolina.

*Officinal Part.*—The Turpentine obtained from the stem by incision (*Terebinthina Canadensis, Canada Balsam*). It occurs in the form of a pale yellow ductile oleo-resin, of the consistence of thin honey, with a peculiar agreeable odour, and a slightly bitter feebly acrid taste; by exposure drying very slowly into a transparent adhesive varnish; solidifying when mixed with a sixth of its weight of magnesia.

*Properties and Uses.*—Terebinthinate stimulant, its action being chiefly directed to mucous surfaces; rarely employed. It is an ingredient in Charta Epispastica, and Collodium Flexile.

*Dose.*—From twenty to thirty grains.

### ABIES EXCELSA, *Lamarck*. THE SPRUCE FIR.

(*Steph. et Church*, vol. ii. t. 75.)

*Habitat.*—Norway, Russia, Germany, Switzerland, and other parts of Europe, also the northern parts of Asia. Cultivated commonly in England.

*Officinal Part.*—The resinous exudation from the stem (*Abietis Resina*); melted and strained (*Pix Burgundica, Burgundy Pitch*); hard and brittle, yet gradually taking the form of the vessel in which it is kept; opaque, varying in colour, but generally dull reddish-brown; of a peculiar somewhat empyreumatic perfumed odour, and aromatic taste. Without bitterness; free from vesicles; gives off no water when heated.

*Properties and Uses.*—Stimulant and rubefacient; only applied in the form of plaster.

*Preparation.*—**Pitch Plaster** (*Emplastrum Picis*).
Take of Burgundy Pitch, twenty-six ounces; Com-

mon Frankincense, thirteen ounces; Resin and Yellow Wax, of each four ounces and a half; Expressed Oil of Nutmeg, one ounce; Olive Oil, two fluid ounces; Water, two fluid ounces. Add the oils and the water to the frankincense, burgundy pitch, resin, and wax, previously melted together; then, constantly stirring, evaporate to a proper consistence.

A mild stimulant application to the chest in chronic coughs and and other pulmonary affections, to the loins in lumbago, &c.

It forms an ingredient in Emplastrum Ferri.

## PINUS PALUSTRIS, *Lambert.* THE SWAMP PINE.
## PINUS TÆDA, *Linn.* THE FRANKINCENSE PINE.

(*Lambert, Gen. Pinus,* t. 16, 17, 20.)

*Habitat.*—The Southern States of North America.

*Officinal Part.*—The concrete turpentine (*Thus Americanum, Common Frankincense*). A softish bright yellow opaque solid, resinous but tough, having the odour of American turpentine.

*Properties and Uses.*—Terebinthinate stimulant, not prescribed internally. It forms an ingredient in Emplastrum Picis.

*Preparations.*—**Oil of Turpentine** (*Oleum Terebinthinæ*). The oil obtained by distillation of the oleoresin (turpentine) of *Pinus palustris,* Lambert, *P. Tæda,* Linn., and sometimes from *P. Pinaster,* Aiton. It is a colourless, limpid, very inflammable fluid, with a strong peculiar odour and hot pungent taste, sparingly soluble in water, moderately so in alcohol, readily in ether, miscible in all proportions in the fixed oils; dissolves resins, fats, and caoutchouc; Sp. Gr. 0·86. Under exposure to the air it absorbs oxygen, and becomes yellowish and somewhat denser. When pure it is neutral to test paper.

*Properties.*—Primarily, stimulant, its action being chiefly directed to mucous surfaces, especially to that of the genito-urinary organs, increasing the quantity of urine, to which it communicates a peculiar violet odour. Secondarily, sedative, antispasmodic, and astringent. In large doses, purgative and anthelmintic. Locally or externally applied, a valuable rubefacient and counter-irritant.

*Therapeutic Uses.*—In typhus and typhoid fevers, and in the advanced stages of fevers of whatever original type, in low adynamic inflammation, especially of the lungs, and in other cases where the vital powers are greatly depressed, it proves valuable as a stimulant. In puerperal fever it has been vaunted as a specific, but on insufficient grounds. In passive hæmorrhages, *e.g.,* hæmoptysis, especially in that connected with phthisis, hæmatemesis, hæmaturia, menorrhagia, and in uterine and hæmorrhoidal hæmorrhage, it exercises considerable powers as an astringent. In hysteria, epilepsy, puerperal and other convulsions, and in tetanus, also in ileus, colica pictonum, and flatulent colic, it proves valuable as an antispasmodic. For the expulsion of ascarides lumbricoides and tænia it acts as an efficient vermifuge. Amongst the other diseases in which it has been used with advantage are purpura hæmorrhagica, cerebral affections attended with depression, biliary concretions (conjoined with ether, it is considered to act as a solvent), the advanced stages of dysentery, gonorrhœa, leucorrhœa, dropsy, cholera, and diseases of the eye, especially syphilitic and rheumatic iritis, and in incipient gangrene of the cornea. As an external application it proves valuable in burns, gangrenous, ill-conditioned, and indolent ulcerations (in these cases it is also given internally), chronic rheumatism, neuralgia, asthma, croup, enlargements of the joints, and local hæmorrhage, as after the extraction of a tooth.

*Dose.*—As a diuretic and astringent, from eight to thirty minims; as a stimulant and antispasmodic, from half a fluid drachm to a drachm; as a purgative and anthelmintic, from half a fluid ounce to one fluid ounce. As a rubefacient or counter-irritant it may be applied in the form of liniment or ointment, or as an epithem, which is readily prepared by placing a piece of calico, soaked in the oil of turpentine, on the skin, and applying over it with slight pressure, a compress of flannel warmed as hot as the patient can bear it. Its action thus applied is speedy and certain.

*Preparations of Oil of Turpentine.*—**Confection of Turpentine** (*Confectio Terebinthinæ*). Take of Oil of Turpentine, one fluid ounce; Liquorice Root, in powder, one ounce; Clarified Honey, two ounces. Rub the oil of turpentine with the liquorice, add the honey, and mix to a uniform consistence.

*Dose.*—From one to two drachms.

**Enema of Turpentine** (*Enema Terebinthinæ*). Take of Oil of Turpentine, one fluid ounce; Mucilage of Starch, fifteen fluid ounces. Mix.

Useful in hysterical and other convulsions, apoplexy, and in all cases where turpentine cannot be administered by mouth. Very serviceable in relieving tympanitis in the advanced stages of fever. Effectual in removing ascarides vermiculares from the rectum.

**Liniment of Turpentine** (*Linimentum Terebinthinæ*). Take of Soft Soap, two ounces; Camphor, one ounce; Oil of Turpentine, sixteen fluid ounces. Dissolve the camphor in the oil of turpentine, then add the soap, rubbing them together until they are thoroughly mixed.

**Liniment of Turpentine and Acetic Acid** (*Linimentum Terebinthinæ Aceticum*). Take of Oil of Turpentine, Acetic Acid, and Liniment of Camphor, of each one fluid ounce. Mix.

Both these liniments are valuable stimulant and rubefacient applications in rheumatic, neuralgic, and other chronic painful affections.

**Ointment of Turpentine** (*Unguentum Terebinthinæ*). Take of Oil of Turpentine, one fluid ounce; Resin, in coarse powder, sixty grains; Yellow Wax and Prepared Lard, of each half an ounce. Mix the ingredients together by the heat of a steam or water bath. Remove the vessel and stir the mixture constantly while it cools.

Stimulant application to indolent and ill-conditioned ulcers.

**Resin** (*Resina*), the residue of the distillation of the turpentines from various species of Pinus, *Linn.*, and Abies, *Lam.* It is translucent, semi-opaque, yellowish, brittle, pulverizable; fracture shining; odour and taste faintly terebinthinate. It is easily fusible, and burns with a dense yellow flame and much smoke. Insoluble in water; soluble in alcohol, ether, and the volatile oils. With wax, fixed oils, and spermaceti it unites by fusion. By distillation it yields oil (*Resin Oil*) and tar.

*Properties and Uses.*—Stimulant. Only employed as an external application. It is an ingredient in several officinal plasters.

*Preparations.*—**Resin Plaster** (*Emplastrum Resinæ*). Take of Resin, half a pound; Lead Plaster, three pounds. To the lead plaster, previously melted with a gentle heat, and gradually, add the resin first melted, and stir them until they are thoroughly mixed.

Local stimulant. Used as a support to injured parts in surgery. It is an ingredient in Emplastrum Opii, Emp. Belladonnæ, Emp. Calefaciens, and Emp. Plumbi Iodidi.

**Ointment of Resin** (*Unguentum Resinæ*). Take of Resin, in coarse powder, eight ounces; Yellow Wax, four ounces; Simple Ointment, sixteen ounces. Melt with a gentle heat; strain the mixture, while hot, through flannel, and stir constantly while it cools.

Stimulant application to indolent and ill-conditioned ulcers, especially to those resulting from burns; and also to blistered surfaces, to keep up a discharge.

## PINUS SYLVESTRIS, *Linn.* Wild Pine or Scotch Fir.

(*Lambert, Gen. Pinus*, t. 1. *Steph. et Church., Med. Bot.*, vol. ii. t. 73.)

*Habitat.*—Highlands of Scotland, Denmark, Norway, and other northern countries of Europe.

*Officinal Part.*—A bituminous liquid (*Pix Liquida, Liquid* or *Wood Tar*), obtained from the wood of *Pinus sylvestris*, Linn., and other pines, by destructive distillation. A thick, viscid, tenacious fluid, of a brownish-black colour, and a well-known peculiar aromatic odour. Water agitated with it acquires a pale-brown colour, sharp empyreumatic taste, and acid reaction.

*Properties.*—Stimulant, its action being chiefly directed to the mucous membranes and the cutaneous surface.

*Therapeutic Uses.*—In cutaneous diseases it has been prescribed, both internally and externally, with success. Used also in typhoid fever, habitual constipation, and in chronic bronchitis. The vapour from heated tar has been found serviceable in phthisis and other chronic pulmonary affections.

*Dose.*—From half a drachm to a drachm, made into pills with flour, three or four times daily.

*Preparations.*—**Ointment of Tar** (*Unguentum Picis liquidæ*). Take of Tar, five ounces, Yellow Wax, two ounces. Melt the wax with a gentle heat, add the tar, and stir the mixture briskly while it cools.

Used as an application in ringworm, psoriasis and other skin diseases, and also to ulcerations.

**Creasote** (*Creasotum*). A product of the distillation of Wood Tar. It is a colourless or slightly yellowish liquid, with a strong empyreumatic odour. It is sparingly dissolved by water, but freely by alcohol, ether, and glacial acetic acid. Specific gravity 1·071. It coagulates albumen. A slip of deal dipped into it, and afterwards into hydrochloric acid, acquires on exposure for a short time to the air a greenish-blue colour. Dropped on white filtering paper and exposed to a heat of 212°, it leaves no translucent stain. It turns the plane of polarisation of a ray of polarised light to the right. It is not solidified by the cold produced by a mixture of hydrochloric acid and sulphate of soda.

*Properties.*—Primarily stimulant, secondarily sedative. Locally applied, irritant and caustic. Antiseptic, in which character it acts by the power it possesses of coagulating albumen.

*Therapeutic Uses.*—In gastric irritation, gastrodynia, and vomiting, unattended with inflammatory action, it exercises a well marked influence. It has also been successfully employed in diarrhœa, passive hæmorrhage, gonorrhœa, and leucorrhœa. It has been recommended in diabetes. Externally, it has been employed in skin diseases, phagedenic and scrofulous ulcerations, bed sores, nævi, erysipelas, and syphilitic tumours. Glanders have been benefited by syringing the nostrils several times daily with a creasote lotion. Applied to a carious tooth, it often relieves toothache; here it acts as a powerful sialogogue. The inhalation of the vapour (*infra*) has been thought useful in chronic bronchitis and other chronic pulmonary affections.

*Dose.*—From one to three minims, in the form of pill or the subjoined mixture.

*Preparations.*—**Creasote Mixture** (*Mistura Creasoti*). Take of Creasote, sixteen minims; Glacial Acetic Acid, sixteen minims; Spirit of Juniper, half a fluid drachm; Syrup, one fluid ounce; Water, fifteen fluid ounces. Mix the creasote with the acetic acid, gradually add the water, and lastly the syrup and spirit of juniper.

*Dose.*—From one to two fluid ounces, three or four times daily. Each fluid ounce contains one minim of creasote.

**Ointment of Creasote** (*Unguentum Creasoti*). Take of Creasote, one fluid drachm; Simple Ointment, one ounce. Mix thoroughly.

A stimulant application to skin diseases and ulcerations.

**Inhalation of Creasote** (*Vapor Creasoti*). Take of Creasote, twelve minims; Boiling Water, eight fluid ounces. Mix the creasote and water in an apparatus so arranged that air may be made to pass through the solution, and may afterwards be inhaled.

## JUNIPERUS COMMUNIS, *Linn.* COMMON JUNIPER.

(*Steph. et Church. Med. Bot.*, vol. iii. t. 141.)

*Habitat.*—Northern parts of Europe, Asia, and America.

*Officinal Part.*—The Fruit (*Juniperi Fructus, Juniper Berries*); about the size of a pea, of a blackish-purple colour, covered by a glaucous bloom; marked superiorly with a tri-radiate groove, inferiorly by bracteal scales, arranged in a stellate form; taste sweetish, terebinthinate; odour agreeable and balsamic. *Active principle*, a volatile oil.

*Properties.*—Stimulant, diuretic, and carminative.

*Therapeutic Uses.*—In asthenic dropsical affections, flatulence, flatulent colic, and spasmodic affections of the bowels, also in chronic gonorrhœa and leucorrhœa, it has been found serviceable.

*Dose.*—From forty grains to two drachms, in infusion; it is best administered in the form of Volatile Oil or Spirit.

*Preparations.*—**Oil of Juniper** (*Oleum Juniperi*). A volatile oil obtained by distillation from the unripe fruit. It is colourless, or a pale greenish-yellow colour, of a sweetish odour, and warm aromatic taste.

*Dose.*—From one to five minims.

**Spirit of Juniper** (*Spiritus Juniperi*). Take of Oil of Juniper, one fluid ounce; Rectified Spirit, forty-nine fluid ounces. Dissolve.

*Dose.*—From thirty minims to one fluid drachm, three or four times daily. It is one fifth the strength of the preparation of the same name in *Brit. Pharm.*, 1864.

## JUNIPERUS SABINA, *Linn.* COMMON SAVINE.

(*Woodville, Med. Bot.*, t. 94.)

*Habitat.*—Central and Southern Europe, Asiatic Russia; cultivated in England.

*Officinal Parts.*—The fresh and dried Tops (*Sabinæ Cacumina*), collected in the spring. *Characters.*—Twigs densely covered with minute imbricated appressed leaves in four rows; odour strong, peculiar, and unpleasant; taste acrid, bitter, resinous, and disagreeable. *Active principle*, a volatile oil (*Oleum Sabinæ*) and an acrid resin.

*Properties.*—Acrid stimulant and emmenagogue; in large doses poisonous.

*Therapeutic Uses.*—In amenorrhœa, leucorrhœa, passive menorrhagia, habitual abortion, and other affections depending upon deficient or depressed action of the uterine system, it has been used with advantage. Externally applied to syphilitic warts and skin diseases.

*Dose.*—From three to ten grains, in infusion. Chiefly prescribed in one of the subjoined formulæ.

*Preparations.*—**Oil of Savine** (*Oleum Sabinæ*). The Volatile Oil obtained by distillation from the fresh Tops of Savine; limpid, colourless, or of a pale-yellow colour, having the peculiar odour of the plant, and bitter acrid taste.

*Dose.*—From one to five minims. This is the best form for internal administration.

**Tincture of Savine** (*Tinctura Sabinæ*). Take of Savine, dried and coarsely powdered, two ounces and a half; Proof Spirit, one pint. Macerate the savine for forty-eight hours in fifteen fluid ounces of the spirit, in a closed vessel, agitating occasionally; then transfer to a percolator, and when the fluid ceases to pass continue the percolation with the remaining five ounces of spirit Afterwards subject the contents of the percolator to pressure, filter the product, mix the liquids, and add sufficient proof spirit to make one pint.

*Dose.*—From twenty to sixty minims.

**Ointment of Savine** (*Unguentum Sabinæ*). Take of Fresh Savine Tops, bruised, eight ounces; White Wax, three ounces; Prepared Lard, sixteen ounces. Melt the lard and the wax together on a water bath, add the savine, and digest for twenty minutes. Then remove the mixture, and express through calico.

Stimulant; much employed for dressing blistered surfaces and setons when it is desired to maintain a free discharge.

(*Non-officinal.*)

**Pinus longifolia,** *Roxb.* (*Royle, Illust.*, t. 85). A native of the Himalaya, at 2,000 to 6,000 feet elevation. Known by the Hindústani names of *Cheersullah, Sarul,* and *Thansa.* The people of Upper India obtain from it tar and turpentine. The former is said to be equal to that obtained by a more refined process in Europe; and the turpentine is stated merely to require attention to render it equal to the imported article. A detail of the process followed by the natives is given in the second volume of the Asiatic Society of Bengal, p. 249. Dr. Hugh Cleghorn (*Journ. Agri.-Hort. Soc. of India,* 1865, vol. xiv. P. i. App. p. 7) furnishes some interesting remarks on the manufacture of tar from this tree, as well as from *P. excelsa* and *P. Deodara.* He speaks of the product being of a superior description, equal in fact to Swedish tar. In an economical point of view, this subject may be worthy of attention. Royle (*Illust.*, vol. i. p. 351) mentions a terebinthinate exudation of this pine, under the names of *Cheer-ke-goond, Birjee,* and *Gunda Biroza.* The last of these names, however, is applied chiefly to Olibanum, the produce of *Boswellia floribunda,* Endl.

**Pinus Deodara,** *Roxb.*— This elegant Himalayan Pine is known by the names of *Deodar* and *Kelon.* According to Dr. T. Thomson (*Hooker's Journ. of Bot.*, 1849, vol. i. p. 96), the term *Deodara,* signifying "God-given," or the "gift of God," is applied to more than one tree, but in Kumaon and Cashmere to *Pinus Deodara* only; at Simla *P. Deodara* is called *Kela* (*Kelon,* Royle); and the sacred name, according to Madden, is given to *Cupressus torulosa,* Lambert. It yields a coarse, very fluid kind of turpentine (*Kelon ká tel,* Hind.), held in much esteem by the natives as an application to ulcers and skin diseases. It appears also to enter largely into their nostrums for the treatment of leprosy (Prof. H. H. Wilson, *Calcutta Med. Phys. Trans.*, vol. i. p. 41). Dr. Gibson regards it as very effectual in this disease when given in large doses. In the 2nd volume of these Transactions, Dr. J. Johnston details a severe case of lepra mercurialis, treated externally and internally with Deodar oil, extracted by heat from the wood. Commenting on this case, Dr. Johnston remarks that the Deodar oil produced the happiest effects by suddenly checking and ultimately curing the disease. A drachm of the oil was as large a dose as the patient's stomach could bear. It always acted as a diaphoretic, and produced no other sensible effects. It was found extremely variable in its action, in some a drachm causing vomiting, whilst in others half an ounce induced only slight nausea. Dr. Johnston extended its use to other skin diseases with advantage. Dr. Royle (*op. cit.* p. 352) states that the leaves and small twigs of the Deodara are also brought down to the plains, being much employed in native medicine. They may, doubtless, possess some mild terebinthinate properties.

# Class II.—Monocotyledones, *vel* Endogenae.

## SMILACEÆ.

### SMILAX OFFICINALIS, *Humb. et Bonpl.* JAMAICA SARSAPARILLA.

*Habitat.*—Central America.

*Officinal Part.*—The dried Root (*Sarsæ Radix, Sarsaparilla*), imported into Great Britain from Jamaica. The roots are usually not thicker than a goosequill, generally many feet in length, reddish-brown, covered with rootlets, and folded in bundles about eighteen inches long; scentless; taste mucilaginous, feebly bitterish, faintly acrid. They contain a small portion of an acrid bitter resin, a trace of volatile oil, and a crystallizable principle, *Smilacine.*

*Properties.*—Alterative tonic.

*Therapeutic Uses.*—In syphilitic and chronic rheumatic affections it has long been held in esteem. It has likewise been employed in chronic affections of the liver, and long standing skin diseases, especially those of a syphilitic character.

*Dose.*—From half a drachm to a drachm of the powdered root.

*Preparations.*—**Decoction of Sarsaparilla** (*Decoctum Sarsæ*). Take of Jamaica Sarsaparilla, cut transversely, two ounces and a half; Boiling water, one pint and a half. Digest the sarsaparilla in the water for an hour, then boil for ten minutes in a covered vessel; cool, and strain, pouring water, if required, over the contents of the strainer, or otherwise making the strained product measure a pint.

*Dose.*—From two to four fluid ounces three or four times daily.

**Compound Decoction of Sarsaparilla** (*Decoctum Sarsæ compositum*). Take of Jamaica Sarsaparilla, cut transversely, two ounces and a half; Sassafras, in chips, a quarter of an ounce; Guaiacum Wood turnings, a quarter of an ounce; Fresh Liquorice Root, bruised, a quarter of an ounce; Mezereon Bark, sixty grains; Boiling Water, one pint and a half. Digest the solid ingredients in the water for an hour; boil for ten minutes in a covered vessel; cool, and strain, pouring water, if required, over the contents of the strainer, or otherwise making the strained product measure a pint.

*Dose.*—From two to four fluid ounces three or four times daily. A more efficient preparation than the preceding.

**Liquid Extract of Sarsaparilla** (*Extractum Sarsæ liquidum*). Take of Jamaica Sarsaparilla, cut transversely, one pound; Water, at 160°, fourteen pints; Rectified Spirit, one fluid ounce. Digest the Sarsaparilla in one half of the water for six hours, and decant the liquor. Digest the residue in the remainder of the water for the same time, express and filter the mixed liquors, and evaporate them by a water bath to seven fluid ounces, or until the specific gravity of the liquid is 1·13. When cold, add the spirit. The specific gravity should be about 1·095.

*Dose.*—From two to four fluid drachms. This is the best form for administration.

(*Non-officinal.*)

**Smilax glabra**, *Roxb.*—The large tuberous roots of this species, indigenous in Sylhet and the adjacent Garrow country, where it is known by the name of *Húrína-shúk China*, are used by the natives, in decoction, in the treatment of syphilitic affections (Roxburgh, *Flor. Indica*, p. 792). The roots of **S. lanceæfolia**, *Roxb.* (*Gútea-shúk China*) are likewise employed in rheumatism. Roxburgh states that the roots of both these species so closely resemble China root, the produce of *Smilax China*, Linn., that they can hardly be distinguished from it. This latter drug is imported largely into India from China, and is to be met with in most bazaars, under the name of *Chob-China*. It is, however, usually worm-eaten and worthless. **Smilax ovalifolia**, *Roxb.* (*Wight, Icones*, vol. iii. t. 809), abounds in the low jungles in the Madras and Malayan Peninsulas. From the similarity of the roots in physical characters to Vera Cruz Sarsaparilla, the Editor, when stationed in Burmah, employed it in hospital practice; but with no very satisfactory results. It was abandoned in favour of the large tuberous roots of another species, very common in the neighbourhood of Mergui, and known to the Burmese by the name of **Tsein-apho.** In botanical characters it approaches closely to *S. prolifera*, Roxb. The results attendant on its use in chronic rheumatism, especially in that connected with secondary syphilis, in cachexia, and in some obstinate forms of skin disease, were very marked. It was employed in decoction (two ounces and a half of the tuberous root to two pints of water, boiled down to one pint), in doses of from two to four fluid ounces, thrice daily. Whether its virtues are impaired by the process of drying and long keeping is uncertain; but to medical officers stationed in Burmah, where it can be procured fresh, it is well deserving of notice as a valuable alterative tonic. It must not be confounded with imported China root, which it much resembles, and which is sold in the bazaars under the Burmese name of *Tsein-apho-taroup*. (*Indian Ann. of Med. Sci.*, 1858, vol. v. p. 580.)

## SCITAMINEÆ.

### ZINGIBER OFFICINALE, *Roscoe*. OFFICINAL GINGER.

(*Rheede, Hort. Mal.*, vol. xi. t. 12; *Roscoe, Scit.*, t. 83.)

*Habitat.*—Cultivated in the tropical portions of both hemispheres.

*Officinal Part.*—The dried Rhizome (*Zingiberis Radix, Ginger*). It occurs in irregular lobed decorticated pieces, three or four inches long, sub-compressed, yellowish-white but not chalky on the surface, with a short mealy fracture, hot taste, and agreeable aroma. Powder, yellowish-white. Its activity resides in a volatile oil and in a soft acrid resin.

*Properties.*—Stimulant, stomachic, and carminative.

*Therapeutic Uses.*—In flatulence, flatulent colic, and spasmodic affections of the bowels, and in chronic rheumatism, it is employed beneficially. As an external or local application it acts favourably, as a stimulant and rubefacient, in some forms of headache, toothache, various affections of the throat, and in shortness of sight dependent upon deficient power in the contractile tissue of the iris (66).

*Dose.*—From ten to twenty grains of the powdered root.

*Preparations.*—**Tincture of Ginger** (*Tinctura Zingiberis*). Take of Ginger, in coarse powder, two ounces and a half; Rectified Spirit, one pint. Macerate the ginger for forty-eight hours, in fifteen fluid ounces of the spirit, in a closed vessel, agitating occasionally;

then transfer to a percolator; and when the fluid ceases to pass, continue the percolation with the remaining five ounces of spirit. Afterwards subject the contents of the percolator to pressure, filter the product, mix the liquids, and add sufficient rectified spirit to make one pint.

*Dose.*—From fifteen minims to one fluid drachm. A useful adjunct to antacid and carminative draughts.

**Strong Tincture of Ginger** (*Tinctura Zingiberis fortior, Essence of Ginger*). Take of Ginger, in fine powder, ten ounces; Rectified Spirit, a sufficiency. Pack the ginger tightly in a percolator, and pour over it carefully half a pint of the spirit. At the expiration of two hours add more spirit, and let it percolate slowly, until one pint of tincture has been collected.

*Dose.*— From five to twenty minims.

**Syrup of Ginger** (*Syrupus Zingiberis*). Take of Strong Tincture of Ginger, six fluid drachms; Syrup, nineteen fluid ounces. Mix with agitation.

*Dose.*—From one to two fluid drachms.

***Infusion of Ginger** (*Infusum Zingiberis*). Take of Ginger, bruised, half an ounce; Boiling Water, ten fluid ounces. Infuse in a covered vessel for one hour and strain.

*Dose.*—From one to two fluid ounces. A useful carminative, especially valuable as being almost invariably available. In catarrhal and rheumatic affections, three ounces of the warm infusion taken at bed time acts favourably as a diaphoretic. It forms likewise an eligible vehicle for stimulant gargles.

Ginger is also an ingredient in Confectio Opii, Confectio Scammonii, Infusum Sennæ, Pilula Scillæ composita, Pulvis Cinnamomi compositus, Pulv. Jalapæ compositus, Pulv. Opii compositus, Pulv. Rhei. compositus, Pulv. Scammonii compositus, Syrupus Rhamni, and Vinum Aloes.

[The rhizome of **Zingiber Zerumbet**, *Roxb.* (*Wight, Icones*, vol. vi. t. 2003), constitutes apparently the *Zerumbad* of Avicenna (*Canon Med.* lib. ii. p. 118), and the *Zerumbet Zedoary* of Ainslie (*Mat. Ind.* vol. i. p. 492), whilst that of **Z. Cassumunar**, *Roxb.* (*Roscoe, Scit.*, t. 85), is the *Turmeric coloured Zeodary* of the latter writer (*Ibid.* p. 493). They both partake in a minor degree in the carminative properties of common ginger, but have no special claims to notice.]

## ELETTARIA CARDAMOMUM, *Maton.* OFFICINAL OF MALABAR CARDAMOM PLANT.

(*Roxb., Corom. Plants*, t. 226, 227.)

*Habitat.*—Mountain ranges of the Western Coast of the Madras Peninsula. Cultivated in Malabar.

*Officinal Part.*—The dried capsules (*Cardamomum, Cardamoms*). The seeds are obtusely angular, corrugated, reddish brown, internally white, with a warm aromatic agreeable taste and odour, contained in ovate-oblong triangular, pale-brown, coriaceous, ribbed pericarps. They contain a volatile oil and an acrid resin. The seeds are best kept in their pericarps, from which they should be separated when required for use, the pericarpial coats being rejected.

*Properties.*—Stimulant, carminative.

*Therapeutic Uses.*—In atonic dyspepsia, and flatulent and spasmodic affections of the bowels, and in case of nervous depression, they prove serviceable.

*Dose.*—From ten to twenty grains of the powdered seed. They are, however, rarely prescribed, excepting in the following form.

*Preparations.*—**Compound Tincture of Cardamoms** (*Tinctura Cardamomi composita*). Take of Cardamom Seeds, freed from the pericarps and bruised, a quarter of an ounce; Caraway Fruit, bruised, a quarter of an ounce; Raisins, freed from their seeds, two ounces; Cinnamon Bark, bruised, half an ounce; Cochineal, in powder, sixty grains; Proof Spirit, one pint. Macerate the solid ingredients, for forty-eight hours, in fifteen fluid ounces of the spirit, in a closed vessel, agitating occasionally; then transfer to a percolator; and when the fluid ceases to pass, continue the percolation with the remaining five ounces of spirit. Afterwards subject the contents of the percolator to pressure, filter the product, mix the liquids, and add sufficient proof spirit to make one pint.

*Dose.*—From half a fluid drachm to two drachms.

Cardamom seeds also form an ingredient in Extractum Colocynthidis compositum, Pulvis Cinnamomum compositus, Pulv. Cretæ aromaticus, Tinctura Gentianæ composita, Tinct. Rhei. and Vinum Aloes. The Compound Tincture enters into Decoctum Aloes compositum, Mistura Ferri aromatica, Mist. Sennæ composita and Tinctura Ferri composita.

[**Elettaria Cardamomum**, var. β. *Thwaites* (*E. major*, Smith), cultivated at Candy, affords the *Ceylon Cardamoms*, which, in medicinal properties and uses, agree closely with the officinal Cardamoms. They consist of a lanceolate-oblong capsule, acutely triangular, more or less curved, with flat or ribbed sides about an inch and a half in length, and a third of an inch in breadth. The pericarp is coriaceous, tough, brownish or yellowish ash coloured, three-celled; the seeds angular, rugged, of a yellowish-red tinge; of a fragrant odour, and spicy taste. It is apparently to this variety of Cardamoms that Ainslie and some other subsequent writers on Indian Materia Medica apply the name Grains of Paradise.]

## CURCUMA LONGA, *Linn.* TURMERIC PLANT.

(*Rheede, Hort. Mal.*, vol. xi. t. 16.)

*Habitat.*—Cultivated throughout the East.

*Officinal Part*—The Root-stock or Tubers (*Curcuma, Turmeric*); occurs either in circular or oval pieces about two inches long and one broad, pointed at one end and marked with annular wrinkles, or in cylindrical pieces two or more inches long, somewhat contorted and tuberculated; yellowish externally; internally, more or less orange-yellow; odour, peculiar and aromatic; taste, aromatic. When chewed, tinges the saliva yellow.

*Properties and Uses.*—Carminative; much used as a condiment. It is officinal only as a chemical test.

*Preparations.*—**Tincture of Turmeric** (*Tinctura Curcumæ*). Take of Turmeric, bruised, one ounce; Proof Spirit, six fluid ounces. Macerate for seven days in a close vessel, and filter.

**Turmeric Paper** (*Charta Curcumæ*). Unsized paper steeped in Tincture of Turmeric, and dried by exposure to the air.

Employed as a test for alkalies, which render it reddish or brownish.

[The Editor has witnessed excellent effects from turmeric employed in the two following modes. 1. in coryza, the fumes of burning turmeric directed into the nostrils; the fumes, which are somewhat irritant, cause a considerable discharge of mucus from the schneiderian membrane, and there is a marked degree of relief of the congestion often so troublesome in these cases. 2. In catarrhal and purulent ophthalmia, when a decoction of turmeric (half ounce of the bruised root to ten ounces of water) proves a very effectual lotion for relieving the burning, and moderating the urgency of the symptoms. Its use in the former mode is noticed in Dr. A. Hunter's report.]

(*Non-officinal.*)

**Curcuma aromatica**, *Salisb.*—*C. Zedoaria*, Roxb.—(*Wight, Icones*, vol. vi. t. 2005.)—Common in many parts of India. Its roots constitute the *Bun-haldi* or *Jungli-haldi* of the Hindústani Materia Medica, the *Round Zedoary* of pharmacologists. It occurs in segments, halves, quarters, or flat sections of a roundish or ovate tuber, marked externally with the remains of fibres; of a pale yellowish or brownish-grey colour, pungent bitter taste, and aromatic odour. Morin (*Journ. de Pharm.*, vol. ix. p. 257) detected in it a volatile oil and a resin, in which whatever activity it may possess doubtless resides. Carminative and tonic properties are assigned to it. The roots of **Curcuma Zedoaria**, *Roscoe* (*C. Zerumbet, Roxb.. Corom. Pl.*, t. 201), are supposed to constitute the *Long Zedoary* of the shops, which agrees nearly with the preceding, excepting in shape, being in pieces about the length of the little finger, about half an inch in diameter, and slightly curved or arched. The roots of **Curcuma Amada**, *Roxb.* (*Roscoe, Scit.*, t. 99),—*Am-haldí*, Hind.,—called also *Mango Ginger* by the English, from its possessing the fragrance of that fruit, are employed by the natives as a carminative and stomachic; but they do not, any more than the roots of the other species, possess in these characters any advantage over ginger. Hence, though perhaps useful in their way, they may safely be set aside. Arrowroot of fair quality is prepared from the tubers of **C. angustifolia**, *Roxb.*, and **C. rubescens**, *Roxb.* (*Roscoe, Scit.*, t. 107), both indigenous Indian plants.

**Alpinia nutans**, *Roscoe* (*Wight, Icones*, vol. vi. t. 2027),—*Púnag-champa*, Beng.,—a native of the Malayan Archipelago, much cultivated in gardens in India, affords a rhizome which is said to have been confounded with Galangal. *The Greater* and *the Lesser Galangal* are supposed to be the produce respectively of **Alpinia Galanga**, *Linn.*, and **Alpinia Chinensis**, *Roscoe*, both natives of countries east of Singapore, whence they are imported into India, and find a place in the native Materia Medica under the name of *Kholinján* (Hind.) Like the Zedoaries, they have long since been discarded in European practice: they possess no properties which are not possessed in an equal degree by ginger. The latter remarks apply equally to the fragrant roots of **Kæmpferia rotunda**, *Linn.* (*Wight, Icones*, vol. vi. t. 2029), and **K. Galanga** (*Ibid.*, vol. iii. t. 899), both of which are employed medicinally by the natives under the names respectively of *Bhú champa*, Hind.; and *Chundú-múla*, Hind., and *Katsjula Kalungú*, Tam. Irvine (*Med. Topog. of Ajmeer*, p. 171) mentions that the natives add *Kholinján* root to bazaar spirit, with the view of rendering the liquor more intoxicating.

**Hedychium spicatum**, *Smith* (*Bot. Mag.*, t. 2300).—A Himalayan plant, the fragrant aromatic root of which constitutes the *Sit-ruttee* or *Káfúr Kuchri* of the bazaars. It is considered by Royle (*Illust.*, vol. i. p. 358) to be very probably the *Sittarittie* or *Lesser Galangal* of Ainslie (*Mat. Ind.*, vol. i. p. 140.) From its sensible properties it may be judged to possess stomachic carminative qualities.

**Amomum xanthioides**, *Wallich.*—This plant inhabits the Malayan Peninsula. Its aromatic seeds, resembling those of the Malabar Cardamom, are sometimes found in the London market. The fruit consists of rounded clusters of an oblong obtuse form, brown-coloured, hairy or prickly capsules arising from a repent stem, containing seeds resembling Malabar Cardamoms, but not so rugose; they are, however, distinguishable by their peculiar aromatic taste and smell. Examined by Mr. D. Hanbury (*Pharm. Journ.*, 1855, vol. xiv. p. 417), they proved identical with the *Bastard Cardamom* sent from Siam. Excellent figures of the fruit have been furnished by Mr. Hanbury. Roxburgh (*Flor. Ind.*, vol. i. p. 45) states that the fruits of **Amomum aromaticum**, *Roxb.*, are collected by the natives of the valleys on the eastern frontier of Bengal, where the plant is indigenous, and are sold for medicinal and other purposes under the name of *Morung Elachi*. He adds that though the capsules differ from those of the *Elettaria Cardamomum* (being ovate, the size of a large nutmeg, rather fleshy and rugose), yet that the seeds are very similar in shape and spicy flavour to the officinal article.

## MUSACEÆ.

(*Non-officinal.*)

**Musa sapientum,** *Linn.* (*Rheede, Hort. Mal.*, vol. i. t. 12–14; *Roxb. Corom. Pl.*, t. 275.)—*the Banana and Plantain*—is extensively cultivated throughout the tropical and warmer portions of the globe, for the sake of its fruit, which forms a valuable article of diet. It is mentioned in this place only on account of its leaves, especially the young and tender ones, which are of a beautifully fine texture, and are in common use in India for dressing blistered surfaces. For this purpose a piece of the leaf, of the required size, smeared with any bland vegetable oil, is applied to the denuded surface, and kept *in situ* by means of a bandage. They are thus employed in the Bombay General European Hospital (*Dr. W. Dymock*); and their use for this purpose is favourably noticed in the reports of Drs. J. Hutchinson, Van Someren, J. Newton, and L. Stewart; the Editor, from several years' experience in their use, can testify to their utility in such cases. They communicate a pleasant soothing sensation, and the blistered surface is generally found to heal satisfactorily in four or five days. For the first two days the upper smooth surface of the leaf is placed next to the skin, and subsequently the under side, until the healing process is complete. As a general rule this is equal, if not superior, to the ordinary mode of dressing blisters with spermaceti ointment, which not unfrequently, especially in tropical countries, where animal fats soon become rancid, gives rise to much irritation. Dr. Van Someren reports that he employs plantain leaf as a substitute for gutta percha tissue in the water dressing of wounds and ulcers, and that it answers well for the purpose. A piece of fresh plantain leaf forms an extemporaneous, cool, and pleasant shade for the eyes, in the various forms of ophthalmia so common in the East. In a hygienic point of view, the preserved fruit deserves notice as a nourishing and antiscorbutic article of diet for long voyages. When carefully prepared, it is agreeable to the taste, much resembling dried figs, is of small cost, and will keep good for a long period.

# AMARYLLIDACEÆ.

## * CRINUM ASIATICUM, *var.* TOXICARIUM, *Herbert.*

(*Wight, Icones,* vol. vi. t. 2021, 2022.)

*Habitat.*—Low humid localities in Bengal, the Concans, and other parts of India; cultivated also in gardens; Ceylon, the Moluccas, and Cochin China.

*Officinal Part.*—The fresh Root (*Crini Radix*); bulbous, with a terminal stoloniferous fusiform portion issuing from the crown of the bulb; with an unpleasant narcotic odour; readily dried in the stove, and reducible to powder after desiccation.

*Properties.*—Emetic; in small doses nauseant and diaphoretic.

*Therapeutic Uses.*—Analogous to those of Squill.

*Preparations.*—**Juice of Crinum** (*Succus Crini; Infusum Crini, Beng. Ph.*) Take of the fresh Root of Crinum, half an ounce; Cold Water, two ounces. Bruise the root in a stone mortar, gradually adding the water. Strain, with pressure, through calico.

*Dose.*—From two to four fluid drachms every twenty minutes, until the desired effect is produced.

**Syrup of Crinum** (*Syrupus Crini*). Take of the fresh Root of Crinum, sliced, eight ounces; Boiling Water, one pint; Refined Sugar, one pound. Macerate the root in the water for two hours, bruise in a mortar, press through calico, add the sugar, and dissolve with the aid of gentle heat.

*Dose*—About two fluid drachms, repeated as required: used as a nauseant and emetic for children.

[The dried sliced roots are also an efficient emetic, but require to be given in double the dose of the recent article. Sir W. O'Shaughnessy remarks (*Bengal Disp.* p. 656) that this is the only indigenous and abundant emetic plant, of which he has experience, which acts without producing griping, purging, or other unpleasant symptoms. In a communication to the Editor, he remarks that it is a good emetic and diaphoretic whenever ipecacuanha is not at hand, but that it should be regarded, not so much as a substitute for that article, as a resource in case of need.]

(*Non-officinal.*)

**Agave Americana,** *Linn.* (*Bot. Mag.,* t. 3654).—An American plant naturalized in most parts of India. Diuretic and alterative properties are assigned to its roots by the Mexicans. Dr. Æ. Ross reports having employed them in this character, in decoction (in the proportion of four ounces to one pint of water), in secondary syphilis, with great apparent benefit. Dr. R. F. Hutchinson regards this remedy as well worthy of further trials; he mentions, also, that a thin slice of the large fleshy leaves constitutes a good poultice.

## HYPOXIDEÆ.

(*Non-officinal.*)

**Curculigo orchioides,** *Gaërtn.* (*Roxb., Corom. Pl.,* t. 13.) The roots of this small low-growing plant, common in most parts of India, are described by Ainslie (*Mat. Ind.* vol. ii. p. 242) as tuberous, wrinkled, about four inches long, having a slightly bitter and mucilaginous taste. How far they constitute a portion of the *Saféd Músli* of the Native Materia Medica (as has been supposed) is undetermined. Dr. Birdwood (*Products of Bombay,* p. 92) agrees with Dr. Royle in referring this drug to *Murdannia scapifolia,* Royle (*Illust.,* t. 95.) Further inquiries are required to determine its botanical source. The roots of *C. orchioides* are held in the highest esteem by the Hindú doctors of Travancore, in gonorrhœa, dysuria, menorrhagia, &c.; and from the unanimous testimony borne by them to their value in these and other allied affections, there is reason for supposing that they exercise some influence on the genito-urinary system generally; but there is no evidence based on European observation as to their value in these cases.

## IRIDEÆ.

### CROCUS SATIVUS, *Linn.* THE SAFFRON CROCUS.

(*Royle, Illust.,* t. 99; *Steph. et Church, Med. Bot.,* vol. ii. t. 101.)

*Habitat.*—Asia Minor; cultivated in France, Spain, and other parts of Europe; also in Cashmere.

*Officinal Part.*—The dried stigma and part of the style (*Crocus, Saffron*). Consists of thread-like styles, each terminated by three long orange-brown stigmas, which are broadest at their summit; has a powerful aromatic odour. Rubbed on the moistened finger, it leaves an intense orange-yellow tint. When pressed between folds of white filtering paper, it leaves no oily stain.

*Properties and Uses.*—Formerly regarded as antispasmodic and emmenagogue; employed at present chiefly as a colouring and flavouring agent.

*Dose.*—From ten to forty grains in infusion or powder.

*Preparations.*—**Tincture of Saffron** (*Tinctura Croci*). Take of Saffron, one ounce; Proof Spirit, one pint. Macerate the saffron for forty-eight hours in fifteen fluid ounces of the spirit, in a closed vessel, agitating occasionally; then transfer to a percolator, and when the fluid ceases to pass, continue the percolation with the remaining five ounces of spirit. Afterwards subject the contents of the percolator to pressure, filter the product, mix the liquids, and add sufficient proof spirit to make one pint.

*Dose.*—From half a fluid drachm to two fluid drachms.

Saffron also forms an ingredient in Decoctum Aloes compositum, Pilula Aloes et Myrrhæ, Pulvis Cretæ Aromaticus, Tinctura Cinchonæ composita, Tinct. Opii Ammoniata, and Tinct. Rhei.

## LILIACEÆ.

### ALOE SOCOTRINA, *Lam.*, AND OTHER UNDETERMINED SPECIES OF ALOE YIELDING SOCOTRINE ALOES.

(*Steph. et Church, Med. Bot.*, vol. ii. t. 110.)

*Habitat.*—Island of Socotra.

*Officinal Part.*—The inspissated juice of the leaf (*Aloe Socotrina, Socotrine Aloes*). It occurs in reddish-brown masses, opaque or translucent at the edges; breaks with an irregular or smooth and resinous fracture; has a bitter taste, and a strong but fragrant odour; dissolves entirely in proof spirit, and during solution exhibits under the microscope numerous minute crystals. Its activity resides in a resin, and in a peculiar principle, *Aloine.*

*Properties.*—In small doses, stomachic tonic; in larger ones, purgative, and indirectly emmenagogue.

*Therapeutic Uses.*—In constipation, especially in that connected with hysteria, or dependent on atony of the intestinal muscular coat, which often supervenes upon fevers and other debilitating diseases, it is a remedy of great value. It likewise proves serviceable in atonic dyspepsia, jaundice, amenorrhœa, and chlorosis. Locally applied, dissolved in glycerine, it acts favourably in skin diseases as a stimulant.

*Dose.*—From two to three grains every second or third day, as a stomachic tonic; from five to ten grains as a purgative. Generally administered in combination with other medicines.

*Preparations.*—**Extract of Socotrine Aloes** (*Extractum Aloes Socotrinæ*). Take of Socotrine Aloes, in small fragments, one pound; Boiling Water, one gallon. Add the aloes to the water, and stir well until they are thoroughly mixed. Set aside for twelve hours; then pour off the clear liquor, strain the remainder, and evaporate the mixed liquors by a water bath or a current of warm air to dryness.

*Dose.*—From two to six grains. It enters into Decoctum Aloes compositum and Extractum Colocynthidis compositum.

**Pill of Socotrine Aloes** (*Pilula Aloes Socotrinæ.*) Take of Socotrine Aloes, in powder, two ounces; Hard Soap, in powder, one ounce; Volatile Oil of Nutmeg, one fluid drachm; Confection of Roses, one ounce. Beat all together until thoroughly mixed.

*Dose.*—From five to ten grains.

**Pill of Aloes and Myrrh** (*Pilula Aloes et Myrrhæ*). Take of Socotrine Aloes, two ounces; Myrrh, one ounce; Saffron, dried, half an ounce; Confection of Roses, two ounces and a half. Triturate the aloes, myrrh, and saffron together, and sift; then add the confection of roses, and beat together into a uniform mass.

*Dose.*—From five to ten grains as a cathartic and emmenagogue.

**Pill of Aloes and Assafœtida** (*Pilula Aloes et Assafœtida*). Take of Socotrine Aloes, in powder, one ounce; Assafœtida, one ounce; Hard Soap, in powder, one ounce; Confection of Roses, one ounce. Beat all together until thoroughly mixed.

*Dose.*—From five to ten grains. Valuable as an antispasmodic and cathartic in hysterical cases.

**Compound Decoction of Aloes** (*Decoctum Aloes compositum*). Take of Extract of Socotrine Aloes, one hundred and twenty grains; Myrrh and Saffron, of each ninety grains; Carbonate of Potash, sixty grains; Extract of Liquorice, one ounce; Compound Tincture of Cardamoms, eight fluid ounces; Water, a sufficiency. Reduce the extract of aloes and myrrh to coarse powder, and put them together with the carbonate of potash and extract of liquorice into a suitable covered vessel with a pint of distilled water; boil gently for five minutes, then add the saffron. Let the vessel with its contents cool, then add the tincture of cardamoms, and covering the vessel closely, allow the ingredients to macerate for two hours; finally, strain through flannel, pouring as much distilled water over the contents of the strainer as will make the strained product measure thirty fluid ounces.

*Dose.*—From half a fluid ounce to two fluid ounces.

This decoction contains four grains of extract of aloes in a fluid ounce, while that of the Pharmacopœia of 1864 contained 5·6 grains, and that of the *Lond. Ph.* contained 3·3 grains.

**Wine of Aloes** (*Vinum Aloes*). Take of Socotrine Aloes, one ounce and a half; Cardamom seeds freed from the pericarps and bruised, eighty grains; Ginger, in coarse powder, eighty grains; Sherry, two pints. Macerate for seven days in a closed vessel, with occasional agitation; filter the liquor, and add sufficient sherry to make two pints.

*Dose.*—From one to two fluid drachms.

**Tincture of Aloes** (*Tinctura Aloes*). Take of Socotrine Aloes, in coarse powder, half an ounce; Extract of Liquorice, one ounce and a half; Proof Spirit, a sufficiency. Macerate the aloes and extract of liquorice in fifteen fluid ounces of the spirit for seven days, in a closed vessel, with occasional agitation, then filter, and add sufficient proof spirit to make one pint.

*Dose.*—From one to two fluid drachms. A good adjunct to purgative and emmenagogue draughts.

**Enema of Aloes** (*Enema Aloes*). Take of Aloes, forty grains; Carbonate of Potash, fifteen grains; Mucilage of Starch, ten fluid ounces. Mix, and rub together.

Useful in hysteria connected with amenorrhœa, and for dislodging ascarides vermiculares from the rectum.

Socotrine Aloes also enters into the composition of Pilula Rhei composita, Tinctura Benzoini composita, and Extractum Colocynthidis compositum.

## ALOE VULGARIS, *Lam.* Common Aloe.

(*Aloe Barbadensis*, Miller.)

(*Steph. et Church, Med. Bot.*, vol. ii. t. 109.)

*Habitat.*—East and West Indies, Northern Africa, and Southern Europe.

*Officinal Part.*—The inspissated juice of the leaf (*Aloe Barbadensis, Barbadoes Aloes*); imported into England from Barbadoes. It occurs in yellowish-brown or dark-brown opaque masses; breaks with a dull conchoidal fracture; has a bitter nauseous taste, and a strong disagreeable odour; dissolves almost entirely in proof spirit, and during solution exhibits under the microscope numerous crystals. Usually imported in gourds. Its activity resides in a resin and a peculiar principle, *Aloine.*

*Properties, Therapeutic Uses, and Dose.*—The same as those of Socotrine Aloes.

*Preparations.*—**Extract of Barbadoes Aloes** (*Extractum Aloes Barbadensis*). Prepared in the same manner as Extract of Socotrine Aloes.

*Dose.*—From two to six grains.

**Pill of Barbadoes Aloes** (*Pilula Aloes Barbadensis*). Take of Barbadoes Aloes, in powder, two ounces; Hard Soap, in powder, one ounce; Oil of Caraway, one fluid drachm; Confection of Roses, one ounce. Beat all together until thoroughly mixed.

*Dose.*—From five to ten grains.

**Pill of Aloes and Iron** (*Pilula Aloes et Ferri*). Take of Sulphate of Iron, one ounce and a half; Barbadoes Aloes, in powder, two ounces; Compound Powder of Cinnamon, three ounces; Confection of Roses, four ounces. Reduce the sulphate of iron to powder, rub it with the aloes and compound powder of cinnamon, and, adding the confection, make the whole into a uniform mass.

*Dose.*—From five to ten grains.

*Other Preparations.*—Barbadoes Aloes may be substituted for Socotrine Aloes in all the preparations given under the latter heading, it having been proved that in their action on the living body the two kinds differ little, if at all.

Barbadoes Aloes forms an ingredient in Pilula Cambogiæ composita, Pilula Colocynthidis composita, Pilula Colocynthidis et Hyoscyami.

## URGINEA SCILLA, *Steinheil.* Officinal Squill.

(*Bot. Mag.*, t. 918.)

*Habitat.*—Shores of the Mediterranean.

*Officinal Part.*—The sliced and dried bulb (*Scilla, Squill*). The bulb is pear-shaped, weighing from half a pound to ten pounds; outer scales membranous, brownish-red or white; inner scales thick, whitish, fleshy, juicy; taste mucilaginous, intensely and disagreeably bitter, somewhat acrid. The dried slices are white or yellowish-white, slightly translucent, scentless, disagreeably bitter, brittle, and easily pulverizable if very dry, but if exposed readily recovering moisture and flexibility. Its activity appears to reside in a peculiar resinous acrid extractive.

*Properties.*—Expectorant and diuretic in small doses; emetic and cathartic in larger ones. In over-doses an irritant poison.

*Therapeutic Uses.*—In the asthenic forms of dropsy, also in chronic bronchitis, asthma, and catarrhal affections, it acts beneficially. It has been advised as an emetic in croup and hooping cough.

*Dose.*—From one to three grains of the powdered bulb as an expectorant and diuretic; from ten to fifteen grains as an emetic.

*Preparations.*—**Tincture of Squill** (*Tinctura Scillæ*). Take of Squill, bruised, two ounces and a half; Proof Spirit, one pint. Macerate the squill for forty-eight hours, with fifteen ounces of the spirit, in a closed vessel, agitating occasionally; then transfer to a percolator; and when the fluid ceases to pass, continue the percolation with the remaining five ounces of the spirit. Afterwards subject the contents of the percolator to pressure, filter the product, mix the two liquids, and add sufficient proof spirit to make one pint.

*Dose.*—From ten to thirty drops. A good adjunct to cough and diuretic draughts.

**Vinegar of Squill** (*Acetum Scillæ*). Take of Squill, bruised, two ounces and a half; Diluted Acetic Acid, one pint; Proof Spirit, one fluid ounce and a half. Macerate the squill in the acetic acid for seven days;

then strain with expression, add the spirit to the strained liquor, and filter.

*Dose.*—From fifteen to forty minims.

**Oxymel of Squill** (*Oxymel Scillæ*).—Take of Vinegar of Squill, one pint; Clarified Honey, two pounds. Mix and evaporate by a water-bath until the product, when cold, shall have a specific gravity 1·32.

*Dose.*—From one half to one fluid drachm.

**Syrup of Squill** (*Syrupus Scillæ*).—Take of Vinegar of Squill, one pint; Refined Sugar, two pounds and a half. Dissolve with the aid of heat.

*Dose.*—From one half to one fluid drachm.

**Compound Squill Pill** (*Pilula Scillæ composita*). Take of Squill, in fine powder, one ounce and a quarter; Ginger, in powder, one ounce; Ammoniacum, in powder, one ounce; Hard Soap, in powder, one ounce; Treacle, by weight, two ounces, or a sufficiency. Mix the powders, add the treacle, and beat into a uniform mass.

*Dose.*—From five to ten grains.

It forms an ingredient also in Pilula Ipecacuanhæ cum Scilla.

(*Non-officinal.*)

**Urginea Indica**, *Kunth*, — *Scilla Indica*, Roxb. —(*Wight, Icones*, vol. vi. t. 2063), inhabits the sandy shores of the peninsular of India. The bulb is described by Roxburgh (*Flor. Indica*, vol. ii. p. 147) as being about the size of a large apple, white, of a taste fully as nauseous and bitter as the officinal squills; and, judging from these physical characters, he considered it probable that it possesses active properties. Examined, however, by Sir W. O'Shaughnessy, the bulbs were found inodorous, nearly tasteless, and devoid of any medicinal activity (*Bengal Disp.*, p. 663). An explanation of this discrepancy is probably to be found in the statement of Mr. Moodeen Sheriff, to the effect that the bulb when quite young and small, not exceeding a lime in size, in doses of ten, fifteen, and twenty grains, acts as a diuretic even more powerfully than the officinal squill, but as it grows larger it loses this property and becomes useless. Mr. Odoy Chund Dutt reports having given an extensive trial to the variety of squills met with in Behar, and found it so useful, even when administered alone, that he seldom had recourse to the European article. Additional evidence of its medicinal activity is furnished by Mr. Kanny Loll Dey (*Ind. Drugs*, p. 104). There can be little doubt that this is a fair substitute for the officinal squill, but the relative strength of the two has yet to be determined. Dr. H. R. Oswald reports that he has used an infusion of the bulbs in anasarcous cases, and that it acts as a diuretic, though not powerfully.

He likewise employed it, in five-grain doses, in bronchial affections, as an expectorant, but with what result is not stated.

**Ledebouria hyacinthoides,** *Roth.* (*Wight, Icones*, vol. vi. t. 2040). The bulbs of this plant, inhabiting sandy plains in many parts of India, resemble squills in general appearance, but are of a smaller size; they possess a bitterish nauseous acrid taste, and are employed by farriers in Southern India for the relief of stranguary, and in fevers occurring in horses (Ainslie, *Mat. Ind.*, vol. i. p. 402). For years they were issued from the Bombay Medical Stores in some of the preparations, in lieu of officinal squill (*Indian. Journ. of Med. Phys. Sci.*, Jan. 18, 1838, p. 9). Sir W. O'Shaughnessy, however, from trials made with them, holds out but little prospect of their being usefully employed in medicine (*Bengal Disp.*, p. 663).

**Aloe Indica,** *Royle* (*A. perfoliata, Roxb.*) and **Aloe litoralis,** *König*, the former inhabiting dry sandy plains in the North-western Provinces, and the latter similar localities on the sea coasts of the Madras Peninsula. According to Pereira (*Mat. Med.* vol. ii. P. ii. p. 193), *A. Indica* is the source, at any rate in part, of the *Indian Aloes* described by him. By inspissating the viscid juice of the leaves of *A. litoralis* collected at Cape Comorin, where the plant is in great abundance, the Editor in 1853 prepared several ounces of excellent aloes, which proved actively purgative in the same doses that the officinal aloe is usually prescribed in. Dr. W. Dymock, of Bombay, corroborates the statement that this plant yields very good aloes, adding that he has tried it both in the fresh and dried state. It appears certain that, with a little care, aloes of good quality might be obtained from this source, in considerable quantities, at a cost far less than that of the imported article. The aloe procurable in the bazaars, mostly imported, is generally of a very inferior description. The freshly expressed juice is in almost universal use as an external refrigerant application to all external or local inflammations.

**Gloriosa superba,** *Linn.* (*Wight, Icones*, vol. vi. t. 2047.)—The root of this handsome climbing plant, common in low jungles throughout India, has active properties assigned to it. Burman (*Flor. Indica*, p. 82), Roxburgh (*Flor. Indica*, vol. ii. p. 143), Ainslie (*Mat. Med. of Hind.*, p. 164), and others, speak of it as violently poisonous, and it finds a place in the List of Indian Poisons published by Dr. Norman Chevers (*Indian Ann. of Med. Sci.*, vol. ii. p. 147); but none of these authorities furnish any details of a case in which its ill effects have been observed. A belief in its poisonous properties is, however, common amongst the natives of all parts of India; and Dr. George Bidie informs the Editor that in Mysore he found *Bish* (*Root of Aconitum ferox*) largely adulterated with the root of this plant. It is very desirable to obtain further information with regard to its properties. In Travancore, a remedy held in esteem in the treatment of gonorrhœa is a white farinaceous powder, obtained from this root by bruising and repeated washing and maceration.

**Asparagus sarmentosus,** *Linn.*—The root of this plant, common throughout India, is sold in the bazaars of Patna under the name of *Utees* (*Irvine, Mat. Med. of Patna*, p. 119); and is supposed to constitute a portion of *Atís* (*Aconitum heterophyllum*, Wall) met with in the shops (*Bengal Disp.*, p. 168). This is confirmed by the report of Dr. R. F. Hutchinson. Its insipid taste is sufficient to distinguish it from the latter, which is intensely and purely bitter. There seems reason for supposing that these roots form a portion of the drug called *Saféd Músli* (see also *Bombax Malabaricum* and *Curculigo orchioides*). The roots of **A. racemosus,** *Willd.* (*Wight, Icones,* vol. vi. t. 2056), and **A. ascendens,** *Roxb.*, are, together with the preceding, employed medicinally by the natives, but they appear wholly unworthy of notice.

## MELANTHACEÆ.

### COLCHICUM AUTUMNALE, *Linn.* OFFICINAL COLCHICUM, or MEADOW SAFFRON.

(*Steph. et Church, Med. Bot.*, vol. ii. t. 70 ; *Engl. Bot.*, t. 133.)

*Habitat.*—Meadows throughout Europe.

*Officinal Parts.*—1. The fresh corm (*Colchici Cormus*), collected about the end of June, stripped of its coats, sliced transversely, and dried at a temperature not exceeding 150°. The fresh corm about the size of a chestnut, flattened where it has an undeveloped bud ; furnished with an outer brown and an inner yellow coat ; internally white, solid, and fleshy; yielding, when cut, a milky, acrid, and bitter juice. Dried slices about a line thick, moderately indented on one, rarely on both sides, firm, flat, whitish, amylaceous. 2. The Seeds (*Colchici Semina*), collected when fully ripe. They are of a reddish-brown colour, about the size of black-mustard seed, very hard, inodorous, of a bitter acrid taste. The activity both of the root and seeds resides in a peculiar crystallizable principle, *Colchicine.*

*Properties.*—Stimulant, its action being chiefly directed on the intestinal canal (hence its cathartic and emetic action), and on the liver (cholagogue), and on the genito-urinary system (diuretic). In gouty and rheumatic affections it appears to exercise an influence *sui generis* as a sedative. In large doses, it is a powerful acro-narcotic poison.

*Therapeutic Uses.*—In gout and rheumatism it is a remedy of established value; but it requires to be prescribed with discrimination, and under certain limitations. Amongst the other morbid states in which it has been employed with benefit are dropsical affections, especially when supervening on scarlet fever or connected with disease of the heart, cystitis and nephritis, and lithic acid deposits in the urine, particularly when these states occur in persons of a gouty diathesis ; senile enlargement of the prostate gland ; gonorrhœa, especially for the prevention of chordee ; rheumatic iritis, jaundice, obstinate constipation, chronic bronchitis, hooping cough, erysipelas, and as an anthelmintic in tænia.

*Dose.*—From two to eight grains of the powdered corm, repeated thrice daily or oftener. It is best given conjoined with aromatics.

*Preparation of the Corm.*—**Extract of Colchicum** (*Extractum Colchici*). Take of Fresh Colchicum Corms, deprived of their coats, seven pounds; crush the corms; press out the juice; allow the feculence to subside, and heat the clear liquid to 212°; then strain through flannel, and evaporate by a water bath, at a temperature not exceeding 160°, until the extract is of a suitable consistence for forming pills.

*Dose.*—From half a grain to two grains every four or six hours.

**Acetic Extract of Colchicum** (*Extractum Colchici Aceticum*). Take of fresh Colchicum Corms, deprived of their coats, seven pounds; Acetic Acid, six fluid ounces. Crush the corms, add the acetic acid, and press out the juice; allow the feculence to subside, and heat the clear liquor to 212°; then strain through flannel, and evaporate by a water bath, at a temperature not exceeding 160°, to the consistence of a soft extract.

*Dose.*—From half a grain to two grains three or four times daily.

**Wine of Colchicum** (*Vinum Colchici*). Take of Colchicum Corms, dried and sliced and bruised, four ounces; Sherry, one pint. Macerate the colchicum in the wine for seven days in a closed vessel, with occasional agitation, press and strain through calico; then add sufficient sherry to make one pint.

*Dose.*—From ten to thirty minims thrice daily or oftener.

*Preparation of the Seeds.*—**Tincture of Colchicum Seed** (*Tinctura Colchici Seminum*). Take of Colchicum Seed, bruised, two ounces and a half; Proof Spirit, one pint. Macerate the colchicum for forty-eight hours, with fifteen ounces of the spirit, in a close vessel, agitating occasionally. Then transfer to a percolator, and, when the fluid ceases to pass, continue the percolation with the remaining five ounces of spirit. Afterwards subject the contents of the percolator to pressure; filter the product; mix the liquids; and add sufficient proof spirit to make one pint.

*Dose.*—From ten to thirty minims three or four times a day. An excellent form for administration, often advantageously conjoined with antacids in gouty and rheumatic cases.

## VERATRUM VIRIDE, *Aiton*. GREEN OR AMERICAN HELLEBORE.

(*Bot. Mag.*, t. 1096; *Bigelow, Amer. Med. Bot.*, vol. ii. t. 33.)

*Habitat.*—East Coast of North America, from Canada to Carolina.

*Officinal Part.* — The rhizome (*Veratri Viridis Radix, Green Hellebore Root*) collected in the autumn, and dried. It consists of a somewhat tunicated top, with a thick hard base, and numerous radicles attached to it. The odour, disagreeable in the recent state, is lost by drying; the taste is at first sweetish, and then bitter, followed by a persistent acrid burning sensation in the mouth.

*Properties.*—Powerful sedative, especially of the circulatory system; in over doses, emetic and powerfully depressant.

*Therapeutic Uses.*—In some acute inflammations, *e.g.*, pneumonia; in acute and chronic rheumatism, gout, neuralgia, asthma, and in cardiac disease attended with increased action, it has been found serviceable. It has also been used in typhoid (enteric) fever, but with doubtful results.

*Dose.*—From one to two grains of the powdered root; it is, however, best administered in the form of Tincture.

*Preparation.*—**Tincture of Green Hellebore** (*Tinctura Veratri Viridis*). Take of Green Hellebore Root, in coarse powder, four ounces; Rectified Spirit, one pint. Macerate the hellebore for forty-eight hours in fifteen fluid ounces of the spirit, in a closed vessel, agitating occasionally; then transfer to a percolator, and, when the fluid ceases to pass, continue the percolation with the remaining five ounces of spirit. Afterwards subject the contents of the percolator to pressure, filter the product, mix the liquids, and add sufficient rectified spirit to make one pint.

*Dose.*—From five to twenty minims, repeated every third or fourth hour till the development of its physiological effects, when it should be discontinued, or the dose diminished.

## ASAGRÆA OFFICINALIS, *Lindley*. SABADILLA, OR CEVADILLA PLANT.

(*Bot. Reg.*, 1839, vol. xxv. t. 33.)

*Habitat.*—Mexico.

*Officinal Part.*—The Seeds (*Sabadillæ Semina, Sabadilla* or *Cevadilla Seeds*). *Characters.*—Fruit about half an inch long, consisting of three light-brown papyraceous follicles, each containing from one to three seeds, which are about a quarter of an inch long, blackish-brown, shining, slightly winged, possessing an intensely acrid bitter persistent taste. Their activity resides in an alkaloid, *Veratria.*

*Properties and Uses.*—Irritant. Has been employed as an anthelmintic, also in rheumatic and neuralgic affections; externally for destroying pediculi; but it is an unsafe and dangerous remedy in any case. The seeds are only officinal as a source of Veratria.

*Preparation.* — **Veratria** (*Veratria*). An Alkaloid, obtained from Cevadilla; not quite pure. *Characters.* —Pale grey; amorphous; without smell; but, even in the most minute quantity, powerfully irritating the nostrils; strongly and persistently bitter, and highly acrid; insoluble in water, sparingly soluble in spirit and ether, and in diluted acids, leaving traces of an insoluble brown resinoid matter. Heated with access of air it melts into a yellow liquid, and at length burns away, leaving no residue. An active poison.

*Dose.*—From one twelfth to one sixth of a grain, in the form of pill. From its highly poisonous nature, it is rarely, if ever, advisable to prescribe it internally.

**Ointment of Veratria** (*Unguentum Veratriæ*). Take of Veratria, eight grains; Prepared Lard, one ounce; Olive Oil, half a fluid drachm. Rub the veratria and the oil together; then mix them thoroughly with the lard.

A useful application in neuralgic, rheumatic, and paralytic cases. The strength of the ointment employed by Dr. Turnbull was from ten to twenty grains or more to one ounce of lard. Care is necessary in its application. If applied to a blistered or denuded surface, or if continued too long on the sound skin, the veratria is apt to become absorbed into the system, and to produce poisonous effects.

(*Non-officinal.*)

**Hermodactyl.**—This drug, which formerly held a high place in the treatment of gout and rheumatism, is still found in some of the bazaars of India, under the Hindústani name of *Súrinjan* (*Súr-renjan*, Ulfaz Udwiyeh, No. 1053). Sir W. O'Shaughnessy (*Bengal Disp.* p. 661) describes two kinds; one bitter (*Súrinjan tulk*), and the other tasteless (*Surinján shírín*). From trials made with the former, he came to the conclusion that it possesses all the properties of colchicum. It has, however, been long discarded from European practice, and no advantage would be gained by re-introducing it, as every effect which could be expected from it is obtainable more readily and eff tually from colchicum. M. Planchon, in his exhaustive treatise on this drug (*Des Hermodactes*, &c., Paris, 4to, 1856), assigns **Colchicum variegatum**, Linn. (*Bot. Mag.*, t. 1028), as its botanical source.

## PALMACEÆ.

(*Non-officinal.*)

**Cocos nucifera**, *Linn.* (*Rheede, Hort. Mal.*, vol. i. t. 1–4; *Roxb., Corom. Pl.*, t. 73).—*Cocoa-nut Tree.*—The product of this most useful of all trees which chiefly claims attention in this place, is the oil obtained by expression from the nucleus or kernel of the fruit. When freshly prepared, it is of a pale-yellowish colour, and almost inodorous, but after a few days it acquires a deeper hue, and a peculiar rancid odour and taste. It solidifies at about 70° F. It consists of a solid fat called *Cocin* or *Cocinine* (a combination of glycerine and cocinic or coco-stearic acid, and of a liquid fat or oleine (*Knapp's Chem. Technology*, 1848, vol. i. p. 468). On account of its cheapness it is much used as a vehicle for liniments, and other external applications; but for this purpose it is inferior to *Ground-nut Oil* (*Arachis hypogœa*) and *Jinjili Oil* (*Sesamum Indicum*). It is thought to have special properties in strengthening the hair; hence it is much in use as a local application in alopecia, and in loss of hair after fevers, and debilitating diseases. It was proposed by the late Dr. Theophilus Thompson (*Proceed. of Royal Society*, 1854, P. iii. p. 41) as a substitute for cod-liver oil; and in this character it has been favourably noticed by Dr. J. H. Warren (*Boston Med. and Surg. Journ.*, vol. iii. p. 377) and others. The substance used in these cases was not the ordinary commercial oil, but the oleine obtained by pressure from the crude oil (in the solid state it is met with in England), refined by being treated with alkalies, and then repeatedly washed with distilled water. In his Lettsomian Lectures, Dr. Thompson gives the result of his treatment with this agent, in 53 cases of phthisis. Of the first 30, 19 were much benefited, in 5 the disease remained stationary, and in the remaining 6 the disease continued to advance. Of the second 23, 15 were materially benefited, 3 remaining stationary, and 5 became worse. Dr. Garrod (*Brit. and For. Med. Chir. Rev.*, Jan. 1856) has shown that it exercises a marked influence, almost equal to cod-liver oil, in increasing the weight of the body. The great disadvantage of its employment experienced by Dr. Thompson, Dr. Garrod, and also by the Editor, who instituted some trials with it, is, that under its prolonged use it is apt to induce disturbance of the digestive organs, and diarrhœa. Its use is favourably noticed in the Report of Drs. Van Someren and Oswald, and Mr. J. Wood. Dr. Shortt reports having successfully employed the fresh "milk," *i.e.* the expressed juice of the grated kernel, in debility, incipient phthisis, and cachectic affections, in doses of from four to eight ounces twice or thrice daily. It has a pleasant taste, and may be used as an excellent substitute for cow's milk in coffee; it may thus be advantageously administered even to children. In large doses it proves aperient, and in some cases actively purgative; hence it is suggested by Mr. Wood as a substitute for castor oil and other nauseous purgatives. The freshly drawn sweet juice of the tree, called *Toddy*, equally with that of the Palmyra Palm, is valuable in the preparation of the Toddy Poultice (see *Borassus flabelliformis*). From this fluid, whether obtained from the Cocoa-nut or Palmyra Palm, a spirit (*Arrack*), vinegar, and an impure kind of sugar (*Jaggery*), are prepared.

**Borassus flabelliformis**, *Linn.* (*Rheede, Hort. Mal.*, vol. i. t. 9, 10; *Roxb. Corom. Pl.*, t. 71, 72.)—*Palmyra Palm.*—This noble and useful palm inhabits dry sandy soils in most parts of India as far as 30° N. Lat. Regarded medicinally, the product most worthy of note is the Toddy, the saccharine juice obtained by the excision of the spadix or young flowering branch, collected before sunrise in considerable quantities, in a vessel attached to the wounded part. This fluid, when freshly drawn, is pleasantly sweet, but rather nauseous, and if taken in doses of about a tumbler full, for several mornings in succession, it acts as a laxative. Left exposed to the air, soon after sunrise vinous fermentation commences, and it becomes converted into arrack, one of the most intoxicating drinks of the country. This arrack, subjected to distillation until it has a Sp. Gr. of ·920, may be employed as Proof Spirit in the preparation of officinal Tinctures and for other pharmaceutical purposes. A very useful stimulant application (*Toddy Poultice*), intended as a substitute for Yeast Poultice, may be prepared by adding freshly drawn toddy to rice flour till it has the consistence of a soft poultice, and subjecting this to heat over a gentle fire, stirring constantly till fermentation commences. This spread on a cloth, and applied to the parts, acts as a valuable stimulant application to gangrenous ulcerations, carbuncles, and indolent ulcers. The Editor has repeatedly seen it employed with satisfactory results. The light-brown cotton-like substance from the outside of the base of the fronds is employed by the Cingalese doctors as a styptic for arresting hæmorrhage from superficial wounds (*Bennett's Ceylon,* p. 92.) The same substance from the cocoa-nut tree is used for a similar purpose by the people of Bengal (*Long. Journ. of Agri.-Hort. Soc. of India,* 1859, vol. xi. p. 351). It is also used in like manner in Travancore. It is reported to act very effectually. This may be worthy of remembrance in cases of accidents occurring in localities where the usual appliances are not at hand.

**Caryota urens**, *Linn.* (*Rheede, Hort Mal.*, vol. i. t. 11.)—*Bastard Sago Tree.*—An excellent spirit is obtained by the fermentation and distillation of the toddy obtained from this elegant Palm, which is not uncommon on the Western coast of the Madras Peninsula. It is well adapted for pharmaceutical purposes. An inferior sort of sago is prepared from the pith. A glass of the freshly drawn toddy, taken early in the morning, acts as a laxative; it is thus much used by the people of Malabar.

**Areca Catechu**, *Linn.* (*Rheede, Hort. Mal.*, vol. i. t. 5–8; *Roxb., Corom. Pl.*, t. 75.) — *Betel Nut* or *Areca Palm.* — The seed of this elegant Palm (*Betel Nut*) is in common use throughout the East as a masticatory, in conjunction with the leaf of Piper Betel and chunam (unslaked lime). It is considered to strengthen the gums, sweeten the breath, and improve the tone of the digestive organs. According to the analysis of Morin (*Journ. de Pharm.*, vol. viii. p. 449) it contains a large proporation of tannic and gallic acids; hence the statement in the Taleef Shereef (p. 92) that it is astringent, is doubtless correct. From it there is prepared in some parts of India an astringent extract, which constitutes one of the varieties of catechu, the *Cachou d'Arec* of Guibourt (*Hist. des Drogues*, vol. iii. p. 375), and the *Betel Nut Catechu*, or *Kassu*, of Pereira (*Mat. Med.*, vol. ii. P. ii. p. 341). It occurs in round, flat cakes, from two to three inches in diameter, from half an inch to an inch in thickness, weighing from two to three ounces, blackish brown internally, inodorous, of a strongly astringent rather bitter taste. It possesses the same properties, and is applicable to the same cases, as officinal Catechu, the produce of *Acacia Catechu*. The seed, reduced to charcoal and powdered, forms an excellent dentifrice. Anthelmintic virtues have been assigned to the nut (*Braithwaite's Retrospect of Med.*, 1863, vol. xlvii. p. 116), but it can hardly have any claim to this character, as, amongst the Hindús and Burmese, who use it habitually as a masticatory, intestinal worms (lumbrici) are almost universally met with. Dr. J. Shortt states that the powdered nut, in doses of ten or fifteen grains every three or four hours, is useful in checking diarrhœa arising from debility. The dry expanded petioles, according to Dr. Bholanauth Bose, serve as excellent ready-made splints for fractures. He considers that they cannot be too highly recommended for hospital use in India generally.

# AROIDEÆ.

(*Non-officinal.*)

**Acorus calamus**, *Linn.* (*Steph. et Church, Med. Bot.*, vol. i. t. 32.) —*Sweet Flag.*—A common plant in moist sites throughout Europe, Asia, and North America. The root-stock or rhizome has long been held in esteem as a stomachic and tonic, and its aromatic bitterness seems to justify its use in these characters. In the dried state it is met with in all the bazaars of India, being one of the most popular remedies of the native practitioners. It appears to be well adapted for those forms of atonic dyspepsia which are attended with flatulence, and Dr. Pereira (*Mat. Med.*, vol. ii. P. i. p. 140) speaks of it as especially serviceable in the dyspepsia of gouty subjects. As an antiperiodic it is favourably noticed by Dr. A. T. Thomson (*Dispensatory*, p. 183); and Prof. Royle (*Mat. Med.*, p. 655) states that he frequently employed it with success in intermittent fevers occurring in natives of India; he prescribed it in conjunction with Bonduc Nut (*Cœsalpinia Bonducella*, Linn.), Chiretta and other bitters. In low adynamic fevers it certainly appears to be an appropriate adjunct to other remedies of the same class. Dr. Æ. Ross speaks of it as an excellent stimulant diaphoretic in these cases; he also reports of it as most serviceable in atonic and choleraic diarrhœa, and as a very useful external application (the powdered rhizome rubbed up with cashew spirit) in chronic rheumatism. His estimate of it in these cases is very high. Its powers as an insectifuge and insecticide, especially in relation to fleas, are noticed in several of the reports received from India. The dose of the dried rhizome in powder is from twenty to forty grains or more, but it is best administered in infusion (dried rhizome, bruised, one ounce; boiling water, ten fluid ounces), in doses of from one and a half to two fluid ounces. The root-stock occurs in pieces of various lengths, about the thickness of the thumb, rather flattened; spongy, and provided with numerous sheath-like ringed appendages; odour, peculiar and aromatic; taste, bitterish and acrid. It contains a volatile oil, in which its virtues reside. It was officinal in the London and Edinburgh Ph., but has been omitted in the British Ph.

**Scindapsus (Pothos) officinalis**, *Schott.* (*Wight, Icones*, vol. iii. t. 778).—The dried and sliced fruit of this plant, common in many parts of India, forms an article of the Indian Materia Medica, under the name of *Gujpipul*, Hind. (*Gudjpepullie*, Taleef Shereef, p. 118, No. 710.) Stimulant, diaphoretic, and anthelmintic virtues are ascribed to it, but our knowledge of its virtues rests solely on native testimony. Dr. Bholanauth Bose reports very highly of the styptic powers of the pressed juice of the petioles of **Colocasia antiquorum**, *Schott.* (*Wight, Icones*, vol. iii. t. 786.) He states that it is capable of arresting even arterial hæmorrhage, and that the wound after its application generally heals by first intention. The roots of **Typhonium orixense,** *Schott* (*Wight, Icones*, vol. iii. t. 806), **Dracontium polyphyllum,** *Linn.* **Colocasia macrorhiza,** *Schott,* **Alocasia montana,** *Schott* (*Wight, Iones*, vol. iii. t. 796), and other plants of this Natural Order, indigenous in India, possess in common considerable acridity in the fresh state, and are employed by the natives as external stimulants or rubefacients in various affections. Any good effect which could be expected from them may, however, be more readily obtained from a mustard poultice. The acrid principle is very volatile; and by the application of heat, or by simple drying, the roots become innocuous or even wholesome as articles of diet. Powerful antispasmodic powers are attributed to the fresh roots of *D. polyphyllum* by the people of Malabar.

## CYPERACEÆ.

**Cyperus rotundus,** *Linn.*—(*Motha*, Hind.)—The roots of this plant, common in moist localities throughout India, are ovoid, of the size of a pigeon's egg, united by a long woody radicle of leafy texture; substance white, friable, and spongy; odour sweet, slightly aromatic; taste bitter, resinous, and balsamic, especially when dry. (*Bengal Disp.*, p. 627.) Stimulant, diaphoretic and diuretic properties are assigned to them; and in the Taleef Shereef (p. 159) they are further described as astringent and vermifuge. They are much in repute amongst the natives of Calcutta as a powerful tonic, and are employed chiefly in disorders of the stomach, and irritable states of the bowels. In the *Calcutta Med. Phys. Trans.*, vol. ii. p. 399, General Hardwick furnishes an account of two cases of cholera which recovered under their use; but how far the disease yielded to the remedy appears extremely doubtful. The roots of **C. pertenuis** (*Nagur-Motha*, Hind.), partake in the aromatic properties of the preceding, and are regarded as diaphoretic and diuretic. Both are of very minor importance.

# GRAMINEÆ.

## SECALE CEREALE, *Linn.* COMMON RYE.

(*Steph. et Church, Med. Bot.*, vol. ii. t. 113.)

*Habitat.*—Cultivated in many parts of Europe.

*Officinal Part.*—The sclerotium (compact mycelium or spawn) of Claviceps purpurea, *Tulasne,* produced within the paleæ of the common rye (*Ergota, Ergot.*) It has the following characters:—Subtriangular, curved, with a longitudinal furrow on the concave side, obtuse at the ends; from one third of an inch to an inch and a half in length; of a violet brown colour on the surface, pinkish within, solid, frangible, fracture short, odour faintly marked, but strong if the powder be triturated with solution of potash. Its activity resides in an extractiform alkaloid, *Secalina.* It likewise contains a fixed oil, which is probably only a bland oil holding a portion of Secalina in solution. It should be kept, dried at 212° F., in well stoppered bottles.

*Properties.*—Stimulant, its action being chiefly directed on the muscular tissue of the uterus and on the genito-urinary system; hence its value as parturifacient and emmenagogue. Astringent properties have also been assigned to it. Taken continuously as an article of food or otherwise, it acts as a poison, inducing two peculiar states of the constitution, denominated respectively gangrenous ergotism and convulsive ergotism.

*Therapeutic Uses.*—In lingering labours depending upon atony or want of muscular contractions of the uterus, it is an agent of established value. In retention of the placenta from the same cause, and in hæmorrhage occurring during labour, it is no less valuable. Amongst other affections of the genito-urinary system in which it has been employed with benefit, are amenorrhœa, leucorrhœa, chlorosis, atonic menorrhagia, hypertrophy of the uterus, retention of urine arising from deficient contractility of the muscular coat of the bladder or from paralysis, incontinence of urine, gonorrhœa, gleet, and spermatorrhœa. It has likewise been found serviceable in atonic hæmaturia and other passive hæmorrhages, chronic diarrhœa, and in certain affections of the eye, characterised by want of power or disturbed accommodation of vision from the organ having been overtasked.

*Dose.*—From twenty to thirty grains of the fresh powder as a parturifacient, repeated once or twice at intervals of twenty or thirty minutes, if required. As an emmenagogue and astringent, from four to six grains twice or thrice daily.

*Preparations.*—**Infusion of Ergot** (*Infusum Ergotæ.*) Take of Ergot, in coarse powder, a quarter of an ounce; Boiling Water, ten fluid ounces. Infuse in a covered vessel for half an hour, and strain.

*Dose.*—From one to two fluid ounces repeated in the same manner as the powder (*ante*). The infusion should be prepared fresh when required.

**Tincture of Ergot** (*Tinctura Ergotæ*). Take of Ergot, in coarse powder, five ounces; Proof Spirit, one pint. Macerate the Ergot for forty-eight hours, in fifteen fluid ounces of the Spirit, in a closed vessel, agitating occasionally; then transfer to a percolator, and, when the fluid ceases to pass, continue the percolation with the remaining five ounces of spirit. Afterwards subject the contents of the percolator to pressure, filter the product, mix the liquids, and add sufficient proof spirit to make one pint.

*Dose.*—From ten minims to one fluid drachm.

**Liquid Extract of Ergot** (*Extractum Ergotæ Liquidum*). Take of Ergot, in coarse powder, one pound; Ether, one pint, or a sufficiency; Distilled Water, three pints and a half; Rectified Spirit, eight fluid ounces. Shake the ether in a bottle with half a pint of the water, and after separation decant the ether. Place the ergot in a percolator, and free it from its oil by passing the washed ether slowly through it. Remove the marc, and digest it in three pints of the water at 160° for twelve hours. Press out, strain, and evaporate the liquor by the heat of a water-bath to nine fluid ounces; when cold, add the spirit. Allow it to stand for an hour to coagulate, then filter. The product should measure sixteen fluid ounces.

*Dose.*—From ten to thirty minims, as a parturifacient.

[Dr. R. Tytler (*Calcutta Med. Phys. Trans.*, 1831, vol. v. p. 441) observed Barley, during its growth in the Upper Provinces of India, affected with a disease very similar to, if not identical with, the Ergot in Rye. The diseased grain is represented as having been extremely poisonous. He noticed an analogous disease in Oats, and occasionally in the spikes of *Holcus spicatus*. It has also been observed in Rice. (See *Journ. Agri.-Hort. Soc. of India*, vol. i. p. 7.]

Mr. M. C. Cooke has met with it in no less than fifteen species of Gramineæ in Great Britain. The Ergot of Wheat has indeed been recommended as superior to that of Rye as a parturifacient.

## SACCHARUM OFFICINARUM, *Linn.* THE SUGAR CANE.

(*Steph. et Church, Med. Bot.*, vol. iii. t. 148.)

*Habitat.*—Cultivated in the tropics of both hemispheres.

*Officinal Part.*—1. Pure Cane Sugar (*Saccharum purificatum, Refined Sugar*) prepared from the juice of the stem. Compact, crystalline, snow-white, dry, scentless, and purely sweet, *Comp.* $C_{24}H_{22}O_{22}$, or $\mathbf{C_{12}H_{22}O_{11}}$. 2. The uncrystallised residue of the refining of sugar (*Theriaca, Treacle*). A thick, brown, fermentable syrup, very sweet; not crystallising by rest or evaporation, Sp. Gr. about 1·40. *Test.*—Nearly free from empyreumatic odour and flavour.

*Properties and Uses.*—Demulcent, nutritive, and dietetic; much employed in disguising the taste of nauseous medicines, and in the formation of syrups, electuaries, confections, and lozenges. Treacle is chiefly employed in making pills; it serves well to give cohesiveness, to preserve the pill-mass soft, to prevent mouldiness, and in some cases to check chemical change. The medicinal virtues of both sugar and treacle are of minor importance.

*Preparation of Sugar.*—**Syrup** (*Syrupus, Syrupus simplex, Edin. Ph.*) Take of Refined Sugar, five pounds; Water, two pints. Dissolve the sugar in the water with the aid of heat; and add, after cooling, as much water as may be necessary to make the weight of the product seven pounds and a half. The specific gravity should be 1·330.

Chiefly used as a flavouring agent.

## HORDEUM DISTICHON, *Linn.* COMMON OR LONG-EARED BARLEY.

(*Woodville. Med Bot.*, vol. v. t. 29.)

*Habitat.*—Cultivated throughout the temperate zone.

*Officinal Part.*—The husked seeds (*Hordeum decorticatum, Pearl Barley*). They are white, rounded, retaining a trace of the longitudinal furrow.

*Properties and Uses.*—Demulcent; much used as a nutritive article of diet for the sick.

*Preparation.*—**Decoction of Barley** (*Decoctum Hordei*). Take of Pearl Barley, two ounces; Water, one pint and a half. Wash the barley in cold water, and reject the washings; boil with the water for twenty minutes in a covered vessel, and strain.

A useful demulcent drink; may be taken *ad libitum* in all cases requiring this class of remedies.

TRITICUM VULGARE, *Villars.* COMMON WHEAT.
(*Steph. et Church, Med. Bot.*, vol. ii. t. 113.)

*Habitat.*—Cultivated in all temperate parts of the globe.

*Officinal Parts.*—1. The grain, ground and sifted (*Tritici Farina, Wheaten Flour*). 2. Starch procured from the seed (*Amylum*). It occurs in white columnar masses. When rubbed in a mortar with a little cold distilled water, it is neither acid nor alkaline to test-paper, and the filtered liquid does not become blue on the addition of solution of iodine. Mixed with boiling water and cooled, it gives a deep-blue colour with iodine.

*Properties and Uses.*—Demulcent, nutritive. Flour forms a soothing local application in erysipelatous and other external inflammations. It is also applied to burnt and excoriated surfaces, in which it acts chiefly by protecting the parts from the air. Internally, flour and water is used as a chemical antidote in poisoning by the preparations of mercury, copper, zinc, silver, and tin, and by iodine. It forms a constituent in linseed and other poultices. Wheaten bread is used in pharmacy in the preparation of pills; soaked in water, it is likewise employed in the form of poultice.

*Preparations.* — **Mucilage of Starch** (*Mucilago Amyli*). Take of Starch, one hundred and twenty grains; Water, ten fluid ounces. Triturate the starch with the water, gradually added; then boil for a few minutes, constantly stirring.

Demulcent; a good vehicle for enemas in dysentery and other bowel affections.

**Glycerine of Starch** (*Glycerinum Amyli*). Take of Starch, one ounce; Glycerine, eight fluid ounces. Rub them together until they are intimately mixed; then transfer the mixture to a porcelain dish, and apply a heat gradually raised to 240°, stirring it constantly until the starch particles are completely broken, and a translucent jelly is formed.

Demulcent application in skin diseases, excoriations, and other local affections.

---

* ORYZA SATIVA, *Linn.* COMMON RICE.

*Habitat.*—Cultivated throughout the tropics.

*Officinal Part.*—1. The husked seeds (*Oryza, Rice*), from one to three lines long, white, translucent, cylindrical, furrowed, obtuse at both ends, brittle. 2. The Flour (*Oryzæ Farina, Rice flour*), procured from the seeds.

*Properties and Uses.*—Analogous to those of wheat, over which it possesses the advantage, in tropical countries, of being generally available at comparatively small cost.

*Preparations.*—**Decoction of Rice** (*Decoctum Oryzæ*). Take of Rice, one ounce; Water, two pints. Boil in a covered vessel for twenty minutes, and strain.

An excellent demulcent refrigerant drink in febrile and inflammatory diseases, dysuria, and other affections requiring this class of remedies. It is rendered more palatable by being acidulated with lime juice, and sweetened with sugar.

**Poultice of Rice** (*Cataplasma Oryzæ*). Take of Rice Flour, a sufficiency; place in an open vessel over the fire, and gradually add Water, constantly stirring until the mass has the required consistency.

This poultice is in constant use in hospital and dispensary practice in India. The Editor, from many years' experience of its use in all cases in which linseed-meal poultices are usually employed in English practice, can testify to its value as a substitute for the latter article.

## *ANDROPOGON (CYMBOPOGON) CITRATUM (67), *D.C.* Lemon Grass.

*Habitat.*—Commonly cultivated in gardens in India; also in Ceylon, upon a larger scale, for the sake of its volatile oil.

*Officinal Part.*—The Volatile Oil (*Oleum Andropogi citrati, Lemon Grass Oil, Oil of Verbena*), obtained by distillation from the fresh plant; of a pale-sherry colour, transparent, extremely pungent taste, and a peculiar fragrant lemon-like odour.

*Properties.*—Stimulant, carminative, antispasmodic, and diaphoretic; locally applied, rubefacient.

*Therapeutic Uses.*—In flatulent and spasmodic affections of the bowels, and in gastric irritability, it is a remedy of value. In cholera it proves serviceable, not only by allaying and arresting the vomiting, but by aiding the process of reaction. Externally applied, it forms an excellent embrocation in chronic rheumatism, neuralgia, sprains, and other painful affections. (68)

*Dose.*—From three to six drops on sugar or in emulsion. For external application it should be diluted with twice its bulk of any bland oil or soap liniment.

## *ANDROPOGON (CYMBOPOGON) NARDUS, *Linn.*

CITRONELLE.

(*Andropogon Martini, Thwaites.*)

*Habitat.*—Madras Peninsula and Ceylon.

*Officinal Part.*—The volatile oil obtained by distillation from the fresh plant. This oil is imported for the use of perfumers into England, from Ceylon and Madras, under the name of *Oil of Citronelle.* It closely assimilates in characters, properties, and uses with the analogous product of *A. citratum,* D.C.

## *ANDROPOGON PACHNODES, *Trin.*

A volatile oil, resembling in general characters the two preceding oils, known by the Hindústani name *Rúsa ka tel,* manufactured in Northern and Central India, is the produce, it is believed, of this species of Andropogon, which is regarded by some botanists as a form of *A. schoenanthus,* Linn., and of *A. Martini,* Roxb. It has obtained considerable repute as an external application in rheumatic, neuralgic, and other painful affections. (69)

(*Non-officinal.*)

**Andropogon muricatus,** *Retz.*—This grass extends throughout India, and is much valued for its fragrant roots (*Khus-khus,* Hind., *Vetti-ver,* Tam.), which form an article of export to Europe, where it is used in perfumery. Antispasmodic, diaphoretic, diuretic, and emmenagogue properties havo been assigned to it; but beyond being a gentle stimulant diaphoretic, it seems to have no just claims to notice as a medicine. An account of the uses to which it has been applied in Europe is given by Pereira (*Mat. Med.,* vol. ii. P. i. p. 132). Its uses in native practice are detailed in the Taleef Shereef, p. 14, No. 47. According to the analysis of Geiger, it contains a resin, a bitter extractive, and a volatile oil. The dose of the powdered root is about twenty grains, or it may be given in infusion (two drachms of the bruised root to ten ounces of boiling water), in doses of an ounce or more. As a medicine, as far as is at present known, it is an article of very minor importance.

**Bambusa arundinacea,** *Schultz.*—In addition to the many important uses to which *the Bamboo* is applied in tropical life, it forms by no means an insignificant article of the Indian Materia Medica. Its supposed virtues are set forth at length in the Taleef Shereef (art. *Bans,* p. 28, No. 114). A belief in the emmenagogue properties of the leaves is common alike in India and China; but neither in this nor in any other character does it appear worthy ol attention as a medicine. In positions where ordinary surgical appliances are not at hand, it is well to bear in mind that, with very little manipulation, splints of any required length or size can be obtained with little delay from the stems of the bamboo. For this purpose the older drier stems are to be preferred, the younger yielding somewhat on pressure. A silicious concretion, *Tabashir* or *Tabasheer*, found in the articulations of the bamboo, merits a brief notice. The most complete account of its varieties, history, formation, and properties has been published by Sir David Brewster (*Philosoph. Trans.*, 1819, and *Edin. Journ. of Science*, vol. viii. p. 286); and in the same paper are embodied some learned remarks by Prof. H. H. Wilson on its nomenclature, and the uses to which it is applied by the natives, drawn from Sanscrit works. Several analyses of it have been made by Smithson, Fourcroy and Vauquelin, John, and Dr. E. Turner. The most recent and complete is that of Prof. T. Thomson, of Glasgow, (*Records of Gen. Science*, Feb. 1836,) who found its constituents to be, in 100 parts, Silica, 90·50; Potash, 1·10; Peroxide of Iron, 0·90; Aluminia, 0·40; Moisture, 4·87; Loss, 2·23. It is highly prized in native practice as a stimulant and aphrodisiac; but from its composition we are warranted in believing that as a medicinal agent it is inert. (*Madras Quart. Journ. of Med.*, April 1862, p. 245.)

## FILICES.

### NEPHRODIUM FILIX MAS, *Richard*. MALE SHIELD FERN.

(*Aspidium Filix mas, Swartz, in Brit. Pharm.*)
(*Hooker, Brit. Ferns*, t. 15.)

*Habitat.*—Woods and shady localities in various parts of Europe, Asia, and Northern Africa.

*Officinal Part.*—The dried rhizome, with the bases of the foot-stalks and portion of the root fibres (*Filix Mas, Male Fern*) collected in the summer. As met with it usually consists of fragments of dried thickened bases of the frond stalks, to which small portions of the rhizome are found adhering; odour feeble, earthy, disagreeable; taste at first sweetish, subsequently bitter and nauseous. The powder, which partakes in the peculiar odour and taste of the dried root, of a greenish yellow colour, should be preserved in well-stoppered bottles. Its activity resides in an oleoresin.

*Properties and Uses.*—Anthelmintic; especially adapted for the treatment of tape-worm.

*Dose.*—From one to three drachms of the freshly prepared powder. But it is far more powerful when administered in the following preparation:

*Preparation.*—**Liquid Extract of Male Fern** (*Extractum Filicis liquidum*). Take of Male Fern, in coarse powder, two pounds; Ether, four pints, or a sufficiency. Pack the male fern closely in a percolator, and pass the ether slowly through it until it passes colourless. Let the ether evaporate on a water-bath, or recover it by distillation, and preserve the oily extract.

*Dose.*—From fifteen to thirty minims in the form of electuary or emulsion, preceded by the action of a purgative. The above preparation has also been designated Ethereal Extract, and Ethereal Oil of Male Fern. It is a most effective preparation.

## FUNGI.

(*Non-officinal.*)

**Polyporus anthelminticus,** *Berkeley.*—Under the Burmese names of **Wa-mo** (*Bamboo Mushroom*), and **Than-mo** (*Worm Mushroom*), this fungus is held in high esteem by the people of the Tenasserim Provinces, where it is indigenous, as an anthelmintic. It was first brought to notice in 1840 by Dr. Packman (*Madras Quart. Med. Journ.*, vol. v. p. 146); and in that journal are the details of four cases, three by Dr. Richmond, and one by Dr. Shaw, which prove that its character as an anthelmintic in cases of lumbrici is worthy of further attention. The dose of the dried fungus is about two drachms, rasped or in powder, given in any convenient vehicle. It produces no sensible effect on the system, but if followed on the third morning by a purgative, the entozoa are expelled in a lifeless state, proving that the remedy has exercised a specific influence on them. Being without taste or smell, children take it readily. In case of the first dose not producing the desired effect, it may be repeated at intervals of two or three days, and the quantity may be increased to three or even four drachms; no injurious effect appears to be produced, however large the dose (*Packman*). It seems well worthy of further trials, though it is to be feared that it never could be obtained in sufficient quantities to come into general use. Amongst the Burmese themselves, its use has in a great measure been superseded, according to the reports of Drs. Marr and Rean, by an imported nostrum which has santonine for a base. For a botanical account of this fungus see *Gardener's Chronicle*, Aug. 18th, 1866.

## LICHENES.

### CETRARIA ISLANDICA, *Achar.* ICELAND MOSS.

(*Steph. et Church. Med. Bot.*, vol. ii. t. 69.)

*Habitat.*—Dry mountainous districts of the northern portions of Europe and America.

*Officinal Part.*—The entire Lichen (*Cetraria, Iceland Moss*).—It is foliacious, lobed, crisp, cartilaginous, brownish-white, paler beneath, bitter and mucilaginous. A strong decoction gelatinises on cooling. It contains a large proportion of starch, and a bitter principle, *Cetrarin* or *Cetraric Acid.*

*Properties.*—Demulcent, nutritive, tonic.

*Therapeutic Uses.*—In scrofulous and scorbutic affections, accompanied by much debility, and also in debility arising from diarrhœa, dysentery, and other exhausting diseases, this lichen in the form of decoction or jelly, proves serviceable as a tonic and nutritive agent. It has likewise been thought valuable in phthisis. Cetrarin has been proposed as an antiperiodic.

*Preparation.*—**Decoction of Iceland Moss** (*Decoctum Cetrariæ*). Take of Iceland Moss, one ounce; Water, one pint. Wash the moss in cold water, to remove impurities; boil it with the distilled water for ten minutes in a covered vessel, and strain, with gentle pressure, while hot; then pour distilled water over the contents of the strainer until the strained product measures a pint.

*Dose.*—From one to three ounces three or four times daily.

[When intended solely as a nutritive, the bitter principle should be removed. This may be effected in two ways; 1, by macerating the lichen in twenty-four times its weight of a weak alkaline solution formed by 1 part of an alkaline carbonate and 375 parts of water; 2, by macerating it in distilled water, and heating the infusion once or twice up to about 180° F. It is then to be boiled in water or milk. When the decoction is sufficiently concentrated, it gelatinises on cooling. It may be flavoured with sugar, lemon peel, wine, or aromatics, and it then forms a nutritious as well as agreeable article of diet for the sick room.]

## ROCCELLA TINCTORIA, *D.C.* Dyer's Orchella Weed.

*Habitat.*—Maritime rocks of Madeira and other islands in the Atlantic, also Coast of South America; a closely allied species, *R. fuciformis,* D.C., occurs in Ceylon and India.

*Officinal Part.*—The entire lichen, from an infusion of which a blue pigment (*Lacmus, Litmus*) is prepared by the action of soda or potash.

*Properties and Uses.*—Litmus is officinal solely as a chemical test.

*Preparations.*—**Tincture of Litmus** (*Tinctura Lacmi*). Take of Litmus, in powder, one ounce; Proof

R 2

Spirit, ten fluid ounces. Macerate for two days in a closed vessel, and filter.

**Blue Litmus Paper.** Unsized Paper steeped in Tincture of Litmus, and dried by exposure to the air.

Employed to detect the presence of acids and acidulous salts, which communicate to it a more or less red tinge.

**Red Litmus Paper.** Unsized Paper steeped in Tincture of Litmus, which has been previously reddened by the addition of a very minute quantity of sulphuric acid, and dried by exposure to the air.

A test for alkalies, which restore to the paper the blue colour of litmus.

[According to Dr. Robert Haines the powdered thallus of *R. tinctoria* and other allied species forms an ingredient in the nostrum called "Goa Powder," which has obtained in some parts of India considerable repute as a remedy in ringworm.]

(*Non-officinal.*)

**Parmelia perlata,** *Ach*, and **P. perforata,** *Ach*. (*Lichen rotundatus, Rottler*, in *Ainslie, Mat. Ind.* vol. ii. p. 170.) This lichen, common on rocks in most parts of the Madras Peninsula, is known by the names *Kulpasi*, Tam., and *Patthar ká phúl*, Hind. Some years since it attracted considerable attention as a diuretic, for which purpose it was first boiled in water, then beaten into a pulp or bruised in a mortar, and placed as a poultice over the renal and lumbar regions. Its efficacy in dropsical affections was attested by Dr. Stevenson, of H. M. 13th Dragoons (*Calcutta Med. Phys. Trans.*, vol. v. p. 430), Dr. W. H. Radford (*Mad. Med. Journ.* 1839, vol. i. p. 18), and others (*Ibid.* 1843, vol. v. p. 389). According to these authorities the application of the lichen poultice was followed by marked diuresis; and dropsical cases which had resisted ordinary means, improved or recovered under its use. Dr. S. Rogers (*Ibid.* vol. i. p. 18), however, states that he tried it extensively at the Madras Native Infirmary, and that in every instance he failed to observe that it produced the least effect upon the kidneys. To test its alleged efficacy, it should be tried in a series of cases simultaneously with another series treated with an ordinary linseed or rice poultice; and the probability is that the continuous application of warmth and moisture by their means respectively would be found nearly equal.

## ALGÆ.

### * GRACILARIA LICHENOIDES, AND G. CONFERVOIDES, *Greville*. CEYLON MOSS.

(*Turner's Fuci*, t 118.)

*Habitat.*—Coast of Ceylon and the islands of the Indian Archipelago.

*Officinal Part.*—The dried plant (*Ceylon Moss*). Occurs in yellowish white or light purple ramifying filaments from one to several inches in length; at the base the larger filaments not exceeding the thickness of a crow quill, the smaller fibres being about as thick as fine sewing thread; consistence cartilaginous, odour resembling sea weed, taste feebly saline. Its virtues reside in a vegetable jelly (*Pectin*), the amount of which in the plant has been found to range from 37 to 78 per cent. [70]

*Properties and Uses.*—Demulcent and nutritive, a light and readily digestible article of diet for invalids and children; useful in dysenteric and other cases characterised by irritation of the intestinal canal.

*Preparation.*—**Decoction of Ceylon Moss** (*Decoctum Gracilaræ*). Take of Ceylon Moss, ground to a fine powder, a quarter of an ounce; Water, two pints. Boil for twenty minutes, and strain.

*Dose.*—May be taken *ad libitum.*

[If milk be substituted for water in the above preparation, it is generally rendered more acceptable to the palate as well as more nourishing. It may be further improved by the addition of cinnamon or other aromatics. By increasing the proportion of the ground moss to half an ounce, the strained solution, on cooling, becomes a firm jelly, which, with the addition of a little wine, sugar, and spices, forms an excellent article of light food for convalescents and sick children.]

*(Non-officinal.)*

**Gillur ka putta.**—Under this Hindústani name there is met with, in Upper India, a dried leaf-like looking substance, which is held in repute as a remedy for bronchocele. It is steeped in cold water during the night, and the infusion drunk in the morning on an empty stomach. Mr. H. Cope, who has published an interesting paper on this substance (*Journ. of Agri.-Hort. Soc. of India*, 1858, vol. x. p. 216), forwarded specimens to Dr. T. Thomson, who regards it as *Laminaria saccharina*, a common seaweed in temperate seas from Britain to Japan. He suggests that it is imported into the Punjaub from the mouth of the Amoor River or thereabouts. Any efficacy it possesses depends upon the iodine contained in it.

# PRODUCTS OF FERMENTATION AND DISTILLATION.

## CEREVISIÆ FERMENTUM. BEER YEAST.

The Ferment obtained in brewing beer. It is viscid, semi-fluid, frothy, exhibiting under the microscope numerous round or oval confervoid cells, which are known by the name of *Torula Cerevisiæ*, but which are really a peculiar condition of *Pennicillia* and other moulds.

*Medical Properties and Uses.*—Stimulant; has been successfully employed in the adynamic forms of fever and dysentery. Its chief use is as an external stimulant in the form of poultice.

*Dose.*—From half an ounce to one ounce.

*Preparation.* — **Yeast Poultice** (*Cataplasma Fermenti*). Take of Beer Yeast, six fluid ounces; Flour, fourteen ounces; Water, heated to 100°, six fluid ounces. Mix the yeast with the water, and stir in the flour. Place the mass near the fire till it rises.

A valuable application to fetid, sloughing, and cancerous ulcerations.

[In India, where yeast is rarely procurable, an efficient substitute for this application is the Toddy Poultice, described in art. *Borassus flabelliformis*.)

## VINUM XERICUM. SHERRY.

A Spanish wine, prepared by fermentation from the juice of the grape. Pale yellowish-brown, containing from seventeen to eighteen per cent. of alcohol.

*Medical Properties and Uses.*—Diffusible stimulant; valuable in many forms of nervous and constitutional debility. It is the menstruum employed in preparing all the officinal wines.

## SPIRITUS VINI GALLICI. SPIRIT OF FRENCH WINE; BRANDY.

Spirit obtained by the distillation of French wine. Pale, or of a very slight brownish-yellow tint; of a peculiar vinous, aromatic odour.

*Medical Properties and Uses.*—Powerful diffusible stimulant, best administered in the following form:

*Preparation.*—**Mixture of the Spirit of French Wine** (*Mistura Spiritus Vini Gallici*). Take of Spirit of French Wine, Cinnamon Water, of each, four fluid ounces; the Yolks of two Eggs; Refined Sugar, half an ounce. Rub the yolks and sugar together, then add the cinnamon water and spirit.

*Dose.*—From one to two fluid ounces, repeated according to circumstances. A valuable stimulant and restorative in the adynamic forms and advanced stages of fever, in exhaustion from uterine and other hæmorrhages, and other cases where the vital powers are greatly depressed.

## ALCOHOL. ABSOLUTE ALCOHOL.

A volatile liquid, $C_4H_6O_2$ or $\mathbf{C_2H_6O}$, obtained by the distillation of Rectified Spirit with Lime. *Characters and Tests.*—Colourless and free from empyreumatic odour. Specific gravity, 0·795. It is entirely volatile by heat, is not rendered turbid when mixed with water, and does not cause anhydrous sulphate of copper to assume a blue colour when left in contact with it.

It is used in chemical analysis.

## SPIRITUS RECTIFICATUS. RECTIFIED SPIRIT.

Alcohol, $C_4H_6O_2$ or $\mathbf{C_2H_6O}$, with sixteen per cent. of water; obtained by the distillation of fermented saccharine fluids. *Characters.*—Colourless, transparent, very mobile and inflammable, of a peculiar pleasant odour, and a strong spirituous burning taste. Burns with a blue flame without smoke. *Tests.* — Specific gravity, 0·838. Remains clear when diluted with distilled water. Odour and taste purely alcoholic. Four fluid ounces with thirty grain-measures of the volumetric solution of nitrate of silver exposed for twenty-four hours to bright light, and then decanted from the black powder which has formed, undergoes no further change when again exposed to light with more of the test.

Principally employed in pharmacy as a menstruum in the preparation of Tinctures.

## SPIRITUS TENUIOR. PROOF SPIRIT.

Take of Rectified Spirit, five pints; Distilled Water, three pints. Mix. *Test.*—Specific gravity, 0·920. Other tests the same as those of Rectified Spirit.

*Medical Properties and Uses.*—Powerful diffusible stimulant; in over doses, poisonous. Proof Spirit, diluted with six or eight times its volume of water, forms an excellent evaporating or refrigerant lotion, much used in febrile, inflammatory, and other affections. It is not administered internally *per se*.

With the exception of the Tinctures of Aconite, Arnica, Assafœtida, Benzoin, Indian Hemp, Capsicum, Castor, Cubebs, Perchloride of Iron, Acetate of Iron, Iodine, Kino, Lavender, Myrrh, Nux Vomica, Opium (Ammoniated), Pyrethrum, Tolu, Green Hellebore, and Ginger, which are directed to be prepared with Rectified Spirit, all the other Officinal Tinctures are prepared with Proof Spirit. Rectified or Proof Spirit is also used largely in other pharmaceutical processes.

[Spirit of the specific gravity of Rectified Spirit, 0·838, or of Proof Spirit, 0·920, may be prepared in India from the fermented juice or Arrack obtained from the Palmyra (*Borassus flabelliformis*) or Cocoa-nut Palms (*Cocos nucifera*), or from Shum-shoo, a spirit manufactured chiefly by the Chinese from rice. The "Mahwa Spirit," obtained by distillation from the flowers of *Bassia latifolia*, is said to be objectionable on account of its peculiar flavour.]

## ÆTHER. ETHER.

### (*Æther Sulphuricus, Edin. et Dubl. Ph.*)

A volatile liquid prepared from alcohol, and containing not less than 92 per cent. by volume of pure ether, $C_4H_5O$ or $\mathbf{C_4H_{10}O}$. *Characters.*—A colourless, very volatile, and inflammable liquid, emitting a strong and characteristic odour, and boiling below 105°. *Tests.*—Specific gravity, 0·735. Fifty measures, agitated with an equal volume of water, are reduced to 45 by an absorption of 10 per cent. It evaporates without residue.

*Medical Properties.*—Powerful diffusible stimulant and antispasmodic. The vapour inhaled is a valuable anæsthetic. Applied and kept in contact with the skin, it acts as a rubefacient. Diluted with water, it forms an evaporating, refrigerant lotion.

*Therapeutic Uses.*—In asthma, spasmodic affections of the bowels, flatulent colic, also in the collapse of cholera, in the advanced stage of fevers, and in most cases where the vital powers are greatly depressed, it proves valuable. Its uses as an anæsthetic are the same as those of chloroform. As an internal remedy it is best administered in the form of Spiritus Ætheris.

*Dose.*—From twenty to sixty minims largely diluted.

Ether is employed in the preparation of Collodium, Collodium flexile, Liquor Epispasticus, and Spiritus Ætheris.

*Preparation.*—**Spirit of Ether** (*Spiritus Ætheris*). Take of Ether, ten fluid ounces; Rectified Spirit, one pint. Mix. Specific gravity, 0·809.

*Medical Properties and Uses.*—The same as Ether, but weaker in operation.

*Dose.*—From thirty minims to a fluid drachm and a half; repeated at short intervals as required.

It enters into the composition of Tinctura Lobeliæ Ætherea.

[Pure Ether, or Ether free from Alcohol and Water, $C_4H_5O$ or $C_4H_{10}O$, specific gravity not exceeding 0·720, is officinal in the British Ph. It is only employed in some pharmaceutical processes.]

## SPIRITUS ÆTHERIS NITROSI. Spirit of Nitrous Ether.

(*Spiritus Ætheris Nitrici, Lond. et Edin. Ph.*)

An alcoholic solution of nitrous ether, $C_4H_5O,NO_3$, or $C_2H_5NO_2$. *Characters.*—Transparent and nearly colourless, with a very slight tinge of yellow, mobile, inflammable, of a peculiar penetrating apple-like odour, and sweetish cooling sharp taste. *Tests.*—Specific gravity, 0·845. It effervesces feebly, or not at all, when shaken with a little bicarbonate of soda. When agitated with solution of sulphate of iron and a few drops of sulphuric acid, it becomes deep olive-brown or black. If it be agitated with twice its volume of saturated solution of chloride of calcium in a closed tube, two per cent. of its original volume will separate in the form of nitrous ether, and rise to the surface of the mixture.

*Medical Properties.*—Stimulant, diaphoretic, diuretic, and antispasmodic.

*Therapeutic Uses.*—In mild febrile and catarrhal affections, coryza, influenza, also in dysuria, and in mild forms of dropsy, it proves serviceable. It is generally given in conjunction with other appropriate remedies. It is often effectual in relieving nausea and flatulence.

*Dose.*—From thirty minims to two fluid drachms.

## CHLOROFORMUM. CHLOROFORM.

Terchloride of Formyle, $C_2HCl_3$ or **$CHCl_3$**. *Characters.* — A limpid colourless liquid, of an agreeable ethereal odour and sweet taste. Dissolves in alcohol and ether in all proportions, and slightly in water, communicating to it a sweetish taste. Burns, though not readily, with a green and smoky flame. *Tests.*—Specific gravity, 1·49. It is not coloured by agitation with sulphuric acid, leaves no residue and no unpleasant odour after evaporation.

*Medical Properties.*—Inhaled in the form of vapour, anæsthetic; taken internally, narcotic, sedative, and antispasmodic; applied externally, undiluted, rubefacient and counter-irritant; diluted, anodyne.

*Therapeutic Uses.*—As an anæsthetic the therapeutic applications are numerous and important. Amongst the chief are, to produce insensibility to pain in surgical operations, to relieve or banish the pains of childbirth, to relax the muscular system so as to allow of the more ready reduction of dislocations, and placing in apposition fractured bones, and by the same means to aid taxis in the reduction of strangulated hernia, and the passage of a catheter in spasmodic stricture of the urethra. Amongst other affections in which anæsthesia, more or less complete, by chloroform vapour, has been found serviceable, are, puerperal and epileptoid convulsions, chorea, tetanus, spasmodic asthma, laryngismus stridulus, ileus, and other spasmodic affections; also in the passage of renal and biliary calculi. The local application of the vapour by means of an appropriate instrument has been found of great service in relieving the pain of cancerous and other painful affections of the uterus and rectum. Internally it has been prescribed with advantage in nausea and gastric irritability, cholera, colica pictonum, cough and dyspnœa of phthisis. Locally or externally, in the form of liniment, it proves useful in various rheumatic and neuralgic affections, sprains, and bruises.

*Dose.*—As an internal remedy, from three to ten minims incorporated with mucilage, yolk of egg, or syrup. As an anæsthetic, the best mode of administration is to commence with small doses, taking care that it is well diluted with atmospheric air, and increasing and repeating the dose according to the degree of anæsthesia which it is desired to produce. A fluid drachm is about the average dose which it is advisable to commence with. In all cases the production of anæsthesia should be conducted with the greatest care and circumspection.

*Preparations.*—**Spirit of Chloroform** (*Spiritus Chloroformi*). Take of Chloroform, one fluid ounce; Rectified Spirit, nineteen fluid ounces. Dissolve. *Test.*—Specific gravity, 0·871.

*Dose.*—From twenty to sixty minims, repeated according to circumstances. This preparation, misnamed *Chloric Ether,* is a popular and justly esteemed remedy, and is much employed as a stimulant, anodyne, and antispasmodic.

**Compound Tincture of Chloroform** (*Tinctura Chloroformi composita*). Take of Chloroform, two fluid ounces; Rectified Spirit, eight fluid ounces; Compound Tincture of Cardamoms, ten fluid ounces. Mix.

*Dose.*—From twenty to sixty minims.

**Liniment of Chloroform** (*Linimentum Chloroformi*). Take of Chloroform and Liniment of Camphor, of each, two fluid ounces. Mix.

A useful application in neuralgic and rheumatic pains, tumours, and other local affections.

## ACETUM. VINEGAR.

(*Acetum Britanicum, Lond. Ph.*)

An acid liquid, prepared from malt and unmalted grain by acetous fermentation. *Characters.* — A liquid of a brown colour and peculiar odour. *Tests.*—Specific gravity, 1·017 to 1·019. 445·4 grains by weight (1 fluid ounce) of it require at least 402 grain measures of the volumetric solution of soda for their neutralization, corresponding to 4·6 per cent. of anhydrous acetic acid. If ten minims of solution of chloride of barium be added to a fluid ounce of the vinegar, and the precipitate, if any, be separated by filtration, a further addition of the test will give no precipitate. Sulphuretted hydrogen causes no change of colour.

*Medical Properties.*—Refrigerant, sedative, and antiseptic.

*Therapeutic Uses.* — In febrile and inflammatory affections, diluted vinegar forms a useful external refrigerant; it is applied also to burns and scalds, hospital gangrene, incipient mammary abscesses, bruises, sprains, and other local affections. It is a direct antidote in poisoning by the alkalies; has been advised also in cases of narcotic poisoning, after the evacuation of the stomach by an emetic or the stomach pump; the fact, however, of its forming a soluble salt with morphia would negative its use in poisoning by opium. The inhalation of the vapour of hot vinegar and water often affords much relief in cynanche tonsillaris, and other forms of sore throat.

*Dose.*—From one to two fluid drachms, in any bland vehicle. A refrigerant drink in fevers is made by adding from one to two fluid ounces of vinegar to a quart of water, and sweetening to taste. As a lotion it should be diluted with about double its bulk of water.

[Vinegar is largely prepared in India from the Toddy or saccharine juice of the Palmyra (*Borassus flabelliformis*) and Cocoa-nut Palm (*Cocos nucifera*), and also from the juice of the Sugar Cane.]

## ACIDUM ACETICUM. Acetic Acid.

An acid liquid prepared from wood by destructive distillation and subsequent purification. 100 parts by weight contain thirty-three parts of the acetic acid $HO,C_4H_3O_3$ or $\mathbf{HC_2H_3O_2}$, corresponding to 28 parts of anhydrous acetic acid, $C_4H_3O_3$ or $\mathbf{C_4H_6O_3}$. *Characters.*—A colourless liquid having a strong acid reaction and a pungent odour. *Tests.*—Specific gravity, 1·044. 182 grains by weight require for neutralization 1000 grain measures of the volumetric solution of soda. It leaves no residue when evaporated, and gives no precipitate with sulphuretted hydrogen, chloride of barium, or nitrate of silver. If a fluid drachm of it mixed with half an ounce of distilled water and half a drachm of pure hydrochloric acid be put into a small flask with a few pieces of granulated zinc, and, while the effervescence continues, a slip of bibulous paper wetted with solution of subacetate of lead be suspended in the upper part of the flask above the liquid for about five minutes, the paper will not become discoloured.

*Medical Properties and Uses*—Analogous to those of Vinegar.

*Dose.*—From five to fifteen drops diluted.

*Preparations.*—**Dilute Acetic Acid** (*Acidum Aceticum dilutum*). Take of Acetic Acid, one pint; Distilled Water, seven pints. Mix. *Tests.*—Specific gravity, 1·006. One fluid ounce requires for neutralization 313 grain-measures of the volumetric solution of soda.

*Dose.*—From one to two fluid drachms.

**Oxymel** (*Oxymel*). Take of Clarified Honey, forty ounces; Acetic Acid, five fluid ounces; Water, five fluid ounces. Liquify the honey by heat, and mix with it the acetic acid and water.

*Dose.*—From one to two fluid drachms; useful as an expectorant in slight catarrhal affections. Added to Decoction of Barley, it forms an agreeable refrigerant drink in febrile and inflammatory affections; it is frequently used as an ingredient in gargles and cough mixtures.

Acetic Acid is an ingredient in Acetum Cantharidis, Extractum Colchici Aceticum, Linimentum Terebinthinæ Aceticum, Liquor Epispasticus, and Oxymel. It is also the acid constituent of the Officinal Acetates and their respective solutions. The Dilute Acid is the menstruum employed in the preparation of Acetum Scillæ.

## ACIDUM ACETICUM GLACIALE. Glacial Acetic Acid.

(*Acidum Aceticum, Edin. Ph.*)

Concentrated acetic aid, corresponding to at least 84 per cent. of anhydrous acid, $C_4H_3O_3$ or $\mathbf{C_4H_6O_3}$. *Characters and Tests.*—It crystallises when cooled to 34°, and remains crystalline until the temperature rises to above 48°. Specific gravity, 1·065 to 1·066, and this is increased by adding ten per cent. of water. At the mean temperature of the air it is a colourless liquid, with a pungent acetous odour. 60 grains by weight mixed with a fluid ounce of distilled water, require for neutralisation at least 990 grain-measures of the volumetric solution of soda. If a fluid drachm of it, mixed with half an ounce of distilled water and half a drachm of pure hydrochloric acid, be put into a small flask with a few pieces of granulated zinc, and while the effervescence continues a slip of bibulous paper wetted with solution of subacetate of lead be suspended in the upper part of the flask above the liquid for about five minutes, the paper will not become dicoloured.

A very powerful caustic and vesicant, only employed as an external application. It has been used locally for the destruction of warts, syphilitic vegetations, nævi materni, and in some obstinate skin diseases. Its application to the skin is followed by rapid vesication; hence it may be employed on an emergency when the preparations of cantharides are not at hand, or where there is reason to fear, as in some affections of the kidneys, that the absorption of cantharidine (from an ordinary blister) might prove injurious.

It is an ingredient in Acetum Cantharidis and Mistura Creasoti.

## ACIDUM CARBOLICUM. Carbolic Acid.

(*Phenic Acid.*)

An acid, $HO,C_{12}H_5O$ or $\mathbf{HC_6H_5O}$, obtained from coal-tar oil by fractional distillation and subsequent purification. *Characters and Tests.*—In colourless acicular crystals, which at a temperature of 95° become an oily liquid, having a strong odour and taste, resembling those of creasote, which it also resembles in many of its characters and properties. Its specific gravity is 1·065; boiling point, 370°. The crystals readily absorb moisture on exposure to the air, and they are thus liquified; the acid, however, is but slightly soluble in water, but it is freely soluble in alcohol, ether, and glycerine. It does not redden blue litmus paper. A slip of deal dipped into it, and afterwards into hydrochloric acid, and then allowed to dry in the air, acquires a greenish-blue colour. It coagulates albumen. It does not affect the plane of polarisation of a ray of polarised light.

*Properties.*—Escharotic stimulant, and rubefacient; is a powerful deodorizing and disinfecting agent.

*Therapeutic Uses.*—In gastric irritability, especially when caused by miasma or sewerage exhalation, it has been found to exercise a sedative action analogous to that of creasote. Locally it has been used with advantage in phagedenic, cancerous, syphilitic, and other obstinate forms of ulceration, in chronic skin diseases, and in ozœna and other diseases attended by fetid discharges. In diphtheria it has been advantageously used, dissolved in glycerine, as a local application.

*Dose.*—From one to three grains largely diluted.

*Preparation.*—**Glycerine of Carbolic Acid** (*Glycerinum Acidi Carbolici*). Take of Carbolic Acid, one ounce; Glycerine, four fluid ounces. Rub them together in a mortar until the acid is dissolved.

A good form for external application. For children and for others with delicate skins the proportion of glycerine requires to be increased.

(*Non-officinal.*)

**Petroleum.** — A bituminous liquid, of the colour and consistence of treacle, which exudes spontaneously from the earth, and is met with on the surface of certain lakes in the neighbourhood of Rangoon, and in the volcanic islands on the Arracan coast. From the researches of Drs. Christison and Gregory (*Trans. of Royal Soc. Edin.*, vol. xiii. p. 1) it is probable that it is a product of destructive distillation, since it contains paraffine and eupion, substances obtained from organic bodies by heat. Its action on the system is that of a terebinthinate stimulant, in which character it has been prescribed internally in doses of about half a fluid drachm suspended in mucilage in rheumatism and gonorrhœa. It is said to act powerfully as a diuretic. A case of Beri-beri, successfully treated by it externally and internally, is recorded by Mr. S. Arokeum (*Madras Quart. Med. Journ.* July 1863, p. 159), but how far the recovery was due in this instance to the petroleum is doubtful. It is a useful external application in skin diseases; and a case of chronic eczema, which had resisted a variety of treatment, local and constitutional, cured by it, is published by Dr. J. W. Mudge (*Ind. Ann. of Med. Sci.*, 1854, vol. ii. p. 450). He used it incorporated with soap in the proportion of a drachm to an ounce. It has also been found useful as an external application in chronic rheumatism.

# Animal Kingdom.

# ANIMAL MATERIA MEDICA.

## ANNELIDA.

### 1. SANGUISUGA OFFICINALIS, *Savigny*. The Green Leech.

### 2. SANGUISUGA MEDICINALIS, *Savigny*. The Speckled Leech.

(*Moquin-Tandon, Med. Zool.*, t. 35, 36.)

*Habitat.*—Europe and certain parts of Northern Africa; collected for use chiefly in Spain, France, Italy, and Hungary.

*Officinal Part.*—The live animal (*Hirudo, Leech*). It has the following characters: Body elongated, two or three inches long, tapering to each end, plano-convex, wrinkled transversely; back olive-green, with six rusty-red longitudinal stripes. 1. Belly olive-green, not spotted; 2. Belly greenish-yellow, spotted with black.

*Medical Properties and Uses.*—Leeches are only employed for the purpose of local abstraction of blood in cases of external inflammation or congestion, and in cases of internal inflammation in which there is a direct capillary connexion between the skin and the internal inflamed part, *e.g.*, pleuritis and peritonitis. They are likewise applicable to those inflammations in which, from any circumstance, it is unadvisable to employ general blood-letting. They are of the greatest importance in the inflammatory affections of infancy and childhood.

The number of leeches required must be regulated by the circumstances of the case: one leech is calculated to draw on an average about a drachm and a half to two drachms of blood, not including that which flows subsequently, which often equals the quantity abstracted by the leech. The Indian leech has been found to draw between four and five times its own weight of blood. (71) In cases of excessive or long-continued hæmorrhage from leech bites, pressure, together with matico, alum, nitrate of silver, or other styptics, may be had recourse to.

[Leeches are procurable, especially during the wet season or monsoon, in most parts of India, in the neighbourhood of tanks, and swamps. They are also bred to a considerable extent in the Deccan (72) and other parts of India. The species or even genus to which the Indian leech belongs has not been determined. Two kinds, a large and a small one, brought from Madras by Dr. F. Day, and deposited by him at the Indian Museum, are apparently new species; the former approaches nearly in character to *Bdella nilotica, Sav.* Those employed in Bombay, according to Dr. H. J. Carter (*Bombay Med. Phys. Trans.*, 1859, vol. iv. N.S., p. xix.), approach nearly to *Hirudo granulosa, Sav.* (73) The subject demands further investigation.]

# INSECTA. INSECTS.

## COLEOPTERA. Beetles.

### CANTHARIS VESICATORIA, *Latreille.* COMMON CANTHARIDES.

(*Stephenson, Med. Zool.*, t. 26, f. 2.)

*Habitat.*—Various parts of Europe, imported in the dried state into England from Russia, Sicily, and Hungary.

*Officinal Part.*—The dried Insect (*Cantharis, Cantharides*). It has the following characters: From eight to ten lines long, furnished with two wing-covers of a shining metallic-green colour, under which are two membranous transparent wings; odour, strong and disagreeable; powder, greyish-brown, containing shining green particles. Free from mites. Its activity resides in a peculiar principle, *Cantharidin.*

*Medical Properties and Uses.*—Administered internally, an acrid stimulant diuretic, its action being chiefly directed on the mucous membrane of the genito-urinary system, and particularly on the neck of the bladder. In over doses, poisonous. Externally applied, a powerful and valuable counter-irritant and vesicant.

*Therapeutic Uses.*—Amongst the diseases in which cantharides have been successfully employed internally are enuresis dependent on atony of the bladder, leucorrhœa, amenorrhœa, albuminaria, some forms of paralysis, epilepsy, dropsical affections of an asthenic type, the chronic stage of hooping cough, and some cutaneous diseases, especially lepra and psoriasis. As an external application in the form of blisters, their therapeutic applications are multifarious and important; *e.g.*, advanced stages of acute inflammation; internal congestions; nervous and spinal affections, as in paralysis, epilepsy and chorea; also in sciatica and other forms of neuralgia; dropsical affections, as in hydrocephalus, hydropericardium, hydrothorax, and hydarthrosis; many acute and chronic diseases of the eye and ear, and arthritic enlargements. The mode of application requires to be regulated by circumstances in each individual case.

*Dose.*—From one to two grains of finely powdered Cantharides in the form of pill; it is, however, more safely and efficiently administered in the form of Tincture.

*Preparations.*—**Tincture of Cantharides** (*Tinctura Cantharidis*). Take of Cantharides, in coarse powder, a quarter of an ounce; Proof Spirit, one pint. Macerate for seven days in a closed vessel, with occasional agitation, strain, press, filter, and add sufficient proof spirit to make one pint.

*Dose.*—From five to twenty minims twice or thrice daily.

**Vinegar of Cantharides** (*Acetum Cantharidis*). Take of Cantharides, in powder, two ounces; Glacial Acetic Acid, two fluid ounces; Acetic Acid, eighteen fluid ounces, or a sufficiency. Mix thirteen fluid ounces of the acetic acid with the glacial acetic acid, and digest the cantharides in this mixture for two hours at a temperature of 200°; then transfer the ingredients, after they have cooled, to a percolator, and when the liquid ceases to pass, pour five fluid ounces of acetic acid over the residuum in the apparatus. As soon as the percolation is complete, subject the contents of the percolator to pressure, filter the product, mix the liquids, and add sufficient acetic acid to make one pint.

Employed only externally as a vesicant.

**Blistering Liquid** (*Liquor Epispasticus, Linimentum Cantharidis, Brit. Ph.*, 1864). Take of Cantharides, in powder, eight ounces; Acetic Acid, four fluid ounces; Ether, a sufficiency. Mix the cantharides and acetic acid; pack them in a percolator, and at the expiration of twenty-four hours pour ether over the contents of the percolator, and allow it to pass slowly through till twenty fluid ounces are obtained. Keep it in a stoppered bottle.

A powerful vesicant, more speedy and energetic in its action than the preceding.

**Blistering Paper** (*Charta Epispastica*). Take of White Wax, four ounces; Spermaceti, one ounce and a half; Olive Oil, two fluid ounces; Resin, three quarters of an ounce; Canada Balsam, quarter of an ounce; Cantharides, in powder, one ounce; Distilled Water, six fluid ounces. Digest all the ingredients, excepting the Canada balsam, in a water-bath for two hours, stirring them constantly, then strain and separate the plaster from the watery liquid. Mix the Canada balsam with the plaster melted in a shallow vessel, and pass strips of paper over the surface of the hot liquid, so that one surface of the paper shall receive a thin coating of plaster.

It may be convenient to employ paper ruled so as to indicate divisions each of which is one square inch.

Warmed and applied to the surface, it acts as a vesicant.

**Plaster of Cantharides** (*Emplastrum Cantharidis*). Take of Cantharides, in powder, twelve ounces; Yellow Wax, Prepared Suet, of each seven ounces and a half; Prepared Lard, six ounces; Resin, three ounces. Liquify the wax, suet, and lard together by a water-bath, and add the resin, previously melted; then introduce the cantharides, mix the whole thoroughly, and continue to stir the mixture while it is allowed to cool.

This preparation is in ordinary use as a blistering agent. Its numerous uses in this character are noticed above.

**Ointment of Cantharides** (*Unguentum Cantharidis, Ceratrum Cantharidis, Lond. Ph.*) Take of Cantharides, Yellow Wax, of each one ounce; Olive Oil, six fluid ounces. Infuse the cantharides in the oil, in a covered vessel, for twelve hours, then place the vessel in boiling water for fifteen minutes, strain through muslin with strong pressure, add the product to the wax previously melted, and stir constantly while the mixture cools.

An irritant dressing for blisters and issues.

**Warm Plaster** (*Emplastrum Calefaciens*). Take of Cantharides, in coarse powder, Expressed Oil of Nutmeg, Yellow Wax, Resin, of each, four ounces; Soap Plaster, three pounds and a quarter; Resin Plaster, two pounds; Boiling Water, one pint. Infuse the cantharides in the boiling water for six hours; squeeze strongly through calico, and evaporate the expressed liquid by a water-bath till reduced to one third. Then add the other ingredients, and melt in a water-bath, stirring well until the whole is thoroughly mixed.

A useful stimulant application to indolent tumours, chronic glandular swellings, and arthritic enlargements.

### *MYLABRIS CICHORII, *Fabr.* TELINI FLY.

*Stephenson, Med. Zool.*, t. 26. f. 5.

*Habitat.*—Southern Europe, extending from Italy through Greece and Egypt to China. It is of common occurrence throughout India.

*Officinal Part.*—The dried Insect (*Mylabris, Telini fly*). It has the following characters: about an inch in length, and a third of an inch broad; the elytra of an obscure yellow, with three large somewhat zigzag transverse bands. The first band is interrupted, and sometimes reduced to three or four spots. Active principle, *Cantharidin.*

*Medical Properties and Uses.*—The same as Cantharis vesicatoria, for which it affords a complete substitute as a vesicant. As an internal remedy it should not be substituted for the Tincture of Cantharides, as the strength and operation of the latter is well ascertained, which is not the case with our present article. It is regarded as more powerful than the European article. (74)

[Other blistering flies exist in many parts of India: thus, in Upper and Central India there have been found **Meloe Trianthema** (so called from its being usually found on *Trianthema decandra*, Roxb.), **Lytta gigus** and **Lytta violacea**; whilst in the Peninsula, especially in the neighbourhood of Pondicherry, are found **Mylabris pustulata** and **M. punctum.** An interesting report on the properties of the two latter species has been published by Dr. Collas, in the "Moniteur Officiel" of Pondicherry, March 2nd, 1855. In addition to these, Mr. Moore, of the India Museum, enumerates **Mylabris Indica,** *Fussl.*, **M. melanura, M. humeralis, M. proxima, M. orientalis, Lytta Assamensis,** and **Epicauta Nipalensis.** But with *M. Cichorii* existing plentifully in most parts of India, the necessity of increasing the number of these vesicant agents is lessened.]

## HYMENOPTERA.

### APIS MELLIFICA, *Linn.* THE HIVE OR HONEY BEE.

*Habitat.*—Various parts of the Old World; domesticated in most parts of the globe.

*Officinal Parts.*—1. (*Mel, Honey.*) A saccharine secretion deposited by the insect in the honeycomb.. When recently separated from the honeycomb it is a viscid translucent liquid, of a brownish-yellow colour, which gradually becomes partially crystalline and opaque. It has a peculiar heavy odour, and a very sweet taste. Boiled with water for five minutes, and allowed to cool, it does not become blue with the solution of iodine. 2. (*Cera flava, Yellow Wax.*) The prepared Honeycomb. Occurs in masses; firm, breaking with a granular fracture; yellow, having an agreeable honey-like odour. Not unctuous to the touch; does not melt under 140°; yields nothing to cold rectified spirit, but is entirely soluble in oil of turpentine. Boiling water in which it has been agitated, when cooled, is not rendered blue by iodine. 3. (*Cera alba, White Wax.*) Yellow Wax, bleached by exposure to moisture, air, and light. Occurs in circular cakes, hard, nearly white, translucent. It is not unctuous to the touch, and does not melt under 150° F.

*Medical Properties and Uses.*—Honey is emollient and slightly laxative, and is often employed as a flavouring agent in cough mixtures and gargles. Wax is also emollient and demulcent, and has occasionally been prescribed in dysentery, diarrhœa, and catarrh; but its chief use is as an ingredient in ointments, plasters, and suppositories.

*Dose.*—Of White Wax from ten to twenty grains suspended in a mixture by aid of mucilage.

*Preparations.*—**Clarified Honey** (*Mel Depuratum*). Take of Honey, five pounds. Melt the honey in a water bath, and strain while hot, through flannel previously moistened with warm water.

Demulcent; forms an ingredient in Oxymel, Oxymel Scillæ, Mel Boracis, Confectio Piperis, Conf. Scammonii, and Conf. Terebinthinæ.

**Simple Ointment** (*Unguentum Simplex*). Take of White Wax, two ounces; Prepared Lard, three ounces; Almond Oil, three fluid ounces. Melt the wax and lard in the oil on a water-bath; then remove the mixture, and stir constantly while it cools.

A useful application for ulcers; used also as the basis of several officinal ointments.

***Ceromel.** Take of Yellow Wax, one ounce; Clarified Honey, four ounces. Mix with the aid of gentle heat, and strain.

A mild stimulant application for indolent and other ulcerations; well adapted for use in India and other tropical countries, where animal fats soon become rancid and unfit for medicinal use.

[Both honey and wax of good quality are obtainable in India.

They are the products of **Apis socialis**, *Latr.*, **A. dorsata**, *Latr.*, **A. nigripennis**, *Latr.*, **A. bicolor**, *Klug.*, and probably of other species.]

## HEMIPTERA.

### COCCUS CACTI, *Linn.* COCHINEAL INSECT.

*Habitat.*—Reared in Mexico and Teneriffe.

*Officinal Part.*—The dried female insect (*Coccus, Cochineal*). Ovate, plano-convex, about two lines long, wrinkled, black or greyish-white; yields, when crushed, a puce-coloured powder. The greyish-white insect quickly becomes black when warmed before the fire.

*Properties and Uses.*—Has had anti-spasmodic and other properties assigned to it on insufficient grounds. Valuable only as a colouring agent.

*Preparation.*—**Tincture of Cochineal** (*Tinctura Cocci*). Take of Cochineal, in powder, two ounces and a half; Proof Spirit, one pint. Macerate for seven days, filter, and add sufficient proof spirit to make one pint.

Cochineal is an ingredient in Tinctura Cardamoni composita and Tinctura Cinchonæ composita.

## PISCES. Fishes.

### ACIPENSER HUSO, *Linn.*, AND OTHER SPECIES OF STURGEON.

*Habitat.*—The Caspian and Black Seas.

*Officinal Part.*—The swimming bladder or sound, prepared and cut into fine shreds (*Ichthyocolla, Isinglass*). It is light, coriaceous, of a whitish colour, semi-transparent, tasteless, inodorous, insoluble in cold water, readily soluble in boiling water, and forms a transparent jelly in cooling. Fifteen grains of isinglass are sufficient to impart a firm consistence to one ounce of water. Many varieties are met with in commerce. (75) Its principal constituent is gelatine.

*Medical Properties and Uses.*—Demulcent, nutritive, much used in the form of jelly as an article of diet for the sick. Used also in solution as a test to distinguish gallic from tannic acid; the latter yielding with it a yellowish-white precipitate, whilst the former remains unaffected.

### GADUS MORRHUA, *Linn.* COMMON COD.

*Habitat.*—Abundant on the coasts of Norway, France, Britain, and Ireland, but especially on the coasts of Newfoundland.

*Officinal Part.*—The Oil extracted from the fresh liver by heat not exceeding 180° F. (*Oleum Morrhuæ, Cod-liver Oil*). Pale yellow, with a slight fishy odour, and bland fishy taste. A drop of sulphuric acid added to a few drops of the oil on a porcelain slab developes a violet colour, which soon passes to a yellowish or brownish-red. In addition to biliary principles, it contains in minute proportions iodine, bromine, chlorine, phosphorus, phosphoric and sulphuric acids, with traces of lime, magnesia, and soda.

*Medical Properties.*—Valuable alterative and nutritive.

*Therapeutic Uses.*—In scrofulous or tubercular affections generally it is a remedy of the greatest value. It has been used with especial benefit in phthisis, rachitis, tabes mesenterica, acute and chronic hydrocephalus, ophthalmia, and in atrophy occurring in scrofulous subjects. It has likewise been used with advantage in anæmic states, especially in neuralgia and sciatica associated with anæmia, obstinate skin diseases, chronic rheumatism, diabetes, epilepsy, chorea, and in dyspepsia characterised by mal-assimilation of food.

*Dose.*—A drachm twice or thrice daily, and increased as the patient is able to bear it. When from any cause it cannot be administered by mouth, it may be given in enema, or may be introduced into the system by means of inunction. The best time for its administration is immediately after a meal.

## *SQUALUS CARCHARIAS, *Linn.* WHITE SHARK.

*Habitat.*—Widely distributed; common in the Indian Seas.

*Officinal Part.*—The Oil extracted from the Liver by heat (*Oleum Squalæ, Shark Liver Oil*); of a fine amber colour, or of the colour of pale brandy. Smell and taste similar to Cod liver oil, but more strongly marked, and more disagreeable. Perfectly limpid at 86° F. When left undisturbed for some time it deposits in considerable quantity a white granular substance, stearine, to which the name of *Squalin* has been applied.

*Medical Properties, Uses, and Doses.*—The same as cod liver oil, for which it may be used as a substitute. It is well adapted for dispensary practice in India. The great objection to it is its nauseous taste, but this might probably be obviated by more care being taken in its preparation.

[Dr. Collas, of Pondicherry, reports very highly of this oil; it is also favourably spoken of by Dr. F. Day (*Proceed. of Zoolog. Soc.*, March 14th, 1865, p. 316); and it has been used with marked advantage in the Leper Hospital at Madras, and elsewhere in the Madras Presidency (*Madras Med. Reports*, 1855, p. 376). Dr. Collas considers that *Squalin* is likely to constitute an important addition to the pharmacy of tropical climates; as, in addition to being itself a valuable application to ulcers and wounds, it is well adapted as a substitute for lard, over which it possesses the great advantages of not becoming rancid, and of having a greater consistence. As a local application to ulcers he directs that the squalin be simply spread on lint, and applied to the affected surface (*Madras Exhibition Cat.* 1857, and *Moquin-Tandon, Med. Zoology*, p. 109). According to Dr. Delattre, some of the active principles are present in larger proportions in the oil of the shark than in that of the cod; it is richer in iodine and in phosphorus, but contains less bromine and sulphur. (*Brit. and For. Med. Chir. Rev.*, Jan. 1860, p. 249.) Some years since; trials were made in India with the liver oil of **Cybium Commersonii**, *Cuv. et Val.* (*Seir Fish*). Although favourably reported of, it does not appear to have come into use. For other remarks on the fish liver oils of India see Dr. G. Bidie (*Madras Quart. Med. Journ.*, vol. v. p. 281). He considers that much of the offensive smell and taste of the Indian oil depends upon the livers being allowed to putrify before the process of extraction is commenced; hence he proposes to prepare it by boiling the fresh livers in water.

## AVES. Birds.

### GALLUS BANKIVA, *Var.* DOMESTICUS, *Temminck.*

#### The Domestic Cock and Hen.

*Habitat.*—Domesticated in all parts of the globe.

*Officinal Parts.*—1. Albumen of the Egg (*Albumen Ovi, White of Egg*); a colourless, glairy, viscid fluid, inodorous, tasteless, coagulated by heat, unaffected by Acetic Acid. 2. The Yolk (*Vitellus Ovi*); a thick oily fluid, opaque, yellow, inodorous, with a bland pleasant taste. Agitated with water it forms a milky emulsion.

*Medical Properties and Uses.*—Emollient, demulcent, nutritive. The albumen is a chemical antidote in poisoning by corrosive sublimate, by the soluble salts of copper and zinc, and by creosote. In cases of poisoning by other acrid metallic salts, it acts as a mechanical antidote, enveloping the poisonous particles, and sheathing the mucous coat of the stomach and intestines. The yolk, in addition to its value as a nutritive article of diet for the sick, is employed in making emulsions, in suspending oils, oleo-resins, and resins.

*Preparation.* — **Solution of Albumen.** Take the White of One Egg; Distilled Water, four fluid ounces. Mix by trituration in a mortar, and filter through clean tow, first moistened with distilled water. This solution must be recently prepared.

Only employed as a chemical test.

The yolk of the egg forms an ingredient in Mistura Spiritus Vini Gallici.

# MAMMALIA.

## CETACEA.

### PHYSETER MACROCEPHALUS, *Linn.* THE SPERM WHALE.

*Habitat.*—The Pacific and Indian Oceans.

*Officinal Part.*—Nearly pure cetine separated, by cooling and purification, from the oil contained in the head (*Cetaceum, Spermaceti*). It is crystalline, pearly-white, glistening, translucent, with little taste or odour, reducible to powder by the addition of a little rectified spirit. Scarcely unctuous to the touch; does not melt under 100°.

*Medical Properties and Uses.*—Demulcent and emollient; rarely employed, excepting as an external application in the form of ointment.

*Preparation.* — **Spermaceti Ointment** (*Unguentum Cetacei.*) Take of Spermaceti, five ounces; White Wax, two ounces; Almond Oil, one pint, or a sufficiency. Melt together with a gentle heat, remove the mixture, and stir constantly while it cools.

Emollient dressing for blistered or excoriated surfaces and ulcerations.

Spermaceti is also an ingredient in Charta Epispastica.

## RUMINANTIA.

### MOSCHUS MOSCHIFERUS, *Linn.* THE MUSK ANIMAL.

*Habitat.*—Thibet and Central India.

*Officinal Part.*—The inspissated and dried secretion from the preputial follicles (*Moschus, Musk*). It occurs in irregular reddish-black rather unctuous grains; having a strong peculiar very diffusible odour, and a bitter aromatic taste; contained in a round or slightly oval membranous sac, about two inches in diameter, covered on the outer side with stiff greyish hairs arranged in a concentric manner around its central orifice.

*Medical Properties.*—Stimulant and antispasmodic.

*Therapeutic Uses.*—In typhus and typhoid fevers, and in the advanced stages of other febrile diseases, in asthenic pneumonia, retrocedent gout, hypochondriasis, and other affections of an asthenic type, it has been found useful as a stimulant. Amongst the spasmodic and nervous affections in which it has been found serviceable are spasmodic asthma, laryngismus stridulus, the chronic stage of hooping cough, infantile convulsions, epilepsy, chorea, and various forms of hysteria, especially sleeplessness. It is, however, rarely used at the present day.

*Dose.*—From five to ten grains, in the form of pills, or suspended in a mixture by the aid of mucilage.

## OVIS ARIES, *Linn.* THE SHEEP.

*Habitat.*—Domesticated in all parts of the globe.

*Officinal Part.*—The internal fat of the abdomen, purified by melting and straining (*Sevum præparatum, Prepared Suet*). A white soft solid, smooth, almost inodorous, fusible at 103°. It is composed principally of *stearine* and *oleine*, with a little *margarine.*

*Medical Properties and Uses.*—Emollient; sometimes added to poultices; occasionally employed as a nutrient.

Prepared suet is an ingredient in Emplastrum Cantharidis and Unguentum Hydragyri.

## BOS TAURUS, *Linn.* THE OX.

*Habitat.*—Domesticated in all parts of the globe.

*Officinal Part.*—The fresh lacteal secretion (*Lac, Milk*); an opaque white emulsive fluid, with a bland sweetish taste, and faint peculiar odour, with numerous globules of fatty matter floating in it.

*Medical Properties and Uses.*—Valuable nutritive and demulcent; of great service as an article of diet, especially in some ulcerated conditions of the stomach. Is useful both as an antidote and as a protecting agent in corrosive and irritant poisoning.

Milk is an ingredient in Mistura Scammonii.

*Preparation.*—**Sugar of Milk** (*Saccharum Lactis*). $C_{24}H_{24}O_{24}$, or $C_{12}H_{24}O_{12}$. Crystallized Sugar, obtained from the whey of cow's milk by evaporation. It occurs usually in cylindrical masses, two inches in diameter, with a cord or stick in the axis, or in fragments of cakes; greyish-white, crystalline on the surface and in its texture, translucent, hard, inodorous, faintly sweet, gritty when chewed.

Doubtfully nutritive, probably inert; employed chiefly as a vehicle for medicinal powders.

**Purified Ox Bile** (*Fel Bovinum Purificatum*). Take of Fresh Ox Bile, one pint; Rectified Spirit, two pints. Mix the bile and the spirit by agitation in a bottle, and set aside for twelve hours until the sediment subsides. Decant the clear solution, and evaporate in a porcelain capsule on a water bath until the residue acquires a suitable consistence for forming pills. *Characters.*—A yellowish green substance of pilular consistence, having a taste partly sweet and partly bitter, soluble in water and in spirit. A solution of one or two grains of it, in about a fluid drachm of water, when treated, first with a drop of freshly made syrup, consisting of one part of sugar and four of water, and then with sulphuric acid cautiously added until the precipitate at first formed is redissolved, gradually acquires a cherry-red colour, which changes in succession to carmine, purple, and violet. Its watery solution gives no precipitate on the addition of rectified spirit.

Laxative; has been found serviceable in dyspepsia, constipation, diarrhœa, and other disorders of the intestinal canal dependent on a deficient supply of bile, which by this means it is intended to supply. In some forms of jaundice, tabes mesenterica, and hypochondriasis, it has been thought useful. It has also been prescribed in epilepsy, delirium tremens, and diabetes, with uncertain results. Externally fresh ox bile has been applied with effect in various forms of hypertrophy, in chronic rheumatism, sprains, and in deafness depending on an accumulation of hardened wax in the meatus.

*Dose.*—From five to ten grains, in the form of pill or in capsules. For external application it should be diluted with six or eight times its weight of any bland oil or spirit of camphor.

## PACHYDERMATA.

### SUS SCROFA, *Linn.* THE HOG.

*Habitat.*—Domesticated in all parts of the globe.

*Officinal Part.*—The fat deprived of its membranes and purified by heat (*Adeps præparatus; Axungia, Edin. Ph.; Prepared Lard*). A soft, white, fatty substance, melting at about 100°; has no rancid odour, dissolves entirely in ether. Distilled water in which it has been boiled, when cooled and filtered, gives no precipitate with nitrate of silver, and is not rendered blue by the addition of solution of iodine. It contains about 62 per cent. of *oleine*, and 38 of *margarine* and *stearine*.

*Medical Properties and Uses.*—Emollient; not prescribed internally. Inunction with lard has been extensively employed in scarlatina, exanthemata, erysipelas, and other external inflammations, bruises, and spains. In the former class of cases, it has been thought to modify existing symptoms in a remarkable degree. It is the basis of many officinal ointments.

**Benzoated Lard**, see *Styrax Benzoin*, p. 133.

[The practitioner in India will do well to bear in mind the strong religious prejudices entertained by the Mohammedans against the swine and any of its products.]

# RODENTIA.

## CASTOR FIBER, *Linn.* THE BEAVER.

*Habitat.*—Canada and Siberia.

*Officinal Part.*—The dried preputial follicles and their secretion (*Castoreum, Castor*). *Characters.*—Follicles in pairs, about three inches long, fig-shaped, firm, and heavy, brown or greyish-black, containing a dry resinous reddish-brown or brown, highly odorous secretion, in great part soluble in rectified spirit and in ether. It contains a volatile oil, an acrid bitter resin, and a crystallizable principle, *Castorin*. Castor is imported into Great Britain from the Hudson's Bay Territory.

*Medical Properties.*—Mild stimulant and antispasmodic.

*Therapeutic Uses.*—In hysterical, nervous, and spasmodic affections, it is a useful addition to other more powerful remedies of the same class. It has been employed with alleged benefit in asthma, dysmenorrhœa, and epilepsy, but its powers given alone are very doubtful.

*Dose.*—From five to ten grains or more, in the form of pills.

*Preparation.*—**Tincture of Castor** (*Tinctura Castorei*). Take of Castor, one ounce; Rectified Spirit, one pint. Macerate for seven days in a closed vessel, with occasional agitation; strain, press, filter, and add sufficient rectified spirit to make one pint.

*Dose.*—From one to two fluid drachms.

*(Non-officinal.)*

**Viverra Zibetha,** *Linn.* (*The Zibeth,* or *Zibeth Civet Cat*). In Southern India, the unctuous odorous secretion of this animal is much employed by the native practitioners, under the name of *Kustúri.* In Travancore there was, and probably is still, an establishment, kept up at the expense of Government, in which these animals were kept and reared for the sake of their secretion, which is used for perfumery as well as for medicinal purposes. Valuable stimulant and aphrodisiac virtues are ascribed to it, but probably it possesses no special powers in these respects. The secretion collects in a shallow pouch, situated between the anus and the genital organs; this pouch communicates with two small sacs, about the size of an almond, the inner surface of which is pierced with a number of small apertures communicating with the glandular secreting follicles. A muscle which covers the whole apparatus, has the power of compressing the secreting follicles as well as the sac, and thus expels the secretion. On being first expelled it is semi-fluid and of a yellow colour, but soon acquires a greater consistence and brown colour. It has a disagreeable ammoniacal odour, and acrid pungent taste.

# Inorganic Kingdom.

# INORGANIC MATERIA MEDICA.

## AQUA.

### Water.

Natural Water, the purest that can be obtained, to be filtered if necessary. *Tests.*—Free from odour, taste, and visible impurity.

*Medical Properties and Uses.*—Diluent and refrigerant, whether taken internally or applied externally. In medicine, surgery, and pharmacy its uses are numerous and important.

*Preparation.*—**Distilled Water** (*Aqua Destillata*) HO or **$H_2O$**.—Take of Water, free from taste and odour, ten gallons. Distil from a copper still, connected with a block-tin worm; reject the first half gallon, and preserve the next eight gallons. *Tests.*—A fluid ounce of it evaporated in a clean glass capsule leaves scarcely a visible residue. It is not affected by sulphuretted hydrogen, oxalate of ammonia, nitrate of silver, chloride of barium, or solution of lime.

Much employed for pharmaceutical purposes.

## CARBON.

*Symbol,* C; *At. weight,* 6; *or* **C=12.**

Carbon is extensively diffused through nature, forming a large portion both of animal and of vegetable substances.

## CARBO LIGNI.

### Wood Charcoal.

Wood charred by exposure to a red heat, with but little access of air. It occurs in the form of black, brittle, porous masses, without taste or smell, very light, and retaining the shape and texture of the wood from which it was obtained. When burned at a high temperature with free access of air, it leaves about two per cent. of ash.

*Medical Properties.*—Antiseptic, deodorizing, and disinfectant.

*Therapeutic Uses.*—In dyspepsia attended with constipation and gastrodynia, in some forms of diarrhœa and dysentery, and in intermittent fevers, it has been employed; in some cases with benefit. It is chiefly employed as an external application in the form of cataplasm. It is also much used as a dentifrice, and is thought to check caries of the teeth.

*Dose.*—From twenty to sixty grains or more.

*Preparation.*—**Charcoal Poultice** (*Cataplasma Carbonis*).—Take of Wood Charcoal in powder, half an ounce; Crumb of Bread, two ounces; Linseed Meal or Rice Flour, one ounce and a half; Boiling Water, ten fluid ounces. Macerate the bread in the water for ten minutes near the fire, then mix, and add the linseed meal or rice flour gradually, stirring the ingredients that a soft poultice may be formed. Mix half the charcoal with this, and sprinkle the remainder on the surface of the poultice.

A valuable application to foul and gangrenous ulcerations, correcting fetor, and stimulating to healthy action.

## CARBO ANIMALIS PURIFICATUS.

### Purified Animal Charcoal.

Animal Charcoal from which the earthy salts have been almost wholly removed by the action of hydrochloric acid. *Characters.*—A black pulverulent substance; inodorous and almost tasteless. Tincture of litmus diluted with twenty times its bulk of water, agitated with it and thrown upon a filter, passes through colourless. When burned at a high temperature with free access of air, it leaves only a slight residue.

*Medical Properties and Uses.*—Deodorizing and antiseptic. It has been employed as an antidote in poisoning by the alkaloids, but with uncertain results; whatever power it possesses is apparently due to its mechanical operation. About half an ounce is regarded as sufficient to counteract the poisonous effects of one grain of strychnia, morphia, or other alkaloid. In pharmacy, and in the arts, it is employed as a decolorizing agent.

*Dose.*—From twenty to sixty grains.

## PHOSPHORUS.

### *Symbol,* P; *At. weight,* 31.

A non-metallic element obtained from bones. *Characters.*—A semi-transparent, colourless, wax-like solid, which emits white vapours when exposed to the air. Specific gravity, 1·83. It is soft and flexible at common temperatures, melts at 110°, ignites in the air at a temperature a little above its melting point, burning with a luminous flame, and producing dense white fumes. Insoluble in water, but soluble in ether, in boiling oil of turpentine, and in bi-sulphide of carbon.

*Medical Properties.*—Stimulant in small, powerful irritant poison in larger doses. One grain and a half has proved fatal.

*Therapeutic Uses.*—In epilepsy, ramollissement of the brain, impotence, phthisis, inveterate skin diseases, cholera, &c., it has been advised; but it is inferior in safety and efficacy to many other remedies.

*Dose.*—About one fortieth part of a grain. It is best administered dissolved in ether or in olive oil, in the proportion of four grains to one ounce of the menstruum. The dose of either, is from five to ten drops twice or thrice daily.

The chief use of Phosphorus is in the oxidized form as Dilute Phosphoric Acid.

## ACIDUM PHOSPHORICUM DILUTUM.

### Diluted Phosphoric Acid.

Phosphoric Acid, $3HO,PO_5$ or $\mathbf{H_3PO_4}$, dissolved in water and corresponding to 10 per cent. by weight of anhydrous phosphoric acid, $PO_5$ or $\mathbf{P_2O_5}$. *Characters.*—A colourless liquid, with a sour taste and strongly acid reaction. Specific gravity, 1·08. With ammonio-nitrate of silver it gives a canary-yellow precipitate, soluble in ammonia and in diluted nitric acid. Evaporated it leaves a residue, which melts at a low red heat, and upon cooling leaves glacial phosphoric acid $HO,PO_5$). *Tests.* — It is not precipitated by sulphuretted hydrogen, chloride of barium, nitrate of silver acidulated with nitric acid, or by the solution of albumen. When mixed with an equal volume of pure sulphuric acid, and then introduced into solution of sulphate of iron, it does not communicate to it a dark colour. Mixed with an equal volume of solution of perchloride of mercury and heated, no precipitate is formed. 355 grains by weight of it poured upon 180 grains of oxide of lead in fine powder leave, by evaporation, a residue (principally phosphate of lead), which, after it has been heated to dull redness, weighs 215·5 grains. Six fluid drachms therefore correspond to 35·5 grains of anhydrous phosphoric acid.

*Medical Properties.*—Tonic, refrigerant, and aphrodisiac in small doses; stimulant, especially of the nervous system, in larger doses; in over doses, poisonous.

*Therapeutic Uses.*—In the advanced stages of typhus and typhoid fevers, scrofulous and calculous affections, diabetes, caries, dropsy, and cardialgia it has been used with alleged benefit.

*Dose.*—From ten to thirty minims properly diluted.

[The hypophosphites of lime, potash, soda, ammonia, and iron have been strongly recommended on the ground that they produce all the beneficial effects of phosphorus, without the irritant and other ill effects which occasionally follow its internal administration. They have been employed in phthisis, anæmia, leucocythemia, dyspepsia, epilepsy, and other affections supposed to be connected with a deficiency of phosphates in the system. The dose of the alkaline hypophosphites is from two to five grains in a bitter infusion, or in the form of syrup.]

## SULPHUR.

*Symbol,* S; *At. weight,* 16; *or* S=32.

Sulphur exists as a natural production in some volcanic countries, especially in Sicily. It likewise abounds in nature in the combined state, forming metallic sulphides. It occurs also in small quantity in many vegetable and animal substances.

## SULPHUR SUBLIMATUM.

### Sublimed Sulphur.

Sulphur prepared from crude or rough sulphur by sublimation. *Characters.*—A slightly gritty powder of a fine greenish-yellow colour; without taste, and without odour unless heated; burning in open vessels with a blue flame and the evolution of sulphurous acid. *Tests.*—Entirely volatilized by heat; does not redden moistened litmus paper. Solution of ammonia, agitated with it, and filtered, does not on evaporation leave any residue.

*Medical Properties.*—Alterative and diaphoretic in small, and mildly aperient in larger doses.

*Therapeutic Uses.*—In scabies and some other cutaneous affections, it is valuable both as an external and an internal remedy. Amongst other diseases in which it has been prescribed internally with advantage are colica pictonum and various forms of lead poisoning, ptyalism and mercurial tremors and palsy, chronic rheumatism, spasmodic asthma, angina pectoris, chronic stage of hooping cough and chronic bronchitis, chorea and scrofula. In hæmorrhoidal affections, in stricture and prolapsus of the rectum, and in chronic dysentery, it forms, from the mildness and peculiarity of its operation, a very eligible aperient.

*Dose.*—From ten to thirty grains as an alterative and diaphoretic; from a drachm to three drachms as an aperient. Sulphur is also often very advantageously employed in the form of aqueous or vapour bath.

*Preparations.* — **Confection of Sulphur** (*Confectio Sulphuris*). Take of Sublimed Sulphur, four ounces; Acid Tartrate of Potash, in powder, one ounce; Syrup of Orange Peel, four fluid ounces. Rub them well together.

*Dose.*—From one to two drachms, once or twice daily.

**Ointment of Sulphur** (*Unguentum Sulphuris*). Take of Sublimed Sulphur, one ounce; Benzoated or Prepared Lard, four ounces. Mix thoroughly.

An effectual application in scabies. It should be thoroughly rubbed into the surface of the body, night and morning, for two days in succession; the patient wearing, during that time, a flannel shirt next to the skin. On the third morning, after a warm bath, the cure will generally be effected. A third day of inunction is occasionally necessary.

## SULPHUR PRÆCIPITATUM.

### Precipitated Sulphur.

Precipitated Sulphur, obtained by decomposing sulphuret of calcium by hydrochloric acid, and washing and drying the precipitate. *Characters.* — A greyish-yellow soft powder free from grittiness, and from the smell of sulphuretted hydrogen. When heated in an open vessel, it burns with a blue flame and the evolution of sulphurous acid. *Tests.* — Entirely volatilized by heat. Under the microscope it is seen to consist of opaque globules without any admixture of crystalline matter. Otherwise it corresponds with sublimed sulphur.

*Medical Properties, Uses, and Dose.*—The same as Sublimed Sulphur.

## SULPHURIS IODIDUM.

### Iodide of Sulphur.

A compound prepared by heating gently in a flask four parts of iodine and one part of sulphur until fusion is effected. *Characters.*—A greyish black solid substance, with a radiated crystalline appearance. It resembles iodine in smell, and in the property of staining the cuticle when applied to it. Soluble in about sixty parts of glycerine; insoluble in water, but decomposed when boiled with it. *Test.*—If 100 grains be thoroughly boiled with water the iodine will pass off in vapour, and about 20 grains of sulphur will remain. It should be kept in well stoppered bottles.

*Properties and Uses.*—Similar to those of iodine.

*Dose.*—Half a grain gradually increased to five grains or more. Rarely employed, except as an external application in the following form.

**Ointment of Iodide of Sulphur** (*Unguentum Sulphuris Iodidi*). Take of Iodide of Sulphur, thirty grains; Prepared Lard, one ounce. Triturate the iodide of sulphur in a porcelain mortar, and gradually add the lard, rubbing them together until the ointment is perfectly smooth and free from grittiness.

A useful application in eczema, lepra, psoriasis, sycosis, and other chronic or obstinate skin diseases.

## ACIDUM SULPHURICUM.

### Sulphuric Acid.

An acid produced by the combustion of sulphur and the oxidation of the resulting sulphurous acid by means of nitrous vapours. It contains 96·8 per cent. by weight of the sulphuric acid, $HO,SO_3$ or $\mathbf{H_2SO_4}$, and corresponds to 79 per cent. of anhydrous sulphuric acid, $SO_3$ or $\mathbf{SO_3}$. *Characters.*—A colourless liquid of oily appearance, intensely acid and corrosive. *Tests.*—Specific gravity, 1·843. It evolves much heat on the addition of water and, when thus diluted, gives a copious precipitate with chloride of barium. 50·6 grains by weight, mixed with an ounce of distilled water, require for neutralization 1000 grain-measures of the volumetric solution of soda. Evaporated in a platinum capsule it leaves little or no residue. When a solution of sulphate of iron is carefully poured over its surface, there is no purple colour developed where the two liquids meet. Diluted with six times its volume of distilled water, it gives no precipitate with sulphuretted hydrogen.

*Medical Properties and Uses.*—Powerful escharotic. The parts touched with it first become white, but they subsequently assume a brownish-black appearance. Taken internally it is a powerful corrosive poison, and is wholly unfitted for internal use. As an escharotic it is inferior to nitric acid.

*Preparations.*—**Diluted Sulphuric Acid** (*Acidum Sulphuricum Dilutum*). Take of Sulphuric Acid, seven fluid ounces; Distilled Water, a sufficiency. Dilute the acid with 77 fluid ounces of the water, and when the mixture has cooled to 60° add more water, so that it shall measure 83½ fluid ounces. *Tests.*—Specific gravity, 1·094. 359 grains by weight (6 fluid drachms) of it require for neutralization 1000 grain-measures of the volumetric solution of soda, corresponding to 10·14 per cent. of anhydrous sulphuric acid. Six fluid drachms therefore correspond to 40 grains of the anhydrous acid.

*Medical Properties.*—Refrigerant, astringent, and tonic.

*Therapeutic Uses.*—In colica pictonum, and in lead poisoning in general, it is valuable both as a prophylactic and as a curative. In passive hæmorrhage from the stomach, lungs, kidneys, or uterus, it proves serviceable, especially in combination with gallic acid. In various forms of diarrhœa, in the profuse perspiration of phthisis, in the exanthemata, in the advanced stages of continued fevers, in some skin diseases, and in syphilitic affections, it has been employed with advantage. In scarlatina and other forms of sore throat it forms an excellent adjunct to gargles.

*Dose.*—From five to thirty minims largely diluted, repeated several times daily.

**Aromatic Sulphuric Acid** (*Acidum Sulphuricum Aromaticum*). Take of Sulphuric Acid, three fluid ounces; Rectified Spirit, two pints; Cinnamon Bark, in coarse powder, two ounces; Ginger, in coarse powder, one ounce and a quarter. Mix the sulphuric acid gradually with the spirit, add the cinnamon and ginger, macerate for seven days, agitating frequently, then filter. *Tests.*—Specific gravity, 0·927. 304·2 grains by weight (6 fluid drachms) require for neutralization 830 grain-measures of the volumetric solution of soda, corresponding to 10·91 per cent. of anhydrous sulphuric acid. Six fluid drachms therefore correspond to 33·2 grains of anhydrous acid.

*Dose.*—From five to thirty minims largely diluted; a useful and agreeable aromatic tonic in passive diarrhœa, perspirations in phthisis, and other exhausting diseases.

## ACIDUM SULPHUROSUM.

### Sulphurous Acid.

Sulphurous acid gas, $SO_2$, dissolved in water, and constituting 9·2 per cent. by weight of the solution. *Characters.*—A colourless liquid, with a pungent sulphurous odour. *Tests.*—Specific gravity, 1·04. It gives no precipitate, or but a very slight one, with chloride of barium, but a copious one if solution of chlorine be also added. 34·7 grains by weight of it, mixed with an ounce of distilled water and a little mucilage of starch, do not acquire a permanent blue colour with the volumetric solution of iodine, until 1000 grain measures of the latter have been added. When evaporated it leaves no residue.

*Medical Properties and Uses.*—Possessed of the power of destroying parasitic vegetable growths, it has been applied with great success in the cure of various forms of tinea, and other skin diseases of vegetable parasitic origin. For this purpose the acid, diluted with two or three times its volume of water, may be applied by compresses of lint, or it may be combined with equal parts of glycerine, and painted over the affected surface. The suffocating character of the vapour renders it unfit for internal administration, unless highly diluted.

*Dose.*—From thirty minims to one fluid drachm.

## CHLORUM.

### Chlorine.

*Symbol*, Cl; *At. weight*, 35·5.

Chlorine exists abundantly in the inorganic kingdom, in union with metals forming metallic chlorides; thus with sodium, as Chloride of Sodium or Common Salt, and with other bases. It is also present as chlorides in both animals and vegetables. At ordinary temperature and pressure it exists in the form of a gas, of a yellowish-green colour, pungent suffocating odour, and astringent taste. It possesses valuable properties as a deodorizer, disinfectant, and antiseptic, and has been used with advantage as an antidote in poisoning by sulphuretted hydrogen and hydrocyanic acid. Inhalation of the diluted gas by means of an appropriate apparatus has been employed in phthisis, chronic bronchitis, and hepatic affections (*vide* Calx Chlorata).

## LIQUOR CHLORI.

### SOLUTION OF CHLORINE.

Chlorine gas dissolved in water. *Characters.*—A yellowish-green liquid, smelling strongly of chlorine, and immediately discharging the colour of a dilute solution of sulphate of indigo. *Tests.*—Specific gravity, 1·003. Evaporated, it leaves no residue. When twenty grains of iodide of potassium dissolved in an ounce of distilled water are added to 439 grains by weight (one fluid ounce) of this preparation, the mixed solution acquires a deep red colour, which requires for its discharge 750 grain-measures of the volumetric solution of hyposulphite of soda, corresponding to 2·66 grains of chlorine.

*Medical Properties.*—Caustic, irritant, and poisonous; largely diluted, stimulant and alterative. Employed chiefly as an external application.

*Therapeutic Uses.*—In scarlatina, typhus fever, and chronic liver affections, it has been employed, but with uncertain results. Locally applied (diluted with eight or more parts of water) it proves useful in various forms of cynanche (as a gargle), aphthæ, stomatitis, cancrum oris, and ptyalism; also in some obstinate skin diseases and foul ulcerations. In the last-named it tends to destroy fetor, and to stimulate to healthy action.

*Dose.*—From ten to thirty minims, largely diluted.

## ACIDUM HYDROCHLORICUM.

### HYDROCHLORIC ACID.

(*Acidum Muriaticum purum, Edin. et Dubl. Ph.*)

Hydrochloric acid gas, $HCl$, dissolved in water, and forming 31·8 per cent. by weight of the solution. *Characters.* — A nearly colourless and strongly acid liquid, emitting white vapours having a pungent odour. *Tests.*—Specific gravity, 1·16. When evaporated to dryness, it leaves no residue. It gives with nitrate of silver a curdy white precipitate, soluble in excess of ammonia, insoluble in nitric acid. 114·8 grains by weight, mixed with half an ounce of distilled water, require for neutralization 1000 grain-measures of the volumetric solution of soda. When diluted with four times its volume of distilled water, it gives no precipitate with solution of chloride of barium, or with sulphuretted hydrogen, and does not tarnish or alter the colour of bright copper foil when boiled with it. If a fluid drachm of it, mixed with half an ounce of distilled water, be put into a small flask with a few pieces of granulated zinc, and while the effervescence continues, a slip of bibulous paper wetted with solution of the subacetate of lead be suspended in the upper part of the flask above the liquid for about five minutes, the paper will not become discoloured.

*Medical Properties and Uses.*—Powerful escharotic and corrosive poison, occasionally applied as an escharotic to phagedenic ulcerations, gangrenous stomatitis, cancrum oris, and warts. Only admissible as an internal remedy in the diluted form.

*Preparation.*—**Diluted Hydrochloric Acid** (*Acidum Hydrochloricum Dilutum, Acidum Hydrochloricum Dilutum,* Edin. Ph.) Take of Hydrochloric Acid, eight fluid ounces; Distilled Water, a sufficiency. Dilute the acid with sixteen ounces of the water, then add more water, so that at a temperature of 60° it shall measure twenty-six and a half fluid ounces. *Tests.*—Specific gravity, 1·052. 345 grains by weight (six fluid drachms) require for neutralization 1,000 grain-measures of the volumetric solution of soda, corresponding to 10·58 per cent. of real acid. Six fluid drachms contain one molecule, or 36·5 grains of hydrochloric acid $HCl$.

*Medical Properties.*—Ant-alkaline, stimulant, tonic.

*Therapeutic Uses.*—In typhus and typhoid fever, in the continued fevers of childhood and scarlatina, in some forms of dyspepsia, in calculous affections, especially in the oxalic acid and phosphatic diatheses, in syphilis, and in the chronic stage of hooping cough, it has been found useful. In phthisis it is an important auxiliary to other treatment. In various forms of cynanche and other affections of the throat and fauces requiring mild stimulant action, it proves a valuable adjunct to gargles. Care is necessary thoroughly to wash out the mouth with water or a weak alkaline solution, after each exhibition of this acid, in order to prevent its injurious action on the teeth.

*Dose.*—From ten to thirty minims, freely diluted.

# IODUM.

## IODINE.

*Symbol*, I; *At. weight*, 127.

Iodine, a non-metallic element, obtained principally from the ashes of sea-weeds. It occurs in the form of laminar crystals of a peculiar odour, dark colour, and metallic lustre, which, when heated, yield a beautiful violet-coloured vapour; very sparingly soluble in water, but freely dissolved by alcohol, by ether, and by a solution of iodide of potassium. The aqueous solution strikes a deep-blue colour with starch. *Tests.*—It sublimes without leaving any residue, and the portion that first comes over does not include any slender colourless prisms emitting a pungent odour. 12·7 grains dissolved in an ounce of water containing 15 grains of iodide of potassium require for complete discoloration 1,000 grain-measures of the volumetric solution of hyposulphite of soda.

*Properties.*—In small doses alterative and tonic, in large doses irritant and poisonous. In long continued doses it induces a peculiar train of irritant symptoms designated Iodism. Externally applied, stimulant and counter-irritant. By chemists it is employed as a test for starch, with which it strikes a deep-blue colour.

*Therapeutic Uses.*—In scrofula and scrofulous affections generally, and in enlargement of the lymphatic glands, abscesses, ulcers, ophthalmia, caries, and arthritic enlargements, occurring in persons of a scrofulous diathesis, it is a remedy of great value, either given internally or locally applied. In phthisis the inhalation of the vapour has been thought useful. Amongst other diseases in which it has been employed with advantage are, bronchocele, chronic hydrocephalus, hydarthrosis, and other dropsical affections, ovarian disease, dysmenorrhœa, enlargement of the prostate gland, hydrocele, chronic affections of the liver and spleen, rheumatism and rheumatic gout, erysipelas, secondary syphilis, and ulcers and skin diseases connected therewith.

*Dose.*—From one eighth to one quarter of a grain, gradually increased to a grain or more, in aqueous solution. It is rarely given alone, the combination with potassium (in the form of Iodide of Potassium) having been found generally the better form of administration.

*Preparations.*—**Tincture of Iodine** (*Tinctura Iodi*). Take of Iodine half an ounce; Iodide of Potassium, a quarter of an ounce; Rectified Spirit, one pint. Dissolve the iodine and the iodide of potassium in the spirit.

*Dose.*—From five to twenty minims twice or thrice daily. It contains one grain of iodine and half a grain of iodide of potassium in forty minims. Valuable as an external application in enlarged glands, diseased joints, chronic skin diseases, and pulmonary affections, applied by means of a camel's-hair brush. It is also extensively used, diluted with three parts of water, as an injection in hydrocele.

**Solution of Iodine** (*Liquor Iodi*). Take of Iodine, twenty grains; Iodide of Potassium, thirty grains; Distilled Water, one fluid ounce. Dissolve.

**Liniment of Iodine** (*Linimentum Iodi*). Take of Iodine, one ounce and a quarter; Iodide of Potassium, half an ounce; Camphor, quarter of an ounce; Rectified Spirit, ten fluid ounces. Dissolve the iodine, iodide of potassium, and camphor in the spirit.

Employed only as an external application in bronchocele, tumours, &c. Its action is that of a vesicant and powerful counter-irritant.

**Ointment of Iodine** (*Unguentum Iodi, Unguentum Iodi Compositum,* Brit. Ph. 1864). Take of Iodine and Iodide of Potassium, of each, thirty-two grains; Proof Spirit, one fluid drachm; Prepared Lard, two ounces. Rub the iodine and the iodide of potassium well together, with the spirit, in a glass or porcelain mortar. Add the lard gradually, and mix thoroughly.

Useful as an external application in the same class of cases as the two preceding preparations.

**Inhalation of Iodine** (*Vapor Iodi*). Take of Tincture of Iodine, one fluid drachm; Water, one fluid ounce. Mix in a suitable apparatus; and, having applied a gentle heat, let the vapour that arises be inhaled.

## BROMUM.

### BROMINE.

*Symbol*, Br; *At. weight*, 80.

Bromine, a liquid non-metallic element obtained from sea-water, and from some saline springs. It is a dark brownish-red, very volatile liquid, with a strong and disagreeable odour. Its specific gravity is 2·966. At the common temperature of the air it gives off red vapours, and at a temperature of 145°·4 it boils. *Test.*—Agitated with solution of soda in such proportion that the fluid remains very slightly alkaline, it forms a colourless liquid, which, if coloured by the further addition of a small quantity of the bromine, forms an orange-coloured compound on the subsequent addition of a cold solution of starch.

*Properties.*—In its pure state caustic and irritant; properly diluted and in small doses, tonic, diuretic, and alterative, its action being chiefly directed on the lymphatic system. Approximates to iodine in its action on the system. Deodoriser and disinfectant.

*Therapeutic Uses.*—Internally in scrofula and scrofulous affections; locally to phagadenic ulcerations, hospital gangrene, erysipelas, and obstinate skin diseases.

*Dose.*—From six to eight minims of a solution of one part of bromine to forty of water. For external application it may be used of a strength varying from five to fifteen grains to one ounce of lard. It is best administered in the form of Bromide of Ammonium or Bromide of Potassium, of which it forms the active ingredient.

## NITROGEN.

*Symbol,* N ; *At. weight,* 14.

Nitrogen, a gas, devoid of colour, odour, and taste, forms about 77 per cent. of atmospheric air. It is a constituent of all animal bodies, and also of many vegetable products. Those which contain it in the largest proportion are considered the most nourishing as articles of diet. In combination with other elements it forms numerous important compounds, *e.g.* Nitric Acid and Ammonia.

## ACIDUM NITRICUM.

### Nitric Acid.

An acid prepared from nitrate of potash or nitrate of soda by distillation with sulphuric acid and water, and containing 70 per cent. by weight of the nitric acid, $HO,NO_5$ or $\mathbf{HNO_3}$, corresponding to 60 per cent. of anhydrous nitric acid, $NO_5$ or $\mathbf{N_2O_5}$. *Characters.*—A colourless liquid, having a specific gravity of 1·42. When exposed to the air, it emits an acrid, corrosive vapour. *Tests.*—If it be poured over copper filings, dense red vapours are immediately formed; but if the acid be mixed with an equal volume of water, and then added to the copper, it gives off a colourless gas, which acquires an orange-red colour as it mixes with the air, and which, if it be introduced into a solution of sulphate of iron, communicates to it a dark-olive brown colour. The boiling point of the acid is 250°. If submitted to distillation the product continues uniform throughout the process. It leaves no residue when evaporated to dryness. Diluted with six times its volume of distilled water, it gives no precipitate with chloride of barium or nitrate of silver. Ninety grains by weight of it mixed with half an ounce of distilled water require for neutralization 1,000 grain-measures of the volumetric solution of soda.

*Medical Properties.*—Powerful escharotic and caustic. It communicates a persistent yellow stain to the cuticle, which is enlivened by alkaline solutions. Taken internally in an undiluted state, it acts as a powerful corrosive poison.

*Therapeutic Uses.*—In phagedenic ulcerations, hæmorrhoidal tumours, primary chancres, warts, and cancrum oris, the application of the pure acid has been found effectual in destroying the affected surface, and in tending to establish a subsequently healthy action. For this purpose it is superior to all the other mineral acids.

*Preparations.*—**Diluted Nitric Acid** (*Acidum Nitricum Dilutum*). Take of Nitric Acid, six fluid ounces; Distilled Water, a sufficiency. Dilute the acid with twenty-four fluid ounces of the water; then add more water, so that at a temperature of 60° it shall measure thirty-one fluid ounces. *Characters and Tests.*—Colourless. Specific gravity, 1·101. 361·3 grains by weight (six fluid drachms) require for neutralization 1,000 grain-measures of the volumetric solution of soda, corresponding to 14·95 per cent. of anhydrous nitric acid. Six fluid drachms, therefore, correspond to fifty-four grains of the anhydrous acid.

*Medical Properties.*—Ant-alkaline, tonic, alterative, and refrigerant. Externally applied, stimulant.

*Therapeutic Uses.*—In syphilis and syphilitic affections, in mercurial cachexia, in chronic diseases of the liver and spleen, in calculous affections, especially those occurring in the phosphatic diathesis, and in chronic inflammation of the bladder and in cystirrhœa, it is a remedy of value. Amongst other diseases in which it has been employed with advantage are dropsy, especially that consequent on hepatic disease, or on the prolonged use of mercury, diabetes, chronic stage of hooping cough, cholera and choleraic diarrhœa, cardialgia and chronic rheumatism. Largely diluted it has been used with advantage as a lotion, in chronic ulcerations, caries, and obstinate skin diseases.

*Dose.*—From ten to thirty minims, freely diluted, twice or thrice daily. The teeth should be carefully protected from the action of the acid, by washing the mouth out with a weak alkaline solution after each dose of the medicine. The strength of a lotion for external use may vary from two to four drachms of the acid to a pint of water.

**Diluted Nitro-hydrochloric Acid** (*Acidum Nitro-hydrochloricum Dilutum*). Take of Nitric Acid, three fluid ounces; Hydrochloric Acid, four fluid ounces; Distilled Water, twenty-five fluid ounces. Mix the acids, and allow them to remain for twenty-four hours in a bottle the mouth of which is partially closed; then add the water in successive portions, shaking the bottle after each addition; and preserve the mixture in a stoppered bottle. *Characters and Tests.* — Colourless. Specific gravity, 1·074. 352·4 grains by weight (six fluid drachms) require for neutralization 920 grain-measures of the volumetric solution of soda.

*Medical Properties.*—Analogous to those of Diluted Nitric Acid.

*Therapeutic Uses.*—In chronic hepatic affections, hepatic dysentery, jaundice, dropsy consequent on disease of the liver or spleen, it proves of great value, both given internally and applied externally in the form of bath, lotion, or epithem. It is also serviceable in calculous affections occurring in the oxalic acid and cystic oxide diatheses, in chronic bronchitis, gangrene of the lungs, scarlatina, typhus and typhoid fever, and secondary syphilitic affections.

*Dose.*—From five to twenty minims, freely diluted, twice or thrice daily. The ordinary proportion for baths and external applications is from six to eight fluid ounces to a gallon of water.

## AMMONIA.

*Symbol,* $NH_3$; *At. weight,* 17.

Ammonia, either in a free or combined state, is diffused extensively throughout the organic and inorganic kingdoms of nature. It exists in minute quantities in atmospheric air; is one of the constituents of urine in man, in which it occurs in combination with phosphoric, hydrochloric, and uric acids. It is also a product of the putrefaction of animal matters. It is a colourless transparent gas, with a powerful pungent odour and acrid alkaline taste. Reddens turmeric paper, which, however, by subsequent exposure to the air, resumes its original colour; evolves white fumes when brought in contact with the vapour of hydrochloric acid. Sp. Gr. 0·59.

## LIQUOR AMMONIÆ FORTIOR.

### Strong Solution of Ammonia.

Ammoniacal gas, $NH_3$, dissolved in water, and constituting 32·5 per cent. of the solution. *Characters.*—A colourless liquid, with a characteristic and very pungent odour, and strong alkaline reaction. *Tests.*—Specific gravity, 0·891. 52·3 grains by weight require for neutralization 1,000 grain-measures of the volumetric solution of oxalic acid. One fluid drachm contains 15·83 grains of ammonia, $NH_3$. When diluted with four times its volume of distilled water, it does not give precipitates with solution of lime, oxalate of ammonia, sulphide of ammonium, or ammonio-sulphate of copper, and, when treated with an excess of nitric acid, is not rendered turbid by nitrate of silver or by chloride of barium.

*Properties.*—Powerful stimulant and irritant; locally applied, caustic and vesicant. Vapour also powerfully stimulant. In over doses, poisonous.

*Therapeutic Uses.*—The same as Liquor Ammoniæ (*infra*).

*Dose.*—From three to ten minims largely diluted.

*Preparations.*—**Solution of Ammonia** (*Liquor Ammoniæ*). Take of Strong Solution of Ammonia, one pint; Distilled Water, two pints. Mix, and preserve in a stoppered bottle. *Tests.*—Specific gravity 0·959. Eighty-five grains by weight require for neutralization 500 grain-measures of the volumetric solution of oxalic acid, corresponding to 10 per cent. by weight of ammonia, $NH_3$. One fluid drachm contains 5·2 grains of ammonia.

*Properties.*—Valuable stimulant, whether employed internally, externally, or in the form of vapour.

*Therapeutic Uses.*—In the advanced stages of febrile and inflammatory diseases, and in other cases, as in cholera, when the vital powers are greatly depressed, it is of great value as a stimulant, especially when conjoined with other remedies of the same class. In the bites of venomous snakes and insects, it is the remedy most to be relied upon, given internally and locally applied. In nervous affections connected with debility it is often beneficial. In syncope and asphyxia, the vapour, properly diluted, proves very advantageous.

*Dose.*—From ten to thirty drops freely diluted.

**Liniment of Ammonia** (*Linimentum Ammoniæ*). Take of Solution of Ammonia, one fluid ounce; Olive Oil, three fluid ounces. Mix together with agitation.

A serviceable stimulant and rubefacient.

Solution of Ammonia enters into the following officinal preparations: Spiritus Ammoniæ Aromaticus, Spiritus Ammoniæ Fœtidus, Linimentum Camphoræ compositum, Linimentum Hydrargyri, and Tinctura Opii Ammoniata.

## AMMONIÆ CARBONAS.

### Carbonate of Ammonia.

*(Ammoniæ Sesquicarbonas, Lond. et Dubl. Ph.)*

Carbonate of Ammonia, $2NH_4O,3CO_2$, or $N_4H_{16}C_3O_8$, a volatile and pungent ammoniacal salt, produced by submitting a mixture of sulphate of ammonia or chloride of ammonium and carbonate of lime to sublimation. *Characters.*—Translucent crystalline masses, with a strong ammoniacal odour, and alkaline reaction; soluble in cold water, more sparingly in spirit. It volatilizes entirely when heated, and is readily dissolved by acids with effervescence. *Tests.*—If diluted nitric acid be added to it in slight excess, and the solution be boiled, it will give no precipitate with chloride of barium or nitrate of silver. Fifty-nine grains dissolved in one ounce of distilled water will be neutralized by 1000 grain-measures of the volumetric solution of oxalic acid.

*Properties.*—Antacid, stimulant, diaphoretic, and expectorant; in larger doses, emetic; in over-doses, poisonous.

*Therapeutic Uses.*—In cardialgia and gastrodynia it often affords speedy relief. In scarlatina, rubeola, erysipelas, urticaria, and in some skin diseases, especially lepra and psoriasis, it is a remedy of great value. In chronic and sub-acute pulmonary affections, it proves serviceable as a stimulant expectorant, especially when given in combination with senega. Hysteria, epilepsy, puerperal insanity, paralysis, glanders, phlegmasia dolens, and asthma are some of the other diseases in which it has been used with advantage. It has been proposed as a remedy in diabetes. It forms a very useful addition to a warm bath in cases of violent cold and rheumatism. The vapour is often effectual in syncope and asphyxia.

*Dose.*—From five to fifteen grains in solution. In doses of thirty grains it acts as an emetic.

*Preparations.*—**Aromatic Spirit of Ammonia** (*Spiritus Ammoniæ Aromaticus*). Take of Carbonate of Ammonia, eight ounces; Strong Solution of Ammonia, four fluid ounces; Volatile Oil of Nutmeg, four fluid drachms; Oil of Lemon, six fluid drachms; Rectified Spirit, six pints; Water, three pints. Mix and distil seven pints. *Test.*—Specific gravity, 0·870.

*Properties and Uses.*—Under the name of *Spirit of Sal Volatile*, this preparation has long enjoyed high and deserved repute as a stimulant in syncope, hysteria, nervous debility, flatulent colic, &c. On account of its pleasant taste and smell, it is generally preferred to Liquor Ammoniæ, to which, though much weaker, it bears a close resemblance in medicinal properties.

*Dose.*—From thirty to sixty minims freely diluted.

It forms an ingredient in Tinctura Guaiaci Ammoniata and Tinctura Valerianæ Ammoniata.

**Fetid Spirit of Ammonia** (*Spiritus Ammoniæ Fœtidus*). Take of Assafœtida, one ounce and a half; Strong Solution of Ammonia, two fluid ounces; Rectified Spirit, a sufficiency. Break the assafœtida into small pieces, and macerate it in a closed vessel in fifteen fluid ounces of the spirit, for twenty-four hours, then distil off the spirit, mix the product with the solution of ammonia, and add sufficient rectified spirit to make one pint.

A valuable stimulant and antispasmodic.

*Dose.*—From half a fluid drachm to one drachm.

## LIQUOR AMMONIÆ ACETATIS.

### SOLUTION OF THE ACETATE OF AMMONIA.

Acetate of Ammonia, $NH_4O,C_4H_3O_3$ or $\mathbf{NH_4,C_2H_3O_2}$, dissolved in water. Take of Acetic Acid, ten fluid ounces; Carbonate of Ammonia, three ounces and a quarter, or a sufficiency; Distilled Water, two pints and a half. Reduce the carbonate of ammonia to powder, and add it gradually to the acetic acid, until a neutral solution is formed, then add the water.

*Properties.*—Refrigerant and diaphoretic.

*Therapeutic Uses.*—In febrile, inflammatory and catarrhal affections, it forms a valuable addition to refrigerant and diaphoretic mixtures. Externally applied, diluted with water, it is employed as a refrigerant lotion, to local inflammations, and as a collyrium in some forms of ophthalmia.

*Dose.*—From two to six fluid drachms, properly diluted, repeated every third or fourth hour.

## LIQUOR AMMONIÆ CITRATIS.

### SOLUTION OF CITRATE OF AMMONIA.

Citrate of Ammonia, $3NH_4O,C_{12}H_5O_{11}$ or $\mathbf{3NH_4.C_6H_5O_7}$, dissolved in water. Take of Citric Acid, three ounces;

Strong Solution of Ammonia, two fluid ounces and three-quarters or a sufficiency; Distilled Water, one pint. Dissolve the citric acid in the water, and add the solution of ammonia until the liquid is neutral to test papers.

*Properties, Uses, and Dose.*—The same as Liquor Ammoniæ Acetatis. Its flavour, however, is more agreeable.

## AMMONIÆ BENZOAS.

### Benzoate of Ammonia.

Benzoate of Ammonia, $NH_4O,C_{14}H_5O_3$ or $\mathbf{NH_4C_7H_5O_2}$, prepared as follows:—Take of Solution of Ammonia, three fluid ounces or a sufficiency; Benzoic Acid, two ounces; Distilled Water, four fluid ounces. Dissolve the Benzoic Acid in three fluid ounces of Solution of Ammonia previously mixed with the water; evaporate at a gentle heat, keeping ammonia in slight excess; and set aside, that crystals may form. *Characters.*—Colourless laminar crystals, soluble in water and alcohol. It gives a bulky yellowish precipitate with persalts of iron. Its aqueous solution, when heated with caustic potash, evolves ammonia; and, if it be not too dilute, when acidulated with hydrochloric acid, it gives a deposit of benzoic acid. *Test.*—When heated it sublimes without any residue.

*Properties.*—Stimulant, especially of the mucous passages of the genito-urinary system.

*Therapeutic Uses.*—In chronic cystitis, cystirrhœa, and in removing phosphatic deposits from the urine, it has been employed with alleged success.

*Dose.*—From ten to twenty grains in solution, twice or thrice daily.

## AMMONIÆ PHOSPHAS.

### Phosphate of Ammonia.

Phosphate of Ammonia, $2NH_4O,HO,PO_5$ or $\mathbf{(NH_4)_2HPO_4}$. Take of Diluted Phosphoric Acid, twenty fluid ounces; Strong Solution of Ammonia, a sufficiency. Add the ammonia to the phosphoric acid until the solution is slightly alkaline, then evaporate the liquid, adding more ammonia from time to time, so as to keep it in slight excess, and when crystals are formed, on the cooling of the solution, dry them quickly on filtering paper placed on a porous tile, and preserve them in a stoppered bottle. *Characters.*—Transparent colourless prisms. Soluble in water, insoluble in rectified spirit. When heated with caustic potash, ammonia is evolved. The aqueous solution gives a yellow precipitate with nitrate of silver. *Tests.*—If twenty grains of this salt be dissolved in water, and solution of ammonio-sulphate of magnesia added, a crystalline precipitate falls, which, when well washed upon a filter with solution of ammonia diluted with an equal volume of water, dried and heated to redness, leaves 16·8 grains of the pyrophosphate of magnesia.

*Properties.*—Stimulant, its action being chiefly directed to the urinary system.

*Therapeutic Uses.*—In diseases, acute and chronic, connected with the uric acid diathesis, especially in some forms of gout, it has been used with advantage.

*Dose.*—From five to twenty grains, thrice daily.

## AMMONII CHLORIDUM.

### CHLORIDE OF AMMONIUM.

(*Ammoniæ Hydrochloras, Brit. Ph.* 1864; *Ammoniæ Murias, Edin. et Dubl. Ph. Sal Ammoniac.*)

Chloride of Ammonium, $NH_4Cl$, may be formed by neutralizing hydrochloric acid with ammonia and evaporating to dryness. It is principally prepared from the impure ammoniacal liquors obtained as secondary products in the manufacture of coal gas and animal charcoal. *Characters.* — Colourless, inodorous, translucent, fibrous masses; tough, and difficult to powder; soluble in water and in rectified spirit. *Tests.*—Its aqueous solution, when heated with caustic potash, evolves ammonia, and when treated with nitrate of silver forms a copious curdy precipitate. When heated it volatilizes without decomposition and leaves no residue.

*Properties.*—In small and continued doses alterative; in larger doses stimulant, its action being chiefly directed on the absorbent system and on glandular structures.

*Therapeutic Uses.*—In chronic affections of the lungs and of the liver and spleen, in dropsy connected with hepatic and ovarian disease, in passive hœmorrhages, especially hæmoptysis, in neuralgic and rheumatic affections of the face, in certain forms of nervous headaches, in amenorrhœa, in hooping cough, and in intermittent and continued fevers, it has been employed internally with advantage. Locally or externally, it has been applied, in solution, to indolent tumours, enlarged glands, incipient mammary abscesses, hydrocele, bruises, sprains, and certain chronic skin diseases.

*Dose.*—From five to fifteen grains in solution, twice or thrice daily, in chronic cases. For the relief of severe neuralgic or rheumatic pain it is best given in doses of half a drachm, repeated every third or fourth hour till two drachms have been exhibited. For an ordinary lotion or wash, the strength may vary from half an ounce to one ounce to ten ounces of water. A freezing mixture (sometimes called an *Ice Poultice*) is prepared by dissolving five ounces of this salt, and an equal quantity of nitrate of potash, in sixteen ounces of water. It is a valuable application, when ice is not procurable.

[Sal Ammoniac, under the Hindústani name *Nausádar* or *Naushádar*, is commonly met with in the bazaars of India, in the form of thick fibrous translucent cakes, inodorous, of a bitter acrid taste, and is obtained from the unburnt extremity of brick-kilns in which the manure of animals, especially that of the camel, is used as fuel. It is always more or less impure, and, when intended for medicinal purposes, requires to be dissolved in boiling water, strained through calico, and the solution evaporated to crystallization.]

## AMMONII BROMIDUM.

### Bromide of Ammonium.

Bromide of Ammonium, $NH_4Br$, occurs in the form of colourless crystals, which become slightly yellow by exposure to the air, and have a pungent saline taste. May be sublimed unchanged by the application of heat. Readily soluble in water; less soluble in spirit. *Test.*—A solution of the salt in water, mixed with mucilage of starch and a drop of an aqueous solution of chlorine, does not exhibit blue but an orange colour.

*Properties.*—Valuable alterative.

*Therapeutic Uses.*—In glandular enlargements, scrofulous ophthalmia, hooping cough, and in many affections in which the ganglionic nervous system is functionally engaged, it has been advantageously employed.

## POTASSIUM.

*Symbol,* K. (*Kalium*); *At. weight,* 39.

Potassium is the metallic base of Potassa or Potash, the Oxide of Potassium (*Symbol,* KO.; *At. Weight,* 47, or **$K_2O$; =94**). Thus oxydized it exists extensively both in the organic and in the inorganic kingdoms of nature, in combination with acids and earths.

## POTASSA CAUSTICA.

### CAUSTIC POTASH; HYDRATE OF POTASSIUM.

(*Potassæ Hydras, Lond. Ph.; Potassa, Edin. Ph.*)

Hydrate of Potash, KO,HO or **KHO**, obtained by subjecting the solution of potash to heat in a silver or iron basin until the residue has the consistence of oil; and then pouring it into moulds. It occurs in the form of hard white pencils, very deliquescent, powerfully alkaline and corrosive. Its solution in water acidulated by nitric acid gives a yellow precipitate with perchloride of platinum, and scanty white precipitates with nitrate of silver and chloride of barium. *Tests.*—Fifty-six grains dissolved in water leave only a trace of sediment, and require for neutralization at least 900 grain-measures of the volumetric solution of oxalic acid. On account of its deliquescence in the air, it requires to be kept in closely stoppered bottles.

*Properties.*—Powerful caustic and escharotic; taken internally, a corrosive poison.

*Therapeutic Uses.*—As an application in hospital gangrene, as a means of destroying superficial nævi materni, of obliterating varicose veins, of removing permanent strictures of the urethra, and of opening scrofulous abscesses, caustic potash has been resorted to with effect. It is also used in making issues. The great objection to its use is its ready deliquescence.

[A mixture of equal parts of Caustic Potash and Lime (Potassa cum Calce) is equally effectual as a caustic, and possesses the advantage over Caustic Potash *per se*, of being far less deliquescent. It is used in the form of paste prepared with spirit.]

## LIQUOR POTASSÆ.

### SOLUTION OF POTASH.

Solution of Potash is obtained by boiling slaked lime (½ part) with carbonate of potash (1 part) dissolved in water (12 parts); when cold the carbonate of lime may be separated by decantation. *Characters.*—A colourless, inodorous, transparent liquid, of extremely acrid caustic taste, powerfully alkaline, saponaceous when rubbed between the fingers, corrodes both animal and vegetable textures. Specific gravity, 1·058. *Tests.*—462·9 grains by weight (1 fluid ounce) require for neutralization 482 grain-measures of the volumetric solution of oxalic acid corresponding to 5·84 per cent. by weight of hydrate of potash, KO,HO or **KHO**. It does not effervesce when added to an excess of diluted hydrochloric acid. Mixed with an equal volume of distilled water it gives no precipitate with lime water or with oxalate of ammonia. When treated with an excess of diluted nitric acid, and evaporated to dryness, the residue forms with water a nearly clear solution, which may be slightly precipitated by chloride of barium and nitrate of silver, but is unaffected, or very slightly affected, by ammonia. One fluid ounce contains 27 grains of hydrate of potash. As it rapidly absorbs carbonic acid from the air, and moreover acts on flint glass, it requires to be kept in well-stoppered bottles of green glass.

*Properties.*—Primarily antacid, secondarily alterative and diuretic. In over-doses poisonous.

*Therapeutic Uses.*—Cardialgia from acidity of the primæ viæ, acute and chronic rheumatism, tubercular affections, especially phthisis, calculous affections connected with the uric acid diathesis, ardor urinæ and irritable states of the bladder arising from an acrid state of the urine, bronchocele, dropsical affections, chronic skin diseases, especially psoriasis and lepra, bronchial congestion and catarrh, and the advanced stages of pneumonia, are amongst the principal diseases benefited by its use.

*Dose.*—From fifteen to sixty minims, freely diluted.

## POTASSÆ CARBONAS.

### CARBONATE OF POTASH.

Carbonate of Potash, KO,$CO_2$ or $\mathbf{K_2CO_3}$, with about 16 per cent. of water of crystallization. Obtained from commercial pearl-ash, the product of lixiviation of wood-ashes, by treating the pearl-ash with its own weight of distilled water, and evaporating the solution so formed to dryness, while it is kept briskly agitated. *Characters.*—A white crystalline powder, alkaline and caustic to the taste, very deliquescent, readily soluble in water but insoluble in spirit, effervescing with diluted hydrochloric acid, and forming a solution with which perchloride of platinum gives a yellow precipitate. *Tests.*—Loses about sixteen per cent. of its weight when exposed to a red heat. When supersaturated with nitric acid, and evaporated to dryness, the residue is almost entirely soluble in water, only a little silica remaining undissolved; and the solution is precipitated only faintly by chloride of barium and nitrate of silver. Eighty-three grains require for neutralization at least 980 grain-measures of the volumetric solution of oxalic acid. In consequence of its ready deliquescence on exposure to the air, it requires to be kept in well stoppered bottles.

*Properties and Uses.*—Analogous to those of Liquor Potassæ, but, being weaker in its action on the system, may be longer continued with safety. It forms in solution, in the proportion of half a drachm to a pint of water, a serviceable alkaline lotion in many skin diseases.

*Dose.*—From ten to thirty grains in solution, or in the form of effervescing draughts with a vegetable acid.

[An impure carbonate of potash is prepared in some parts of India by the incineration of the leaves of the palm and plantain. In its crude state it is unsuited for medicinal purposes. Potash is said also to constitute a great portion of the ashes of *Achyranthes aspera, Lin.*]

## POTASSÆ BICARBONAS.

### BICARBONATE OF POTASH.

Bicarbonate of Potash, $KO,HO,2CO_2$ or $\mathbf{KHCO_3}$ obtained by passing a stream of carbonic acid gas (generated by action of dilute hydrochloric acid on marble) through a solution of carbonate of potash to saturation. *Characters.*—Colourless right rhombic prisms, not deliquescent, of a saline feebly alkaline taste, not corrosive. Diluted hydrochloric acid causes strong effervescence, forming a solution with which perchloride of platinum gives a yellow precipitate. *Tests.*—Fifty grains exposed to a low red heat leave thirty-four and a half grains of a white residue, which require for exact saturation 500 grain-measures of the volumetric solution of oxalic acid.

*Properties and Uses.*—Similar to those of the carbonate of potash, but weaker in operation.

*Dose.*—From ten to forty grains or more. For effervescing draughts, twenty grains of the bicarbonate of potash = fourteen grains of citric acid, or fifteen grains of tartaric acid.

*Preparation.*—**Effervescing Solution of Potash** (*Liquor Potassæ Effervescens, Potash Water*). Take of Bicarbonate of Potash, thirty grains; Water, one pint. Dissolve the bicarbonate of potash in the water, and filter the solution; then pass into it as much pure washed carbonic acid gas (obtained by the action of sulphuric acid on chalk, or as above,) as can be retained under a pressure of seven atmospheres. Keep the solution in bottles securely closed, to prevent the escape of the compressed gas. *Characters.*—Effervesces strongly when the containing vessel is opened, carbonic acid gas escaping. The liquid is clear and sparkling, and has an agreeable acidulous taste. *Tests.*—Ten fluid ounces, after being boiled for five minutes, require for neutralization 150 grain-measures of the volumetric solution of oxalic acid. Five fluid ounces evaporated to one-fifth, and twelve grains of tartaric acid added, yield a crystalline precipitate, which, when dried, weighs not less than 12 grains.

## POTASSA SULPHURATA.

### SULPHURATED POTASH.

(*Potassii Sulphuretum, Lond. et Edin. Ph.; Hepar Sulphuris, Dubl. Ph.*)

Sulphurated Potash, obtained by the fusion of carbonate of potash and sublimed sulphur. *Characters.*—Solid greenish fragments, liver-brown when recently broken, alkaline, and acrid to the taste, readily forming with water a yellow solution, which has the odour of sulphuretted hydrogen, and evolves it freely when excess of hydrochloric acid is dropped into it, sulphur being at the same time deposited. The acid fluid, when boiled and filtered, is precipitated yellow by perchloride of platinum, and white by chloride of barium. *Tests.*—About three fourths of its weight are dissolved by rectified spirit.

*Properties.*—Stimulant; its action being chiefly directed on the cutaneous system (diaphoretic) and on the bronchial mucous surface (expectorant). In large doses it is an acro-narcotic poison.

*Therapeutic Uses.*—In obstinate skin diseases, chronic bronchitis, and catarrhal affections, croup, atonic dyspepsia, and chronic rheumatism, it has been prescribed internally with advantage. Externally applied in the form of baths, lotion, and ointment, it is a valuable remedy in scabies and other skin diseases.

*Dose.*—From three to five grains, gradually increased to ten grains or more, in solution or in the form of pill with soap. For lotions the proportion may range from one to two drachms to a pint of water; and for baths, from three to four ounces to thirty gallons of water.

*Preparation.*—**Ointment of Sulphurated Potash** (*Unguentum Potassæ Sulphuratæ*). Take of Sulphurated Potash, thirty grains; Prepared Lard, one ounce. Triturate the sulphurated potash in a porcelain mortar, and gradually add the lard, rubbing them together until the ointment is perfectly smooth and free from grittiness. This ointment, when used, should be recently prepared.

## POTASSÆ SULPHAS.

### SULPHATE OF POTASH.

Sulphate of Potash, $KO,SO_3$ or $\mathbf{K_2SO_4}$, obtained, by neutralization with carbonate of potash, from the impure bisulphate of potash, which constitutes the residue of the process for the manufacture of nitric acid. It exists in a native state in both the inorganic and the organic kingdoms. *Characters.*—Colourless, hard, six-sided prisms terminated by six-sided pyramids, which decrepitate strongly when heated, and are sparingly soluble in water; insoluble in alcohol. *Tests.*—Its solution, acidulated with hydrochloric acid, is precipitated white by chloride of barium, and yellow by perchloride of platinum. Neutral to test paper. Its solution is not affected by oxalate of ammonia.

*Properties.*—Mild aperient, lactifuge? In over-doses poisonous.

*Therapeutic Uses.*—In dyspeptic and hepatic affections, especially jaundice, in gastric remittent fever, albuminuria, and for hæmorrhoidal subjects, it is well adapted as an aperient, on account of the mildness of its action; otherwise it does not possess any special advantages over other remedies of the same class.

*Dose.*—From fifteen to sixty grains, generally given combined with rhubarb.

Sulphate of Potash forms an ingredient in Pulvis Ipecacuanhæ compositus, Pilula Colocynthidis composita, and Pil. Colocynthidis et Hyoscyami.

## POTASSÆ CHLORAS.

### CHLORATE OF POTASH.

Chlorate of Potash, $KO,ClO_5$, or $\mathbf{KClO_3}$, obtained by passing a stream of chlorine gas (generated by the action of hydrochloric acid on the black oxide of manganese) through a mixture of carbonate of potash, slaked lime, and water, and subsequent boiling. On filtration and evaporation the crystals separate. *Characters.*—Colourless rhomboidal crystalline plates, with a cool saline taste, sparingly soluble in cold water. It explodes when triturated with sulphur. *Tests.*—By heat it fuses, gives off oxygen gas, and leaves a white residue (chloride of potassium), which readily forms with water a neutral solution, and which is precipitated white by nitrate of silver, and yellow by perchloride of platinum.

*Properties.*—Refrigerant, diuretic, alterative.

*Therapeutic Uses.*—In typhoid fever, scarlatina, and the exanthemata generally, and in supervening dropsical affections, it is a remedy of great value. Amongst the other diseases in which it has been prescribed internally with advantage, are chronic bronchitis, phthisis, cholera, choleraic diarrhœa, jaundice, mercurial, syphilitic and other forms of cachexia, diphtheria, and scurvy, As a local or external application in cancrum oris, aphthæ, and aphthous ulceration, various forms of cynanche, ptyalism, gonnorrhœa and leucorrhœa (in the form of injection), and scrofulous and syphilitic ulcerations, it exercises a beneficial iufluence.

*Dose.*—From ten to twenty grains in solution. As a refrigerant drink in fevers, a drachm dissolved in a pint of water may be used. As a local application, the strength of the solution may range from one to two drachms to a pint of water.

*Preparation.*—**Chlorate of Potash Lozenges** (*Trochisci Potassæ Chlorates*). Take of Chlorate of Potash, in powder, three thousand six hundred grains (8 oz. 100 grs.); Refined Sugar, in powder, twenty-five ounces; Gum Acacia, in powder, one ounce; Mucilage of Gum Acacia, two fluid ounces; Distilled Water, one fluid ounce, or a sufficiency. Mix the powders and add the mucilage and water to form a proper mass. Divide into 720 lozenges, and dry these in a hot-air chamber with a moderate heat. Each lozenge contains five grains of chlorate of potash.

*Dose.*—From one to six lozenges.

## POTASSÆ NITRAS.

### NITRATE OF POTASH. SALTPETRE.

Nitrate of Potash, $KO,NO_5$ or $\mathbf{KNO_3}$, obtained by solution and evaporation from the impure nitrate of commerce, which exists in a natural state in the soil in many parts of India and other portions of the globe. It occurs in the form of white crystalline masses or fragments of striated six-sided prisms, colourless, of a peculiar cool saline taste. Thrown on the fire it deflagrates; warmed in a test tube with sulphuric acid and copper filings, it evolves ruddy fumes. Its solution acidulated with hydrochloric acid gives a yellow precipitate with perchloride of platinum. *Tests.*—Its solution is not affected by chloride of barium or nitrate of silver.

*Properties*—Refrigerant, diuretic, and diaphoretic, when administered in solution freely diluted; irritant if given in the solid form or in concentrated solution; in the latter forms, poisonous in large doses. Externally applied in solution, refrigerant.

*Therapeutic Uses.*—Febrile and inflammatory affections, acute and chronic rheumatism, hæmorrhage accompanied by vascular excitement, scurvy, purpura hæmorrhagica, dropsical affections, dysmenorrhœa, gonorrhœa, leucorrhœa, and some forms of dyspepsia.

are the diseases in which it has been chiefly employed internally. As a local application it has been used in solution, as a collyrium in acute forms of ophthalmia, as a gargle in cynanche, and as a cold refrigerant lotion, for which purpose it should be combined with an equal quantity of chloride of ammonium. Inhalation of the fumes of bibulous paper soaked in a saturated solution of the nitrate, and dried, often affords marked relief in asthma and other spasmodic coughs.

*Dose.*—From ten to thirty grains in solution in the proportion of about eight grains to a fluid ounce of any bland fluid.

[Under the Hindústani name *Shora,* Nitrate of Potash is to be obtained in most of the bazaars of India, but often in a very impure state. To fit it for internal use it should be purified by dissolving it in boiling water, removing the scum, and, after the liquid has been allowed to settle, straining it through a hempen cloth, and setting aside to crystallize. Dr. Stevenson has published an interesting account of its manufacture at Tirhoot (*Bengal Asiat. Journ.* 1833, vol. ii. p. 23.)

## POTASSÆ PERMANGANAS.

### Permanganate of Potash.

Permanganate of Potash, $KO,Mn_2O_7$ or $\mathbf{KMnO_4}$, occurs in the form of dark-purple, slender, prismatic crystals, inodorous, with a sweet astringent taste, soluble in water. A single small crystal suffices to form with an ounce of water a rich purple solution, which, when mixed with a little rectified spirit and heated, becomes yellowish-brown. The crystals heated to redness decrepitate, evolve oxygen gas, and leave a black residue, from which water extracts potash, recognised by its alkaline reaction and by its giving when acidulated with hydrochloric acid, a yellow precipitate with perchloride of platinum. *Tests.*—Entirely soluble in cold water. Five grains dissolved in water require for complete decoloration a solution of forty-four grains of granulated sulphate of iron acidulated with two fluid drachms of diluted sulphuric acid.

*Properties.*—Alterative? Powerful local deodorizer and antiseptic.

*Therapeutic Uses.*—In diabetes it has been employed with doubtful result. Externally applied in the form of lotion (*infra*), or in powder mixed with an equal weight of finely powdered chalk, to cancerous and ill-conditioned ulcers, to correct the fetor of discharges from mucous surfaces, and as a gargle in ulceration of the tonsils and throat.

*Dose.*—From one to three grains in solution largely diluted.

*Preparation.* — **Solution of Permanganate of Potash** (*Liquor Potassæ Permanganatis*). Take of

Permanganate of Potash, four grains; Distilled Water, one fluid ounce. Dissolve.

This solution is analogous to, but weaker than Condy's Disinfecting Fluid. It is a valuable deodoriser; but in order to develope its powers in this character, it is requisite to place it in contact with the source of the offensive odour. The strength of a solution for external application ranges from one to two fluid drachms to ten fluid ounces of water.

*Dose.*—From two to four fluid drachms.

## POTASSÆ TARTRAS.

### Tartrate of Potash.

Tartrate of Potash, $2KO,C_8H_4O_{10}$ or $\mathbf{K_2C_4H_4O_6}$, obtained by neutralizing acid tartrate of potash with carbonate of potash. It occurs in the form of small colourless four or six sided prisms. Heated with sulphuric acid it forms a black tarry fluid, evolving inflammable gas and the odour of burned sugar. Hydrochloric acid, added sparingly to its solution, causes the separation of a white crystalline precipitate of cream of tartar. *Tests.*—Entirely dissolved by its own weight of water. 113 grains, heated to redness till gas ceases to be evolved, leave an alkaline residue, which requires for exact saturation 1000 grain-measures of the volumetric solution of oxalic acid.

*Properties.*—Diuretic in small, and purgative in large doses.

*Therapeutic Uses.*—In dyspeptic and hepatic affections, attended with slightly increased or febrile action, it is employed advantageously as a purgative. In lithiasis it is employed with the view of rendering the urine alkaline.

*Dose.*—As a diuretic, from forty grains to a drachm and a half; as a purgative, from two drachms to half an ounce or more, in solution.

## POTASSÆ TARTRAS ACIDA.

### Acid Tartrate of Potash.

(*Potassæ Bitartras, Lond., Edin., and Dubl. Ph. Bitartrate of Potash, Cream of Tartar.*)

Acid Tartrate of Potash, $KO,HO,C_8H_4O_{10}$, or $\mathbf{KHC_4H_4O_6}$. An acid salt obtained from the crude tartar which is deposited during the fermentation of grape juice. *Characters.*—A gritty white powder, or fragments of cakes crystallized on one surface; of a pleasant acid taste, sparingly soluble in water, insoluble in spirit. Heated in a crucible, it evolves inflammable gas and the odour of burned sugar, and leaves a black residue of carbon and carbonate of potash. This effervesces with dilute hydrochloric acid, and forms a solution which, when filtered, gives a yellow precipitate with perchloride of platinum, and when neutralized by ammonia is rendered slightly turbid by oxalic acid. *Tests.*—188 grains, heated to redness till gas ceases to be evolved, leave an alkaline residue, which requires for exact saturation 1000 grain-measures of the volumetric solution of oxalic acid.

*Properties.* — Refrigerant, diuretic, laxative; in large doses, hydragogue-cathartic.

*Therapeutic Uses.*—In febrile and inflammatory affections, a solution (in the proportion of about an ounce to a gallon of water), flavoured to taste, forms a useful and agreeable refrigerant drink. In dropsical affections, especially when partaking of an acute or active character, in albuminuria, hepatitis, dysentery, beri-beri, and hæmorrhoidal affections, it proves a valuable adjunct to other purgatives and diuretics.

*Dose.* —From twenty to forty grains, largely diluted as a refrigerant and diuretic, from one to two drachms as an aperient, and from three to six drachms as a hydragogue-cathartic.

Acid Tartrate of Potash forms an ingredient in Pulvis Jalapæ compositus and Confectio Sulphuris.

## POTASSÆ CITRAS.

### CITRATE OF POTASH.

Citrate of Potash, $3KO,C_{12}H_5O_{11}$ or $\mathbf{K_3C_6H_5O_7}$, obtained by decomposing carbonate of potash with citric acid. *Characters.*—A white powder of saline, feebly acid taste, deliquescent, and very soluble in water. Heated with sulphuric acid it forms a brown fluid, gives off an inflammable gas, and evolves the odour of acetic acid. Its solution, mixed with a solution of chloride of calcium, remains clear till it is boiled, when a white precipitate separates, readily soluble in acetic acid. Its solution, acidulated with hydrochloric acid, gives a yellow precipitate with perchloride of platinum. *Test.*—102 grains, heated to redness till gas ceases to be evolved, leave an alkaline residue, which requires for exact saturation 1000 grain-measures of the volumetric solution of oxalic acid. On account of its deliquescence when exposed to the air, it requires to be kept in well stoppered bottles.

*Properties and Uses.*—An excellent refrigerant and diuretic in febrile and inflammatory affections. As under its use the urine becomes alkaline, it is adapted for lithiasis, and for acid states of that secretion.

*Dose.*—From twenty to forty grains in solution, three or four times daily.

## POTASSÆ ACETAS.

### Acetate of Potash.

Acetate of Potash, $KO,C_4H_3O_3$ or $\mathbf{KC_2H_3O_2}$, obtained by decomposing carbonate of potash with acetic acid. *Characters.*—White, foliaceous, satiny masses, very deliquescent; with an aqueous solution of which tartaric acid causes a crystalline precipitate, sulphuric acid the disengagement of acetic acid, and a dilute solution of perchloride of iron strikes a blood-red colour. *Tests.*—Neutral to test paper, entirely soluble in rectified spirit. Its solution is unaffected by sulphide of ammonium.

*Properties.*—Alterative, mild and efficient diuretic; in large doses purgative; rarely employed in the latter character.

*Therapeutic Uses.*—Dropsical affections, acute rheumatism, chronic diseases of the skin, gonorrhœa, and visceral and glandular enlargement, are the diseases in which it has proved most useful.

*Dose.*—From twenty to forty grains, three or four times daily, as a diuretic and alterative; from two to three drachms as a purgative.

## POTASSII IODIDUM.

### Iodide of Potassium.

Iodide of Potassium, KI. It occurs in colourless, generally opaque, cubic crystals, readily soluble in water, and in a less degree in spirit. It commonly has a feeble alkaline reaction; its solution mixed with mucilage of starch, gives a blue colour on the addition of a minute quantity of solution of chlorine. It gives a crystalline precipitate with tartaric acid. *Tests.*—The addition of tartaric acid and mucilage of starch to its watery solution does not develope a blue colour. Does not brown on addition of tartaric acid. Solution of nitrate of silver added in excess forms a yellowish-white precipitate, which, when agitated with ammonia, yields by subsidence a clear liquid in which excess of nitric acid causes no turbidity.

Its aqueous solution is only faintly precipitated by the addition of saccharated solution of lime.

*Properties.*—Valuable alterative, stimulant of the absorbent system, diuretic; locally applied, irritant.

*Therapeutic Uses.*—Analogous to those of Iodine; valuable in secondary syphilitic affections, especially of the bones and periosteum, in scrofulous affections, especially those of the eye, and in the advanced stages of inflammation, for the absorption of effusions and deposits. Amongst other diseases in which it proves effectual, are chronic inflammation and enlargement of the liver, enlargement of the spleen, dropsical affections, hydarthrosis, hydrocephalus, gout, rheumatism, chronic bronchitis, tabes mesenterica, bronchocele, saturnine and mercurial poisoning, and certain neuralgic and nervous affections, especially when connected with a syphilitic taint. Externally applied, it aids its internal administration in the absorption of effusions and deposits, and proves valuable in many forms of skin disease and obstinate ulceration.

*Dose.*—From two to ten grains, twice or thrice daily, in solution.

*Preparations.*—**Ointment of Iodide of Potassium** (*Unguentum Potassii Iodidi*). Take of Iodide of Potassium, sixty-four grains; Carbonate of Potash, four grains; Water, one fluid drachm; Prepared Lard, one ounce. Dissolve the iodide of potassium and carbonate of potash in the water, and mix thoroughly with the lard.

Iodide of Potassium forms also an ingredient in Linimentum Iodi, Liquor Iodi, Tinctura Iodi, and in Unguentum Iodi.

**Liniment of Iodide of Potassium and Soap** (*Linimentum Potassii Iodidi cum Sapone*). Take of Hard Soap, cut small, and Iodide of Potassium, of each, one ounce and a half; Glycerine, one fluid ounce; Oil of Lemon, one fluid drachm; Water, ten fluid ounces. Dissolve the soap in seven fluid ounces of the water by the heat of a water-bath. Dissolve the iodide of potassium and glycerine in the remainder of the water, and mix the two solutions together. When the mixture is cold, add the oil of lemon and mix the whole thoroughly.

Both the above preparations are eligible modes of applying the remedy externally.

## POTASSII BROMIDUM

### Bromide of Potassium.

Bromide of Potassium, KBr. It occurs in colourless cubical crystals, with no odour, but a pungent saline taste, readily soluble in water, less soluble in spirit. Its aqueous solution gives a white crystalline precipitate with tartaric acid. When its solution in water is mixed with a little chlorine, ether agitated with it, on rising to the surface, exhibits a red colour. *Tests.*—Ten grains require for complete decomposition 840 grain-measures of the volumetric solution of nitrate of silver. A solution of this salt, mixed with mucilage of starch and a drop of an aqueous solution of chlorine, does not exhibit a blue, but an orange colour.

*Properties.*—Similar to those of the Iodide of Potassium, but exercising a powerfully sedative action on the generative system and sexual functions (anaphrodisiac). It likewise exercises an anæsthetic influence on mucous membranes generally, but especially those of the pharynx and larynx; hence it is valuable in preparing patients for laryngoscopic examinations and operations. Externally applied, stimulant.

*Therapeutic Uses.*—In nymphomania, priapism, chordee, some forms of spermatorrhœa, menorrhagia and other affections, as in epilepsy and hysteria, dependent upon or connected with undue sexual excitement, it is a remedy of great value. It has likewise been employed in scrofulous affections, enlargements of the spleen and liver, amenorrhœa, gonorrhœa, incontinence of urine in children, asthma and spasmodic coughs, hypertrophy of the heart, and obstinate skin diseases.

*Dose.*—From five to thirty grains, in solution, or in the form of pill.

## SODIUM.

*Symbol,* Na. (*Natrium*) ; *At. weight,* 23.

Sodium, the metallic base of Soda, is of a soft waxy consistence, malleable, of a silvery lustre, rapidly oxydizes on exposure to the air, and burns with a brilliant yellow flame. Fuses at 207°7. Specific gravity, 0·97. It decomposes water, and dissolves with the evolution of hydrogen as caustic soda. It exists largely throughout nature in the form of common salt (NaCl). It is a constituent of many animal fluids.

## SODA CAUSTICA.

### Caustic Soda. Hydrate of Soda.

Hydrate of Soda, NaO,HO, or **NaHO**, with some impurities, obtained by evaporating Solution of Soda to dryness in a silver basin, and subsequent fusion. *Characters.*—Hard greyish-white fragments of cakes, very alkaline and corrosive. It imparts a yellow colour to flame, and its solution in water acidulated by nitric acid gives (owing to impurities) scanty white precipitates with nitrate of silver and chloride of barium, and no precipitate with perchloride of platinum. *Tests.*—Forty grains dissolved in water leave scarcely any sediment, and require for neutralization about 900 grain-measures of the volumetric solution of oxalic acid. Being deliquescent on exposure to the air, it requires to be kept in well stoppered green glass bottles.

*Properties and Uses.*—Caustic and escharotic, employed in the same cases and in the same manner as Caustic Potash, over which it possesses the advantage of being less deliquescent, and consequently more manageable.

## LIQUOR SODÆ.

### Solution of Soda.

Solution of Soda is obtained by treating a boiling solution of Carbonate of Soda with slaked lime, and decanting the precipitated carbonate of lime; Soda remains in solution. *Characters.*—A clear transparent fluid, inodorous, of a powerfully alkaline taste. *Tests.*—Specific gravity, 1·047. One fluid ounce requires for neutralization 470 grain-measures of the volumetric solution of oxalic acid. It does not effervesce when added to an excess of dilute hydrochloric acid, nor give a precipitate with solution of lime or oxalate of ammonia. When it is treated with an excess of diluted nitric acid, and evaporated to dryness, the residue forms with water a clear solution, which, owing to impurities, may be rendered turbid by chloride of barium and by nitrate of silver, but not by ammonia. One fluid ounce contains 18·8 grains of the hydrate of soda. It requires to be kept well stoppered in bottles of green glass.

*Properties and Uses.*—Analogous to those of Liquor Potassæ, applicable especially to certain forms of dyspepsia connected with biliary derangement.

*Dose.*—From ten drops to a fluid drachm, freely diluted.

Solution of Soda is employed in the preparation of Caustic Soda.

## SODÆ CARBONAS.

### Carbonate of Soda.

Carbonate of Soda, $NaO,CO_2+10HO$, or $\mathbf{Na_2CO_3.10HO}$. Obtained from the ashes of marine plants, or produced by chemical decomposition of sulphate of soda. *Characters.* —Transparent colourless laminar crystals of a rhombic shape, efflorescent, with a harsh alkaline taste and strong alkaline reaction. It imparts a yellow colour to flame, and dissolves with effervescence in diluted hydrochloric acid, forming a solution which does not precipitate with perchloride of platinum. By heat it undergoes aqueous fusion, and then dries up, losing sixty-three per cent. of its weight. *Tests.*—When nitric acid is added in excess, only a slight precipitate is occasioned by chloride of barium or nitrate of silver. One hundred and forty-three grains require for neutralization at least 960 grain-measures of the volumetric solution of oxalic acid.

*Properties and Uses.*—Analogous to those of the bicarbonate of soda, but more irritant in its action.

*Dose.*—From five to thirty grains in solution. For preparing effervescing draughts, twenty grains are saturated by about nine grains and three quarters of Citric Acid, ten grains and a half of Tartaric Acid, and two and a half fluid drachms of Lemon Juice.

*Preparation.*—**Dried Carbonate of Soda** (*Sodæ Carbonas Exsiccata*).—Take of Carbonate of Soda, eight ounces. Expose the carbonate of soda in a porcelain capsule to a rather strong sand heat until the liquid which first forms is converted into a dry cake; and, having rubbed this to powder, enclose it in a stoppered bottle.

*Dose*—From three to ten grains.

[Considerable quantities of impure Carbonate of Soda are prepared in India by the incineration of *Salicornia Indica,* Willd., *S. brachiata,* Roxb., *Suaeda nudiflora,* Willd., and probably of other allied species. It is known by the Hindústani name of *Khar-suji* or *Suji-khar,* and is not to be confounded with another impure salt called *Saji-mitti,* which is a mineral product obtained from the soil in the district of Monghyr and other parts of Bengal. It contains from 40 to 50 per cent. of carbonate of soda, traces of sulphate of soda, organic matter, clay, sand, and oxide of iron. The Bengal Ph. (p. 360) contains directions for the preparation of carbonate of soda from this earth, but it is very doubtful if it could be manufactured at a less cost than the article imported from Europe. For an account of the soda soils of Baramahal see a paper by Capt. Campbell, *Bengal Asiat. Trans.,* 1841, vol. x. p. 159.]

## SODÆ BICARBONAS.

### Bicarbonate of Soda.

Bicarbonate of Soda, NaO, HO, 2CO , or **$NaHCO_3$**. Prepared by passing a stream of carbonic acid gas (generated by the action of hydrochloric acid on fragments of marble) through a mixture of one part of the carbonate and one and a half parts of the dried carbonate of soda to saturation. *Characters.*—In powder or small opaque irregular scales, white, of a saline not unpleasant taste. Imparts a yellow colour to flame. Dissolves with much effervescence in diluted hydrochloric acid, forming a solution in which perchloride of platinum causes no precipitate. *Tests.* — When acidulated with nitric acid, its solution scarcely precipitates with chloride of barium or nitrate of silver. Eighty-four grains exposed to a red heat leave fifty-three grains of an alkaline residue, which requires for neutralization 1000 grain-measures of the volumetric solution of oxalic acid.

*Properties.*—Primarily antacid, secondarily alterative.

*Therapeutic Uses.*—In acidity of the primæ viæ, and in cardialgia, diarrhœa, flatulence, and vomiting connected therewith, it is a remedy of great value. In lithiasis, rheumatism, albuminuria, and in purpura hæmorrhagica it has also been found useful. In some chronic skin diseases, especially those of a papular and scaly character, it has been employed successfully, both internally and externally, in the form of baths, lotions, and ointments.

*Dose.*—From fifteen to forty grains in solution.

*Preparations.* — **Effervescing Solution of Soda** (*Liquor Sodæ Effervescens, Aqua Sodæ Effervescens, Soda Water*). Take of Bicarbonate of Soda, thirty grains; Water, one pint. Dissolve the bicarbonate of soda in the water, and filter the solution; then pass into it as much pure washed carbonic acid gas, obtained by the action of sulphuric acid on chalk, as can be introduced with a pressure of seven atmospheres. Keep the solution in bottles securely closed, to prevent the escape of the compressed gas. *Characters.*—Effervesces strongly when the containing vessel is opened, carbonic acid gas escaping. The liquid is clear and sparkling, and has an agreeable acidulous taste. *Tests.* —Ten fluid ounces, after being boiled for five minutes, require for neutralization 178 grain-measures of the volumetric solution of oxalic acid.

A well-known antalkaline and refrigerant. It is not to be confounded with ordinary Soda Water, which is a solution of carbonic acid in water.

**Effervescent Citro-tartrate of Soda** (*Sodæ Citrotartras Effervescens*). Take of Bicarbonate of Soda, in powder, seventeen ounces; Tartaric acid in powder, eight ounces; Citric Acid, in powder, six ounces. Mix the powders thoroughly, place them in a dish or pan of suitable form heated to between 200° and 220°, and when the particles of the powder begin to aggregate, stir them assiduously until they assume a granular form; then, by means of suitable sieves, separate the granules of uniform and most convenient size, and preserve the preparation in well-closed bottles.

An agreeable and useful refrigerant.

*Dose.*—From half a drachm to two drachms in solution.

**Bicarbonate of Soda Lozenges** (*Trochisci Sodæ Bicarbonatis*). Take of Bicarbonate of Soda, in powder, three thousand six hundred grains (8 oz. 100 grs.); Refined Sugar, in powder, twenty-five ounces; Gum Acacia, in powder, one ounce; Mucilage of Gum Acacia, two fluid ounces; Distilled Water, one fluid ounce. Mix the powders, and add the mucilage and water to form a proper mass. Divide into 720 lozenges, and dry these in a hot-air chamber with a moderate heat.

*Dose.*—From one to six lozenges. Each lozenge contains five grains of bicarbonate of soda.

## SODÆ BIBORAS.

### BIBORATE OF SODA. BORAX.

Borax, $NaO,2BO_3+10HO$ or $Na_2B_4O_7.10H_2O$. in a crude state, is produced by spontaneous evaporation of water on the shore of certain lakes in Thibet and other parts of the East. It is likewise made artificially by boiling together in proper proportions boracic acid and carbonate of soda. *Characters.*—Transparent colourless crystals, sometimes slightly effloresced, with feebly alkaline reaction; insoluble in rectified spirit, soluble in 12 parts of cold and half a part of boiling water. A hot saturated solution, when acidulated with any of the mineral acids, lets fall, as it cools, a scaly crystalline deposit (boracic acid), the solution of which in spirit burns with a green flame. *Test.*—191 grains dissolved in ten fluid ounces of distilled water require for saturation 1,000 grain-measures of the volumetric solution of oxalic acid.

*Properties.*—Refrigerant, diuretic, emmenagogue, parturifacient? and lithontriptic; locally applied, stimulant.

*Therapeutic Uses.*—In chlorosis, amenorrhœa, dysmenorrhœa, and some forms of uterine hæmorrhage, it has been used with alleged benefit. It has likewise been prescribed internally in dropsical affections, epilepsy, puerperal diarrhœa, puerperal affections, and to promote uterine contractions in tedious labours; but as in all these cases it has been given conjoined with other powerful remedies, it is difficult to determine the amount of influence exerted by it. A weak solution injected into the bladder has been found a powerful solvent of lithic acid deposits. As a local application it proves valuable in aphthæ, aphthous ulceration, ptyalism, sore or cracked nipples, and gangrene, and in various forms of skin disease, in which it is especially effectual in allaying pruritus.

*Dose.*—From twenty to forty grains.

*Preparations.*—**Borax Honey** (*Mel Boracis*). Take of Borax, in fine powder, sixty-four grains; Clarified Honey, one ounce. Mix.

A valuable local application to aphthæ, and some other affections of the mouth.

**Glycerine of Borax** (*Glycerinum Boracis*). Take of Borax, in powder, one ounce; Glycerine, four fluid ounces. Rub them together in a mortar until the borax is dissolved.

A useful application in some skin diseases.

[The Borax (*Sohágá*, Hind.) met with in the bazaars of India is brought from Thibet, Assam, and Nepaul. If necessary, it may be purified by boiling one pound of it with one drachm of quick lime in three pints of water, straining through cloth, and evaporating to crystallization.]

## SODÆ PHOSPHAS.

### PHOSPHATE OF SODA OR RHOMBIC PHOSPHATE OF SODA.

Phosphate of Soda, $2NaO,HO,PO_5+24HO$, or $\mathbf{Na_2HPO_4.12H_2O}$. exists in a natural state both in the organic and inorganic kingdoms. May be prepared for medicinal purposes by neutralizing a solution of the superphosphate of lime (obtained by the action of sulphuric acid on bone-ash) with carbonate of soda. It occurs in the form of transparent colourless rhombic prisms, terminated by four converging planes, efflorescent, tasting like common salt. *Tests.*—It imparts a yellow colour to flame. Its solution gives a yellow precipitate with nitrate of silver, soluble in ammonia and in nitric acid; and with chloride of barium it yields a white precipitate soluble in nitric acid. Heated to dull redness it loses sixty-three per cent. of its weight, leaving a residue, which, when dissolved in water, gives with chloride of barium a precipitate soluble in diluted nitric acid. Acidulated with hydrochloric acid, sulphuretted hydrogen gives no precipitate.

*Properties.* — Mild and efficient purgative; in small doses, alterative.

*Therapeutic Uses.*—In febrile and inflammatory affections, also in constipation, especially in children, it is well adapted as a purgative, both from the mildness of its operation and its slightly disagreeable taste. It has also been thought peculiarly adapted for diabetic patients. In lithiasis it is recommended from the solvent power it exercises over lithic acid deposits. It has been also thought useful in cholera.

*Dose.*—From two drachms to one ounce as a purgative; from twenty to forty grains as an alterative. As its taste is little distinguishable from that of common salt, it may be given in the same manner as the latter, dissolved in soup or gruel.

## SODII CHLORIDUM.

### Chloride of Sodium. Common Salt.

Chloride of Sodium, NaCl, exists extensively in both kingdoms of nature, forming upwards of 2·5 per cent. of the waters of the ocean. It exists also in large quantities in the solid form as Rock Salt, and in solution in brine springs. From these sources it is prepared by various processes. *Characters.*—Small white crystalline grains, or transparent cubic crystals, with a purely saline taste, imparting a yellow colour to flame, soluble in water. The solution is not precipitated by perchloride of platinum, but gives with nitrate of silver a white precipitate, soluble in ammonia, but insoluble in nitric acid.

*Properties.*—In small continued doses it promotes appetite, and assists the processes of digestion and assimilation (peptic); in large doses, in solution, it acts as an emetic and purgative. Anthelmintic. Locally applied, rubefacient.

*Therapeutic Uses.*—In some forms of dyspepsia, infantile diarrhœa, intermittent fevers, hæmoptysis, and phthisis, salt has been employed with alleged benefit. It forms an important ingredient in the so-called "saline treatment" of cholera. It is a chemical antidote in poisoning by nitrate of silver. Heated salt, in the form of an epithem, has been found useful in scrofulous glandular enlargements, and diseases of the joints.

*Dose.*—From ten to twenty grains or more as a peptic; from half an ounce to one ounce as a purgative; from an ounce and a half to two ounces, dissolved in tepid water, as an emetic. Baths of the strength of sea-water may be prepared by dissolving salt in water in the proportion of one pound of salt to every three gallons of water.

[The drug *Kala Nimuk* (*Black Salt*), called also *Bit-loban*, held in high esteem by the natives of India, is nothing more than an impure chloride of sodium containing a little sulphuret of iron. Its mode of preparation is given in the Taleef Shereeff (p. 167). Its medicinal uses amongst the natives are multifarious, and from the evidence of Dr. Henderson (*Tilloch's Phil. Mag.*, 1802,

p. 206), and Mr. Twining (*Diseases of Bengal*, vol. i. p. 507), there is reason to believe that in chronic enlargements of the spleen and liver, the result of malarious poisoning, it possesses considerable powers. The Editor has elsewhere (*Madras Quart. Med. Journ.*, *April* 1862, p. 239,) given an account of its other medicinal uses. A rough analysis of it was made some years since by Mr. Accum (*Asiat. Researches*, vol. xi. p. 193).]

## LIQUOR SODÆ CHLORATÆ.

### SOLUTION OF CHLORINATED SODA.

A mixed solution of hypochlorite of soda, chloride of sodium, and bicarbonate of soda. A colourless alkaline liquid, with astringent taste and feeble odour of chlorine. *Tests.*—It decolorizes sulphate of indigo. It effervesces with hydrochloric acid, evolving chlorine and carbonic acid, and forming a solution which is not precipitated by perchloride of platinum. Specific gravity, 1·103. Seventy grains by weight, added to a solution of twenty grains of iodide of potassium in four fluid ounces of water, and acidulated with two fluid drachms of hydrochloric acid, require for the discharge of the brown colour which the mixture assumes, 500 grain-measures of the volumetric solution of hyposulphite of soda. It is not precipitated by oxalate of ammonia.

*Properties.*—Stimulant, tonic, and antiseptic; externally applied, stimulant, astringent, and deodorizing.

*Therapeutic Uses.*—In typhus and typhoid (enteric) fevers, in scarlet fever, and in the advanced stages of febrile and inflammatory affections, and in the exanthemata generally, when they assume a low adynamic form, it is a remedy of great value. In intermittent fevers, and in the mesenteric affections of children, it has also been employed with alleged good effects. As a local or external application it proves valuable in aphthous, scorbutic, and mercurial ulceration of the gums, in various forms of cynanche, especially in that which accompanies scarlet fever, in fetid discharges from the vagina, meatus auditorius and other passages, in several obstinate skin diseases, especially when of a syphilitic origin, and in phagedenic ulcerations. In the latter class of cases it is effectual not only in removing fetor, but in stimulating to healthy action. It is an antidote in poisoning by sulphuretted hydrogen, the hydrosulphides, and hydrocyanic acid.

*Dose.*—From ten to thirty minims, largely diluted. For a gargle it may be diluted with fifteen, and for a lotion with ten or fifteen parts of water.

*Preparation.*—**Chlorine Poultice** (*Cataplasma Sodæ Chloratæ*). Take of Solution of Chlorinated Soda, two fluid ounces; Rice flour, four ounces; Boiling Water, eight fluid ounces. Add the rice flour gradually to the water, stirring constantly; then mix in the solution of chlorinated soda.

A valuable application to phagedenic and fetid ulcers and obstinate skin diseases.

## SODÆ ARSENIAS.

### Arseniate of Soda.

Arseniate of Soda, $2NaO,HO,AsO_5+14HO$, or $\mathbf{Na_2HAsO_4.7H_2O}$. is obtained by fusing a mixture of arsenious acid (10 parts) with nitrate (8½ parts) and carbonate of soda (5½ parts), treating the fused mass, when cold, with water, and crystallizing the arseniate of soda from the solution. It occurs in colourless transparent prisms, soluble in water; the solution is alkaline, giving white precipitates with chloride of barium and chloride of calcium, and a liver-brown precipitate with nitrate of silver, soluble in nitric acid; acidulated with hydrochloric acid, sulphuretted hydrogen should on boiling give a yellow precipitate. *Tests.*—Heated to 300°, it loses 40·38 per cent. of its weight. An aqueous solution of ten grains of the residue, treated with 53 grain-measures of the volumetric solution of soda, continues to give a precipitate with the volumetric solution of nitrate of silver until 1613 measures of the latter have been added.

*Properties and Uses.*—Alterative and tonic, analogous to those of arsenious acid and liquor arsenicalis, but less irritating.

*Dose.*—From one sixteenth to one eighth of a grain. It is best administered in the form of the subjoined Solution:—

*Preparation.* — **Solution of Arseniate of Soda** (*Liquor Sodæ Arseniatis*). Take of Arseniate of Soda (rendered anhydrous by a heat not exceeding 300°), four grains; Distilled Water, one fluid ounce. Dissolve.

*Dose.*—From five to ten minims, gradually increased. Each fluid drachm contains half a grain of the anhydrous arseniate of soda.

## SODÆ ACETAS.

### Acetate of Soda.

Acetate of Soda, $NaO,C_4H_3O_3+6HO$, or $\mathbf{NaC_2H_3O_2.3H_2O}$. Obtained by decomposing carbonate of soda with acetic acid. *Characters.*—Transparent colourless crystals, soluble in water, forming a solution neutral to test paper. *Tests.*—The solution when dilute, is not precipitated by chloride of barium, but by nitrate of silver and subnitrate of mercury; becomes deep-brown red on addition of perchloride of iron.

*Properties.*—Diuretic in small, and purgative in large doses.

*Therapeutic Uses.*—Analogous to those of acetate of potash, over which it possesses the advantage of not being deliquescent.

*Dose.*—From twenty to forty grains as a diuretic, from one to four drachms as a purgative.

## SODÆ SULPHAS.

### SULPHATE OF SODA.

### (*Glauber's Salt.*)

Sulphate of Soda, $NaO,SO_3+10HO$, or $Na_2SO_4.10H_2O$. may be obtained from the residue left in the manufacture of hydrochloric acid, by neutralizing it with carbonate of soda, dissolving in water and evaporating to crystallization. *Characters.* — Transparent oblique prisms; has a saline and bitter taste; effloresces on exposure to the air; soluble in water, insoluble in spirit. Exposed to heat in a porcelain crucible it loses 55·9 per cent. of water. Heated with solution of potash no odour of ammonia is evolved, and no precipitate is formed on addition of perchloride of platinum. Imparts a yellow colour to flame. *Test.*—Fifty grains of it dissolved in distilled water, and acidulated with hydrochloric acid, give, on addition of chloride of barium, a white precipitate, which, when washed and dried, weighs 72·2 grains.

*Properties and Uses.* — Purgative, corresponding closely with sulphate of magnesia.

*Dose.*—From half an ounce to one ounce of the crystallized salt, in solution. Of the anhydrous or effloresced salt, half of these quantities suffices.

[Sulphate of Soda exists largely in the soil in Oude, and many other parts of India, and is sold in the bazaars in dirty-brown crystalline masses, under the Hindustani names of *Khari mutti* and *Khari nún.* An account of this product is furnished by Dr. Spry (*Calcutta Med. Phys. Soc. Trans.*, vol. viii. p. 1, App. p. 16), who gives directions for its purification, and fitting the sulphate of soda, of which it contains a very large per-centage, for medicinal use. For this purpose all that is required is to dissolve it in boiling water, strain through calico, and evaporate to crystallization. In the elevated district of the Doab, in North-western India, an efflorescence on the soil is frequently met with, and is distinguished by the name of *Reh.* Two samples of this were examined by Prof. H. B. Medlicott

(*Journ. Agri.-Hort. Soc. of India*, 1863, vol. xiii. p. 2); one of them contained 96 per cent. of sulphate of soda, and 4 of the chloride of sodium, the proportion in the other specimen being relatively 76 and 24 per cent.]

## SODA TARTARATA.

### TARTARATED SODA.

(*Sodæ et Potassæ Tartras, Brit. Ph.* 1864; *Potassio-Tartrate of Soda; Rochelle Salt.*)

Tartarated Soda, $NaO,KO,C_8H_4O_{10}+8HO$, or $\mathbf{NaKC_4H_4O_6.4H_2O}$. obtained by neutralizing acid tartrate of potash with carbonate of soda. *Characters.*—It occurs in colourless transparent prisms or halves of prisms of the right rhombic order, generally eight-sided; tasting like common salt. *Tests.*—Heated with sulphuric acid it blackens, evolving inflammable gases and the odour of burnt sugar. It imparts a yellow colour to flame. Easily soluble in cold water. A strong solution gives a crystalline precipitate with a small quantity of acetic or hydrochloric acid. 141 grains, heated to redness till gas ceases to be evolved, leave an alkaline residue, which requires for neutralization 1000 grain-measures of the volumetric solution of oxalic acid.

*Properties.*—Diuretic in small, and purgative in large doses.

*Therapeutic Uses.*—In febrile and inflammatory affections and in the puerperal state it is well adapted for a purgative by the mildness of its action. In gouty and rheumatic cases and in lithiasis it proves serviceable from the alkaline reaction it exercises on the urine.

*Dose.*—From twenty to forty grains as a diuretic; from two drachms to one ounce as a purgative, in simple solution, or in the state of effervescence,—prepared by dissolving two drachms of the Tartarated Soda, and forty grains of Bicarbonate of Soda, in half a pint of water, and adding to it thirty grains of Tartaric Acid. The saline ingredients are sold in shops in separate packets under the name of *Seidlitz Powders.*

## SODÆ VALERIANAS.

### VALERIANATE OF SODA.

Valerianate of Soda, $NaO,C_{10}H_9O_3$, or $\mathbf{NaC_5H_9O_2}$, obtained by saturating valerianic acid (generated by distilling sulphuric acid with bichromate of potash and fousel oil) with solution of soda. It occurs in dry white masses without alkaline reaction, entirely soluble in rectified spirit, and giving out a powerful odour of valerian on the addition of diluted sulphuric acid.

*Properties and Uses.*—Stimulant and antispasmodic, resembling valerian in its action, and applicable to the same class of cases.

*Dose.*—From half a grain to three grains. It is rarely employed, excepting in the preparation of the valerianate of zinc.

## LITHIUM.

*Symbol*, L.; *At. weight*, 7.

Lithium, the metallic base of the alkali Lithia, which exists solely in the inorganic kingdom, and forms a constituent in many mineral waters. It is a white metal; fuses at 356°. Sp. Gr. 0·59.

## LITHIÆ CARBONAS.

### CARBONATE OF LITHIA.

Carbonate of Lithia, $LO,CO_2$, or $\mathbf{L_2CO_3}$. A white powder or minute crystalline grains, alkaline in reaction, soluble in 100 parts of cold water, insoluble in alcohol. *Tests.*—It dissolves with effervescence in hydrochloric acid; and the solution leaves a residue of chlriode of lithium, which communicates a purplish red colour to the flame of a spirit lamp, and redissolved in water yields a precipitate with phosphate of soda. Ten grains of the salt neutralized with sulphuric acid, and afterwards heated to redness, leave 14·86 grains of dry sulphate of lithia; which, when redissolved in distilled water, yields no precipitate with oxalate of ammonia or solution of lime.

*Properties.*—Diuretic, exercising a well-marked alkaline influence on the urine. It is a ready solvent of lithic acid deposits.

*Therapeutic Uses.*—In gout and other affections occurring in connexion with the lithic acid diathesis, it has been used with benefit.

*Dose.*—From three to six grains, freely diluted in simple or aërated water.

*Preparation.*—**Effervescing Solution of Lithia** (*Liquor* vel *Aqua Lithiæ effervescens*, *Lithia Water*). Take of Carbonate of Lithia, ten grains; Water, one pint. Mix in a suitable apparatus, and pass into it as much pure washed carbonic acid gas, obtained by the action of sulphuric acid on chalk, as can be introduced with a pressure of seven atmospheres. Keep the solution in bottles securely closed, to prevent the escape of the compressed gas. *Characters.*—Effervesces strongly when the containing vessel is opened, carbonic acid gas escaping. The liquid is clear and sparkling, and has an agreeable acidulous taste. *Test.*—Half a pint of it, evaporated to dryness, yields five grains of a white solid residue, answering to the tests for carbonate of lithia.

*Dose.*—From five to ten fluid ounces.

## LITHIÆ CITRAS.

### CITRATE OF LITHIA.

Citrate of Lithia, $3LO,C_{12}H_5O^{11}$, or $\mathbf{L_3C_6H_5O_7}$, obtained by the action of citric acid in solution on carbonate of lithia. *Characters.*—A white amorphous powder, deliquescent, and soluble in water without leaving any residue. Heated to redness it blackens, evolving inflammable gas; and the residue, neutralized by hydrochloric acid, yields with rectified spirit a solution which burns with a purple red flame. *Tests.*—Twenty grains of the salt, burned at a low red heat with free access of air, leave 10·6 grains of white residue.

*Properties and Uses.*—Similar to those of the carbonate of lithia, but is thought to be less irritant in its action.

*Dose.*—From five to ten grains.

## CALCIUM.

*Symbol,* Ca; *At. weight,* 20; *or* **Ca=40.**

Calcium, the metallic base of the alkaline earth Lime, exists extensively, variously combined, in the mineral, vegetable, and animal kingdoms. It is a yellowish metal of Sp. Gr. 1·578; melts at a red heat.

## CALCII CHLORIDUM.

### CHLORIDE OF CALCIUM.

Chloride of Calcium, CaCl or $\mathbf{CaCl_2}$, may be formed by neutralizing hydrochloric acid with carbonate of lime, filtering, evaporating until it becomes solid, and finally drying the salt at about 400°. It occurs in white agglutinated masses, dry, but very deliquescent, evolves no chlorine or hypochlorous acid on the addition of hydrochloric acid, and is entirely soluble in twice its weight of water, also in alcohol. *Test.*—The aqueous solution is not precipitated by the addition of lime water.

*Properties.*—Stimulant, its action being chiefly directed on the lymphatic glandular system. In large doses it is an acro-narcotic poison.

*Therapeutic Uses.*—In scrofula and scrofulous affections, in chronic skin diseases, especially in lupus, eczema, and impetigo, and in some ovarian affections, it has been used with apparent advantage.

*Dose.*—From ten to twenty grains, in solution.

## CALX.

### LIME. QUICKLIME.

Lime, an alkaline earth, CaO, with some impurities, obtained by calcining chalk or limestone so as to expel carbonic acid. It occurs in compact masses of a whitish colour, which readily absorb water, and which, when rather less than their weight of water is added, crack and fall into powder with the development of much heat. The powder obtained by this process of slaking, when agitated with distilled water, gives, after filtration, a clear solution, which has an alkaline reaction, and yields a white precipitate with oxalate of ammonia. *Tests.*—The powder obtained by slaking, dissolves without much residue and without effervescence, in diluted hydrochloric acid, and if the solution thus formed be evaporated to dryness, and the residue redissolved in water, only a very scanty precipitate forms on the addition of saccharated solution of lime.

*Preparations.*—**Slaked Lime** (*Calcis Hydras, Hydrate of Lime,* CaO,HO or $\mathbf{CaH_2O_2}$) is prepared as follows: Take of Lime recently burned, two pounds; Water, one pint. Place the lime in a metal pot, pour the water upon it, and when vapour ceases to be disengaged cover the pot with its lid, and set it aside to cool. When the temperature has fallen to that of the atmosphere, put the slaked lime on an iron-wire sieve, and by gentle agitation cause the fine powder to pass through the sieve, rejecting what is left. Put the powder into a well-stopped bottle, and keep it excluded as much as possible from the air. Slaked lime should be recently prepared; it requires 700 parts of water for solution.

*Properties.*—Caustic and escharotic; rarely employed however. excepting when conjoined with caustic potash. Internally administered, a corrosive poison. It is in common use as a masticatory amongst all classes throughout the East, in conjunction with betel nut (*Areca Catechu*) and betel leaf (*Chavica Betle*). When used for any lengthened period it considerably modifies the natural condition of the mucous covering of the mouth, and alters the appearance of the tongue so as to render it useless or fallacious as a means of diagnosis in disease. Its use in moderate quantities does not appear to act prejudicially on the system, but, when largely indulged in, it lays the foundation of much visceral disease.

**Solution of Lime, Lime Water** (*Liquor Calcis*). Take of Slaked Lime two ounces; Water, one gallon. Put the lime into a stoppered bottle containing the water, and shake well for two or three minutes. After twelve hours the excess of lime will have subsided, and the clear solution may be drawn off with a syphon as it is required for use, or transferred to a green glass bottle furnished with a well ground stopper. *Test.*—Ten fluid ounces require for neutralization at least 200 grain-measures of the volumetric solution of oxalic acid.

*Properties.*—Antacid, alterative, astringent.

*Therapeutic Uses.*—In acidity of the primæ viæ, and in dyspepsia, and diarrhœa connected therewith, it is a remedy of much value. Milk with a small proportion of lime water has been found of great service as an article of diet in ulceration of the stomach, also in scrofula and phthisis. As a solvent of urinary calculi it was formerly held in much repute, but is inferior in this respect to the salts of lithium. In poisoning by the mineral and oxalic acids it acts as a chemical antidote. Locally applied to various forms of ulcerations and skin disease.

*Dose.*—From one to four fluid ounces twice or thrice a day. It is best administered in milk.

**Saccharated Solution of Lime** (*Liquor Calcis Saccharatus*). Take of Slaked Lime one ounce; Refined Sugar, in powder, two ounces; Distilled water, one pint. Mix the lime and the sugar by trituration in a mortar. Transfer the mixture to a bottle containing the water; and having closed this with a cork, shake it occasionally for a few hours. Finally separate the clear solution with a syphon, and keep it in a stoppered bottle. *Tests.*—Specific gravity, 1·052. One fluid ounce requires for neutralization 254 grain-measures of the volumetric solution of oxalic acid, which corresponds to 7·11 grains of lime in one fluid ounce.

*Properties and Uses.*—Analogous to those of Solution of Lime. It is thought to be especially adapted for the obstinate dyspepsia of gouty subjects, and chronic diarrhœa of children.

*Dose.*—From fifteen to sixty minims in water, twice or thrice daily.

**Liniment of Lime** (*Linimentum Calcis*). Take of Solution of Lime, two fluid ounces; Olive Oil, two fluid ounces. Mix together with agitation.

This liniment, commonly known as *Carron Oil*, is a valuable application to burns and scalds. It is also applied to blistered surfaces, to hasten the healing process, and to some forms of skin disease.

## CALCIS CARBONAS PRÆCIPITATA.

### Precipitated Carbonate of Lime.

Carbonate of Lime, $CaO,CO_2$, or $\mathbf{CaCO_3}$, obtained by the action of carbonate of soda on chloride of calcium. *Characters.*—A white amorphous powder, insoluble in water, dissolving in hydrochloric acid with effervescence. The solution, when neutralised by ammonia, is copiously precipitated on the addition of oxalate of ammonia. *Test.*—With diluted nitric acid it gives a clear solution, which, if perfectly neutral and deprived of carbonic acid by boiling, is not precipitated by saccharated solution of lime added in excess, or by the solution of nitrate of silver.

*Properties and Uses.*—Similar to those of solution of lime. It is an ingredient in Trochisci Bismuthi.

*Dose.*—From ten to sixty grains.

## CRETA PRÆPARATA.

### Prepared Chalk.

Prepared Chalk obtained from native chalk, friable carbonate of lime, by elutrition, and afterwards dried in small masses, which are usually of a conical form. *Characters.*—A white amorphous powder, effervescing with acids, and dissolving with only a slight residue in dilute hydrochloric acid. This solution, when supersaturated with solution of ammonia, gives, upon the addition of oxalate of ammonia, a copious white precipitate. *Test.*—The salt formed by dissolving the prepared chalk in hydrochloric acid, if rendered neutral by evaporation to dryness and redissolved in water, gives only a very scanty precipitate on the addition of saccharated solution of lime.

*Properties.*—Antacid, astringent, absorbent.

*Therapeutic Uses.*—In diarrhœa connected with acidity of the primæ viæ, and in the advanced stages of bronchitis, attended with colliquative sweats and diarrhœa, it proves serviceable; chiefly employed in the form of Chalk Mixture (*infra*). Finely powdered chalk, sprinkled over ulcers, burns, excoriations, ulcerations, and skin diseases, &c., when accompanied by an acrid irritating discharge, often acts beneficially by absorbing the discharge, and thus preventing the extension of the disease. The surface should at the same time be covered with an emollient poultice.

*Dose.*—From ten to sixty grains or more.

**Chalk Mixture** (*Mistura Cretæ*).—Take of Prepared Chalk, a quarter of an ounce; Gum Acacia, in powder, a quarter of an ounce; Syrup, half a fluid ounce; Cinnamon Water, seven fluid ounces and a half. Triturate the chalk and gum acacia with the cinnamon water, then add the syrup and mix.

*Dose.*—From one to two fluid ounces. Its efficacy is generally increased by the addition of Pulvis Cretæ Aromaticus.

**Aromatic Chalk Powder** (*Pulvis Cretæ Aromaticus, Confectio Aromatica,* Lond. Ph.)—Take of Cinnamon Bark, in powder, four ounces; Nutmeg, in powder, Saffron, in powder, of each, three ounces; Cloves, in powder, one ounce and a half; Cardamom Seeds, in powder, one ounce; Refined Sugar, in powder, twenty-five ounces; Prepared Chalk, eleven ounces. Mix them thoroughly, pass the powder through a fine sieve, and finally rub it lightly in a mortar. Keep it in a stoppered bottle.

*Dose.*—From ten to sixty grains. For children from five to ten grains.

**Aromatic Chalk Powder with Opium** (*Pulvis Cretæ Aromaticus cum Opio*). — Take of Aromatic Chalk Powder, nine ounces and three quarters; Opium, in powder, a quarter of an ounce. Mix them thoroughly, and pass the powder through a fine sieve. Keep it in a stoppered bottle.

*Dose.*—From five to forty grains; must be regulated by the quantity of opium it is desired to administer. Forty grains contain one grain of opium.

## CALX CHLORATA.

### Chlorinated Lime. Chloride of Lime.

Chlorinated Lime, a product obtained by exposing slaked lime to the action of chlorine gas as long as the latter is absorbed. It possesses bleaching and disinfecting properties. It occurs in the form of a dull-white powder, with a feeble odour of chlorine; the effective portion is soluble in water. The solution evolves chlorine copiously upon the addition of oxalic acid, and deposits at the same time oxalate of lime. *Tests.*—Ten grains, mixed with thirty grains of iodide of potassium, and dissolved in four fluid ounces of water, produce, when acidulated with two fluid drachms of hydrochloric acid, a reddish solution, which requires for the discharge of its colour at least 850 grain-measures of the volumetric solution of hyposulphite of soda, corresponding to 30 per cent. of chlorine liberated by hydrochloric acid.

*Properties and Uses.*—Valuable stimulant, antiseptic, and deodoriser, employed in the same class of cases as Liquor Sodæ Chloratæ and Liquor Chlori.

*Dose.*—From one to five grains in solution. The strength of ointments for external application may range from twenty to forty grains to an ounce of lard, of lotions from forty grains to half an ounce to a pint of water, and of gargles from a drachm and a half to two drachms to a pint of water; the solutions to be filtered.

*Preparation.*—**Solution of Chlorinated Lime** (*Liquor Calcis Chloratæ*). Take of Chlorinated Lime, one pound; Distilled Water, one gallon. Mix well the water and the chlorinated lime by trituration in a large mortar, and, having transferred the mixture to a stoppered bottle, let it be well shaken several times for the space of three hours. Pour the contents of the bottle on a calico filter, and let the solution which passes through be preserved in a stoppered bottle. *Tests.*—Specific gravity, 1·035. One fluid drachm mixed with twenty grains of iodide of potassium dissolved in four fluid ounces of water, when acidulated with two fluid drachms of hydrochloric acid, gives a red solution, which requires for the discharge of its colour 500 grain-measures of the volumetric solution of hyposulphite of soda.

*Properties and Uses.*—Analogous to those of Liquor Sodæ Chloratæ.

*Dose.*—From ten to thirty drops freely diluted.

**Inhalation of Chlorine** (*Vapor Chlori*). Take of Chlorinated Lime, two ounces; Water (Cold), a sufficiency. Put the powder into a suitable apparatus; moisten it with the water, and let the vapour that arises be inhaled.

This application has been used with benefit in bronchitic and hepatic affections.

## CALCIS PHOSPHAS.

### Phosphate of Lime.

Phosphate of Lime, $3CaO, PO_5$, or $\mathbf{Ca_3P_2O_8}$, prepared by dissolving bone-ash in hydrochloric acid, precipitating with ammonia, and drying at a temperature not exceeding 212° F. *Characters.*—A light white amorphous powder, insoluble in water, but soluble without effervescence in dilute nitric acid. The solution continues clear when an excess of acetate of soda is added to it, but lets fall a white precipitate on the addition both of a little oxalate of ammonia, and of perchloride of iron. *Tests.*—Ten grains dissolve perfectly and without effervescence in diluted hydrochloric acid. The solution yields with ammonia a white precipitate, which is insoluble in boiling solution of potash, and when washed and dried weighs ten grains.

*Properties.*—Alterative, antacid.

*Therapeutic Uses.*—In scrofula and scrofulous affections, rachitis, mollities ossium, ununited fractures, intermittent fevers, and in chronic syphilitic ulcerations, it has been employed, but with doubtful results.

*Dose.*—From ten to twenty grains. It is an ingredient in Pulvis Antimonialis.

## MAGNESIUM.

*Symbol*, Mg ; *At. weight*, 12 ; *or* **Mg = 24.**

Magnesium, the metallic base of Magnesia; of a brilliant, silver-white colour, hard and ductile. Sp. gr. 1·743. Burns in oxygen, or in air, with brilliant light to Magnesia, MgO. Combined with sulphuric acid, magnesia forms a constituent of sea water and many mineral springs. It exists likewise to a considerable extent in certain limestones, and is present, though in small proportion, in animal solids and fluids, especially the urine. It is also found in the vegetable kingdom.

## MAGNESIA.

### Magnesia.

*(Magnesia Usta, Dubl. Ph.)*

Magnesia, MgO, obtained by subjecting carbonate of magnesia to a heat sufficient to expel the carbonic acid it contains. *Characters.*—A white powder, insoluble in water, but readily dissolved by acids without effervescence. Its solution in hydrochloric acid, when neutralized by ammonia, and mixed with a solution of chloride of ammonium gives a copious crystalline precipitate when phosphate of soda is added to it. *Tests.*—Dissolved in nitric acid, neutralized with ammonia, and mixed with a solution of chloride of ammonium, it does not give any precipitate with oxalate of ammonia or chloride of barium.

*Properties.*—Antacid and laxative.

*Therapeutic Uses.*—In acidity of the primæ viæ, cardialgia, gastric irritation, it proves valuable. It is also useful in the diarrhœa of children connected with acidity, and in the dyspepsia of gouty subjects. It is a chemical antidote in poisoning by the mineral acids, and by oxalic acid.

*Dose.*—From ten to twenty grains as an antacid; from a drachm to three drachms as a laxative. For children the dose is from two to ten grains, according to age. It is best administered in some aromatic water.

## MAGNESIA LEVIS.

### Light Magnesia.

Light Magnesia, MgO obtained by subjecting light carbonate of magnesia to a heat sufficient to expel the carbonic acid it contains. It is a bulky white powder, differing from the preceding preparation only in its greater levity, the volumes corresponding to the same weight being to each other in the ratio of three and a half to one.

*Properties, Uses, and Doses.*—The same as Magnesia.

Light magnesia is an ingredient in Pulvis Rhei Compositus.

## MAGNESIÆ CARBONAS.

### Carbonate of Magnesia.

(*Magnesiæ Carbonas ponderosum, Dubl. Ph.*)

Basic Carbonate of Magnesia, $3(MgO,CO_2) + MgO + 5HO$ or $3(MgCO_3).MgO.5H_2O$, exists in a native state in the mineral kingdom in magnesian limestone as carbonates. For medicinal use it is prepared by decomposing sulphate of magnesia by a solution of carbonate of soda. *Characters.*—A white granular powder, which dissolves with effervescence in the diluted mineral acids, yielding solutions which, when first treated with chloride of ammonium, are not disturbed by the addition of an excess of solution of ammonia, but yield a copious crystalline precipitate upon the addition of phosphate of soda. *Tests.*—With excess of hydrochloric acid it forms a clear solution in which chloride of barium causes no precipitate. Another portion of the solution supersaturated with ammonia gives no precipitate with oxalic acid. Fifty grains calcined at a red heat are reduced to twenty-two.

*Medical Properties and Uses.*—The same as those of Magnesia.

*Dose.*—From five to twenty grains as an antacid; from twenty to sixty grains as a laxative.

*Preparation.*—**Solution of Carbonate of Magnesia, Fluid Magnesia** (*Liquor Magnesiæ Carbonatis*), prepared by saturating a solution of carbonate of magnesia with carbonic acid. It is a clear colourless liquid, free from any bitter taste. *Test.*—A fluid ounce of it, evaporated to dryness, yields a white solid residue, which after being calcined weighs not less than five grains. This residue is insoluble in water, and answers to the tests for magnesia.

*Dose.*—From one to two fluid ounces. An eligible form for administering magnesia as an antacid.

Carbonate of Magnesia is an ingredient in Trochisci Bismuthi.

## MAGNESIÆ CARBONAS LEVIS.

### LIGHT CARBONATE OF MAGNESIA.

Light Carbonate of Magnesia, $3(MgO,CO_2) + MgO + 5HO$ or $\mathbf{3(MgCO_3).MgO.5H_2O}$. *Characters.*—A very light powder, which, when examined under the microscope, is found to be partly amorphous with numerous slender prisms intermixed. The other characters and tests are the same as those of carbonate of magnesia.

*Properties, Uses, and Doses.*—The same as Carbonate of Magnesia.

## MAGNESIÆ SULPHAS.

### SULPHATE OF MAGNESIA.

Sulphate of Magnesia, $MgO,SO_3 + 7HO$ or $\mathbf{MgSO_4.7H_2O}$, is a constituent of sea-water, and is likewise found in many mineral springs, as those of Epsom; hence its common name, *Epsom Salts*. It is obtained by various processes, either from the bittern of sea water left after the crystallization of common salt, or by the action of sulphuric acid on magnesian limestone. *Characters.*—Minute colourless and transparent rhombic prisms, possessing a bitter taste. It readily dissolves in water, and the solution gives copious white precipitates with chloride of barium, as also with a mixed solution of ammonia, chloride of ammonium, and phosphate of soda. *Tests.*—Its aqueous solution at ordinary temperatures is not precipitated by oxalate of ammonia. The precipitate given by carbonate of soda, when obtained from a boiling solution of one hundred grains of the salt, should, when well washed, dried, and heated to redness, weigh 16·26 grains.

*Properties.*—Purgative, refrigerant, diuretic.

*Therapeutic Uses.*—In febrile and inflammatory diseases, and in constipation attended by increased vascular action, especially in persons of robust plethoric habit, it is peculiarly adapted, by the refrigerant or sedative nature of its operation as a purgative. It is an antidote in poisoning by the salts of lead and barytes.

*Dose.*—From two drachms to one ounce as a purgative, in solution in some aromatic water, in compound infusion of roses, or in an infusion of senna.

*Preparation.*—**Enema of Sulphate of Magnesia** (*Enema Magnesiæ Sulphatis; Enema Catharticum, Edin. et Dubl. Ph.*) Take of Sulphate of Magnesia, one ounce; Olive Oil, one fluid ounce; Decoction of Rice, fifteen fluid ounces. Dissolve the sulphate of magnesia in the decoction of rice, add the oil, and mix.

A useful purgative enema.

Sulphate of Magnesia is also an ingredient in Mistura Sennæ composita.

## ALUMINUM.

*Symbol*, Al; *At. weight*, 13·75; or **Al=27·5.**

Aluminum is the metallic base of the earth Alumina ($Al_2O_3$), which, combined with silica in the form of clay, exists in nature in immense abundance. It is likewise a constituent of felspar, granite, porphyry, and other ancient unstratified rocks, and of the slate or shale used in the manufacture of alum. Aluminum is a white malleable metal, of sp. gr. 2·6.

## ALUMEN.

### Alum. Ammonia-Alum.

A double Sulphate of Ammonia and Alumina, $NH_4O,SO, Al_2O_3,3SO_3+24HO$ or $NH_4Al(SO_4)_2.12H_2O$, prepared by various processes from aluminous shale. It occurs in the form of colourless transparent crystalline masses, exhibiting the faces of the regular octahedron, and having an acid sweetish astringent taste. Its aqueous solution gives with caustic potash a white precipitate soluble in an excess of the reagent, and the mixture evolves ammonia when heated. *Test.*—The aqueous solution gives an immediate precipitate with chloride of barium; it does not acquire a blue colour from the addition of yellow prussiate of potash, as does iron-alum. Potash-alum contains potassium instead of ammonium.

*Properties.*—Astringent, styptic, and antiseptic.

*Therapeutic Uses.*—In passive hæmorrhages, atonic diarrhœa, infantile cholera, catarrhal affections of the stomach, colica pictonum, hooping cough, and bronchorrhœa, it has been administered internally with benefit. Amongst the diseases in which it is used as a local application are catarrhal ophthalmia, ophthalmia neomatorum, ophthalmia tarsi, and ecchymosis of the eye (as a collyrium); various forms of cynanche, relaxation of the uvula, scorbutic ulceration of the gums (as a gargle); in leucorrhœa, gonorrhœa, menorrhagia, prolapsus of the uterus and rectum (as an injection); and ulcerations, especially those attended with profuse discharge, exuberant granulations, and hospital gangrene, in the form of lotion or powder.

*Dose.*—From ten to twenty grains. It is best given conjoined with aromatics. For external or local application the strength may range from four to ten grains to the ounce of fluid.

*Preparation.* — **Dried Alum** (*Alumen exsiccatum*). Take of Alum four ounces. Heat the alum in a porcelain dish or other suitable vessel till it liquefies, then raise and continue the heat till aqueous vapour ceases to be disengaged, and the salt has lost 47 per cent. of its weight. Reduce the residue to powder, and preserve it in a well-stopped bottle.

*Properties.*—Similar to alum, but more powerful. It is a mild escharotic.

*Dose.*—From five to fifteen grains.

[In most of the bazaars of India, alum (potash-alum) in a more or less impure state is sold under its Hindústani name, *Phitkari.* It may be rendered fit for medicinal purposes by dissolving it in water, and evaporating the solution so as to obtain crystals. It forms the principal constituent, conjoined with peroxide of iron, of

*Salajet* or *Alum Earth of Nepal,* which forms an important article of the Native Materia Medica. It is probably a form of iron-alum. For an account of this drug and its uses see a paper by the Editor (*Madras Quart. Med. Journ.*, vol. iv. p. 239). Another aluminous earth, named *Pah,* was sent from Scinde by Dr. Stocks; examined by Dr. Haines (*Bombay Med. Phys. Trans.*, 1857, vol. iii. p. 159) it was pronounced to be a variety of feather alum, in which the potassa is replaced by protoxide of iron. Another earth from the same locality, called *Met* or *Meth,* examined by Dr. Haines, was found to contain 13·16 per cent. of alumina and 17·80 per cent. of peroxide of iron (*Ibid.*, p. 160). Alum exists largely in the soil in many parts of India, and is prepared for commerce in Cutch (M^cMurdo, *Bombay Lit. Trans.*, vol. ii. p. 210), Scinde (Vicary, *Lond. Geolog. Soc. Trans.*, 1847, vol. i. p. 341), the Punjaub (Jameson, *Bengal Asiat. Trans.*, 1843, vol. xii.), Behar (Sherwill, *Ibid.*, 1846, vol. xv. p. 58), and elsewhere.

## ARSENICUM.

### Arsenic.

*Symbol,* As; *At. weight,* 75.

Arsenic exists in the mineral kingdom in combination with Sulphur as *Orpiment* and *Realgar,* with Oxygen as *Arsenious Acid,* and with metals as *Arsenides.* The arsenious acid of commerce is chiefly obtained by roasting the last-named ores in a reverberatory furnace. Arsenicum is readily obtained by deoxydation of arsenious acid. It has a steel-grey colour, and volatilizes at 356° without fusion. Sp. gr. 5·85.

## ACIDUM ARSENIOSUM.

### Arsenious acid.

(*Arsenicum Album. White Arsenic.*)

Arsenious Acid, $AsO_3$ or $As_2O_3$, an anhydrous acid obtained by roasting arsenical ores and purifying by sublimation. It occurs in the form of a heavy white powder, or in sublimed masses which usually present a stratified appearance caused by the existence of separate layers differing from each other in degrees of opacity. When slowly sublimed in a glass tube it forms minute brilliant and transparent octahedral crystals. It is sparingly soluble in water, and its solution gives with ammonio-nitrate of silver a canary-yellow precipitate insoluble in water, but readily soluble in ammonia and in nitric acid. Sprinkled on a red-hot coal, it emits an alliaceous odour. *Tests.*—It is entirely volatilised at a temperature not exceeding 400°. Four grains of it, dissolved in boiling water with eight grains of bicarbonate of soda, discharge the colour of 808 grain-measures of the volumetric solution of iodine.

*Properties.*—Alterative, tonic, antiperiodic; in large doses, powerfully poisonous.

*Therapeutic Uses.*—Amongst the diseases in which White Arsenic has been used with most success are those of an intermittent or periodic type, as ague, neuralgia, and spasmodic affections, *e.g.*, tic douloureux, hemicrania, chorea, epilepsy, hooping cough, and spasmodic asthma; and chronic skin diseases, including leprosy. It has likewise been employed with benefit in chronic rheumatism, cancer, uterine congestion and menorrhagia, snake-bites, chronic catarrhal affections, and plethoric states of the system with determination of blood to the head. Locally, it has been applied to cancerous and other malignant ulcerations; but the practice is objectionable, from the danger which might result from the absorption of the metal into the system.

*Dose.*—From one twentieth to one twelfth of a grain, as an alterative; from one twelfth to one eighth of a grain, as an antiperiodic. It is best in all cases to commence with the smaller doses, and cautiously to increase them as circumstances may require. It is generally most advantageously administered in the form of Solution.

*Preparations.*—**Arsenical Solution** (*Liquor Arsenicalis, Liquor Potassæ Arsenitis,* Lond. Ph.; *Fowler's Solution*). Take of Arsenious Acid, eighty grains; Carbonate of Potash, eighty grains; Compound Tincture of Lavender, five fluid drachms; Distilled Water, a sufficiency. Place the arsenious acid and the carbonate of potash in a flask with ten ounces of the water, and apply heat until a clear solution is obtained. Allow this to cool; then add the compound tincture of lavender, and as much distilled water as will make the bulk one pint. *Characters.*—A reddish liquid, alkaline to test paper, and having the odour of lavender. *Tests.*—Specific gravity, 1·009. After being acidulated with hydrochloric acid, it gives with sulphuretted hydrogen a yellow precipitate, which is brightest when the arsenical solution has been previously diluted. 441·5 grains by weight (1 fluid ounce) boiled for five minutes with ten grains of bicarbonate of soda, and when cold diluted with six fluid ounces of water to which a little mucilage of starch has been added, does not give with the volumetric solution of iodine a permanent blue colour until 808 grain-measures have been added; corresponding to four grains of arsenious acid in one fluid ounce.

*Properties and Therapeutic Uses.*—Those of Arsenious Acid.

*Dose.*—Five drops three times daily, in water, at or immediately after a meal. In the majority of cases this is the best form for administering Arsenic. Each fluid drachm contains half a grain of arsenious acid.

**Hydrochloric Solution of Arsenic** (*Liquor Arsenici Hydrochloricus*). Take of Arsenious Acid, in powder, eighty grains; Hydrochloric Acid, two fluid drachms; Distilled Water, a sufficiency. Boil the arsenious acid with the hydrochloric acid and four ounces of the water until it is dissolved, then add distilled water to make the bulk up to one pint. *Characters.*—A colourless liquid, having an acid reaction. *Tests.* — Specific gravity, 1·009. Sulphuretted hydrogen gives at once a bright yellow precipitate. 441·5 grains by weight (1 fluid ounce), boiled for five minutes with twenty grains of bicarbonate of soda, and then diluted with six fluid ounces of distilled water to which a little mucilage of starch has been added, does not give with the volumetric solution of iodine a permanent blue colour until 808 grain-measures have been added; corresponding to four grains of arsenious acid in one fluid ounce.

*Properties and Therapeutic Uses.*—Those of arsenious acid.

*Dose.*—From two to eight minims.

**Arseniate of Soda.** *See* SODA.

**Arseniate of Iron.** *See* IRON.

[Three forms of Arsenic are met with commonly in the Indian bazaars: 1. Arsenious Acid, or White Arsenic (*Saféd sumbul,* Hind.); 2. Yellow Sulphuret, or Orpiment (*Hartal* (76), Hind.); and, 3. Red Sulphuret, or Realgar (*Mainsil,* Hind.) The use of arsenic by the Hindús in leprosy, intermittent fevers, and other affections is of great antiquity. It is also largely used for criminal purposes. For some interesting remarks on this subject see Dr. Norman Chevers, Manual of Med. Jurisprudence for Bengal, 1856, p. 69, *seq.* From the statements made in this valuable work it appears that the greater portion of the white arsenic imported into Calcutta is from the Persian Gulf, a small portion only from Europe; yellow arsenic of a superior quality from Oude, an inferior kind from Rangoon, and the red arsenic from the territories of Oude. The trade seems to be entirely in the hands of the natives. The quantity imported through the Calcutta Custom-house in five years (1850–55) was upwards of 786 maunds = 7,860 lbs.

# ANTIMONIUM.

## ANTIMONY.

*Symbol*, Sb (*Stibium*) ; *At. weight*, 122.

Antimony exists, principally in combination with sulphur or with oxygen, in various parts of the globe ; as sulphide, chiefly in Cornwall, some parts of Hungary, France, and Borneo ; as oxide, in Bohemia and Saxony. The metal is bluish-white, lustrous, and brittle. Sp. gr., 6·715. It fuses above redness. It is much used in making alloys.

# ANTIMONIUM NIGRUM.

## BLACK ANTIMONY.

(*Prepared Sulphuret of Antimony, Brit. Ph.* 1864.)

Black antimony, a native sulphide of antimony, $SbS_3$ or $\mathbf{Sb_2S_3}$, purified from siliceous matter by fusion, and afterwards reduced to fine powder. A greyish-black crystalline powder. It dissolves almost entirely in boiling hydrochloric acid, as chloride $SbCl_3$, with the evolution of sulphuretted hydrogen.

It is employed only in the preparation of Antimonii Sulphuratum and Liquor Antimonii Chloridum.

# ANTIMONII OXIDUM.

## OXIDE OF ANTIMONY.

Oxide of Antimony, $SbO_3$ or $\mathbf{Sb_2O_3}$, obtained by decomposing a solution of chloride of antimony by the addition of water, and treating the precipitate so obtained with carbonate of soda. *Characters*.—A greyish-white powder, fusible at a low red heat, insoluble in water, but readily dissolved by hydrochloric acid. *Tests*.—The solution is precipitated as an orange-coloured sulphide by sulphuretted hydrogen; dropped into distilled water, it gives a white deposit ; entirely soluble in tartaric acid.

*Properties*.—Emetic, laxative, diaphoretic, and expectorant.

*Therapeutic Uses*.—In febrile and inflammatory diseases, catarrhal affections, and chronic skin diseases, it is employed with advantage.

*Dose*.—From one to four grains.

*Preparations.*—**Antimonial Powder** (*Pulvis Antimonialis*). Take of Oxide of Antimony, one ounce; Phosphate of Lime, two ounces. Mix thoroughly.

*Properties and Therapeutic Uses.*—The same as those of the Oxide.

*Dose.*—From three to ten grains.

Oxide of Antimony is employed also in the preparation of Tartarated Antimony.

## ANTIMONIUM SULPHURATUM.

### SULPHURATED ANTIMONY.

(*Antimonii Oxysulphuretum, Lond. Ph.; Antimonii Sulphuretum aureum, Edin. Ph.; Antimonii Sulphuretum præcipitatum, Dubl. Ph.*)

Sulphide of Antimony, $SbS_3$, or $\mathbf{Sb_2S_3}$, with a small and variable amount of oxide of antimony, $SbO_3$ or $\mathbf{Sb_2O_3}$. *Characters.*—An orange-red powder, readily dissolved by caustic potash or soda, also by hydrochloric acid with the evolution of sulphuretted hydrogen and the separation of a little sulphur. Boiled in water with acid tartrate of potash, the resulting solution is precipitated orange-red with sulphuretted hydrogen. *Tests.*—Sixty grains of this preparation, dissolved in hydrochloric acid and dropped into water, give a white precipitate, which, when washed and dried, weighs about 53 grains.

*Properties.*—Alterative, diaphoretic, and emetic.

*Therapeutic Uses.*—In chronic skin diseases, glandular swellings, secondary syphilis, and chronic rheumatism, it has been employed as an alterative and diaphoretic, but with doubtful success.

*Dose.*—From one to five grains as an alterative; from ten to twenty grains as an emetic.

Sulphurated Antimony forms one of the ingredients in Pilula Hydrargyri Subchloridi composita.

[Sulphuret of Antimony is sold in the bazaars of India under the Hindústani names of *Súrma, Anjan,* and *Kuhl*. It was employed in remote antiquity, as it is at the present day, by Asiatic females, for painting the eyebrows and eyelids (Royle, *Antiquity of Hindoo Med.*, p. 100). It does not appear to be administered internally (Irvine, *Mat. Med. of Patna*, p. 96), nor is it enumerated by Dr. Norman Chevers amongst the articles used in Bengal for poisoning purposes. Under the name *Soormee* (*Súrmí*) Prof. Royle considers that a sulphuret of lead is often included; but a specimen of *Safed Soormah* from Scinde, examined by the late Dr. R. Haines of Bombay, proved on analysis to be sulphate of strontia; whilst another, a lighter and softer variety, known by the same name, was found to be only fibrous gypsum (*Bombay Med. and Phys. Trans.*, 1857, vol. iii. p. 158.)]

## ANTIMONII TERCHLORIDI LIQUOR.

### Solution of Terchloride of Antimony.

A solution of Black Antimony, in hydrochloric acid. *Characters.*—A heavy liquid usually of a yellowish-red colour. A little of it dropped into water gives a white precipitate of oxy-chloride of antimony, formerly known as Powder of Algaroth; this, treated with sulphuretted hydrogen, becomes orange-coloured. *Tests.*—Specific gravity, 1·47. One fluid drachm, mixed with a solution of a quarter of an ounce of tartaric acid in four fluid ounces of water, forms a clear solution, which, if treated with sulphuretted hydrogen, gives an orange precipitate, weighing, when washed and dried at 212°, at least 22 grains.

*Properties.*—A powerful caustic and escharotic. Not prescribed internally.

It is employed in the preparation of the Oxide of Antimony.

## ANTIMONIUM TARTARATUM.

### Tartarated Antimony. Tartar Emetic.

(*Antimonii Potassio-Tartras, Lond. Ph.*)

Tartarated Antimony, Tartrate of Antimony and Potash $KO,SbO_3,C_8H_4O_{10}+2HO$, or $\mathbf{KSbC_4H_4O_7.H_2O}$. obtained by the action of acid tartrate of potash on oxide of antimony. *Characters.*—Colourless transparent crystals exhibiting triangular facets, soluble in water, and less so in proof spirit. It decrepitates and blackens upon the application of heat. Its solution in water gives with hydrochloric acid a white precipitate, which is not formed if tartaric acid be previously added. *Tests.*—Twenty grains dissolve without residue in a fluid ounce of distilled water at 60°, and the solution gives with sulphuretted hydrogen an orange precipitate which, when washed and dried at 212°, weighs 9·91 grains.

*Properties.*—Emetic, diaphoretic, expectorant. In small doses, alterative; in large or long continued doses, poisonous. Locally applied, counter-irritant.

*Therapeutic Uses.*—In febrile and inflammatory affections generally it is a valuable means of reducing morbid vascular action. It is of especial use in acute inflammations of the lungs and thoracic viscera, in croup, laryngitis, the early stage of hooping cough, catarrhs, influenza, hepatitis, acute hydrocephalus, acute rheumatism, hydarthrosis, delirium tremens, epilepsy, and other affections connected with or dependant upon plethora; and in purulent ophthalmia, and other eye diseases characterised by inflammatory action. It is also a ready and effectual agent in evacuating the stomach when in an overloaded state.

*Dose.*—From one-sixteenth to one-eighth of a grain as an alterative, from one-eighth to one quarter of a grain as a diaphoretic and expectorant, and from one to four grains (in solution) as an emetic.

*Preparations.*—**Antimonial Wine** (*Vinum Antimoniale*). Take of Tartarated Antimony, forty grains; Sherry, one pint. Dissolve.

*Dose.*—From ten to thirty drops as a diaphoretic and expectorant; nauseant in doses of from one to two fluid drachms; emetic in doses of half an ounce, or in doses of two drachms repeated every ten minutes until it operates. As an emetic for children, from thirty to sixty drops, but for young children generally, ipecacuanha is preferable. Each fluid ounce contains two grains of tartarated antimony.

**Ointment of Tartarated Antimony, Tartar Emetic Ointment** (*Unguentum Antimonii Tartarati*). Take of Tartarated Antimony, in fine powder, a quarter of an ounce; Simple Ointment, one ounce. Mix thoroughly.

A valuable counter-irritant, producing after a few applications a pustular eruption. Amongst the diseases in which it has been most employed are chronic bronchitis, asthma, phthisis and other pulmonary diseases, acute meningitis, hydarthrosis and other chronic affections of the joints, tic douloureux and other forms of neuralgia, and to the spine in some forms of paralysis and the chronic stage of hooping cough. Its employment in all cases requires much caution, on account of the occasional violence of its operation locally, and the danger of absorption of the salt into the system.

## BISMUTHUM.

### Bismuth.

*Symbol,* Bi; *At. weight,* 210.

Bismuth exists generally in the metallic state nearly pure, more rarely in combination with sulphur and with oxygen, in various portions of the globe, especially in Cornwall, Saxony, Bohemia. and some parts of the United States.

## BISMUTHUM PURIFICATUM.

### PURIFIED BISMUTH.

Metallic Bismuth submitted to fusion with nitrate of potash. It occurs in the form of a crystalline metal of a reddish-white colour. It fuses at 507°, and crystallizes in large hollow cubes. *Tests.*—Dissolved in a mixture of equal volumes of nitric acid and distilled water it forms a solution of nitrate of bismuth, which by evaporation yields colourless crystals which are decomposed on addition of water, giving a white precipitate. If the mother liquor from which the crystals have been separated be added to solution of carbonate of ammonia, the precipitate formed is free or nearly so from colour.

It is only officinal as the basis of the following preparations.

## BISMUTHI SUBNITRAS.

### SUBNITRATE OF BISMUTH.

(*Bismuthum Album, Brit. Ph.* 1864; *Bismuthi Nitras, Lond. Ph.*

Subnitrate of Bismuth, $BiO_3,NO_5,2HO$ or $\mathbf{BiNO_4.H_2O}$. obtained by the action of water on nitrate of bismuth. *Characters.*—A heavy white powder in minute crystalline scales, blackened by sulphuretted hydrogen. *Tests.*—Insoluble in water, but soluble in nitric acid mixed with half its volume of distilled water, forming a solution which, poured into water, gives a white precipitate; insoluble in tartaric acid, and blackened by sulphuretted hydrogen. With sulphuric acid, diluted with an equal bulk of water the liquid turns brown on addition of sulphate of iron.

*Properties.*—Astringent, sedative, alterative.

*Therapeutic Uses.*—In atonic dyspepsia, gastralgia, gastrodynia, pyrosis, ulceration of the stomach, atonic diarrhœa, and the advanced stage of dysentery, it is often very serviceable. Locally it has been applied, with occasional success, to chronic cutaneous affections, fissures of the anus, nipples, or lips; also in leucorrhœa and gleet.

*Dose.*—From five to twenty grains twice or thrice daily.

*Preparations.*—**Bismuth Lozenges** (*Trochisci Bismuthi*). Take of Subnitrate of Bismuth, fourteen hundred and forty grains; Carbonate of Magnesia, four ounces; precipitated Carbonate of Lime, six ounces; Refined Sugar, twenty-nine ounces; Gum Acacia, in powder, one ounce; Mucilage of Gum Acacia, two fluid ounces; Rose Water, a sufficiency. Mix the dry ingredients, then add the mucilage, and form the whole into a proper mass with rose water. Divide the mass into 720 lozenges, and dry these in a hot-air chamber with a moderate heat.

Each lozenge contains two grains of subnitrate of bismuth.

*Dose.*—From three to ten lozenges may be taken daily.

**Ointment of Subnitrate of Bismuth** (*Unguentum Bismuthi Subnitratis*). Take of Subnitrate of Bismuth, two drachms; Simple Ointment, one ounce. Mix thoroughly.

A useful local application in the class of affections mentioned above.

## BISMUTHI CARBONAS.

### Carbonate of Bismuth.

Carbonate of bismuth $2(BiO_3,CO_2),HO$ or $2(Bi_2CO_5)H_2O$. obtained by the action of carbonate of ammonia on a solution of purified bismuth in nitric acid. *Characters.*—A white powder blackened by sulphuretted hydrogen; insoluble in water, but soluble with effervescence in nitric acid. *Tests.*—When added to sulphuric acid coloured with sulphate of indigo, the colour of the latter is not discharged. If to nitric acid mixed with half its volume of distilled water as much carbonate of bismuth be added as the acid will dissolve, one volume of this solution poured into twenty volumes of water will yield a white precipitate. The nitric acid solution gives no precipitate with diluted sulphuric acid, nor with solution of nitrate of silver.

*Properties and Therapeutic Uses.*—Similar to those of the subnitrate.

*Dose.*—From five to twenty grains.

## LIQUOR BISMUTHI ET AMMONIÆ CITRATIS.

### Solution of Citrate of Bismuth and Ammonia.

Take of Purified Bismuth, four hundred and thirty grains; Nitric Acid, two fluid ounces; Citric Acid, two ounces; Solution of Ammonia, Distilled Water, of each a sufficiency. Mix the nitric acid with an ounce of distilled water, and add the bismuth in successive portions. When effervescence has ceased, apply for ten minutes a heat approaching that of ebullition, and decant the solution from any insoluble matter that may be present. Evaporate the solution until it is reduced to two fluid ounces, then add the citric acid previously dissolved in four ounces of distilled water, and afterwards the solution of ammonia in small quantities at a time until the precipitate formed is redissolved, and the solution is neutral or slightly alkaline to test-paper. Dilute with distilled water to the volume of one pint. *Characters.*—A colourless solution with a saline and slightly metallic taste. Specific gravity, 1·122. Neutral or slightly alkaline to test paper; mixes with water without change; heated with solution of potash it evolves ammonia, and yields a white precipitate. *Tests.*—Hydrochloric acid added to it gives a white precipitate which is soluble in excess of the reagent. Three fluid drachms of the solution mixed with an ounce of distilled water, and treated with sulphuretted hydrogen in excess, yield a black precipitate, which, collected, washed and dried, weighs 9·92 grains.

*Dose.*—From thirty minims to one fluid drachm. One fluid drachm contains three grains of oxide of bismuth.

## ZINCUM.

### ZINC.

*Symbol,* Zn; *At. weight,* 32·5; or **Zn=65.**

Zinc exists in the mineral kingdom, variously combined, but chiefly with sulphur in the form of sulphuret (*Blende*), and with carbonic acid as an impure carbonate (*Calamine*). It is obtained chiefly from the Mendip Hills and Alston Moor in Great Britain, and from Belgium and Silesia. It exists also in India and China. Zinc is a hard bluish metal, which fuses at 773°. Specific gravity, 6·8 to 7. Soluble in most acids.

## ZINCUM GRANULATUM.

### Granulated Zinc.

Granulated zinc is obtained by subjecting zinc of commerce to fusion, and pouring the fused metal in a thin stream into cold water. It is employed in the preparation of chloride and sulphate of zinc.

## ZINCI OXIDUM.

### Oxide of Zinc.

Oxide of Zinc, ZnO, obtained by subjecting carbonate of zinc to a red heat till the whole of the carbonic acid is evolved. *Characters.*—A soft, nearly white, tasteless, and inodorous powder, becoming pale yellow when heated; and forming with diluted sulphuric acid a solution which is not precipitated by sulphuretted hydrogen, but is precipitated white by sulphide of ammonium. *Tests.*—Dissolves without effervescence in diluted nitric acid, forming a solution which is not affected by chloride of barium or nitrate of silver, and gives with carbonate of ammonia a white precipitate which dissolves entirely without colour in an excess of the reagent.

*Properties.*—Tonic, sedative, and antispasmodic. In large doses, emetic and purgative. Locally applied, astringent.

*Therapeutic Uses.*—Similar to those of the Sulphate of Zinc, It has been highly spoken of as a means of subduing the nervous symptoms of dipsomania.

*Dose.*—From two to four grains, gradually increased to ten grains or more.

*Preparation.* — **Ointment of Zinc** (*Unguentum Zinci*). Take of Oxide of Zinc, in very fine powder, eighty grains; Simple Ointment, one ounce. Add the oxide of zinc to the ointment, previously melted with a gentle heat, and stir the mixture constantly while it cools.

A useful application in many chronic skin diseases, bed sores, excoriations, ophthalmia tarsi, and scrofulous coryza and ozæna.

## ZINCI CARBONAS.

### Carbonate of Zinc.

Carbonate of Zinc, $ZnO,CO_2+2ZnO+3HO$ or $\mathbf{ZnCO_3\,2(ZnO).3H_2O}$. obtained by decomposing sulphate of zinc with carbonate of soda. *Characters.*—White, tasteless, inodorous, insoluble in water; soluble, with effervescence and without residue, in diluted nitric acid, forming a solution which gives a white precipitate with sulphide of ammonium. *Tests.*—Its solution in dilute nitric acid is not precipitated by chloride of barium or nitrate of silver, and gives with carbonate of ammonia a white precipitate entirely soluble, without colour, in an excess of the reagent.

*Properties and Therapeutic Uses.*—Analogous probably to those of the oxide. Employed principally as an external application, either in powder or in the form of ointment.

*Dose.*—From two to eight grains.

*Preparation.*—***Ointment of Carbonate of Zinc** (*Unguentum Zinci Carbonatis*). Take of Carbonate of Zinc, two drachms; Simple Ointment, ten drachms. Mix thoroughly.

This is introduced as a substitute for Ceratum Calaminæ, Lond. Ph. It is a very useful application to burns, scalds, excoriations, and superficial ulcerations.

The Carbonate is employed in the preparation of the Oxide and Acetate of Zinc.

## ZINCI ACETAS.

### Acetate of Zinc.

Acetate of Zinc, $ZnO,C_4H_3O_3+2HO$, or $\mathbf{Zn2(C_2H_3O_2).2H_2O}$. obtained by the action of acetic acid on carbonate of zinc. *Characters.*—Thin, translucent, and colourless crystalline plates, of a pearly lustre, with a sharp unpleasant taste, soluble in water; precipitated pure white by sulphuretted hydrogen; evolving acetic acid when decomposed by sulphuric acid. *Tests.*—A dilute aqueous solution is not affected by chloride of barium or nitrate of silver; and when slightly acidulated with hydrochloric acid, is not precipitated by sulphuretted hydrogen. After it has been boiled for a few minutes with a little nitric acid, it yields with ammonia a white precipitate, entirely soluble, without colour, in an excess of the reagent.

*Properties and Therapeutic Uses.*—Analogous to those of the Sulphate. Chiefly employed in solution (in the proportion of from two to four grains to an ounce of water) as an injection in gonorrhœa, gleet, and leucorrhœa; as a lotion in eczema and other chronic skin diseases; and as a collyrium in ophthalmia, especially in that of infants and children.

*Dose.*—From one to two grains, gradually increased, as a tonic and antispasmodic; from ten to twenty grains as an emetic.

## ZINCI VALERIANAS.

### Valerianate of Zinc.

Valerianate of Zinc, $ZnO,C_{10}H_9O_3$ or **$Zn2(C_5H_9O_2)$**. obtained by decomposing sulphate of zinc with valerianate of soda. *Characters.* — Brilliant white pearly tabular crystals, with a feeble odour of valerianic acid and a metallic taste; scarcely soluble in cold water or in ether; soluble in hot water and alcohol. Heated to redness in an open crucible it leaves a residue which, when dissolved in diluted sulphuric acid, yields with ammonia a precipitate which entirely dissolves in an excess of the reagent, and the resulting solution gives a white precipitate with sulphide of ammonium. *Tests.*—Its solution in hot water is not precipitated by chloride of barium. Heated with dilute sulphuric acid, it gives a distillate, which, when mixed with a solution of acetate of copper, does not immediately affect the transparency of the fluid, but forms after a little time, oily drops, which gradually pass into a bluish-white crystalline deposit.

*Properties.*—Nervine tonic and antispasmodic.

*Therapeutic Uses.*—Epilepsy, chorea, hysteria, and neuralgia are the affections in which it has been principally employed.

*Dose.*—From half a grain to one grain, gradually increased to three grains, twice or thrice daily.

## ZINCI CHLORIDUM.

### Chloride of Zinc.

Chloride of Zinc, $ZnCl$ or **$ZnCl_2$**, obtained by the action of hydrochloric acid on granulated zinc, purifying the solution by the addition of solution of chlorine and of carbonate of zinc, and evaporating till it assumes a solid form. *Characters.* — Colourless opaque rods or tablets, very deliquescent and caustic; soluble almost entirely in water, alcohol, and ether. Its aqueous solution is precipitated white by sulphide of ammonium and by nitrate of silver; but, if first acidulated with hydrochloric acid, it is not affected by sulphuretted hydrogen. *Tests.*—Its solution in water is not affected by chloride of barium or oxalate of ammonia, and is not tinged blue by yellow or red prussiate of potash. Ammonia throws down a white precipitate entirely soluble in an excess of the reagent.

*Properties.*—Powerful escharotic. Given internally in small doses largely diluted, it is regarded as a nervine tonic, but it is rarely employed. In its pure state, a corrosive poison. Its powers as a deodorizer are considerable.

*Therapeutic Uses.*—In cancerous and other malignant ulcerations it has been applied as a caustic, but with no special results beyond those obtained from the use of other articles of the same class. In gonorrhœa and gonorrhœal ophthalmia, a very weak solution (one grain to the ounce of fluid) has been employed locally.

*Dose.*—From half a grain to one grain or more, largely diluted.

*Preparation.* — **Solution of Chloride of Zinc** (*Liquor Zinci Chloridi*). Take of Granulated Zinc, one pound; Hydrochloric Acid, forty-four fluid ounces; Solution of Chlorine, a sufficiency; Carbonate of Zinc, half an ounce, or a sufficiency; Distilled Water, one pint. Mix the hydrochloric acid and water in a porcelain dish, add the zinc, and apply a gentle heat to promote the action until gas is no longer evolved. Boil for half an hour, supplying the water lost by evaporation, and allow the product to cool. Filter it into a bottle, and add solution of chlorine by degrees, with frequent agitation until the fluid acquires a permanent odour of chlorine. Add the carbonate of zinc, in small quantities at a time, and with renewed agitation, until a brown sediment appears. Filter the liquid into a porcelain basin, and evaporate until it is reduced to the bulk of two pints.

This solution, popularly known as *Sir William Burnett's Disinfecting Fluid*, is a valuable deodorizer. Taken internally, in an undiluted state, it acts as a powerful corrosive irritant poison.

## ZINCI SULPHAS.

### SULPHATE OF ZINC.

Sulphate of Zinc, $ZnO,SO_3+7HO$ or $ZnSO_4.7H_2O$. *Characters.*—Colourless transparent prismatic crystals, with a strong metallic styptic taste. Its solution in water gives white precipitates with chloride of barium and sulphide of ammonium. *Tests.*—Its aqueous solution is not tinged purple by tincture of galls; and when acidulated with sulphuric or hydrochloric acid gives no precipitate with sulphuretted hydrogen. It yields with ammonia, as well as with a carbonate of ammonia, a white precipitate, which is entirely soluble, without colour, in an excess of the reagent.

*Properties.* — Tonic, astringent, and antispasmodic. Valuable emetic; in over doses, poisonous. Locally applied, astringent and stimulant; in a dried or anhydrous state, caustic.

*Therapeutic Uses.*—In chorea, epilepsy, spasmodic asthma, the chronic stages of hooping cough, angina pectoris, intermittent fever, hysteria connected with debility, in chronic dysentery and diarrhœa, and in atonic menorrhagia, it has been employed with advantage. As a local application, in solution, it proves useful as an injection in gonorrhœa and leucorrhœa, as a collyrium in various forms of ophthalmia, as a lotion in ulcers and some chronic skin diseases, and as an electuary in aphthous and other ulcerations of the mouth and fauces.

*Dose.*—From one to two grains, gradually increased to five grains or more, as a tonic and antispasmodic; from ten to thirty grains as an emetic. In the last character it is very valuable in cases of poisoning, as it speedily operates without causing subsequent depression.

[Zinc (*Dasta*, Hind.) and some of its salts are known in the East, but are apparently little employed in medicine. The name *Tútenague*, by which Chinese zinc was known in commerce, is evidently derived from the Tamul *Tantanagum.* The common name, *tutty*, of impure oxide of zinc, is apparently of Eastern origin, as *tútia* (*Tutum*, Tam.) is in common use in India and Persia, being applied to an ore of zinc imported from the latter (Royle, *Antiquity of Hindoo Med.*, p. 100). Heyne (*Tracts on India*, p. 166) gives the process by which the natives prepare with zinc, a salt, which they term *Tutanag passom*, and which they prescribe with great confidence in gonorrhœa, spermatorrhœa, leucorrhœa, and hæmorrhoids. The dose appears to be from one to four grains. Dr. Heyne states that he employed it, combined with valerian, in an obstinate case of epilepsy, with the best effect. It is apparently an impure oxide of zinc.]

## CADMIUM.

*Symbol,* Cd ; *At. weight,* 56 ; or **Cd.=112.**

Cadmium occurs naturally as Sulphide of Cadmium in the majority of zinc ores. When freed from the latter, it is a white metal, malleable and ductile, fuses at 442°, and has a specific gravity of 8·7.

## CADMII IODIDUM.

### Iodide of Cadmium.

Iodide of Cadmium, CdI or $\mathbf{CdI_2}$, may be formed by direct combination of Iodine and Cadmium in the presence of Water. *Characters.*—Flat micaceous crystals, white, of a pearly lustre, which melt when heated to about 600°, forming an amber-coloured fluid. At a dull red heat, violet-coloured vapours are given off. It is anhydrous and permanent in the air; freely soluble in water and in rectified spirit, and the solution reddens litmus paper. *Tests.*—The aqueous solution gives a yellow precipitate with sulphuretted hydrogen or sulphide of ammonium, which is insoluble in excess of the latter; the solution also gives a white gelatinous precipitate with excess of solution of potash, the filtrate from which is unaffected by sulphide of ammonium. Ten grains dissolved in water and nitrate of silver added in excess give a precipitate which, when washed with water and afterwards with half an ounce of solution of ammonia, and dried, weighs 12·5 grains.

*Properties and Uses.*—Not prescribed internally. Externally applied it acts as a stimulant, and is applicable to the same class of cases, as the iodide of lead over which it possesses the advantage of not producing yellow discoloration of the skin.

*Preparation.*—**Ointment of Iodide of Cadmium** (*Unguentum Cadmii Iodidi*). Take of Iodide of Cadmium, in fine powder, sixty-two grains; Simple Ointment, one ounce. Mix thoroughly.

A useful application in scrofulous glandular enlargements and some obstinate skin diseases.

## PLUMBUM. LEAD.

*Symbol,* Pb; *At. weight,* 103·5; *or* **Pb.=207.**

Lead exists in the mineral kingdom, variously combined, but principally with sulphur, as a native sulphide called *Galèna.* It is a bluish-white metal, malleable and soft: fuses at 617°. Specific gravity, 11·36. Its great solvent is nitric acid.

## PLUMBI OXIDUM.

### OXIDE OF LEAD.

*Lythargyrum, Brit. Ph.,* 1864.

Oxide of Lead, PbO, obtained by subjecting melted lead to the continued action of a current of heated air. *Characters.*—In heavy scales of a pale brick-red colour, soluble in diluted nitric and acetic acids; either solution, when neutral, giving a copious yellow precipitate with iodide of potassium. *Tests.*—It dissolves without effervescence in diluted nitric acid; and the solution, when supersaturated with ammonia, and then cleared by filtration, does not exhibit a blue colour.

*Properties.*—Imperfectly known; supposed to be irritant. The continued inhalation of its vapour produces poisonous effects. It is only employed externally in the form of plaster.

*Preparation.*—**Lead Plaster** (*Emplastrum Plumbi*). Take of Oxide of Lead, in fine powder, four pounds; Olive Oil, one gallon; Water, three pints and a half. Boil all the ingredients together gently by the heat of a steam-bath, and keep simmering for four or five hours, stirring constantly until the product acquires a proper consistence for a plaster, and adding more water during the process, if necessary.

This, under its popular name, Diachylon Plaster, is in common use in surgery as strapping for retaining in apposition the edges of wounds, and for other purposes. It forms an ingredient in Emplastrum Resinæ, Emp. Saponis, Emp. Ferri, Emp. Galbani, and Emp. Hydrargyri.

## PLUMBI CARBONAS.

### Carbonate of Lead.

Carbonate of Lead. A soft heavy white powder, blackened by sulphuretted hydrogen, insoluble in water, soluble with effervescence in diluted acetic acid, forming a solution which is precipitated yellow by iodide of potassium, and white by sulphuric acid. *Tests.*—Dissolves in acetic acid without leaving any residue; and the solution, when treated with excess of sulphuretted hydrogen, boiled and filtered, gives no precipitate with oxalate of ammonia.

*Properties and Uses.*—Astringent when locally applied, either in the form of powder or ointment, to excoriations, superficial ulcerations, and other skin affections. Not administered internally.

*Preparation.*—**Ointment of Carbonate of Lead** (*Unguentum Plumbi Carbonatis*). Take of Carbonate of Lead, in fine powder, sixty-two grains; Simple Ointment, one ounce. Mix thoroughly.

## PLUMBI ACETAS.

### Acetate of Lead.

Acetate of Lead, $PbO,C_4H_3O_3+3HO$, or $\mathbf{Pb2(C_2H_3O_2).3H_2O}$. obtained by the action of acetic acid on oxide of lead, and evaporating the solution to crystallization. *Characters.* — White crystalline masses slightly efflorescent, having an acetous odour, and a sweet astringent taste. Its solution in water slightly reddens litmus, gives a yellow precipitate with iodide of potassium, and is precipitated white by sulphuric acid, acetic acid being set free. *Tests.* —Its solution in distilled water is clear, or has only a slight milkiness, which disappears on the addition of acetic acid. Thirty-eight grains dissolved in water require for complete precipitation 200 grain-measures of the volumetric solution of oxalic acid.

*Properties.*—Astringent and sedative. In over doses, poisonous.

*Therapeutic Uses.*—In hæmoptysis, hæmatemesis, hæmaturia, menorrhagia, and other internal hæmorrhages, it is a remedy of great power. It is also valuable in various forms of diarrhœa, especially choleraic, the advanced stages of dysentery, ulceration of the stomach, and bronchorrhœa. It has likewise been employed in aneurism of the aorta, hypertrophy of the heart, epilepsy, and incarcerated hernia. Externally, in solution, it forms an astringent sedative application to inflamed or excoriated surfaces, skin diseases, and some forms of ophthalmia; and in the form of injection in gonorrhœa, gleet, and leucorrhœa.

*Dose.*—From one to five grains or more in the form of pill.

*Preparation.*—**Pill of Lead and Opium** (*Pilula Plumbi cum Opio*). Take of Acetate of Lead, in fine powder, thirty-six grains; Opium, in fine powder, six grains; Confection of Roses, six grains. Beat them into a uniform mass.

*Dose.*—From four to eight grains. Eight grains of the mass contain one grain of opium.

**Compound Lead Suppositories** (*Suppositoria Plumbi composita*). Take of Acetate of Lead, thirty-six grains; Opium, in powder, twelve grains; Benzoated Lard, forty-two grains; White Wax, ten grains; Oil of Theobroma, eighty grains. Melt the wax and oil of theobroma with a gentle heat, then add the other ingredients previously rubbed together in a mortar, and having mixed them thoroughly, pour the mixture while it is fluid into suitable moulds of the capacity of fifteen grains; or the fluid mixture may be allowed to cool, and then be divided into twelve equal parts, each of which shall be made into a conical or other convenient form for a suppository.

Each suppository contains one grain of opium; a valuable application in dysentery, and other affections of the pelvic viscera in which astringents and opiates are indicated.

**Ointment of Acetate of Lead** (*Unguentum Plumbi Acetatis*). Take of Acetate of Lead, in fine powder, twelve grains; Benzoated Lard or Simple Ointment, one ounce. Mix thoroughly.

A useful application to skin affections characterized by irritation.

## PLUMBI SUBACETATIS LIQUOR.

### SOLUTION OF SUBACETATE OF LEAD.

Subacetate of Lead, $2PbO,C_4H_3O_3$ or $\mathbf{PbC_2H_3O_2}$, dissolved in water. *Characters.*—A dense clear colourless liquid, with alkaline reaction and sweet astringent taste, becoming turbid by exposure to the air, and forming with mucilage of gum acacia an opaque white jelly. Sulphuric acid in excess gives a white precipitate, acetic acid being set free. *Tests.*—Specific gravity, 1·26. 413·3 grains by weight (six fluid drachms) require for perfect precipitation 810 grain-measures of the volumetric solution of oxalic acid.

*Properties.*—Sedative and astringent; not administered internally.

*Therapeutic Uses.*—To inflamed and erysipelatous surfaces, inflamed glands, painful bruises and sprains, inflamed hæmorrhoids, pruritus pudendi, and other external affections attended with increased vascular action, the diluted solution (*infra*) is an effectual application.

*Preparations.*—**Dilute Solution of Subacetate of Lead** (*Liquor Plumbi Subacetatis dilutus*). Take of Solution of Subacetate of Lead, two fluid drachms; Rectified Spirit, two fluid drachms; Distilled Water, nineteen fluid ounces and a half. Mix, and filter through paper. Keep the clear solution in a stoppered bottle.

**Ointment of the Subacetate of Lead** (*Unguentum Plumbi Subacetatis*). Take of Solution of Subacetate of Lead, six fluid ounces; Camphor, sixty grains; White Wax, eight ounces; Olive Oil, one pint. Melt the wax with sixteen ounces of the oil by the heat of a water bath; remove the vessel, and, as soon as the mixture begins to thicken, gradually add the solution of subacetate of lead, and stir the mixture constantly until it cools; then add the camphor dissolved in the rest of the oil, and mix thoroughly.

A useful cooling application in the class of cases enumerated above.

## PLUMBI NITRAS.

### Nitrate of Lead.

Nitrate of lead, $PbO,NO_5$ or **Pb2(NO )**. obtained by the action of nitric acid on the oxide of lead. It occurs in the form of colourless octahedral crystals which are nearly opaque, permanent in the air, of a sweetish astringent taste, soluble in water and in alcohol. *Test.*—The aqueous solution is precipitated black by sulphuretted hydrogen, white by diluted sulphuric acid, and yellow by iodide of potassium. Added to sulphate of indigo it discharges the colour.

*Properties and Uses.*—Not administered internally. In solution (from ten to forty grains to a fluid ounce of water) it forms an astringent lotion serviceable in sore and fissured nipples, excoriations, and other cutaneous affections. Its solution, in the proportion of a drachm to a fluid ounce of water, constitutes *Ledoyen's Disinfecting Fluid*, which possesses considerable power as a deodoriser. It is employed in the preparation of the Iodide of Lead.

## PLUMBI IODIDUM.

### Iodide of Lead.

Iodide of lead, PbI or **$PbI_2$**, obtained by the decomposition of nitrate of lead by iodide of potassium. It occurs in the form of a deep yellow golden powder or glittering yellow scales, inodorous, tasteless, very sparingly soluble in cold water, but readily so in boiling water; soluble in acetic acid and in alcohol. *Test.*—When heated, it first evolves a yellow and afterwards a violet vapour, leaving a residue which, when dissolved in nitric acid, possesses all the characters of a solution of lead.

*Properties.*—Alterative; externally applied stimulant.

*Therapeutic Uses.*—In scrofulous affections and in chronic enlargement and other affections of the spleen, it has been successfully employed; but it is very rarely prescribed internally. Its principal use is as an application to glandular tumours and skin diseases. It communicates a yellow stain to the cuticle.

*Preparations*—**Iodide of Lead Plaster** (*Emplastrum Plumbi Iodidi*). Take of Iodide of Lead, one ounce; Soap Plaster, Resin Plaster, of each, four ounces. Add the iodide of lead in fine powder to the plasters previously melted, and mix them intimately.

**Ointment of Iodide of Lead** (*Unguentum Plumbi Iodidi.*)—Take of Iodide of Lead, in fine powder, sixty-two grains; Simple Ointment, one ounce. Mix thoroughly.

## FERRUM.

### Iron.

*Symbol*, Fe; *At. weight*, 28; or **Fe=56.**

Iron is diffused very widely throughout nature, both in the organic and in the inorganic kingdoms. It exists most extensively in the latter, variously combined, but chiefly with oxygen (*hæmatite, magnetic iron ore, &c.*) with sulphur (*iron pyrites*), and as protocarbonate of iron

## FERRUM REDACTUM.

### Reduced Iron.

(*Pulvis Ferri, Dubl. Ph.*)

Metallic Iron, with a variable amount of magnetic oxide of iron, obtained by passing hydrogen gas through peroxide of iron contained in a gun-barrel, and exposed to a red heat. *Characters.* — A fine greyish-black powder, strongly attracted by the magnet, and exhibiting metallic streaks when rubbed with firm pressure in a mortar. It dissolves in hydrochloric acid with the evolution of hydrogen, and the solution gives a light-blue precipitate with yellow prussiate of potash. *Test.*—Ten grains, added to an aqueous solution of fifty grains of iodine and fifty grains of iodide of potassium, and digested in a small flask at a gentle heat, leave not more than five grains undissolved, which should be entirely soluble in hydrochloric acid.

*Properties.*—Valuable tonic, acting, like all other ferruginous preparations, principally on the blood, which under its use exhibits an increased proportion of hæmatin and globulin; emmenagogue.

*Therapeutic Uses.*—In anæmia; and in chlorosis, amenorrhœa, chorea, enlargement of the spleen, and other affections characterized by anæmia, it is a remedy of the greatest value.

*Dose.*—From one to five grains twice or thrice daily, at or immediately after a meal.

*Preparation.* — **Reduced Iron Lozenges** (*Trochisci Ferri Redacti*). Take of Reduced Iron, seven hundred and twenty grains; Refined Sugar, in powder, twenty-five ounces; Gum Acacia, in powder, one ounce; Mucilage of Gum Acacia, two fluid ounces; Distilled Water, one fluid ounce or a sufficiency. Mix the iron, sugar, and gum, and add the mucilage and water to produce the proper consistence. Divide into 720 lozenges, and dry these in a hot-air chamber with a moderate heat

Each lozenge contains one grain of reduced iron.

## FERRI OXIDUM MAGNETICUM.

### MAGNETIC OXIDE OF IRON.

### (*Ferri Oxidum Nigrum, Edin. Ph.*)

Magnetic Oxide of Iron, $Fe_3O_4$, combined with about twenty per cent. of water of hydration, and containing some peroxide of iron. *Characters.* — Brownish-black, destitute of taste, strongly attracted by the magnet. It dissolves without effervescence in hydrochloric acid diluted with half its volume of water, and the solution thus obtained gives blue precipitates with the red and yellow prussiate of potash. When a small quantity is heated in a dry test tube by the flame of a lamp, a deposit of moisture takes place in the cool part of the tube. *Tests.*—Twenty grains dissolved in hydrochloric acid continue to give a blue precipitate with the red prussiate of potash until eighty-three grain measures of the volumetric solution of bichromate of potash have been added.

*Properties and Uses.*—Similar to those of Ferrum Redactum.

*Dose.*—From five to ten grains.

## FERRI PEROXIDUM HYDRATUM.

### HYDRATED PEROXIDE OF IRON.

### (*Ferri peroxidum, Brit. Ph.* 1864; *Ferri Sesquioxidum, Lond. Ph.*; *Ferri Oxidum Rubrum, Ferrugo, Edin. Ph.*)

Hydrated Peroxide of Iron, $Fe_2O_3$,HO, or **$Fe_2O_3.H_2O$**. obtained by subjecting moist peroxide of iron to a temperature not exceeding 212° until it ceases to lose weight, and then reducing it to powder. *Characters.*—A reddish-brown powder, destitute of taste, and not magnetic. *Tests.*—It dissolves completely, though slowly, with the aid of heat, in hydrochloric acid diluted with half its volume of water, and the solution gives a copious precipitate with the yellow, but none with the red prussiate of potash. Heated to dull redness in a test tube it gives off moisture.

*Properties.*—Tonic, emmenagogue, anthelmintic.

*Therapeutic Uses.*—In addition to anæmic states of the system, in which it is very effectual, it has been employed with advantage in general debility, neuralgia, chorea, advanced stages of hooping cough, laryngismus stridulus, spasmodic asthma, mercurial tremors, and amenorrhœa.

*Dose.*—From five to thirty grains or more.

*Preparation.* — **Chalybeate Plaster** (*Emplastrum Ferri*). Take of Hydrated Peroxide of Iron, in fine powder, one ounce; Burgundy Pitch, two ounces; Lead Plaster, eight ounces. Add the peroxide of iron to the Burgundy pitch and lead plaster, previously melted together; and stir the mixture constantly till it stiffens on cooling.

Spread on leather, it forms a good support and protection to the subjacent parts.

## FERRI PEROXIDUM HUMIDUM.

### Moist Peroxide of Iron.

(*Ferri Peroxidum Hydratum, Brit. Ph.* 1864.)

Moist Peroxide of Iron is the hydrated peroxide with about 86 per cent. of uncombined water. *Characters.*—A soft moist pasty mass, of a reddish-brown colour. Dissolves readily in diluted hydrochloric acid without the aid of heat, and the solution gives a copious blue precipitate with the yellow, but not with the red prussiate of potash. *Test.*—A little of it dried at 212° until it ceases to lose weight, gives off moisture when heated to dull redness in a test tube.

*Properties and Uses.*—Employed only as an antidote in cases of arsenical poisoning.

*Dose.*—A tablespoonful every five or ten minutes. About twelve parts are required for every part of arsenic swallowed.

## FERRI CARBONAS SACCHARATA.

### Saccharated Carbonate of Iron.

Carbonate of Iron, $FeO,CO_2$ or $\mathbf{FeCO_3}$, mixed with peroxide of iron and sugar, and the carbonate forming at least fifty-seven per cent. of the mixture; obtained by decomposing sulphate of iron with carbonate of ammonia, washing the precipitate, adding sugar to it and drying.

*Characters.*—Small coherent lumps of a grey colour, with a sweet very feeble chalybeate taste. It dissolves with effervescence in warm hydrochloric acid diluted with half its volume of water, and the solution gives but a very slight precipitate with chloride of barium. *Tests.*—Twenty grains, dissolved in excess of hydrochloric acid and diluted with water, continue to give a blue precipitate with the red prussiate of potash until at least 330 grain-measures of the volumetric solution of bichromate of potash have been added.

*Properties.*—Valuable chalybeate tonic, devoid of astringency.

*Therapeutic Uses.*—Similar to those of Ferri Peroxidum.

*Dose.*—From five to twenty grains or more.

*Preparation.*—**Pill of Carbonate of Iron** (*Pilula Ferri Carbonatis*). Take of Saccharated Carbonate of Iron, one ounce; Confection of Roses, a quarter of an ounce. Beat them into a uniform mass.

*Dose.*—From five to ten grains twice daily.

## FERRI PHOSPHAS.

### PHOSPHATE OF IRON.

Phosphate of Iron, $3FeO,PO_5$ or $Fe_3P_2O_8$, partially peroxidized; obtained by decomposing sulphate of iron with phosphate of soda. *Characters.*—A slate-blue amorphous powder, insoluble in water, soluble in hydrochloric acid. The solution yields a precipitate with both the yellow and red prussiate of potash, that afforded by the latter being the more abundant; and when treated with tartaric acid and an excess of ammonia, and subsequently with the solution of ammonio-sulphate of magnesia, lets fall a crystalline precipitate. *Tests.*—When the salt is digested in hydrochloric acid upon a strip of pure copper, a dark deposit does not form on the metal. Twenty grains, dissolved in hydrochloric acid, continue to give a blue precipitate with red prussiate of potash until 250 grain-measures of the volumetric solution of bichromate of potash have been added.

*Properties.*—Chalybeate tonic.

*Therapeutic Uses.*—In addition to anæmic and debilitated states of the system generally, it has been employed with alleged effect in rachitis, diabetes, ramollissement of the brain, and cancer.

*Dose.*—From five to ten grains. It is best given in the form of syrup.

*Preparation.*—**Syrup of Phosphate of Iron** (*Syrupus Ferri Phosphatis*). Take of Granulated Sulphate of Iron, two hundred and twenty-four grains; Phosphate of Soda, two hundred grains; Acetate of Soda, seventy-four grains; Dilute Phosphoric Acid, five fluid ounces and a half; Refined Sugar, eight ounces; Distilled Water, eight fluid ounces. Dissolve the sulphate of iron in four ounces of the water, and the phosphate and acetate of soda in the remainder; mix the two solutions, and, after careful stirring, transfer the precipitate to a calico filter, and wash it with distilled water till the filtrate ceases to be affected by chloride of barium. Then press the precipitate strongly between folds of bibulous paper, and add to it the dilute phosphoric acid. As soon as the precipitate is dissolved, filter the solution, add the sugar, and dissolve without heat. The product should measure exactly twelve fluid ounces.

*Dose.*—From one to two fluid drachms or more. Each fluid drachm contains one grain of the phosphate of iron.

## FERRI SULPHAS.

### SULPHATE OF IRON.

Sulphate of Iron, $FeO,SO_3+7HO$ or $\mathbf{FeSO_4.7H_2O}$, obtained by subjecting iron wire to the action of dilute sulphuric acid, and evaporating the solution to crystallization. *Characters.*—Oblique rhombic prisms, of a pale greenish-blue colour and styptic taste; insoluble in rectified spirit, soluble in water. The aqueous solution is clear, gives a white precipitate with chloride of barium, a blue one with the red, and a nearly white or light-blue one with the yellow prussiate of potash. *Test.*—It gives no precipitate with sulphuretted hydrogen when previously acidulated.

*Properties.*—Powerful chalybeate tonic; astringent, emmenagogue, antiperiodic, and anthelmintic. In large doses, poisonous. Locally applied, astringent, stimulant.

*Therapeutic Uses.*—Anæmia and anæmic states generally, chlorosis, amenorrhœa, leucorrhœa, ulcer of the stomach, splenic enlargement, intermittent fevers, periodical hemicrania, hypochondriasis, chronic stage of hooping cough, and tænia, are the affections in which it has been principally administered internally. Locally it has been applied to erysipelatous surfaces, chancres, hæmorrhoids attended with discharge, prolapsus of the rectum, cancer of the uterus, &c.

*Dose.*—From one to five grains or more, twice or thrice daily.

*Preparations.*—**Dried Sulphate of Iron** (*Ferri Sulphas Exsiccata*). Take of Sulphate of Iron, four ounces. Expose it in a porcelain or iron dish to a moderate heat, which may be finally raised to 400°, until aqueous vapour ceases to be given off. Reduce the residue to a fine powder, and preserve it in a stoppered bottle.

*Dose.*—From half a grain to two grains in the form of pill. Three grains are equal to $4\frac{8}{10}$ of the crystallized Sulphate of Iron.

**Compound Iron Mixture** (*Mistura Ferri composita*). Take of Sulphate of Iron, twenty-five grains; Carbonate of Potash, thirty grains; Myrrh, Refined Sugar, of each, sixty grains; Spirit of Nutmeg, four fluid drachms; Rose Water, nine fluid ounces and a half. Reduce the myrrh to powder, add the carbonate of potash and sugar, and triturate them with a small quantity of the rose water so as to form a thin paste, then gradually add more rose water and the spirit of nutmeg, continuing the trituration and further addition of rose water until about eight fluid ounces of a milky liquid is formed, then add the sulphate of iron dissolved in the remainder of the rose water, mix them together thoroughly, and preserve the mixture as much as possible from contact with the air.

*Dose*—From one to two fluid ounces twice or thrice daily; a very eligible chalybeate tonic in anæmia, amenorrhœa, and chlorosis.

## FERRI SULPHAS GRANULATA.

### Granulated Sulphate of Iron.

This salt differs only from the sulphate in the mode of preparation, occurring in small granular crystals of a pale greenish blue colour. In other respects it corresponds in character and tests with sulphate of iron. Its properties, uses, and doses correspond with those of the latter salt.

## LIQUOR FERRI PERSULPHATIS.

### Solution of Persulphate of Iron.

Take of Sulphate of Iron, eight ounces; Sulphuric Acid, Nitric Acid, of each, six fluid drachms; Distilled Water, twelve fluid ounces, or a sufficiency. Add the sulphuric acid to ten ounces of the water, and dissolve the sulphate of iron in the mixture with the aid of heat. Mix the nitric acid with the remaining two ounces of the water, and add the dilute acid to the solution of the sulphate of iron. Concentrate the whole by boiling, until, by the sudden disengagement of ruddy vapours, the liquid ceases to be black, and acquires a red colour. A drop of the solution is now to be tested with red prussiate of potash; and, if a blue precipitate forms, a few additional drops of nitric acid should be added, and the boiling renewed, in order that the whole of the sulphate may be converted into persulphate of iron. When the solution is cold, make the quantity eleven fluid ounces by the addition, if necessary, of distilled water. *Characters.*—A dense solution of a dark-red colour, inodorous and very astringent, miscible in all proportions with alcohol and water. Diluted with ten volumes of water it gives a white precipitate with chloride of barium, and a blue precipitate with yellow, but not with red, prussiate of potash. *Tests.*—Specific gravity, 1·441. One fluid drachm diluted with two ounces of distilled water gives, upon the addition of an excess of solution of ammonia, a precipitate, which, when well washed and incinerated, weighs 11·44 grains.

*Properties and Uses.*—Not prescribed internally. It is employed in the preparation of Ferri et Ammoniæ Citras, Ferri et Quiniæ Citras, Ferri Oxidum Magneticum, Ferri Peroxidum Humidum, Ferrum Tartaratum, and Tinctura Ferri Acetatis.

*Preparation.*—**Tincture of Acetate of Iron** (*Tinctura Ferri Acetatis*). Take of Solution of Persulphate of Iron, two fluid ounces and a half; Acetate of Potash, two ounces; Rectified Spirit, a sufficiency. Dissolve the acetate of potash in ten fluid ounces, and add the persulphate of iron to eight fluid ounces of the spirit; then mix the two solutions in a two-pint bottle, and shake them well together, repeating the agitation several times during an hour. Put the tincture, with the precipitated salt contained in it, upon a filter, and when the liquid has ceased to run through, put as much rectified spirit upon the filter as will make the filtered product measure one pint.

*Dose.*—From five to thirty minims.

## LIQUOR FERRI PERCHLORIDI FORTIOR.

### STRONG SOLUTION OF PERCHLORIDE OF IRON.

(*Liquor Ferri Perchloridi, Brit. Ph.* 1864.)

An aqueous solution of the Perchloride of Iron obtained by the action of hydrochloric acid on iron wire. *Characters.* —An orange-brown solution, with a strong styptic taste; miscible with water and rectified spirit in all proportions. Diluted with water it is precipitated white by nitrate of silver, and blue by yellow prussiate of potash, but not at all by red prussiate of potash. *Tests.*—Specific gravity, 1·338. A fluid drachm of it diluted with two fluid ounces of water gives, upon the addition of an excess of solution of ammonia, a reddish-brown precipitate, which, when well washed and incinerated, weighs 15·62 grains.

*Properties.*—Powerful astringent and styptic.

*Therapeutic Uses.*—Aneurisms, varicose veins, and nævi materni have been successfully treated by injections of this solution. The practice is not unattended with danger. It has also been applied with advantage in cases of hospital gangrene, fungous tumours, uterine polypi, hæmorrhoids, purulent ophthalmia, onychia, and as a means of arresting hæmorrhage. For internal use the diluted solution or tincture is preferable.

*Dose.*—From two to six drops in syrup or water.

*Preparations.* — **Solution of the Perchloride of Iron** (*Liquor Ferri Perchloridi*). Take of Strong Solution of Perchloride of Iron, five fluid ounces; Distilled Water, fifteen fluid ounces. Mix.

*Dose.*—From ten to thirty minims.

**Tincture of Perchloride of Iron** (*Tinctura Ferri Perchloridi*). Take of Solution of Perchloride of Iron, five fluid ounces; Rectified Spirit, fifteen fluid ounces. Mix, and preserve in a stoppered bottle. *Test.*—Specific gravity, 0·992. This tincture has one fourth of the strength of Tinctura Ferri Sesquichloridi, *Dub.*

*Properties.*—Similar to those of Liquor Ferri Perchloridi. Internally administered it is valuable tonic and diuretic.

*Therapeutic Uses.*—In atonic hæmorrhages, chronic exhausting discharges, diabetes, enuresis, retention of urine from spasmodic stricture of the urethra, albuminuria, diphtheria, erysipelas, purpura hæmorrhagica, and in the profuse perspiration of phthisis, it has often been found effectual. Locally it has been applied to control hæmorrhage, as that from leech bites, and as a stimulant to foul ulcers.

*Dose.*—From ten to thirty minims or more.

[The above is the process for its preparation directed by the British Pharmacopœia; but it has been reported by the Medical Storekeeper at Madras to be objectionable, inasmuch as the solution invariably deposits a brown precipitate. This was not the case with the Tincture as prepared according to the London Pharmacopœia, which has been found to keep unchanged in tropical climates, and which is, therefore, to be preferred. It is as follows: Take of Sesquioxide (Hydrated Peroxide) of Iron, six ounces; Hydrochloric Acid, one pint; Rectified Spirit, three pints. Mix the sesquioxide of iron with the acid, and digest in a sand bath, frequently shaking. Lastly, add the spirit to the liquid when cold, and strain. The dose is the same as that of the corresponding preparation in the British Pharmacopœia.]

## FERRI IODIDUM.

### Iodide of Iron.

Iodide of Iron, FeI or **$FeI_2$**, with about 18 per cent. of water of crystallization, and a little oxide of iron. *Characters.*—Crystalline, green with a tinge of brown, inodorous, deliquescent, soluble in water, forming a slightly green solution, which gradually deposits a rust-coloured sediment, and acquires a red colour. *Test.*—It gives a copious blue precipitate with the red prussiate of potash, and one of a similar colour with mucilage of starch, on the addition of a minute quantity of chlorine.

*Properties.*—Valuable alterative tonic and emmenagogue.

*Therapeutic Uses.*—In scrofulous and tubercular affections generally, especially when conjoined with an anæmic state of the system, it is a remedy of much value. It has likewise been used with advantage in amenorrhœa, dysmenorrhœa, leucorrhœa, chlorosis, diabetes, and secondary syphilitic affections.

*Dose.*—From two to five grains or more.

*Preparations.*—**Syrup of Iodide of Iron** (*Syrupus Ferri Iodidi*). Take of Fine Iron Wire, one ounce; Iodine, two ounces; Refined Sugar, twenty-eight ounces; Distilled Water, thirteen fluid ounces. Prepare a syrup by dissolving the sugar in ten ounces of the water with the aid of heat. Digest the iodine and the iron wire in a flask, at a gentle heat, with the remaining three ounces of the water, till the froth becomes white; then filter the liquid while still hot into the syrup, and mix. The product should weigh two pounds eleven ounces, and should have the specific gravity 1·385.

*Dose.*—From one half to one fluid drachm. One fluid drachm contains four grains and a half of the Iodide.

**Pill of Iodide of Iron** (*Pilula Ferri Iodidi*).—Take of Fine Iron Wire, forty grains; Iodine, eighty grains; Refined sugar, in powder, seventy grains; Liquorice Root, in powder, one hundred and forty grains; Distilled Water, fifty minims. Agitate the iron with the iodine and the water in a strong stoppered ounce phial, until the froth becomes white. Pour the fluid upon the sugar in a mortar, triturate briskly, and gradually add the liquorice.

*Dose.*—From three to ten grains or more. Three grains contain one grain of the Iodide.

## LIQUOR FERRI PERNITRATIS.

### Solution of Pernitrate of Iron.

Pernitrate of Iron in solution, prepared by dissolving iron wire in nitric acid, and diluting with distilled water. *Characters.*—A clear liquid of a reddish-brown colour, slightly acid and astringent to the taste; gives a blue precipitate with the yellow prussiate of potash. When to a little of it, placed in a test tube, half its volume of pure sulphuric acid is added, and then a solution of sulphate of iron is poured on, the whole assumes a dark-brown colour. *Tests.*—Specific gravity, 1·107. One fluid drachm, treated with an excess of solution of ammonia, gives a precipitate which, when washed, dried, and incinerated, weighs 2·6 grains. It gives no precipitate with the red prussiate of potash.

*Properties and Uses.*—Similar to those of Liquor Ferri Perchloridi; especially serviceable as an astringent in diarrhœa.

*Dose.*—From ten to forty minims, freely diluted.

## FERRI ARSENIAS.

### Arseniate of Iron.

Arseniate of Iron, $3FeO, AsO_5$, partially peroxidized, prepared by decomposing sulphate of iron by arseniate of soda. *Characters.*—A tasteless amorphous powder of a green colour, insoluble in water, but readily dissolved by hydrochloric acid. This solution gives a copious light-blue precipitate with the yellow prussiate of potash, and a still more abundant one of a deeper colour with the red prussiate of potash.

A small quantity, boiled with an excess of caustic soda and filtered, gives, when exactly neutralized by nitric acid, a brick-red precipitate, on the addition of solution of nitrate of silver. *Tests.*—The solution in hydrochloric acid, when diluted, gives no precipitate with chloride of barium. Twenty grains, dissolved in an excess of hydrochloric acid diluted with water, continue to give a blue precipitate with the red prussiate of potash until at least seventeen measures of the volumetric solution of bichromate of potash have been added.

*Properties.*—Alterative tonic, supposed to possess the combined properties of iron and arsenic.

*Therapeutic Uses.*—In chronic skin diseases, especially those of a herpetic and squamous character, it is a remedy of considerable power. It has also been employed in elephantiasis, leprosy, cancer, and lupus.

*Dose.*—From one sixteenth to one half of a grain, in the form of pill. Externally it may be applied in the form of ointment, in the proportion of twenty grains to one ounce of simple ointment.

## FERRI ET AMMONIÆ CITRAS.

### Citrate of Iron and Ammonia.

(*Ferri Ammonio-Citras, Dubl. Ph.*)

Citrate of Iron and Ammonia, a combination of peroxide of iron and ammonia with citric acid. *Characters.*—Thin transparent scales of a deep red colour, slightly sweetish and astringent in taste. It feebly reddens litmus paper; is soluble in water, but almost insoluble in rectified spirit. Heated with solution of potash it evolves ammonia, and deposits peroxide of iron. The alkaline solution from which the iron has separated does not, when slightly supersaturated with acetic acid, give any crystalline deposit. *Test.*—When incinerated with exposure to air, it leaves not less than twenty-seven per cent. of peroxide of iron.

*Properties.*—A mild and valuable chalybeate tonic.

*Therapeutic Uses.*—In debility after exhausting diseases, and in the anæmic states of childhood, tabes mesenterica, and tubercular affections generally, it is especially adapted by the mildness and unirritating nature of its operation.

*Dose.*—From five to ten grains twice or thrice daily.

*Preparation.*—**Wine of Citrate of Iron** (*Vinum Ferri Citratis*). Take of Citrate of Iron and Ammonia, one hundred and sixty grains; Sherry or Orange

Wine, one pint. Dissolve, and let the solution remain for three days in a closed vessel, shaking it occasionally; afterwards filter.

*Dose.*—From one to four fluid drachms.

## FERRI ET QUINIÆ CITRAS.

### CITRATE OF IRON AND QUININE.

Citrate of Iron and Quinine, a combination of citric acid, peroxide of iron, protoxide of iron, and quinia. *Characters.*—Thin scales, of a greenish golden-yellow colour, somewhat deliquescent, and entirely soluble in cold water. The solution is very slightly acid, and is precipitated reddish-brown by solution of soda, white by solution of ammonia, blue by the yellow and red prussiates of potash, and greyish-black by tannic acid. The taste is bitter as well as chalybeate. *Tests.*—When burned with exposure to air, it leaves a residue which, when moistened with water, is not alkaline to test paper. Fifty grains dissolved in a fluid ounce of water, and treated with a slight excess of ammonia, give a white precipitate, which, when collected on a filter and dried, weighs eight grains. The precipitate is almost entirely soluble in pure ether, and, when burned, leaves but a minute residue.

*Properties and Uses.*—Similar to those of the Citrate of Iron and Ammonia, but more potent as a tonic; antiperiodic; well adapted for the treatment of splenic enlargements.

*Dose.*—From five to ten grains, twice a day or oftener.

## FERRUM TARTARATUM.

### TARTRATED IRON.

(*Ferri Potassio-Tartras, Lond. Ph.; Ferrum Tartarizatum, Edin. and Dubl. Ph.*)

Tartrated Iron, a compound of peroxide of iron and potash with tartaric acid. *Characters.*—Thin transparent scales of a deep garnet colour; slightly sweetish and astringent in taste; soluble in water, and sparingly soluble in spirit. The aqueous solution, when acidulated with hydrochloric acid, gives a copious blue precipitate with the yellow, but none with the red prussiate of potash. When the salt is boiled with solution of soda, peroxide of iron separates, but no ammonia is evolved; and the filtered solution, when slightly acidulated by acetic acid, gives, as it cools, a crystalline deposit. *Tests.*—By incinerating fifty grains of it at a red heat, washing what is left with distilled water, and again incinerating, a residue of peroxide of iron is obtained, weighing 15 grains.

*Properties and Uses.*—Similar to those of the Citrate of Iron and Ammonia; anthelmintic.

*Dose.*—From five to ten grains, in solution.

## MISTURA FERRI AROMATICA.

### Aromatic Mixture of Iron.

Take of Pale-Cinchona Bark, in powder, one ounce; Calumba Root, in coarse powder, half an ounce; Cloves, bruised, quarter of an ounce; Fine Iron Wire, half an ounce; Compound Tincture of Cardamoms, three fluid ounces; Tincture of Orange Peel, half a fluid ounce; Peppermint Water, a sufficiency. Macerate the cinchona bark, calumba root, cloves, and iron with twelve fluid ounces of the peppermint water in a closed vessel, for three days, agitating occasionally; then filter the liquid, adding as much peppermint water to the filtrate as will make the product measure twelve and a half fluid ounces; to this add the tinctures, and preserve the mixture in a well stopped bottle.

*Dose.*—From one to two fluid ounces, twice or thrice daily, as a mild chalybeate tonic.

## VINUM FERRI.

### Wine of Iron. Steel Wine.

Take of fine Iron Wire, one ounce; Sherry, one pint. Macerate for thirty days in a closed vessel, the iron being almost, but not quite, wholly immersed in the wine, and the vessel frequently shaken, and the stopper removed; then filter.

*Dose.*—From one to four fluid drachms. A very eligible mild chalybeate tonic, well adapted for children and women.

[The natives of India have a great variety of ways of preparing iron for medicinal uses. Two of these processes are given by Dr. Heyne (*Tracts on India*, p. 167), but neither requires any particular notice. In both, the resulting compound appears to be an impure oxide. Their value as tonics is well known. An impure sulphate is sold in almost every bazaar, and may be rendered fit for medicinal use by dissolving in water acidulated with sulphuric acid, filtering and evaporating to crystallization.]

## CUPRUM.

### Copper.

*Symbol*, Cu ; *At. weight*, 31·75 ; **Cu=63·5**

Copper exists extensively through the mineral kingdom, sometimes native, but generally combined with sulphur (as *Copper Pyrites and Copper Glance*), and with oxygen (as *Red and Black Oxide*). It is the only metal of a red colour ; malleable, ductile, and of Sp. gr. 8·9 ; melts at 1996°. Its chief solvent is nitric acid Pure copper foil is employed as a test for arsenic, nitrate of silver, and mercury.

## CUPRI SULPHAS.

### Sulphate of Copper.

Sulphate of Copper, $CuO,SO_3+5HO$ or $\mathbf{CuSO_4,5H_2O}$, may be obtained by heating sulphuric acid and copper together, dissolving the soluble product in hot water, and evaporating the solution until crystallization takes place on cooling. *Characters.*—A blue crystalline salt, in oblique rhombic prisms, soluble in water, forming a pale blue solution which strongly reddens litmus. The aqueous solution gives with chloride of barium a white precipitate insoluble in hydrochloric acid, and a maroon-red precipitate with yellow prussiate of potash. *Test.*—If an aqueous solution of the salt be mixed with twice its volume of solution of chlorine, and solution of ammonia be added, the precipitate formed by the first addition of the ammonia will be dissolved by a further and sufficient addition of the alkali, and a violet blue solution will be produced, leaving nothing undissolved.

*Properties.*—Tonic, astringent, emetic; in large doses an irritant poison. Locally applied in substance to a denuded or granulating surface, mildly caustic, styptic, and in solution stimulant.

*Therapeutic Uses.*—In chronic dysentery and diarrhœa it is a remedy of great value; in chorea, epilepsy, and obstinate hysteria, it has also been found useful. Locally it has been applied in solution in gonorrhœa, leucorrhœa, purulent ophthalmia, chronic skin diseases; weak, irritable, and indolent ulcerations; superficial hæmorrhage; and, in substance, to cancrum oris, aphthous ulcerations, exuberant granulations, and granular conjunctivitis.

*Dose.*—From a quarter of a grain to two grains as a tonic and astringent, and from four to twelve grains as an emetic. As a collyrium or injection, the strength may vary from two to ten grains to the ounce of fluid.

[Hindú practitioners place much reliance on some of their rudely prepared salts of copper, which for the most part are obtained by the action of tamarind, lime, or other vegetable acid juice on metallic copper. None of them seem to deserve attention. The sulphate (*Nīl tutiya,* Hind.) is met with in most bazaars, generally of fair quality. It may be further purified, if required, by dissolving in water, filtering and evaporating to crystallization.]

## HYDRARGYRUM.

### MERCURY.

*Symbol,* Hg; *At. weight,* 100; *or* **Hg=200.**

Mercury is found native, but chiefly as persulphide or cinnabar; it is the only metal which retains its fluidity at ordinary temperatures; brilliantly lustrous, and easily divisible into spherical globules. Boils at 662°, and volatilizes at a heat below that of visible redness, leaving no residue. Sp. gr. 13·59. Chief solvents, nitric and sulphuric acids.

*Properties.*—In the metallic state apparently inert, as large quantities of it have been swallowed without producing any sensible physiological effects. Occasionally, however, when subjected to the action of the intestinal secretions, it forms with them combinations possessed of powerful properties. Persons much exposed to the vapour of mercury are subject to a peculiar train of nervous affections, which not unfrequently prove fatal. When rubbed into the skin, or administered internally in a state of minute subdivision, it acts energetically on the system; one of the most uniform and well marked effects being a swollen and ulcerated condition of the gums, attended with copious salivation, and a peculiar odour of the breath, which, in the aggregate, form the state known as mercurial ptyalism. In general terms mercury may be described as alterative, cholagogue, purgative, and sialogogue; but further remarks on these properties and on its therapeutic uses are reserved for individual mercurial preparations.

*Preparations.* — **Mercurial Pill, Blue Pill** (*Pilula Hydrargyri*). Take of Mercury, two ounces; Confection of Roses, three ounces; Liquorice Root, in fine powder, one ounce. Rub the mercury with the confection of roses, until metallic globules are no longer visible; then add the liquorice, and mix the whole well together.

*Properties.*—Valuable alterative, cholagogue, and aperient.

*Therapeutic Uses.*—For syphilis and syphilitic affections, and for inflammatory and other states of the system where mercurials are indicated, and in which rapid operation is not an object, it is especially adapted. In dyspepsia attended with hepatic derangement, it forms an excellent adjunct to other purgatives and cholagogues.

*Dose.*—From two to three grains twice or thrice daily as an alterative; from five to eight grains as a purgative. Three grains of the pill contain one grain of mercury.

**Mercury with Chalk** (*Hydrargyrum cum Cretâ*). Take of Mercury, by weight, one ounce; Prepared Chalk, two ounces. Rub the Mercury and Chalk in a porcelain mortar until metallic globules cease to be visible to the naked eye, and the mixture acquires a uniform grey colour. *Characters.*—A powder of a light-grey colour; free from grittiness; insoluble in water; hydrochloric acid dissolves the chalk with effervescence, leaving the mercury in a finely divided state. *Tests.*—The solution formed with hydrochloric acid is not precipitated by the addition of chloride of tin.

*Properties and Therapeutic Uses.*— Similar to those of Pilula Hydrargyri, but milder in operation. It is especially adapted for those diseases of infants in which mercurials are indicated.

*Dose.*—From five to fifteen grains for adults; from two to four grains for children. Generally given in combination with other remedies. Three grains contain one grain of mercury.

**Ointment of Mercury, Mercurial Ointment** (*Unguentum Hydrargyri*). Take of Mercury, one pound; Prepared Lard, one pound; Prepared Suet, one ounce. Rub them together until metallic globules cease to be visible.

*Properties and Therapeutic Uses.*—Analogous to those of Pilula Hydrargyri as a constitutional remedy, the mode of administration being by means of the skin, in place of, as in the case of mercurial pill, by the stomach. Inunction with it over an extended or denuded surface, or for a prolonged time, induces salivation; hence it has been used as an adjunct to other forms of mercury administered internally, when the object has been speedily to affect the system. In cases where mercurials are necessary, and, from irritability of the stomach or other causes, they cannot be exhibited internally, inunction of this ointment may be substituted. As a local remedy it has been applied to syphilitic ulcers, enlargement of the joints, and also to tumours of various kinds, with the view of stimulating the absorbents, and thus obtaining their resolution.

It forms an ingredient in Linimentum Hydrargyri, Suppositoria Hydrargyri, and Unguentum Hydrargyri compositum.

**Compound Ointment of Mercury** (*Unguentum Hydrargyri compositum*). Take of Ointment of Mercury, six ounces; Yellow Wax, Olive Oil, of each, three ounces; Camphor, one ounce and a half. Melt the wax with a gentle heat, and add the oil; then, when the mixture is nearly cold, add the camphor in powder, and the ointment of mercury, and mix the whole thoroughly together.

**Liniment of Mercury, Mercurial Liniment** (*Linimentum Hydrargyri*). Take of Ointment of

Mercury, one ounce; Solution of Ammonia, one fluid ounce; Liniment of Camphor, one fluid ounce. Liquify the ointment of mercury in the liniment of camphor with a gentle heat, then add the solution of ammonia gradually, and mix with agitation.

*Properties and Uses.*—Analogous to those of Ointment of Mercury, but more stimulant in its operation.

**Mercurial Plaster** (*Emplastrum Hydrargyri*). Take of Mercury, three ounces; Olive Oil, one fluid drachm; Sublimed Sulphur, eight grains; Lead Plaster, six ounces. Heat the Oil, and add the sulphur to it gradually, stirring until they unite; with this mixture triturate the mercury until globules are no longer visible, then add the lead plaster, previously liquified, and mix the whole thoroughly.

A useful application in hydarthrosis, buboes, tumours, and syphilitic rheumatism.

**Plaster of Ammoniacum with Mercury**. *See* AMMONIACUM.

**Mercurial Suppositories** (*Suppositoria Hydrargyri*). Take of Ointment of Mercury, sixty grains; Benzoated Lard, White Wax, of each, twenty grains; Oil of Theobroma, eighty grains. Melt the benzoated lard, wax, and oil of theobroma with a gentle heat, then add the ointment of mercury, and having mixed all the ingredients thoroughly, without applying more heat, immediately pour the mixture, before it has congealed, into suitable moulds of the capacity of fifteen grains; or the fluid mixture may be allowed to cool, and then be divided into twelve equal parts, each of which shall be made into a conical or other convenient form for a suppository.

Each suppository contains five grains of mercurial ointment. Mercury may by this means be introduced into the system when from any cause it cannot be administered by mouth; or may be used, in addition to internal administration, when it is desired to bring the system speedily under the influence of the remedy.

## HYDRARGYRI OXIDUM RUBRUM.

### RED OXIDE OF MERCURY.

(*Hydrargyri Nitrico-oxidum, Lond. Ph.; Red Precipitate.*)

The Oxide of Mercury, HgO or **HgO**, obtained by decomposing the nitrate by heat. *Characters.*—An orange-red powder, readily dissolved by hydrochloric acid, and yielding a solution which, with caustic potash added in excess, gives a yellow precipitate, and with solution of ammonia a white precipitate. *Tests.*—Entirely volatilized by a heat under redness, being at the same time decomposed into mercury and oxygen. If this be done in a test tube no orange vapours are perceived.

*Properties.* — Irritant and escharotic. Not administered internally.

*Preparation.*—**Ointment of Red Oxide of Mercury** (*Unguentum Hydrargyri Oxidi Rubri, Unguentum Hydrargyri Nitrico-Oxidi, Lond. Ph.*) Take of Red Oxide of Mercury, in very fine powder, sixty-two grains; Yellow Wax, quarter of an ounce; Oil of Almonds, three quarters of an ounce. Melt the wax at a gentle heat, mix the oil with it, and when the mixture is nearly cold, add the oxide of mercury, and mix the whole thoroughly together.

A valuable local application to indolent syphilitic ulcerations, the ulcerations of rupia, and some obstinate skin diseases, and in ophthalmia tarsi, and chronic conjunctivitis.

## HYDRARGYRI SULPHAS.

### Sulphate of Mercury. Persulphate of Mercury.

Sulphate of Mercury, $HgO,SO_3$ or $\mathbf{HgSO_4}$, obtained by the action of sulphuric acid on mercury. A white crystalline heavy powder rendered yellow by affusion of water; entirely volatilized by heat.

*Properties.*—Escharotic; only employed in the preparation of calomel and corrosive sublimate.

## HYDRARGYRI SUBCHLORIDUM.

### Subchloride of Mercury.

(*Hydrargyri Chloridum, Lond. Ph.; Calomelas, Brit. Ph.* 1864; *Calomel.*)

Subchloride of Mercury, $Hg_2Cl$ or $\mathbf{Hg_2Cl_2}$, obtained by submitting to sublimation a mixture of sulphate of mercury, mercury, and chloride of sodium. *Characters.*—A dull white, heavy, and nearly tasteless powder, rendered yellowish by trituration in a mortar; insoluble in water, spirit, or ether. Digested with solution of potash, it becomes black; and the clear solution, acidulated with nitric acid, gives a copious white precipitate with nitrate of silver. *Tests.*—Entirely volatilized by a sufficient heat. Warm ether which has been shaken with it in a bottle leaves, on evaporation, no residue.

*Properties.*—Antiphlogistic, purgative, cholagogue; in small doses, alterative, sialagogue, anthelmintic.

*Therapeutic Uses.*—In acute sthenic, inflammatory, and febrile affections generally, it has been extensively employed as an antiphlogistic; and though less reliance is placed on it now in this character than formerly, still in the early stages of this class of diseases it is valued for the sake of its purgative operation. Amongst the other diseases in which it has been employed with more or less benefit are cholera, jaundice, biliary derangement, dysentery, dropsical affections, neuralgia, tetanus, hydrocephalus, apoplexy, cephalagia, some forms of deafness, obstinate skin diseases, periostitis, and most affections of a syphilitic origin.

*Dose.*—From one to two grains, frequently repeated, as an alterative; from two to six grains or more as a purgative, its operation being aided by other remedies of the same class. It is occasionally employed in the form of fumigation; for this purpose from twenty to thirty grains suffice, applied by means of an appropriate apparatus.

*Preparations.*—**Compound Pill of Subchloride of Mercury** (*Pilula Hydrargyri Subchloridi composita*; *Pilula Calomelanos composita, Brit. Ph.* 1864.) Take Subchloride of Mercury, Sulphurated Antimony, of each, one ounce; Guaiacum Resin, in powder, two ounces; Castor Oil, one fluid ounce, or a sufficiency. Triturate the subchloride of mercury with the antimony, then add the guaiacum resin and castor oil, and beat the whole into a uniform mass.

An excellent alterative in syphilitic, hepatic, and other affections, in doses of from five to ten grains daily. It has long enjoyed a popular reputation under the name *Plummers' Pill.*

**Ointment of Subchloride of Mercury** (*Unguentum Hydrargyri Subchloridi; Ung. Calomelanos. Brit. Ph.* 1864.) Take of Subchloride of Mercury, eighty grains; Prepared Lard, one ounce. Mix thoroughly.

A valuable application in many skin diseases, especially in those of a syphilitic origin.

**Black Mercurial Lotion** (*Lotio Hydrargyri nigra*). Take of Subchloride of Mercury, thirty grains; Solution of Lime, ten fluid ounces. Mix.

Much employed as a local application to chancres and other syphilitic ulcerations.

## HYDRARGYRI PERCHLORIDUM.

### PERCHLORIDE OF MERCURY.

(*Hydrargyri Bichloridum, Lond. Ph.; Hydrargyri Corrosivum Sublimatum, Brit. Ph.* 1864; *Sublimatus Corrosivus, Edin. Ph.; Corrosive Sublimate.*)

Perchloride of Mercury, HgCl or $HgCl_2$, obtained by submitting to distillation a mixture of sulphate of mercury, chloride of sodium, and black oxide of manganese. *Characters.* — In heavy colourless masses of prismatic crystals, possessing a highly acrid metallic taste; more soluble in alcohol, and still more so in ether, than in water. Its aqueous solution gives a yellow precipitate with caustic potash, a white precipitate with ammonia, and a curdy white precipitate with nitrate of silver. *Test.*—When heated, it sublimes without decomposing, or leaving any residue.

*Properties.*—In small and continued doses it is a valuable alterative, stimulating the urinary, cutaneous, and salivary secretions; in large doses, powerful irritant poison. Locally applied in substance, mildly caustic; in solution, stimulant.

*Therapeutic Uses.*—In constitutional syphilis, and in eruptions, epilepsy, ophthalmia, cynanche, rheumatism and other affections connected therewith, it is a remedy of established value. Amongst the other diseases in which it has been employed are hydrocephalus, dropsical affections, glandular enlargements, hemeralopia, and hepatic affections. Locally, in solution, it has been used in gonorrhœa, gleet, and leucorrhœa, (as an injection,) in various forms of ophthalmia (as a collyrium), and in many obstinate skin diseases (as a lotion or wash), It is an effectual destroyer of pediculi. Its application to too extended a surface is objectionable, from danger of the absorption of the mercury.

*Dose.*—From one-sixteenth to one-eighth of a grain, twice or thrice daily, in solution. For external application, the strength of the solution varies from one-half grain to two or three grains to an ounce of distilled water.

[The natives of India are acquainted with several mercurial preparations, which they use extensively in the treatment of disease. For the most part they employ impure chlorides prepared by very crude processes. Two of these, *Rassapuspum* and *Shavirum*, have been examined by Sir W. O'Shaughnessy (Bengal Pharm., p. 342): the first he found to be a sub-chloride, and the latter a perchloride of mercury. They are evidently unsafe, and, as repeated experience has shown, highly irritant; they should never be employed in medicine. For a further account of the mercurial preparations known to the natives of India, consult Ainslie's *Materia Medica of Hindoostan*, p. 105, and Heynes' *Tracts on India*.]

*Preparations.*—**Solution of Perchloride of Mercury** (*Liquor Hydrargyri Perchloridi*). Take Perchloride of Mercury and Chloride of Ammonium, of each, ten grains; Distilled Water, one pint. Dissolve.

*Dose.*—From thirty minims to one fluid drachm; each fluid ounce contains half a grain of the perchloride of mercury.

**Yellow Mercurial Lotion** (*Lotio Hydrargyri flava*). Take of Perchloride of Mercury, eighteen grains; Solution of Lime, ten fluid ounces. Mix.

A serviceable application in many syphilitic affections.

## HYDRARGYRUM AMMONIATUM.

### AMMONIATED MERCURY.

(*Hydrargyri Ammonio-Chloridum, Lond. Ph.*; *Hydrargyri Præcipitatum Album, Edin. Ph.*)

Ammoniated Mercury, $NH_2Hg_2Cl$ or $\mathbf{NH_2HgCl}$, obtained by the action of ammonia on a solution of corrosive sublimate. *Characters.*—An opaque white powder, on which cold water, alcohol, and ether have no action. *Tests.*—Digested with caustic potash, it evolves ammonia, acquiring a pale-yellow colour; and the fluid, filtered, and acidulated with nitric acid, gives a white precipitate with nitrate of silver. Boiled with a solution of chloride of tin it becomes grey by reduction of globules of metallic mercury. Entirely volatilized at a heat under redness.

*Properties and Uses.*—Stimulant. Only used externally in the form of ointment. In large doses, poisonous.

*Preparation.*—**Ointment of Ammoniated Mercury, White Precipitate Ointment** (*Unguentum Hydrargyri Ammoniati; Ung. Præcipitati Albi*). Take of Ammoniated Mercury, sixty-two grains; Simple Ointment, one ounce. Mix thoroughly.

A useful stimulant application in many chronic skin diseases, ophthalmia tarsi, and chronic conjunctivitis. It is also useful in destroying pediculi.

## HYDRARGYRI IODIDUM VIRIDE.

### GREEN IODIDE OF MERCURY.

*(Hydrargyri Iodidum, Lond. Ph.)*

Green Iodide of Mercury, $Hg_2I$ or $\mathbf{Hg_2I_2}$, obtained by triturating together Iodine and Mercury, with the addition of rectified spirit, until metallic globules are no longer visible, and the mixture assumes a green colour. The product thus obtained should be dried in a dark room, on filtering paper, by simple exposure to the air, and preserved in an opaque bottle. *Characters.*—A dull-green powder insoluble in water, which darkens in colour upon exposure to light. *Tests.*—When gradually heated in a test tube, it yields a yellow sublimate, which upon friction becomes red, while globules of metallic mercury are left in the bottom of the tube. Entirely volatilized by a heat under redness. When it is shaken in a tube with ether, nothing is dissolved.

*Properties.*—Alterative and stimulant; in large doses, an irritant poison.

*Therapeutic Uses.*—In syphilis, whether primary or secondary, occurring in persons of a scrofulous diathesis, it is a remedy of much value. It is used also with benefit in lepra, psoriasis and other obstinate skin diseases, neuralgia, and chronic affections of the liver.

*Dose.*—From one to three grains in the form of pill. For ointments the strength may vary from fifteen to twenty grains to an ounce of simple ointment.

## HYDRARGYRI IODIDUM RUBRUM.

### RED IODIDE OF MERCURY.

*(Hydrargyri Biniodidi, Edin. Ph.)*

Red Iodide of Mercury, $HgI$ or $\mathbf{HgI_2}$, obtained by decomposing corrosive sublimate by iodide of potassium. *Characters.*—A crystalline powder of a vermillion colour, becoming yellow when gently heated over a lamp on a sheet of paper; almost insoluble in water, dissolving sparingly in alcohol, but freely in ether, or in an aqueous solutionof iodide of potassium. *Tests.*—When digested with solution of soda it assumes a reddish-brown colour, and the fluid, cleared by filtration and mixed with solution of starch gives a blue precipitate on being acidulated with nitric acid. Entirely volatilized by a heat under redness, and entirely soluble in ether.

*Properties and Uses.*—Analogous to those of Hydrargyri Iodidum Viride, but more energetic in its operation, approaching nearer to corrosive sublimate. Externally applied it has been found effectual in causing the absorption of goitre, and also of elephantoid swellings.

*Dose.*—One sixteenth of a grain, gradually increased to a quarter of a grain, in the form of pill, or dissolved in alcohol.

*Preparation.*—**Ointment of Red Iodide of Mercury** (*Unguentum Hydrargyri Iodidi Rubri*). Take of Red Iodide of Mercury, in very fine powder, sixteen grains; Simple Ointment, one ounce. Mix thoroughly.

A powerfully stimulant application to glandular swellings, tumours, bronchocele, and chronic skin diseases.

## LIQUOR HYDRARGYRI NITRATIS ACIDUS.

### ACID SOLUTION OF NITRATE OF MERCURY.

A Solution of Mercury in Nitric Acid. *Characters.*—A colourless and strongly acid solution, which gives a yellow precipitate with solution of potash added in excess. If a crystal of sulphate of iron be dropped into it, in a little time the salt of iron, and the liquid in its vicinity, acquire a dark colour. *Tests.*—Specific gravity, 2·246. Does not give any precipitate when a little of it is dropped into hydrochloric acid diluted with twice its volume of water.

*Properties.*—Powerful caustic and escharotic. Never given internally.

*Therapeutic Uses.*—In cancerous and malignant ulcers, and in some obstinate skin diseases, it has been employed locally with advantage, but it is too powerful in its action for ordinary cases.

*Preparation.*—**Ointment of Nitrate of Mercury, Citrine Ointment** (*Unguentum Hydrargyri Nitratis, Unguentum Citrinum, Edin. Ph.*) Take of Mercury, by weight, four ounces; Nitric Acid, twelve fluid ounces; Prepared Lard, fifteen ounces; Olive Oil, thirty-two fluid ounces. Dissolve the mercury in the nitric acid with the aid of a gentle heat; melt the lard in the oil, by a steam or water bath, in a porcelain vessel capable of holding six times the quantity; and, while the mixture is hot, add the solution of mercury, also hot, mixing them thoroughly. If the mixture do not froth up, increase the heat till this occurs. Keep it stirred until it is cold.

A very useful stimulant application in chronic diseases of the skin, to foul, indolent, and phagedenic ulcerations, and to ophthalmia tarsi and other affections of the eyelids. In many cases, especially in children and persons with delicate skins, the milder ointment is to be preferred.

**Milder Ointment of Nitrate of Mercury** (*Unguentum Hydrargyri Nitratis Mitius, Lond. Ph.*) Take of Ointment of Nitrate of Mercury, one ounce; Lard, seven ounces. Mix thoroughly. To be used freshly prepared.

## ARGENTUM. *Symbol*, Ag; *At. weight*, 108.

### SILVER.

Silver is extensively diffused throughout the mineral kingdom, occurring either in an almost pure state (*Native Silver*), or variously combined with sulphur (as *Silver-glance*), chlorine, &c. In its metallic state it is apparently inert. It is a white lustrous metal of sp. gr. 10·53. It melts at 1873°. Its chief solvent is nitric acid.

## ARGENTUM PURIFICATUM.

### REFINED SILVER.

Pure metallic silver. *Test.*—If ammonia be added in excess to an acid solution of the metal in nitric acid, the resulting fluid exhibits neither colour nor turbidity.

## ARGENTI NITRAS.

### NITRATE OF SILVER.

Nitrate of Silver, $AgO,NO_5$ or $\mathbf{AgNO_3}$, obtained by dissolving refined silver in nitric acid. *Characters.*—Colourless tabular right rhombic prisms, or white cylindrical rods; soluble in distilled water, and in rectified spirit. The solution gives with hydrochloric acid a curdy white precipitate, which darkens by exposure to light, and is soluble in solution of ammonia. A small fragment heated on charcoal with the blow-pipe, first melts, and then deflagrates, leaving behind a dull-white coating of metallic silver. *Tests.*—Ten grains dissolved in two fluid drachms of distilled water give with hydrochloric acid, a precipitate, which, when washed and thoroughly dried, weighs 8·44 grains. The filtrate when evaporated by a water bath leaves no residue.

*Properties.*—Tonic, anti-spasmodic, and sedative. In large doses, a corrosive poison. Externally applied, in substance, caustic and escharotic; in solution, stimulant.

*Therapeutic Uses.*—The principal diseases in which it has been administered internally with benefit are, the advanced stages of dysentery, diarrhœa, dyspepsia attended with gastralgia and pyrosis, cholera, ulceration of the stomach, chorea, epilepsy, the chronic stage of hooping cough, spasmodic asthma, hysterical headaches, and mercurial palsy. Externally it is a valuable application in hydarthrosis, chronic arthritis, erysipelas, chancres, and indolent, foul, and phagedenic ulcerations. Locally it has been applied in solution as an injection in gonorrhœa, gleet, leucorrhœa, catarrhal inflammation of the bladder, croup, diphtheria, aphonia, aphthous ulceration of the mouth, and cynanche maligna, and many obstinate skin diseases. In substance it has been applied to the urethra in stricture and in spermatorrhœa, and to the pustules in smallpox to prevent "pitting." In solution it also forms a valuable collyrium in various forms of ophthalmia. Applied in substance to poisoned wounds, as dissection wounds, the bites of rabid animals or snakes, so as thoroughly to cauterize the surface, it acts as a preventitive to further ill effects.

*Dose.*—From one sixth to one third of a grain or more, reduced to fine powder, and administered in the form of pill. The strength of solution for external or local application varies from two to ten grains or more to one ounce of distilled water.

## ARGENTI OXIDUM.

### Oxide of Silver.

Oxide of Silver, AgO or **$Ag_2O$**, obtained by decomposing nitrate of silver with solution of lime. *Characters.*—A brown powder, which at a low red heat gives off oxygen, and is reduced to the metallic state. It dissolves completely in nitric acid without the evolution of any gas, forming a solution which has the characters of nitrate of silver. *Test.*—29 grains heated to redness leave 27 grains of metallic silver.

*Properties.*—Analogous to those of the nitrate, but milder in its operation, and may be continued longer than the nitrate without danger of producing blue discoloration of the skin. Anthelmintic.

*Therapeutic Uses.*—In dyspepsia, gastralgia, gastrodynia, pyrosis, ulceration of the stomach, and hæmatemesis it has been found very beneficial. In atonic hæmorrhages and menorrhagia it has been used with advantage. Locally it has been applied to syphilitic and other obstinate ulcerations, ulceration of the cornea, ophthalmia tarsi, &c.

*Dose.*—From half a grain to two grains, twice or thrice daily, in the form of pill. The strength of ointments for external use varies from thirty to forty grains to an ounce of simple ointment.

# Articles and Solutions employed in Chemical Testing.

## ARTICLES AND SOLUTIONS EMPLOYED IN CHEMICAL TESTING.

**Alcohol. Absolute Alcohol.**—*Vide* p. 263.

**Benzol,** $C_{12}H_6$ or $C_6H_6$.—A colourless volatile liquid, obtained from coal tar. Specific gravity 0·85.

**Boracic Acid,** $BO_3,3HO$ or $HBO_2H_2O$.—*Tests*.—Soluble in alcohol. The solution burns with a green flame.

**Chloride of Barium,** $BaCl,2HO$ or $BaCl_2.2H_2O$.

**Copper Foil.**—Pure metallic copper, thin and bright.

**Gold, Fine.**—Gold, free from metallic impurities.

**Hyposulphite of Soda,** $NaO,S_2O_2+5HO$ or $Na_2H_2S_2O_4.4H_2O$.—*Test*.—24·8 grains decolorize 100 measures of the volumetric solution of iodine.

**Indigo,** $C_{16}H_5NO_2$ or $C_8H_5NO$.—A blue pigment prepared from various species of Indigofera, *Linn.*

**Isinglass.**—*Vide* p. 279.

**Litmus.**—*Vide* p. 259.

**Oxalic Acid, Purified,** $2HO,C_4O_6+4HO$ or $H_2C_2O_4.2H_2O$.—Take of Oxalic Acid of commerce, one pound; Boiling Distilled Water, thirty fluid ounces. Dissolve, filter the solution, and set it aside to crystallize. Pour off the liquor, and dry the crystals by exposure to the air on filtering paper placed on porous bricks. *Test*.—It is entirely decomposed and volatilized by a heat above 320°.

**Oxalate of Ammonia,** $2NH_4O,C_4O_6+2HO$ or $(NH_4)_2C_2O_4.H_2O$.—Take of Purified Oxalic Acid, one ounce; Boiling Distilled Water, eight fluid ounces; Carbonate of Ammonia, a sufficiency. Dissolve the oxalic acid in the water, neutralize the solution at a boiling temperature, filter it while still hot, and set it by that crystals may form as it cools.

**Plaster of Paris.**—Native sulphate of lime, $CaO,SO_3+2HO$ or $CaSO_4.2H_2O$, deprived of water by heat.

**Platinum Black.**—Platinum in a state of minute division, obtained by adding excess of carbonate of soda and some sugar to solution of perchloride of platinum, and boiling until a black precipitate is formed which is washed and dried.

**Red Prussiate of Potash**, $K_3Fe_2C_{12}N_6$ or $K_6Fe_2C_{12}N_{12}$.—*Test.* — Its aqueous solution gives no precipitate with persulphate of iron.

**Sulphate of Copper, Anhydrous**, $CuO,SO_3$ or $CuSO_4$.—Sulphate of copper deprived of its water by a heat of 400°. *Characters.*— A yellowish white powder, which becomes blue when moistened with water.

**Sulphide of Iron**, $FeS$ or $FeS$.—Produced by applying the end of a rod of iron, heated to a white heat at a blacksmith's forge, to the end of a roll of sulphur, and allowing the sulphide of iron as it is formed to run into a vessel of water; or, by heating in a covered crucible 56 parts of iron-filings with 32 parts of sulphur.

**Sulphuretted Hydrogen**, $HS$ or $H_2S$.—Take of Sulphide of Iron, half an ounce; Water, four fluid ounces; Sulphuric Acid, a sufficiency. Place the sulphide of iron and the water in a gas-bottle closed with a cork perforated by two holes, through one of which passes air-tight a funnel tube of sufficient length to dip into the water, and through the other a tube for giving exit to the gas. Through the former pour from time to time a little of the acid, so as to develope the sulphuretted hydrogen as it may be required.

**Tin, Granulated.**—Grain tin, reduced to small fragments by fusing and pouring into cold water.

**Turmeric.**—*Vide* p. 231.

**Yellow Prussiate of Potash.**—$K_2FeC_6N_3+3HO$ or $K_4FeC_6N_6.3H_2O$. *Tests.*—Its aqueous solution precipitates deep-blue with persulphate of iron, brick-red with sulphate of copper, and white with acetate of lead.

---

## TEST SOLUTIONS.

**Solution of Acetate of Copper.**—Take of Subacetate of Copper of Commerce, in fine powder, half an ounce; Acetic Acid, one fluid ounce; Distilled Water, a sufficiency. Dilute the acid with half a fluid ounce of the water; digest the subacetate of copper in the mixture at a temperature not exceeding 212° with repeated stirring, and continue the heat until a dry residue is obtained. Digest this in four ounces of boiling distilled water, and by the addition of more of the water make up the solution to five fluid ounces. Filter it.

**Solution of Acetate of Potash.**—Take of Acetate of Potash, half an ounce; Distilled Water, five fluid ounces. Dissolve and filter.

**Solution of Acetate of Soda.**—Take of Acetate of Soda, half an ounce; Distilled Water, five fluid ounces. Dissolve and filter.

**Solution of Albumen.**—*Vide* p. 231.

**Solution of Ammonio-Nitrate of Silver.**—Take of Nitrate of Silver, in crystals, quarter of an ounce; Solution of Ammonia, half a fluid ounce, or a sufficiency; Distilled Water, a sufficiency. Dissolve the nitrate of silver in eight fluid ounces of the water, and to the solution add the ammonia until the precipitate first formed is nearly dissolved. Filter, and then add distilled water, so that the bulk may be ten fluid ounces.

**Solution of Ammonio-Sulphate of Copper.**—Take of Sulphate of Copper, in crystals, half an ounce; Solution of Ammonia, a sufficiency; Distilled Water, a sufficiency. Dissolve the sulphate of copper in eight fluid ounces of the water, and to the solution add the ammonia until the precipitate first formed is nearly dissolved. Clear the solution by filtration, and then add distilled water, so that the bulk may be ten fluid ounces.

**Solution of Ammonio-Sulphate of Magnesia.**—Take of Sulphate of Magnesia, one ounce; Chloride of Ammonium, half an ounce; Solution of Ammonia, half a fluid ounce; Distilled Water, a sufficiency. Dissolve the sulphate of magnesia and chloride of ammonium in eight fluid ounces of the water, and to the solution add the ammonia, and as much distilled water as will make up the bulk to ten fluid ounces. Filter, if necessary.

**Solution of Boracic Acid.**—Take of Boracic Acid, fifty grains; Rectified Spirit, one fluid ounce. Dissolve and filter.

**Solution of Bromine.**—Take of Bromine, ten minims; Distilled Water, five fluid ounces. Place the bromine in a bottle furnished with a well fitting stopper; pour on the water, and shake several times. Keep it excluded from the light.

**Solution of Carbonate of Ammonia.** — Take of Carbonate of Ammonia, in small pieces, half an ounce; Distilled Water, ten fluid ounces. Dissolve and filter.

**Solution of Chloride of Ammonium.**—Take of Chloride of Ammonium, one ounce; Distilled Water, ten fluid ounces. Dissolve and filter.

**Solution of Chloride of Barium.**—Take of Chloride of Barium, in crystals, one ounce; Distilled Water, ten fluid ounces. Dissolve and filter.

**Solution of Chloride of Calcium.**—Take of Chloride of Calcium, one ounce; Distilled Water, ten fluid ounces. Dissolve and filter.

**Solution (Saturated) of Chloride of Calcium.**—Take of Chloride of Calcium, four ounces; Distilled Water, five fluid ounces. Dissolve and filter.

**Solution of Per-chloride of Gold.**—Take of Fine Gold, reduced by a rolling machine to a thin lamina, sixty grains; Nitric Acid, one fluid ounce and a half; Hydrochloric Acid, seven fluid ounces; Distilled Water, a sufficiency. Place the gold in a flask with the nitric acid and six fluid ounces of the hydrochloric acid, first mixed with four fluid ounces of the water, and digest until it is dissolved. Add to the solution the additional fluid ounce of hydrochloric acid, evaporate at a heat not exceeding 212° until acid vapors cease to be given off, and dissolve the chloride of gold thus obtained in five fluid ounces of distilled water. The solution should be kept in a stoppered bottle.

**Solution of Proto-chloride of Tin.**—Take of Granulated Tin, one ounce; Hydrochloric Acid, three fluid ounces; Distilled Water, a sufficiency. Dilute the acid in a flask with one fluid ounce of the water, and, having added the tin, apply a moderate heat until gas ceases to be evolved. Add as much of the water as will make up the bulk to five fluid ounces, and transfer the solution, together with the undissolved tin, to a bottle with an accurately ground stopper.

**Solution of Gelatine.**—Take of Isinglass, in shreds, fifty grains; Warm Distilled Water, five fluid ounces. Mix and digest for half an hour on a water bath with repeated shaking, and filter through clean tow moistened with distilled water.

**Solution of Iodate of Potash.**—Take of Iodine, fifty grains; Chlorate of Potash, fifty grains; Nitric Acid, eight minims; Distilled Water, ten fluid ounces and a half. Rub the iodine and chlorate of potash together in a fine powder; place the mixture in a Florence flask, and, having poured upon it half an ounce of the water acidulated with the nitric acid, digest at a gentle heat until the colour of the iodine disappears. Boil for one minute; then transfer the contents of the flask to a capsule, and evaporate to perfect dryness at 212°. Finally dissolve the residue in the remaining ten ounces of distilled water; filter the solution, and keep it in a stoppered bottle.

**Solution of Iodide of Potassium.**—Take of Iodide of Potassium, one ounce; Distilled water, ten fluid ounces. Dissolve and filter.

**Solution of Oxalate of Ammonia.**—Take of Oxalate of Ammonia, half an ounce; Warm Distilled Water, one pint. Dissolve and filter.

**Solution of Perchloride of Platinum.**—Take of Thin Platinum Foil, quarter of an ounce; Nitric Acid, a sufficiency; Hydrochloric Acid, a sufficiency; Distilled Water, seven fluid ounces. Mix a fluid ounce of the nitric acid with four fluid ounces of the hydrochloric acid and two fluid ounces of the water; pour the mixture into a small flask containing the platinum, and digest at a gentle heat, adding more of the acids mixed in the same proportion, should this be necessary, until the metal is dissolved. Transfer the solution to a porcelain dish, add to it a fluid drachm of hydrochloric acid, and evaporate on a water bath, until acid vapours cease to be given off. Let the residue be dissolved in the remaining five ounces of distilled water. Filter and preserve it in a stoppered bottle.

**Solution of Phosphate of Soda.**—Take of Phosphate of Soda, in crystals, one ounce; Distilled Water, ten fluid ounces. Dissolve and filter.

**Solution of Red Prussiate of Potash.**—Take of Red Prussiate of Potash, in crystals, a quarter of an ounce; Distilled Water, five fluid ounces. Dissolve and filter.

**Solution of Sulphate of Indigo.**—Take of Indigo, dry and in fine powder, five grains; Sulphuric Acid, ten fluid ounces. Mix the indigo with a fluid drachm of the sulphuric acid in a small test tube, and apply the heat of a water bath for an hour. Pour the blue liquid into the remainder of the acid, agitate the mixture, and, when the undissolved indigo has subsided, decant the clear liquid into a stoppered bottle.

**Solution of Sulphate of Iron.**—Take of Granulated Sulphate of Iron, ten grains; Boiling Distilled Water, one fluid ounce. Dissolve and filter. This solution should be recently prepared.

**Solution of Sulphate of Lime.**—Take of Plaster of Paris, quarter of an ounce; Distilled Water, one pint. Rub the plaster of Paris in a porcelain mortar for a few minutes with two ounces of the water; introduce the mixture thus obtained into a pint bottle containing the rest of the water; shake well several times, and allow the undissolved sulphate to subside. When this has occurred, filter.

**Solution of Sulphide of Ammonium.**—Take of Solution of Ammonia, five fluid ounces. Put three fluid ounces of the ammonia into a bottle, and conduct into this a stream of sulphuretted hydrogen so long as the gas continues to be absorbed; then add the remainder of the ammonia, and transfer the solution to a green-glass bottle furnished with a well-ground stopper.

**Solution of Tartaric Acid.**—Take of Tartaric Acid, in crystals, one ounce; Distilled Water, eight fluid ounces; Rectified Spirit, two fluid ounces. Dissolve the tartaric acid in the water, add the rectified spirit, and preserve the solution in a stoppered bottle.

**Solution of Yellow Prussiate of Potash.**—Take of Yellow Prussiate of Potash, in crystals, quarter of an ounce; Distilled Water, five fluid ounces. Dissolve and filter.

---

## TEST SOLUTIONS FOR VOLUMETRIC ESTIMATIONS.

The processes for volumetric estimations may be performed either with British or with metrical weights and measures; and the solutions are so arranged that they will be of the same strength, and the same indications will be obtained in using them, whichever system is employed, without the *necessity* of altering any of the figures by which the quantities of the substances tested, or of the test solutions required in the process, are expressed.

According to the British system, the quantities of the substances to be tested are expressed in grains by weight, whilst the quantities of the test solutions employed in testing are expressed in grain-measures, — the grain-measure being the volume of a grain of distilled water.

According to the metrical system, the quantities of the substances to be tested are expressed in grammes by weight, whilst the quantities of the test solutions employed in testing are expressed in cubic centimetres,—the cubic centimetre being the volume of a gramme of distilled water.

As the cubic centimetre bears the same relation to the gramme that the grain-measure bears to the grain, the one system may be substituted for the other with no difference in the results, excepting that, by the metrical system, all the quantities will be expressed in relation to a weight (the gramme) which is nearly fifteen times and a half (15·432) as great as the British grain.

In practice it will be found convenient, in substituting metrical for British weights and measures, to reduce the values of all the numbers to one tenth, by moving the decimal points. The quantities indicated in the Pharmacopœia, which in grains and grain-measures can be conveniently used, would be found inconveniently large if the same numbers of grammes and cubic centimetres were employed.

The following apparatus is required in the preparation and use of these solutions.

For British weights and measures:—

1. A flask which, when filled to a mark on the neck, contains exactly 10,000 grains of distilled water at 60°. The capacity of the flask is, therefore, 10,000 grain-measures.

2. A graduated cylindrical jar which, when filled to 0, holds 10,000 grains of distilled water, and is divided into 100 equal parts.

3. A burette. A graduated glass tube which, when filled to 0, holds 1,000 grains of distilled water, and is divided into 100 equal parts. Each part, therefore, corresponds to 10 grain-measures.

For metrical weights and measures:—

1. A glass flask which, when filled to a mark on the neck, contains one litre or 1,000 cubic centimetres.

2. A graduated cylindrical jar which, when filled to 0, contains one litre (1,000 cubic centimetres), and is divided into 100 equal parts.

3. A burette. A graduated tube which, when filled to 0, holds 100 cubic centimetres, and is divided into 100 equal parts.

(One cubic centimetre is the volume of one gramme of distilled water at 4° C.* 1,000 cubic centimetres equal one litre, or $1\frac{3}{4}$ (1·763) imperial pint.)

Volumetric solutions, before being used, should be shaken, in order that they may be throughout of uniform strength. They should also be preserved in stoppered bottles. All measurements should be made at 60°.

**Volumetric Solution of Bichromate of Potash** (Bichromate of Potash, $KO,2CrO_3 = 147·5$ or $\mathbf{K_2Cr_2O_7 = 295}$). Take of Bichromate of Potash, 147·5 grains; Distilled Water, a sufficiency. Put the bichromate of potash into the 10,000 grain flask, and, having half filled the flask with water, allow the salt to dissolve; then dilute the solution with more water until it has the exact bulk of 10,000 grain-measures. 1,000 grain-measures of this solution contain 14·75 grains of the bichromate of potash.

**Volumetric Solution of Hyposulphite of Soda** (Hyposulphite of Soda crystallised, $NaO,S_2O_2+5HO=124$ or $\mathbf{Na_2H_2S_2O_4.4H_2O=248}$). Take of Hyposulphite of Soda in crystals, 280 grains; Distilled Water, a sufficiency. Dissolve the hyposulphite of soda in 10,000 grain-measures of water. Fill a burette with this solution, and drop it cautiously into 1,000 grain-measures of the volumetric solution of iodine, until the brown colour is just discharged. Note the number of grain-measures ($n$) required to produce this effect; then put 8,000 grain-measures of the same solution into a graduated jar, and augment this quantity by the addition of distilled water until it amounts to $\frac{8000\times1000}{n}$ grain-measures. If, for example, $n=950$ the 8,000 grain-measures of solution should be diluted to the bulk of $\frac{8000\times1000}{950}=8,421$ grain-measures. 1,000 grain-measures of this solu-

* It is customary to make the measurements with metrical apparatus at 60° Fahr.

tion contain 24·8 grains of the hyposulphite of soda, and correspond to 12·7 grains of iodine.

**Volumetric Solution of Iodine** (Iodine, I=127). Take of Iodine, 127 grains; Iodide of Potassium, 180 grains; Distilled Water, a sufficiency. Put the iodide of potassium and the iodine into the 10,000 grain flask, fill the flask to about two-thirds its bulk with distilled water, gently agitate until solution is complete, and then dilute the solution with more water until it has the exact volume of 10,000 grain-measures. 1,000 grain-measures of this solution contain 12·7 grains of iodine.

**Volumetric Solution of Nitrate of Silver** (Nitrate of Silver, $AgO,NO_5$=170 or **$AgNO_3$=170**). Take of Nitrate of Silver 170 grains; Distilled Water, a sufficiency. Put the nitrate of silver into the 10,000 grain flask, and, having half filled the flask with water, allow the salt to dissolve; then dilute the solution with more water until it has the exact bulk of 10,000 grain-measures. The solution should be kept in an opaque stoppered bottle. 1,000 grain-measures of this solution contain 17·0 grains of nitrate of silver.

**Volumetric Solution of Oxalic Acid** (Crystallized Oxalic Acid, $2HO,C_4O_6+4HO$=126 or **$H_2C_2O_4.2H_2O$=126**). Take of Purified Oxalic Acid in crystals, quite dry, but not effloresced, 630 grains; Distilled Water, a sufficiency. Put the oxalic acid into the 10,000 grain flask, fill the flask to about two thirds of its bulk with water, allow the acid to dissolve, and then dilute the solution with more water until it has the exact volume of 10,000 grain-measures. 1,000 grain-measures of this solution contain 63 grains of oxalic acid.

**Volumetric Solution of Soda** (Hydrate of Soda, NaO,HO=40 or **NaHO=40**). Take of Solution of Soda, a sufficiency; Distilled Water, a sufficiency. Fill a burette with the solution of soda, and cautiously drop this into 63 grains of purified oxalic acid dissolved in about two ounces of water, until the acid is exactly neutralized as indicated by litmus. Note the number of grain-measures ($n$) of the solution used, and having then introduced 9,000 grain-measures of the solution of soda into a graduated jar, augment this quantity by the addition of water, until it becomes $\frac{9000 \times 1000}{n}$ grain-measures. If, for example, $n$=930, the 9,000 grain-measures should be augmented to $\frac{9000 \times 1000}{930}$=9,677 grain-measures. 1,000 grain-measures of this solution contain 40 grains of hydrate of soda.

# CLASSIFIED CATALOGUE

OF

# INDIAN MEDICINAL PRODUCTS

Derived from the Organic Kingdom, indicating those which are more or less analogous to articles officinal in the British Pharmacopœia, and for which they may be employed as substitutes.

---

§ distinguishes officinal Indian Products contained in the British Pharmacopœia.

† in the Non-officinal List indicates those most worthy of attention.

= indicates articles possessing analogous properties.

---

## ALTERATIVES AND ALTERATIVE TONICS.

| Indian Products. | | British Officinal Articles. |
|---|---|---|
| OFFICINAL. | | |
| Calotropis gigantea, *R. Br.*, ,, procera, *R. Br.*, (Root-bark,) p. 141. (*Mudar.*) | | |
| Gynocardia odorata, *R. Br.*, (Seeds,) p. 26. (*Chaulmúgra.*) | | |
| §Hemidesmus Indicus, *R. Br.*, (Root,) p. 140. (*Hemidesmus Root.*) | = | Dulcamara, p. 179, and Sarsaparilla, p. 226. |
| Hydrocotyle Asiatica, *Linn.*, (Leaves,) p. 107. (*Indian Hydrocotyle, or Pennywort.*) | | |

| Indian Products. | British Officinal Articles. |
|---|---|
| **Non-officinal.** | |
| Agave Americana, *Linn.*, (Root,) p. 234. | |
| †Bryonia epigæa, *Rottl.*, (Root,) p. 96. | |
| †Cinnamomum glanduliferum, *Meissn.*, (*Sassafras of Nepal.*) †Cinnamomum parthenoxylon, *Meissn.*, (Root,) p. 196. = | Sassafras Root, p. 192. |
| Clerodendron serratum, *Blume*, (Root,) p. 164. | |
| †Echium, sp. of, (*Gouzabán*, Hind.,) p. 158 - - - - - = | Sarsaparilla, p 226, and Pareira Brava, p. 7. |
| †Eclipta prostrata, *Linn.*, (Root,) p. 128 = | Taraxacum, p. 123. |
| †Ehretia buxifolia, *Roxb.*, (Root,) p. 158 = | Elm bark, p. 123. |
| Euphorbia antiquorum, *Linn.*, (Inspissated juice,) p. 204. | |
| †Hydnocarpus inebrians, *Vahl.*, (Oil of seeds,) p. 27. | |
| Ichnocarpus frutescens, *R.Br.*, (Root,) p. 138. - - - - - = | Sarsaparilla, p. 226. |
| Panax pseudo-ginseng, *Wall.*, (Root,) p. 108. | |
| †Smilax glabra, *Roxb.*, † „ lanceæfolia, *Roxb.*, † „ ovalifolia, *Roxb.*, † „ sp. of (*Tsein-apho*, Burm.) (Root,) p. 227-8 = | Jamaica Sarsaparilla, p. 226. |

## ANTHELMINTICS.

| Indian Products. | British Officinal Articles. |
|---|---|
| **Officinal.** | |
| Garcinia pictoria, *Roxb.*, (Gum-resin,) p. 30. (*Indian or Mysore Gamboge.*) = | Siam Gamboge, p. 80. |
| §Mallotus Philippiensis, *Müll.*, (Glands of capsules,) p. 202. (*Kamala.*) - = | Kousso, p. 82, Male Fern, p. 257. |
| Mucuna pruriens, *D.C.*, (Hairs of legumes,) p. 73. (*Cowhage.*) | |
| §Punica Granatum, *Linn.*, (Root-bark,) p. 93. (*Pomegranate Root-bark.*) - = | Filix Mas., Male Fern. p. 257. |
| **Non-officinal.** | |
| Alstonia scholaris, *R. Br.*, (Bark,) p. 137. | |
| Areca Catechu, *Linn.*, (*Betel nuts*,) p. 247. | |

| Indian Products. | | British Officinal Articles. |
|---|---|---|
| †Aristolochia bracteata, *Retz.*, (Juice,) p. 199. | = | Quassia, p. 49. |
| Asclepias curassavica, *Linn.*, (Juice of leaves,) p. 142. | | |
| †Azadirachta Indica, *Juss.*, (Oil of seeds,) p. 54. | | |
| †Butea frondosa, *Roxb.*, (Seeds,) p. 79. †Carica Papaya, *Linn.*, (Juice of fruit,) p. 97. | = | Santonica, Santonin, p. 122. |
| Clerodendron infortunatum, *Linn.*, (Juice,) p. 164. | | |
| Cucurbita Pepo, *Linn.*, C. maxima, *Duch.*, (Seeds,) p. 96–7. | | |
| Gardenia campanulata, *Roxb.*, (Fruit,) p. 118. | | |
| †Gisekia pharnaceoides, *Linn.*, (Plant,) p. 183. | | |
| Holarrhena antidysenterica, *R. Br.*, ,, pubescens, *Wall.*, (Seeds,) p. 138. | | |
| †Mangifera Indica, *Linn.*, (Seeds) p. 59. | = | Santonica, Santonin, p. 122. |
| †Melanorrhœa usitatissima, *Wall.*, (Juice,) p. 60. | | |
| Melia Azedarach, *Linn.*, (Root-bark,) p. 55. | | |
| Ophioxylon serpentinum, *Linn.*, (Root,) p. 139. | | |
| Peganum Harmala, *Linn.*, (Seeds,) p. 49. | | |
| †Polyporus anthelminticus, *Berk.*, (Dried fungus,) p. 258. | | |
| Quisqualis Indica, *Linn.*, (Fruit,) p. 90. | | |
| †Vernonia anthelmintica, *Willd.*, (Seeds,) p. 126. | = | Santonica, Santonin, p. 122. |

## ANTIDOTES TO SNAKE BITES, &c.

| NON-OFFICINAL. | |
|---|---|
| Achyranthes aspera, *Linn.*, (Flowering spike,) p. 184. | [*Note.*—The drugs of this class have no distinct representatives in the British Pharmacopœia, and with the exception of *Aristolochia Indica*, |
| †Aristolochia Indica, *Linn.*, (Leaves,) p. 198. | |
| Bragantia Wallichii, *R. Br.*, (Plant,) p. 199. | |

C C 2

| Indian Products. | British Officinal Articles. |
| --- | --- |
| Dæmia extensa, *R. Br.*, (Plant,) p. 142.<br>Eupatorium Ayapana, *Vent.*, (Plant,) p. 127.<br>Euphorbia neriifolia, *Linn.*, (Root,) p. 204.<br>Gymnema sylvestre, *R. Br.*, (Plant,) p. 143.<br>Leucas aspera, *Spreng.*, (Plant,) p. 169.<br>Notonia corymbosa, *D.C.*, (Juice,) p. 126.<br>†Ophiorrhiza Munghos, *Linn.*, (Plant,) p. 118.<br>Ophioxylon serpentinum, *Linn.*, p. 139.<br>Salvadora Wightiana, *Planch.*, (Fruit,) p. 170.<br>Strychnos colubrina, *Linn.*, (Wood,) p. 145.<br>Trichodesma Indicum, *R. Br.*, (Plant,) p. 158. | are probably not worthy of much confidence. All of them are inferior in efficacy to Liquor Ammoniæ, and alcoholic stimulants.] |

## ANTIPERIODICS AND FEBRIFUGES.

| Officinal. | |
| --- | --- |
| Aconitum heterophyllum, *Wall.*, (Root,) p. 4. (*Atis*) - - - -<br>Alstonia scholaris, *R. Br.*, (Bark,) p. 137. (*Alstonia Bark*) - - -<br>Azadirachta Indica, *Juss.*, (Bark,) p. 54. (*Nim Bark*) - - - -<br>Berberis Asiatica, *D.C.*, and other sp., (Root-bark,) p. 12. (*Indian Barberry*) - - - -<br>Cæsalpinia Bonducella, *Linn.*, (Seeds,) p. 68. (*Bonduc Nuts*) - -<br>Papaver somniferum, *Linn.*, (Cryst. Principle,) p. 22. (*Narcotine*) - - -<br>§Piper nigrum, *Linn.*, p. 205. (*Black Pepper*) - - - - -<br>Soymida febrifuga, *Juss.*, (Bark,) p. 55. (*Rohun Bark*) - - - -<br>§Strychnos Nux Vomica, *Linn.*, (Seeds and alkaloid,) p. 143. (*Nux Vomica* and *Strychnia*) - - -<br>Toddalia aculeata, *Pers.*, (Root-bark), p. 47. (*Toddalia Root*) - - | All these articles have been employed as substitutes for Cinchona and its alkaloids. Although none of them are so uniformly effectual as that drug, many of them are useful antiperiodics, and capable, in uncomplicated cases, of controlling or subduing malarious paroxysmal fevers. |

| Indian Products. | British Officinal Articles. |
|---|---|
| NON-OFFICINAL. | |
| Acorus Calamus, *Linn.*, (Rhizome,) p. 249. | |
| Adansonia digitata, *Linn.*, (Bark,) p. 36. | |
| Aristolochia Indica, *Linn.*, (Root,) p. 198 = | Serpentaria Root, p. 197. |
| ,, bracteata, *Retz*, (Root,) p. 199. | |
| †Cæsalpinia coriaria, *Willd.*, (Legumes,) p. 79. | |
| †Cedrela Toona, *Roxb.*, (Bark,) p. 56. | |
| Clerodendron infortunatum, *Linn.*, (Juice,) p. 164. | |
| Corydalis Govaniana, *Wall.*, (Cryst. Principle,) p. 23. | |
| Eurycoma longifolia, *Jack.*, (Root,) p. 50. | |
| Fagræa fragrans, *Roxb.*, (Bark,) p. 146. | |
| Ficus oppositifolia, *Roxb.*, (Bark,) p. 249. | |
| Geniosporum prostratum, *Benth.*, p. 169. | |
| †Holarrhena antidysenterica, *R. Br.*, (Bark,) p. 138. (*Conessi Bark*) = | Cinchona Bark, p. 109-115. |
| †Hymenodictyon excelsum, *Wall.*, (Bark,) p. 117 = | Ditto. |
| Justicia Gendarussa, *Linn.*, (Plant,) p. 162. | |
| Kadagaroganie (*Tam.*,) p. 160. | |
| Michelia Champaca, *Linn.*, (Bark,) p. 6. | |
| Nauclea ovalifolia, *Roxb.*, (Bark,) p. 117. | |
| Plumbago Zeylanica, *Linn.*, (Root,) p. 170. | |
| Roylea elegans, *Wall.*, (Plant), p. 168. | |
| Salix tetrasperma, *Roxb.*, (Bark,) p. 213. | |
| Strychnos colubrina, *Linn.*, (Wood,) p. 145. | |
| †Thevetia neriifolia, *Juss.*, (Bark,) p. 138. | |

## ANTISCORBUTICS.

| | |
|---|---|
| OFFICINAL. | |
| Citrus Bergamia, *Risso*, (Juice of fruit,) p. 45. (*Lime Juice*) = | Lemon Juice, p. 44. |

| Indian Products. | | British Officinal Articles. |
|---|---|---|
| **Non-officinal.** | | |
| Feronia Elephantum, *Corr.*, (Ripe fruit,) p. 48. (*Wood-apple.*) | | |
| Musa sapientum, *Linn.*, (Fruit,) p. 233. (*Plantain and Banana.*) | | |
| Phyllanthus Emblica, *Linn.*, (Fruit,) p. 204. | | |

## ANTISPASMODICS.

| Indian Products. | | British Officinal Articles. |
|---|---|---|
| **Officinal.** | | |
| Andropogon citratum, *D.C.*, and other species, (Volatile oil,) p. 255. (*Lemon Grass Oil, Rúsa ka tel, &c.*) | = | Oil of Cajuput, p. 90. |
| §Cannabis sativa, *Linn.*, (Flowering tops,) p. 216.) (*Indian Hemp.*) | | |
| Carum (Ptychotis) Ajowan, *D.C.*, (Fruit and volatile oil.) p. 99. (*Ajwain* or *Omum*) - - | = | Oils of Lavender, Peppermint, Dill, Caraway, &c. |
| Datura alba, *Linn.*, and D. fastuosa, *Linn.*, (Leaves and seeds,) p. 175-7. (*Dhatura*) - - - | = | Stramonium, p. 174, and Belladonna, p. 171. |
| §Ferula Asafœtida, *Linn.*, (Gum resin,) p. 102. (*Assafœtida.**) | | |
| §Nicotiana Tabacum, *Linn.*, (Leaves,) p. 178. (*Tobacco Leaves.*) | | |
| §Papaver somniferum, *Linn.*, (Inspissated juice,) p. 15. (*Patna Garden and Malwa Opium*) - - | = | Smyrna or Turkey Opium, p. 15. |
| **Non-officinal.** | | |
| Artemisia Indica, *Willd.*, (Plant,) p 126. | | |
| Blumea balsamifera, *D.C.*, (Plant,) p. 128. | | |
| Dracontium polyphyllum, *Linn.*, (Plant,) p. 250. | | |
| †Euphorbia neriifolia, *Linn.*, (Juice of leaves,) p. 204. - - - | = | Lobelia ? p. 128. |
| †Gardenia gummifera, *Linn.*, - - ; †Gardenia lucida, *Roxb.*, - - } (Resin,) p. 118. | | |

* Though doubtfully classed as an Indian product, assafœtida of good quality is met with in bazaars throughout India.

| Indian Products. | | British Officinal Articles. |
|---|---|---|
| Gynandropsis pentaphylla, *D.C.*, (Plant,) p. 25. | | |
| †Hyoscyamus insanus, *Stocks*, (Plant,) p. 177. | | |
| †Justicia Adhatoda, *Linn.*, (Inspissated juice,) p. 162. | | |
| Lobelia nicotianæfolia, *Heyne*, (Plant,) p. 129. | | |
| †Nardostachys Jatamansi, *D.C.*, (Root,) p. 120. Valeriana Hardwickii, *Wall.*, (Root,) p. 120. | = | Valerian, p. 119, Sumbul Root, ? p. 106. |
| Viverra Zibetha, *Linn.*, (Odorous secretion,) p. 286 | = | Castor, p. 285. |

## ASTRINGENTS.

| Indian Products. | | British Officinal Articles. |
|---|---|---|
| **Officinal.** | | |
| Acacia Catechu, *Linn.*, (Extract from wood,) p. 62. (*Black Catechu*) | = | Pale Catechu, p. 117. |
| §Ægle Marmelos, *Corr.*, (Fruit,) p. 46. (*Bela, Bael.*) | | |
| Butea frondosa, *Roxb.*, (Inspissated juice,) p. 73. (*Bengal Kino*) | = | Kino, p. 70. |
| Diospyros Embryopteris, *Pers.*, (Extract,) p. 131. (*Gab.*) | = | Catechu, p. 117. |
| §Pterocarpus Marsupium, *D.C.*, (Inspissated juice,) p. 70. (*Kino.*) | | |
| Punica Granatum, *Linn.*, (Rind of fruit,) p. 93. (*Pomegranate Bark*) | = | Oak Bark, p. 209. |
| **Non-officinal.** | | |
| †Acacia Arabica, *Willd.*, and other species, (Bark,) p. 77. (*Babul Bark*) | = | Oak Bark, p. 209. |
| †Areca Catechu, *Linn.*, (Extract from fruit,) p. 249. (*Betel Nut Catechu*) | = | Catechu, p. 117. |
| †Cæsalpinia coriaria, *Linn.*, (Legumes,) p. 79. (*Divi-divi.*) | | |
| †Cæsalpinia Sappan, *Linn.*, (Wood,) p. 79. (*Sappan wood*) | = | Logwood, p. 67. |
| Casuarina muricata, *Roxb.*, (Bark,) p. 217. | | |
| †Cassia auriculata, *Linn.*, (Bark,) p. 78. | = | Oak Bark, p. 209. |

| Indian Products. | | British Officinal Articles. |
|---|---|---|
| Cordia angustifolia, *Roxb.*, (Bark,) p. 158 | | |
| †Eucalyptus resinifera, *Smith*, (Gum,) p. 71.) (*Botany Bay Kino*) | = | Kino, p. 70. |
| Feronia Elephantum, *Corr.*, (Unripe fruit,) p. 48. | = | Bael, p. 40. |
| †Garcinia Mangostana, *Linn.*, (Pericarp,) p. 31.) | | |
| †Holarrhena antidysenterica, *R. Br.* – †Holarrhena pubescens, *Wall.*, – Bark and Seeds, p. 138. | | |
| Lawsonia alba, *Lam.*, (Leaves,) p. 87. | | |
| Mangifera Indica, *Linn.*, (Seeds,) p. 59. | | |
| Múcherus, (Gum.,) p. 36. | | |
| Odina Wodier, *Roxb.*, (Bark,) p. 60. | | |
| Phyllanthus Emblica, *Linn.*, (Dried fruit,) p. 204. | = | Oak Galls, p. 209. |
| Phyllanthus Emblica, *Linn.*, (Extract from wood,) p. 204. | = | Catechu, p. 62, 117. |
| Pistacia Khinjuk, *Stocks*, (Galls,) p. 59. (*Gúl-i-pista*) | = | Oak Galls, p. 209. |
| Psidium pomiferum, *Linn.*, and P. pyriferum, *Linn.*, (Bark,) p. 92. | | |
| Rhus succedanea, *Linn.*, (Galls,) p. 59. (*Kakra-singhi*) | = | Oak Galls, p. 209. |
| Syzigium Jambolanum, *D.C.*, (Bark,) p. 92. | | |
| Tamarindus Indica, *Linn.*, (Seeds,) Appendix, No. 29. | | |
| Tamarix Gallica, *Linn.*, and T. orientalis, *Vahl.*, (Galls,) p. 29. – Terminalia Chebula, *Retz.*, (Fruit and galls,) p. 89 | = | Oak Galls, p. |
| Terminalia tomentosa, *W. et A.* (Bark,) p. 89. | | |

## CARMINATIVE AND STOMACHICS.

| Officinal. | | |
|---|---|---|
| Andropogon citratum, *D.C.*, and other species, (Volatile oil,) p. 255. (*Lemon-grass Oil, &c.*) | = | Oil of Cajuput, p. 90. |

| Indian Products. | | British Officinal Articles. |
|---|---|---|
| Anethum Sowa, *Roxb.*, (Fruit,) p. 101. (*Sowa*, Hind) | = | Common Dill, p. 100. |
| Carum (Ptychotis) Ajowan, *D.C.*, (Fruit, p. 99. (*Ajwain* or *Omum*). | = | Caraway, p. 98; Coriander, p. 101; Anise, Dill, &c. The volatile oil is also an efficient substitute for the oils of Thyme, Peppermint, &c. |
| §Caryophyllus aromaticus, *Linn.*, (Flower buds,) p. 91. (*Cloves*) | = | Pimento, p. 92. |
| §Elettaria Cardamomum, *Maton*, (Fruit,) p. 230. (*Cardamoms.*) | | |
| Fœniculum Panmorium, *D.C.*, (Fruit,) p. 100. (*Panmuhuri*, Hind) | = | Common Fennel, p. 100. |
| §Myristica officinalis, *Linn.*, (Kernels,) p. 189. (*Nutmegs.*) | | |
| §Piper nigrum, *Linn.*, (Fruit,) p. 200. (*Black Pepper.*) | | |
| §Zingiber officinale, *Roscoe*, (Rhizome,) p. 228. (*Ginger.*) | | |
| NON-OFFICINAL. | | |
| †Acorus Calamus, *Linn.*, (Rhizome,) p. 249. | | |
| Alpinia nutans, *Rosc.*, and other species, (Rhizome,) p. 232. | | |
| Amomum aromaticum, *Roxb.*, (Fruit), p. 233<br>Amomum xanthioides, *Wall.*, (Fruit,) p. 232 | = | Cardamoms, p. 230. |
| †Anisomeles Malabarica, *R. Br.*, (Leaves,) p. 168. | | |
| †Anisomeles ovata, *R. Br.*, (Plant and volatile oil), p. 168. | | |
| Artemisia Indica, *Willd.*, (Plant,) p. 126. | | |
| Blumea balsamifera, *D.C.*, (Plant,) p. 128. | | |
| Carum (Ptychotis) Roxburghianum, *Benth.*, (Fruit,) p. 108 | = | Caraway, p. 98. |
| Chavica Betle, *Miquel*, (Juice of leaves,) p. 208. | | |
| Chavica officinarum, *Miquel*, (Fruit,) p. 20<br>Chavica Roxburghii, *Miquel*, (Fruit,) p. 208. (*Long Pepper*) | = | Black Pepper, p. 228. |

| Indian Products. | | British Officinal Articles. |
|---|---|---|
| Chrysanthemum Roxburghii, *Desv.*, (Flowers,) p. 127 | = | Chamomile Flowers, p. 121. |
| Cinnamomum iners, *Reinw.*, ,, Zeylanicum *var.* Cassia, *Nees*, (Inner bark,) p. 195. (*Cassia Bark, Cassia lignea.*) | = | Cinnamon, p. 194. |
| Cinnamomum Tamala, and C. eucalyptoides, *Nees*, (Leaves,) p. 196 | | |
| Coleus aromaticus, *Benth.*, (Juice,) p. 168. | | |
| Cratæva religiosa, *Forst.*, (Leaves,) p. 25. | | |
| Curcuma Amada, *Roxb.*, ,, aromatica, *Salisb.*, ,, Zedoaria, *Roscoe*, (Rhizomes,) p. 232. (*Zedoary.*) | | |
| Cuminum Cyminum, *Linn.*, (Fruit,) p. 108. (*Cumin seeds*) | = | Coriander, 101; Dill, p. 100, &c. |
| Cyperus pertennis, *Linn.*, and C. rotundus, *Linn.*, (Root,) p. 250. | | |
| Eupatorium Ayapana, *Vent.*, (Plant,) p. 127. | | |
| Feronia Elephantum, *Corr.*, (Leaves,) p. 48. | | |
| Hedychium spicatum, *Smith*, (Root,) p. 232. | | |
| Kæmpfera Galanga, *Linn.*, ,, rotunda, *Linn.*, (Root,) p. 232. | | |
| †Micromeria capitellata, *Benth.*, (Plant,) p. 168 | = | Peppermint, p. 166. |
| Murraya (Bergera) Königii, *Linn.*, (Bark and leaves,) p. 49. | | |
| Nigella sativa, *var.* Indica, *D.C.*, (Fruit,) p. 5. | | |
| Solanum Jacquini, *Willd.*, (Plant,) p. 181. | | |
| Vernonia anthelmintica, *Willd.*, (Seeds,) p. 126. | | |
| Withania (Puneeria) coagulans, *Dun.*, (Dried fruit,) p. 181. | | |
| Withania (Physalis) somnifera, *Dun.*, (Root,) p. 182. | | |
| Zanthoxylum alatum, *Roxb.*, and other species (Fruit,) p. 48. | | |
| Zingiber Cassumunar, *Roxb.*, ,, Zerumbet, *Roxb.*, (Rhizome,) p. 229. | = | Ginger, p. 228. |

| Indian Products. | British Officinal Articles. |
| --- | --- |
| **DEMULCENTS AND EMOLLIENTS.** | |
| OFFICINAL. | |
| Abrus precatorius, *Linn.*, (Root,) p. 74. (*Indian Liquorice*) = | Liquorice Root, p. 75. |
| Gracilaria lichenoides, *Grev.*, (Dried plant), p. 261. (*Ceylon Moss*) | |
| Hibiscus esculentus, *Linn.*, (Capsules,) p. 35. (*Edible Hibiscus, Okra.*) | |
| Oryza sativa, *Linn.*, (Husked seed,) p. 254. (*Rice*) = | Pearl Barley, p. 253. |
| Oryza sativa, *Linn.*, (Seed, ground and sifted,) p. 254. (*Rice flour*) = | Wheaten flour, p. 254. |
| Plantago Ispaghula, *Roxb.*, (Seeds,) p. 182 (*Ispaghúl Seeds.*) | |
| NON-OFFICINAL. | |
| Amarantus spinosus, *Linn.*, (Leaves,) p. 184. | |
| Canarium commune, *Linn.*, (Kernels,) p. 52. = | Sweet Almonds, p. 83. |
| Clitorea ternatea, *Linn.*, (Root-bark,) p. 80. | |
| Cordia latifolia, *Roxb.*, and C. Myxa, *Linn.*, (Dried fruit,) p. 157. (*Sebestens*) = | Prunes, p. 86. |
| Curculigo orchioides, *Gœrtn.*, (Roots,) p. 235. | |
| Gmelina parvifolia, *Roxb.*, (Leaves,) p. 164. | |
| Ocimum pilosum, *Linn.*, ,, gratissimum, *Linn.*, (Seeds), p. 167. | |
| †Pedalium Murex, *Linn.*, (Plant and seeds,) p. 151. | |
| Pyrus Cydonia, *Linn.*, (Seeds,) p. 86. | |
| Saféd Músli, p. 36. | |
| Sesamum Indicum, *Linn.*, (Leaves,) p. 151. | |
| †Terminalia Catappa, *Linn.*, (Kernels,) p. 89. = | Sweet Almonds, p. 83. |
| Tiaridium Indicum, *Lehm.*, (Leaves,) p. 158. | |
| Trichodesma Zeylanica, *R. Br.*; (Plant,) p. 158. | |

| Indian Products. | British Officinal Articles. |
|---|---|
| **FIXED OILS.** | |
| OFFICINAL. | |
| Arachis hypogæa, *Linn.*,(Oil of seeds,) p. 74. (*Ground Nut Oil*) = | Olive Oil, p. 133. |
| Garcinia purpurea, *Roxb.*, (Concrete oil,) p. 31. (*Kokum Butter*) = | Theobroma Oil ?, p. 36. |
| NON-OFFICINAL. | |
| †Aleurites triloba, *Forst.*, (Oil,) p. 203. (*Belgaum Walnut Oil*) = | Linseed Oil. |
| Anacardium occidentale, *Linn.*, (Oil,) p. 59. (*Cashew Nut Oil.*) | |
| †Bassia butyracea, *Roxb.*, (Concrete oil,) p. 131. (*Fulwa Butter*) = | Theobroma Oil ?, p. 36. |
| Bassia latifolia, *Roxb.*, (Concrete oil) } p, 130. | |
| Bassia longifolia, *Linn.*, (Concrete oil) } p, 130. | |
| Calophyllum Inophyllum, *Linn.*, (Oil,) p. 32. | |
| Canarium commune, *Linn.*, (Oil,) p. 52. = | Almon Oil, p. 84. |
| Cocos nucifera, *Linn.*, (Oil,) p. 247. (*Cocoa Nut Oil.*) | |
| Moringa pterygosperma. *Gærtn.*, (Oil,) p. 61. | |
| †Sesamum Indicum, *Linn.*, (Oil,) p. 151. (*Jinjili Oil*) = | Olive Oil, p. 133. |
| †Terminalia Catappa, *Linn.*, (Oil,) p. 89. (*Country Almond Oil*) = | Almond Oil, p. 84. |
| **GUMS.** | |
| NON-OFFICINAL. | |
| Acacia Arabica, *Willd.*, (Gum,) p. 62. | |
| „ Farnesiana, *Willd.*, (Gum,) p. 77. | |
| „ Lebbek, *Willd.*, (Gum,) p. 77. | |
| Anacardium occidentale, *Linn.*, (Gum,) p. 59. | |
| Cochlospermum Gossypium, *D.C.*, (Gum,) p. 27. (*Kutira Gum*) = | Tragacanth ? p. 75. |
| Feronia Elephantum, *Corr.*, (Gum,) p. 48, 62. (*Wood-apple Gum*) = | Gum Acacia, p. 61. |
| Odina Wodier, *Roxb.*, (Gum,) p, 60. | |

| Indian Products. | | British Officinal Articles. |
|---|---|---|
| **DIAPHORETICS AND SUDORIFICS.** | | |
| OFFICINAL. | | |
| Andropogon citratum, *D.C.*, and other sp. (Volatile Oil,) p. 255. (*Lemon-grass Oil, Rúsa ka tel, &c.*) | = | Oil of Cajuput, 90. |
| Berberis Asiatica, *D.C.*, and Sp., (Root-bark,) p. 12. (*Indian Barberry.*) | | |
| Calotropis gigantea, *R. Br.*, ,, procera *R. Br.* (*Mudar*) (Root-bark,) p. 141. | = | Ipecacuanha, p. 115. |
| Crinum Asiaticum, *var.* toxicarium, *Herb.*, (Bulb,) p. 234. (*Crinum Root.*) | | |
| §Hemidesmus Indicus, *R. Br.*, (Root,) p. 140. (*Hemidesmus Root.*) | | |
| §Papaver somniferum, *Linn.*, (Inspissated juice,) p. 16. (*Patna Garden, or Malwa Opium.*) | = | Smyrna or Turkey Opium, p. 15. |
| Tylophora asthmatica, *W. et A.*, (Leaves,) p.142. (*Tylophora Leaves.*) | = | Ipecacuanha, p. 115. |
| §Zingiber officinale, *Roscoe*, (Rhizome,) p. 228. (*Ginger.*) | | |
| NON-OFFICINAL. | | |
| Acorus calamus, *Linn.*, (Rhizome,) p, 249. (*Sweet Flag.*) | | |
| Andropogon muricatus, *Retz*, (Root,) p. 256. | | |
| †Anisochilus carnosum, *Benth.*, (Plant,) p. 169. | | |
| †Anisomeles Malabarica, *R. Br.* †Anisomeles ovata, *R. Br.* (Leaves,) p.167. | | |
| Blumea balsamifera, *D.C.*, (Plant,) p.128. | | |
| †Celastrus paniculata, *Willd.*, (Oil of seeds,) p. 56. (*Oleum Nigrum.*) | | |
| Cyperus pertenuis, *Linn.*, (Root,) p. 250. | | |
| Cyperus rotundus, *Linn.*, (Root,) p. 250. | | |
| Eupatorium Ayapana, *Vent.*, (Plant,) p.127. | | |
| Justicia Gendarussa, *Linn.*, (Plant,) p.162. | | |
| Meriandra strobilifera, *Benth.*, (Leaves,) p. 169. | | |
| Moringa pterygosperma, *Gærtn.*, (Root,) p. 61 | = | Armoracia, p. 61. |
| Ocimum basilicum, *Linn.*, Ocimum sanctum, *Linn.*, (Leaves,) p. 167. | | |

| Indian Products. | British Officinal Articles. |
|---|---|
| †Plumbago Zeylanica, *Linn.*, (Root,) p.170. | |
| Scindapsus (Pothos) officinalis, (Fruit,) p. 250. | |

## DIURETICS.

| Indian Products. | British Officinal Articles. |
|---|---|
| **Officinal.** | |
| §Cissampelos Pareira, *Linn.*, (Root,) p. 7. (*Pareira Brava.*) | |
| Crinum Asiaticum, *var.* toxicarium, *Herb.*, (Bulb,) p. 224. (*Crinum Root.*) = | Squill, p. 240. |
| Dipterocarpus lævis, *Ham.*, (Balsam. exud.,) p. 32. (*Gurjun Balsam, Wood Oil*) = | Copaiba, p. 63 |
| §Hemidesmus Indicus, *R.Br.* (Root,) p. 140. (*Hemidesmus Root.*) | |
| **Non-officinal.** | |
| †Achyranthes aspera, *Linn.*, (Leaves,) p.184. | |
| Euphorbia Nivulia, *Linn.*, (Inspissated juice,) p. 204. | |
| Herpestis Monniera, *H. B. et. K.* (Plant,) p. 161. | |
| Hibiscus esculentus, *Linn.*, (Capsules,) p.35. | |
| †Hygrophila spinosa, *T.And.*, (Plant,) p.162. | |
| †Ledebouria hyacinthoides, *Roth.*, (Bulb,) p. 242. = | Squill, p. 240. |
| Luffa amara, *Roxb.*, (Plant,) p. 97. | |
| †Moringa pterygosperma, *Gærtn.*, (Root,) p. 61. = | Armoracia, p. 23. |
| Parmelia perlata and P. perforata, *Ach.*, p. 260. | |
| †Pedalium Murex, *Linn.*, (Plant,) p. 151. | |
| Phyllanthus Niruri, *Linn.*, (Plant,) p. 205. | |
| Phyllanthus urinaria, *Linn.*, (Plant,) p. 205. | |
| †Santalum album, *Linn.*, (Volatile oil,) p. 197. (*Sandal Wood Oil*) = | Copaiba, p. 63. |
| Solanum Jacquini, *Willd.*, ,, nigrum, *Linn.*, (Plant,) p. 181. | |
| Tribulus lanuginosus, *Linn.*, (Fruit,) p. 38. | |
| Urginea Indica, *Kunth.*, (Bulb,) p. 241. (*Indian Squill*) = | Squill, p. 240. |
| Withania (Physalis) somnifera, *Dun.*, (Root,) p. 182. | |

## EMETICS.

| Indian Products. | British Officinal Articles. |
|---|---|
| **Officinal.** | |
| Calotropis gigantea, *R. Br.* - Calotropis procera, *R. Br.* (*Mudar.*) - } (Root-bark,) p. 141. } = | Ipecacuanha, p. 115. |
| Crinum Asiaticum, *var.* toxicarium, *Herb.* (Bulb,) p. 234. (*Crinum Root*) - - - - } = | Squill, p. 240. |
| Sinapis juncea, *Linn.*, (Powdered seed,) p. 25. (*Rai*, or *Indian Mustard*) - - - - } = | Mustard, p. 24. |
| Tylophora asthmatica, *W. et A.*, (Leaves,) p. 142. (*Tylophora Leaves.*) } = | Ipecacuanha, p. 115. |
| **Non-officinal.** | |
| †Acalypha Indica, *Linn.*, (Juice,) p. 205. | |
| Bassia latifolia, *Roxb.*, ,, longifolia, *Roxb.*, { (Residue of seeds after expression of oil,) p. 141. | |
| †Ficus oppositifolia, *Roxb.*, (Seeds and Fruit,) p. 217. | |
| †Ficus polycarpa, *Roxb.*, (Seeds and fruit,) p. 217. | |
| †Ledebouria hyacinthoides, *Kunth*, (Bulb,) p. 242 - - - } = | Squill, p. 240. |
| Randia dumetorum, *Linn.*, (Fruit,) p. 118. | |
| Secamone emetica, *R. Br.*, (Plant,) p. 142. | |
| †Urginea Indica, *Kunth*, (Bulb,) p. 241. (*Indian Squill*) - - - } = | Squill, p. 240. |
| Withania (Puneeria) coagulans, *Dun*, (Fruit,) p. 181. | |

## EMMENOGOGUES.

| Indian Products. | British Officinal Articles. |
|---|---|
| **Non-officinal.** | |
| †Aloe Indica, *Royle*, - † ,, litoralis, *König*, - } (Inspissated juice,) p. 242 } = | { Barbadoes and Socotrine Aloes, p. 236–9. |
| Andropogon muricatus, *Retz*, (Root,) p. 256. | |
| †Aristolochia bracteata, *Retz*, (Root,) p. 199. | |
| ,, Indica, *Linn.*, (Root,) p. 198. | |
| ,, tomentosa, *Blume*, (Plant,) p. 199. | |
| Blumea balsamifera, *D.C.*, (Plant,) p. 128. | |

| Indian Products. | | British Officinal Articles. |
|---|---|---|
| Carica Papaya, *Linn.*, (Seeds,) p. 98. | | |
| Peganum Harmala, *Linn.*, (Seeds,) p. 49. | | |
| †Plumbago rosea, *Linn.*, (Root,) p. 169. | | |
| Ruta angustifolia, *Pers.*, (Plant,) p. 40 | = | Rue, p. 39. |
| Sesamum Indicum, *Linn.*, (Seeds,) p. 150. | | |

## EXPECTORANTS.

| | | |
|---|---|---|
| OFFICINAL. | | |
| Crinum Asiaticum, *var.* toxicarium, *Herb.*, (Bulb,) p. 234. (*Crinum Root*) | = | Squill, p. 240. |
| Tylophora asthmatica, *W. et A.*, (Leaves,) p. 142. (*Tylophora Leaves*) | = | Ipecacuanha, p. 115. |
| NON-OFFICINAL. | | |
| †Acalypha Indica, *Linn.*, (Juice,) p. 205 | = | Senega Root, p. 27. |
| †Anisochilus carnosum, *Benth.*, (Juice,) p. 169. | | |
| †Balsamodendron Mukul, *Hooker*, - - †Balsamodendron pubescens, *Stocks*, (*Bdellium Gúgul*) - - - (Gum-resin,) p. 53. | = | Myrrh, p. 51. |
| Blumea balsamifera, *D.C.*, (Plant,) p. 128. | | |
| Boerhaavia diffusa, *Linn.*, (Plant,) p. 185. | | |
| Dæmia extensa, *R. Br.*, (Plant,) p. 142. | | |
| †Dorema aureum, *Stocks*, (Gum-resin,) p. 108 - - - - | = | Ammoniacum, p. 103. |
| †Justicia Adhatoda, *Linn.*, (Inspissated juice,) p. 162. (*Bakas*, Hind) - | = | Senega Root, p. 27. |
| Ledebouria hyacinthoides, *Roth.*, (Bulb,) p. 242 - - - | = | Squill, p. 240. |
| †Liquidambar Altingia, *Blume*, (Balsam,) p. 88 - - - - | = | Liquid Storax, p. 87. |
| Polygala crotalarioides, *Ham* - - - Polygala telephioides, *Willd.* - - - (Plant,) p. 29. | = | Senega Root? p. 27. |
| Ocimum basilicum, *Linn.*, ,, sanctum, *Linn.*, (Plant,) p. 167. | | |
| Solanum Jacquini, *Willd.*, (Plant,) p. 181. | | |
| Urginea Indica, *Kunth*, (Bulb,) p. 241. (*Indian Squill*) - - - | = | Squill, p. 240. |

| Indian Products. | British Officinal Articles. |
|---|---|

## INSECTICIDES AND INSECTIFUGES.

| Indian Products. | British Officinal Articles. |
|---|---|
| OFFICINAL. | |
| Anamirta Cocculus, *W. et A.*, (Fruit,) p. 9. (*Cocculus Indicus.*) | |
| NON-OFFICINAL. | |
| †Acorus Calamus, *Linn.*, (Rhizome,) p. 249. | |
| Aplotaxis auriculata, *D.C.*, (Root,) p. 127. | |
| Azadirachta Indica, *Juss.*, (Oil of seeds,) p. 54. | |
| Vernonia anthelmintica, *Willd.*, (Seeds,) p. 126. | |

## LACTIFUGES.

| Indian Products. | British Officinal Articles. |
|---|---|
| NON-OFFICINAL. | |
| †Chavica Betle, *Miquel*, (Leaves,) p. 208. | |
| †Jasminum Sambac, *Aiton*, (Flowers,) p. 136. | |
| Meriandra strobilifera, *Benth.*, (Plant,) p. 169. | |

## LACTAGOGUES.

| Indian Products. | British Officinal Articles. |
|---|---|
| NON-OFFICINAL. | |
| †Ricinus communis, *Linn.*, (Leaves,) p. 202. (*Castor Oil leaves.*) | |
| Jatropha Curcas, *Linn.*, (Leaves,) p. 203. (*English Physic Nut leaves.*) | |

## MYDRIATICS.

| Indian Products. | British Officinal Articles. |
|---|---|
| OFFICINAL. | |
| Datura alba, *Linn.*, (Extract of leaves,) p. 176. (*Extract of Datura.*) - = | Extract of Belladonna, p. 171. |
| NON-OFFICINAL. | |
| Scopolia lurida, *Dun.*, (Leaves,) p. 181, = | Belladonna, p. 171. |

| Indian Products. | | British Officinal Articles. |
|---|---|---|
| **NARCOTICS, SEDATIVES, AND ANODYNES.** | | |
| OFFICINAL. | | |
| Aconitum ferox, *Wall.*, and other species, (Root,) p. 3. (*Bikh* or *Bish*) | = | Aconite or Monkshood, p. 1. |
| §Cannabis sativa, *Linn.*, (Flowering tops,) p. 216. (*Indian Hemp.*) | | |
| Datura alba, *Linn.*, (Leaves and seeds,) p. 175. (*Datura*) - - | = | Stramonium, p. 174, and Belladonna, p. 171. |
| §Nicotiana Tabacum, *Linn.*, (Leaves,) p. 178. (Tobacco leaves.) - - | | |
| Papaver somniferum, *Linn.*, (Inspissated juice,) p. 15. (*Malwa* or *Patna Garden Opium*) - - | = | Smyrna or Turkey Opium, p. 15. |
| NON-OFFICINAL. | | |
| Aplotaxis auriculata, *D.C.*, (Root,) p. 127. | | |
| Celsia Coromandeliana, *Vahl.*, (Juice,) p. 161. | | |
| †Hyoscyamus insanus, *Stocks*, (Plant,) p. 180. | | |
| Meconopsis aculeata, *Royle*, ,, Nipalensis, *D.C.*, (Roots,) p. 22. | | |
| Santalum album, *Linn.*, (Wood,) p. | | |
| Withania, (Physalis) somnifera, *Dun.*, p. 182. | | |

## NUTRITIVES.

| Indian Products. | | British Officinal Articles. |
|---|---|---|
| OFFICINAL. | | |
| Gracilaria lichenoides, *Greville*, (Dried Plant,) p. 260. (*Ceylon Moss*) - | = | Iceland Moss, p. 258. |
| Squalus Carcharias, *Linn.*, (Liver Oil,) p. 280. (*Shark Liver Oil*) - | = | Cod Liver Oil, p. 279. |
| NON-OFFICINAL. | | |
| Cocos nucifera, *Linn.*, (Oleine,) p. 247. (*Cocoa Nut Oleine*) - - - ; Cybium Commersonii, *Cuv. et Val.*, (Liver Oil,) p. 281. (*Seir Liver Oil*) | = | Cod Liver Oil, p. 279. |

| Indian Products. | British Officinal Articles. |
|---|---|
| **PARTURIFACIENTS.** | |
| OFFICINAL. | |
| §Cannabis sativa, *Linn.*, (Flowering tops,) p. 216. (*Indian Hemp*) - = | Ergot, p. 251. |
| NON-OFFICINAL. | |
| Aristolochia bracteata, *Retz*, (Root,) p. 199. | |
| Chavica Roxburghii, *Miquel*, (Root,) p. 218. | |
| Ophioxylon serpentinum, *Linn.*, (Root,) p. 139. | |
| †Ergot of Barley and Rice? p. 253. | |
| **PURGATIVES.** | |
| OFFICINAL. | |
| §Cassia lanceolata, *Forsk*, (Leaves,) p. 65. (*Indian or Tinnivelly Senna.*) = | Alexandrian Senna, p. 65. |
| §Cassia Fistula, *Linn.*, (Pulp of pods,) p. 65. (*Cassia Pulp.*) | |
| §Croton Tiglium, *Linn.*, (Oil of seeds,) p. 201. (*Croton Oil*) - - - = | Elaterium, p. 95. |
| Garcinia pictoria, *Roxb.*, (Gum-resin,) p. 30. (*Indian or Mysore Gamboge*) = | Siam Gamboge, p. 30. |
| Pharbitis Nil, *Choisy*, (Seeds,) p. 155. (*Kaladana*) - - - = | Jalap, p. 152. |
| §Ricinus communis, *Linn.*, (Oil of seeds,) p. 202. (*Castor Oil.*) | |
| §Tamarindus Indica, *Linn.*, (Pulp of fruit,) p. 64. (*Tamarind Pulp.*) | |
| NON-OFFICINAL. | |
| Acalypha Indica, *Linn.*, (Juice of leaves), p. 205. | |
| Agati grandiflora, *Desv.*, (Leaves,) p. 78. | |
| †Aleurites triloba, *Forst.*, (Oil of seeds,) p. 203 - - - - = | Castor oil, p. 202. |
| Alhagi Maurorum, *Tourn.*, (Saccharine exud.,) p. 80 - - - = | Manna, p. 136. |
| †Aloe Indica, *Royle*, - Aloe litoralis, *König*, - (Inspissated juice,) p. 242 - - = | Barbadoes and Socotrine Aloes, p. 236–9. |

| Indian Products. | | British Officinal Articles. |
|---|---|---|
| †Argemone Mexicana, *Linn.*, (Oil of seeds,) p. 22 | = | Castor oil, p. 202. |
| Baliospermum montanum, *Müll.*, (Oil of seeds,) p. 201 | = | Croton oil, p. 201. |
| Berthelotia lanceolata, *D.C.*, (Leaves,) p. 126 | = | Senna, p. 65. |
| Cassia alata, *Linn.*, and other Sp., (Leaves,) p. 77–8 | = | Senna, p. 65. |
| Cassia alata, *Linn.*, (Extract from leaves,) p. 78. | = | Extract of Colocynth, p. 94. |
| †Clitorea ternatea, *Linn.*, (Seeds,) p. 80. | | |
| Croton oblongifolius, *Roxb.*, Croton Pavana, *Ham.*, (Oil of seeds,) p. 201. | = | Croton oil, p, 202. |
| †Cucumis Hardwickii, *Royle*, †Cucumis trigonus, *Roxb.*, (Pulp of fruit,) p. 95. | = | Colocynth, p. 94. |
| Gardenia campanulata, *Roxb.*, (Fruit,) p. 118. | | |
| Ipomœa, Sp. of, (*Shapussando or Lal-dana, Hind,*) p. 157. | | |
| †Ipomœa Turpethum, *R. Br.*, (Root and resin,) p. 156. | | |
| Jatropha Curcas, *Linn.*, (Oil of seeds,) p. 203. | | |
| Kadagaroganie, *Tam.*, (Root,) p. 161. | | |
| Mirabilis Jalapa, *Linn.*, (Root,) p. 184. | | |
| Rheum Emodi, *Wall.*, and other Sp., (Root,) p. 187. (*Indian or Himalayan Rhubarb*) | = | Chinese or Turkey Rhubarb, p. 185. |
| Salvadora Wightiana, *Planch,* (Fruit,) p. 170. | | |
| †Terminalia Chebula, *Retz.*, (Fruit,) p. 88. | | |
| Trichosanthes nervifolia, *Linn.*, (Extract of fruit,) p. 96 | = | Elaterium, p. 95. |

## REFRIGERANTS.

| Officinal. | | |
|---|---|---|
| Citrus Bergamia, *Risso,* (Juice of fruit,) p. 45. (*Lime Juice*) | = | Lemon juice, p. 44. |
| §Tamarindus Indica, *Linn.*, (Pulp of fruit,) p. 64. (*Tamarind Pulp.*) | | |

| Indian Products. | | British Officinal Articles. |
|---|---|---|
| NON-OFFICINAL. | | |
| Adansonia digitata, *Linn.*, (Pulp of fruit,) p. 36. | | |
| Aloe Indica, *Royle*, ,, litoralis, *Kön.*, (Fresh juice locally applied,) p. 242. | | |
| †Borassus flabelliformis, *Linn.*, †Cocos nucifera, *Linn.*, (Saccharine juice submitted to acetous fermentation,) p. 248. | = | Vinegar, p. 264. |
| †Cicer arietinum, *Linn.*, (Acid juice,) p. 80. | | |
| Hibiscus Rosa sinensis, *Linn.*, (Petals,) p. 36. | | |
| Santalum album, *Linn.*, (Powdered wood, locally,) p. 197. | | |

## RUBEFACIENTS AND COUNTER-IRRITANTS.

| Indian Products. | | British Officinal Articles. |
|---|---|---|
| OFFICINAL. | | |
| Andropogon citratum, *D.C.*, and other species, (Volatile oil), p. 255–6. (*Lemon-grass oil. Rúsa-ka-tel.*) | = | Oil of Cajuput, p. 90. |
| §Capsicum fastigiatum, *Blume*, (Fruit,) p. 180. (*Capsicum.*) | | |
| §Croton Tiglium, *Linn.*, (Oil of seeds,) p. 200. (*Croton Oil*) | = | Ipecacuanha, p. 115, and Tartar Emetic, p. 350. |
| §Myristica officinalis, *Linn.*, (Expressed oil,) p. 189. (*Expressed oil of Nutmeg.*) | | |
| §Piper nigrum, *Linn.*, (Unripe berries,) p. 205. (*Black Pepper.*) | | |
| Sinapis juncea, *Linn.*, (Powdered seeds), p. 25. (*Rai, or Indian Mustard*) | = | Mustard, p. 23. |
| NON-OFFICINAL. | | |
| Anacardium occidentale, *Linn.*, (Acrid oil,) p. 59.. | | |
| †Anisomeles Malabarica, *R. Br.*, (Oil of leaves), p. 168. | | |
| Argyreia speciosa, *Choisy*, (Leaves,) p. 157. | | |
| Baliospermum (Croton) montanum *Müll*, (Oil of seeds,) p. 201 | = | Croton oil, p. 200. |
| †Chavica Betle, *Miquel*, (Leaves,) p. 208. | | |

| Indian Products. | British Officinal Articles. |
|---|---|
| Chavica officinarum, *Miquel*, (Dried fruit,) p. 208.<br>† ,, Roxburghii, *Miquel*, (Fruit, *Long Pepper*,) p. 208 - - | = Black Pepper, p. 205. |
| Croton oblongifolius, *Roxb.*, - -<br>Croton Pavana, *Ham.* } (Oil of seeds,) p. 201. | = Croton Oil, p. 200. |
| Euphorbia antiquorum, *Linn.*, - -<br>Euphorbia Tirucalli, *Linn.*, - } (Milky juice), p. 204. | |
| †Gynandropsis pentaphylla, *D.C.*, (Leaves,) p. 25. | |
| Jatropha curcas, *Linn.*,<br>,, glandulifera, *Roxb.*, - - - } (Oil of seeds,) p. 203–4. | |
| Moringa pterygosperma, *Gœrtn.*, (Root,) p. 61 - - - | = Armoracia, p. 23. |
| Myrica sapida, *Wall.*, (Bark,) p. 217. | |
| †Myristica Malabarica, *Lam.*, (Concrete oil,) p. 190 - - - | = Expressed oil of Nutmeg, p. 189. |
| †Plumbago rosea, *Linn.*,<br>,, Zeylanica, *Linn.*, - - } (Root-bark,) p. 168–9.<br>†Salvadora Wightiana, *Planch*, (Root-bark,) p. 170 - - - | = Mezereon Bark, p. 188. |
| Semecarpus Anacardium, *Linn.*, (Acrid oil,) p. 60. | |
| †Vateria Indica, *Linn.*, (Concrete oil,) p. 33. | |

## SIALAGOGUES.

| Non-officinal. | |
|---|---|
| †Chrysanthemum Roxburghii, *Desv.*, (Root,) p. 127. | = Pellitory Root, p. 125. |
| †Hyperanthera pterygosperma, *Gœrtn.*, (Root,) p. 61. | = Armoracia, p. 23. |
| Plumbago rosea, *Linn.*, -<br>,, Zeylanica, *Linn.*, } (Root,) p. 170. | |
| †Solanum Jacquini, *Willd.*, (Seeds,) p. 181. | |

| Indian Products. | British Officinal Articles. |
|---|---|

## STIMULANTS.

| Indian Products. | | British Officinal Articles. |
|---|---|---|
| **Officinal.** | | |
| Andropogon citratum, *D.C.*, and other sp., (Volatile oil,) p. 255. (*Lemon-grass oil, Rúsa ka tel, &c.*) | = | Oil of Cajuput, p. 90. |
| §Cannabis sativa, *Linn.*, (Flowering tops,) p. 216. (*Indian Hemp.*) | | |
| **Non-officinal.** | | |
| Anacardium occidentale, *Linn.*, (Spirit distilled from the fruit, *Cashew Spirit*,) p. 59;<br>†Bassia latifolia, *Roxb.*, Bassia longifolia, *Linn.*, (Spirit distilled from the flowers, *Mahwa Spirit*,) p. 130;<br>†Borassus flabelliformis, *Linn.*, †Caryota urens, *Linn.*, †Cocos nucifera, *Linn.*, (Spirit obtained from saccharine juice or Toddy,) p. 247–8. (*Arrack.*) | = | Wine, Brandy, and Proof and Rectified Spirit, p. 262–4. |
| Celastrus paniculata, *Willd.*, (Oil of seeds,) p. 56. ("*Oleum nigrum.*") | | |
| †Nardostachys Jatamansi, *D.C.*, (Root,) p. 120 | = | Valerian Root, p. 119. |
| Peganum Harmala, *Linn.*, (Seeds,) p. 49. | | |
| Rubia cordifolia, *Linn.*, (Root,) p. 118. | | |
| Salix capræa, *Linn.*, (Distil. water of flowers,) p. 213. | | |
| Salvadora Wightiana, *Planch*, (Root,) p. 170. | | |
| †Vitex Negundo, *Linn.*, † " trifolia, *Linn.*, (Leaves), p. 167. | | |

*See also* CARMINATIVES and ANTISPASMODICS.

| Indian Products. | British Officinal Articles. |
|---|---|
| ***Special stimulant applications in affections of the Eye.*** | |
| Argemone Mexicana, *Linn.*, (Juice,) p. 22.<br>†Berberis Lycium, *Royle*, and Sp., (Extract,) p. 13.<br>Cassia Absus, *Linn.*, ,, auriculata *Linn.*, } (Powdered seeds,) p. 78. | |
| ***Ditto in Skin Diseases.*** | |
| Argemone Mexicana, *Linn.*, (Oil of seeds,) p. 22.<br>Bignonia xylocarpa, *Roxb.*, (Oil,) p. 150.<br>†Cassia alata, *Linn.*, ,, occidentalis, *Linn.*, ,, Sophora, *Linn.*, ,, Tora, *Linn.*, } (Leaves,) p. 78.<br>Ficus Bengalensis, *Linn.*, (Juice,) p. 217.<br>Petroleum, p. 270.<br>†Pinus Deodara, *Linn.*, (Oil,) p. 225.<br>†Pongamia glabra, *Vent.*, (Oil of seeds,) p. 79.<br>Rhinacanthus communis, *Nees.*, (Seeds,) p. 163.<br>Santalum album, *Linn.*, (Powdered wood,) p. 197.<br>Thespesia populnea, *Corr.*, (Juice of fruit,) p. 35.<br>Tiaridium Indicum, *Lehm.*, (Leaves,) p. 158. | |
| ***To Ulcers, Abscesses, &c.*** | |
| Argemone Mexicana, *Linn.*, (Juice,) p. 22.<br>†Azadirachta Indica, *Juss.*, (Leaves,) p. 43. (*Nim Poultice.*)<br>†Borassus flabelliformis, *Linn.*, (Toddy,) p. 248. (*Toddy Poultice*) } = | Yeast Poultice, p. 262. |
| Eupatorium Ayapana, *Vent.*, (Leaves,) p. 127. | |

| Indian Products. | | British Officinal Articles. |
|---|---|---|
| †Gardenia gummifera, *Linn.*, (Resin,) p. 118. (*Dikamali Gum.*) | | |
| †Hydrocotyle Asiatica, *Linn.*, (Leaves,) p. 107. | | |
| Mirabilis Jalapa, *Linn.*, (Leaves,) p. 184. | | |
| †Myristica Malabarica, *Lam.*, (Concrete oil,) p. 190. | | |
| Vitex Negundo, *Linn.*, „ trifolia, *Linn.*, } (Leaves,) p. 163. | | |

*In Rheumatism, &c., see* RUBEFACIENTS.

## STIMULANTS, TEREBINTHINATE.

| Indian Products. | | British Officinal Articles. |
|---|---|---|
| OFFICINAL. | | |
| Boswellia floribunda, *Endl.*, (Gum resin,) p. 52. (*Olibanum.*) | | |
| §Canarium commune, *Linn.*, (Resin,) p. 51. (*Elemi.*) | | |
| Dipterocarpus lævis, *Ham.*, (Balsam. exud.,) p. 32. (*Gurjun Balsam, Wood Oil* - - - - -) | = | Copaiba, p. 63. |
| NON-OFFICINAL. | | |
| Ailanthus Malabarica, *D. C.* (Gum resin,) p. 50. | | |
| †Balsamodendron Mukul, *Hook.*, „ pubescens, *Stocks*, } (Gum-resin,) p. 53. (*Bdellium.*) | = | Myrrh, p. 51. |
| Calophyllum Inophyllum, *Linn.*, (Resin,) p. 32. | | |
| Canarium strictum, *Roxb.*, (Resin,) p. 53. | = | Burgundy pitch, p. 218. |
| †Dorema aureum, *Stocks*, (Gum resin?) p. 108. - - - - - | = | Ammoniacum, p. 103. |
| †Pinus Deodara, *Roxb.*, „ longifolia, *Roxb.*, } (Products of distillation, &c., p. 225.) | = | Tar and Turpentine, pp. 219–22. |
| Pistacia Khinjuk, *Stocks*, „ Cabulica, *Stocks*, } (Resin,) p. 59. | = | Mastich, p. 58. |
| Shorea robusta, *Roxb.*, (Resin,) p. 33 Vateria Indica, *Linn.*, (Resin,) p. 33 | = | Pine Resin, p. 221. |

| Indian Products. | British Officinal Articles. |
|---|---|
| **STYPTICS.** | |
| NON-OFFICINAL. | |
| †Borassus flabelliformis, *Linn.*, - †Cocos nucifera, *Linn.*, - - } Downy substance from the base of the fronds, p. 248 - - } = | Matico leaves, p. 207. |
| †Colocasia antiquorum, *Schott.*, (Juice,) p. 250. | |
| Hopea odorata, *Roxb.*, (Powdered resin,) p. 33. | |
| **ASTRINGENT TONICS.** | |
| OFFICINAL. | |
| Alstonia scholaris, *R. Br.*, (Bark,) p. 137. (*Alstonia Bark.*) | |
| Azadirachta Indica, *Juss.*, (Bark,) p. 54. (*Nim Bark*) - - Soymida febrifuga, *Juss.*, (Bark,) p. 55. (*Rohun Bark*) - - } = | Cinchona, p. 109–15. |
| NON-OFFICINAL. | |
| †Cedrela Toona, *Roxb.*, (Bark,) p. 55 = | Cinchona, p. 109–15. |
| Diospyros melanoxylon, *Roxb.*, (Bark,) p. 132. | |
| Flacourtia Cataphracta, *Roxb.*, (Leaves, &c.), p. 27. | |
| †Holarrhena antidysenterica, *R. Br.*, (Bark), p. 137. (*Conessi Bark*) - } = | Cinchona, p. 109–15. |
| Holarrhena pubescens, *Wall.*, (Bark,) p. 138. | |
| †Hymenodictyon excelsum, *Wall.*, (Bark), p. 117. - - - } = | Cinchona, p. 109–15. |
| Mimusops Elengi, *Linn.*, (Bark,) p. 131. | |
| †Nauclea ovalifolia, *Roxb.*, (Bark,) p. 117. | |
| Rhus succedanea, *Linn.*, (Galls,) p. 59. (*Kakra-singhi*) - - - } = | Oak Galls, p. 209. |
| Terminalia Chebula, *Retz*, (Unripe fruit,) p. 89. (*Black Myrobalans.*) | |
| Xylocarpus Granatum, *Kön.*, (Bark,) p. 56. | |
| *See also* ASTRINGENTS. | |

| Indian Products. | British Officinal Articles. |
|---|---|
| **BITTER AND AROMATIC TONICS.** | |
| OFFICINAL. | |
| Aconitum heterophyllum, *Wall.*, (Root,) p. 4. (*Atis.*) | |
| Andrographis paniculata, *Nees*, (Stalk and roots,) p. 161. (*Kariyát*) = | Quassia, p. 49. |
| Berberis Asiatica, *D.C.*, and other species, (Root-bark,) p. 12. (*Indian Barberry.*) | |
| Cæsalpinia Bonducella, *Linn.*, (Seeds,) p. 68. (*Bonduc nuts.*) | |
| §Cissampelos Pareira, *Linn.*, (Root,) p. 7. (*Pareira Brava.*) | |
| Coptis Teeta, *Wall.*, (Root,) p. 4. (*Coptis or Mishmi Teeta.*) | |
| Narcotine, p. 22. | |
| §Ophelia Chirata, *D.C.*, (Dried plant,) p. 148. (*Chiretta*) = | Gentian Root, p. 147. |
| §Strychnos Nux Vomica, *Linn.*, (Seeds,) p. 143. (*Nux Vomica.*) | |
| Tinospora cordifolia, *Miers*, (Root and stems,) p. 9. (*Gulancha*) = | Calumba Root, p. 6. |
| Toddalia aculeata, *Pers.*, (Root-bark,) p. 47. (*Toddalia Bark*) = | Cusparia Bark, p. 40. |
| NON-OFFICINAL. | |
| Acorus Calamus, *Linn.*, (Rhizome,) p. 249. | |
| Ailanthus excelsa, *D.C.*, (Bark,) p. 50. | |
| †Antiaris saccidora, *Nimmo*, (Seeds,) p. 217. | |
| †Aristolochia Indica, *Linn.*, (Root,) p. 198 = | Serpentaria Root, p. 197. |
| Artemisia Indica, *Willd.*, (Plant,) p. 126. | |
| †Brucea (Nima) Quassioides, *Ham.*, (Root,) p. 50 = | Quassia, p. 49. |
| †Chrysanthemum Roxburghii, *Desv.* (Flowers), p. 127 = | Chamomile flowers, p. 121. |
| Cicendia hyssopifolia, *W. et A.*, (Plant,) p. 150 = | Gentian root, p. 147. |

| Indian Products. | British Officinal Articles. |
|---|---|
| Clerodendron infortunatum, *Linn.*, (Plant,) p. 164. | |
| Cocculus villosus, *D.C.*, (Stems,) p. 11. | |
| Cordia latifolia, *Roxb.*, ,, Myxa, *Linn.*, } (Bark,) p. 157. | |
| Corydalis Govaniana, *Wall.*, (Cryst. principle,) p. 23. | |
| †Coscinium fenestratum, *Colebr.*, (Stems,) p. 10 - - - } = | Calumba Root, p. 6. |
| Cratæva religiosa, *Forst.*, (Leaves), p. 25. | |
| Cyperus pertenuis, *Linn.*, ,, rotundus, *Linn.*, } (Roots), p. 250. | |
| Erythræa Roxburghii, *G. Don*, (Plant,) p. 150. | |
| Eupatorium Ayapana, *Vent.*, (Plant,) p. 127. | |
| †Exacum bicolor, *Roxb.*, † ,, pedunculatum, *Linn.*, † ,, tetragonum, *Roxb.*, } (Roots,) p. 149 } = | Gentian Root, p. 147. |
| Ficus oppositifolia, *Roxb.*, (Bark,) p. 217. | |
| †Gentiana Kurroo, *Royle*, (Root,) p. 149 = | Gentian Root, p. 147. |
| Luffa amara, *Roxb.*, (Plant,) p. 97. | |
| Mesua ferrea, *Linn.*, (Bark and root), p. 32. | |
| Michelia Champaca, *Linn.*, (Bark,) p. 6 = | Cascarilla Bark, p. 199. |
| †Ophelia angustifolia, *D. Don*, † ,, densifolia, *Gris.*, † ,, elegans, *Wight*, } (Dried plant,) p. 149 } = | Chiretta, p. 148. |
| Ophiorrhiza Munghos, *Linn.*, (Root,) p. 118. | |
| Ophioxylon serpentinum, *Linn.*, (Root,) p. 138. | |
| †Picrorrhiza kurroa, *Royle*, (Root,) p. 160. | |
| Rhazya stricta, *Dec.*, (Leaves and stems,) p. 138. | |
| Sida acuta, *Burm.*, (Root,) p. 35.) | |
| Thalictrum foliolosum, *D.C.*, (Root,) p. 5. | |
| Tinospora crispa, *Miers*, (Stems,) p. 11. | |

| Indian Products. | | British Officinal Articles. |
|---|---|---|
| Trichosanthes cordata, *Roxb.*, (Root,) p. 96. | | |
| ,, nervifolia, *Linn.*, (Plant,) p. 96. | | |
| ,, palmata, *Roxb.*, (Rind of fruit,) p. 96. | | |

## VESICANTS.

| | | |
|---|---|---|
| **Officinal.** | | |
| Mylabris Cichorii, *Fabr.*, (Dried insect,) p. 277. (*Telini Fly*) - - | = | Cantharides, p. 274. |
| Sinapis juncea, *Linn*, (Seeds,) p. 25. (*Rai, or Indian mustard*) - - | = | Mustard, p. 23. |
| **Non-officinal.** | | |
| Epicauta Nipalensis, Lytta Assamensis, ,, gigas, ,, violacea, Meloe Trianthema, Mylabris punctum, ,, pustulata, and other species, (Dried insect,) p. 277 - - | = | Cantharides, p. 274. |
| Plumbago rosea, *Linn.*, ,, Zeylanica, *Linn.*, (Root-bark,) p. 168-9. Salvadora Wightiana, *Planch*, (Root-bark,) p. 170 - - - | = | Mezereon Bark, p. 188. |

*See also* Rubefacients and Counter-irritants.

## MISCELLANEOUS.

| | | |
|---|---|---|
| Achyranthes aspera, *Linn.*, (Plant,) p. 184. - - - - | = | Yields on incineration a large proportion of potash. |
| Aconitum ferox, *Wall.*, and other species, (Root,) p. 3. (*Bikh or Bish*) | = | As a source of Aconitia. |
| Areca Catechu, *Linn.*, (Unexpanded petioles), p. 249 - - - - Bambusa arundinacea, *Schultz*, (Stems,) p. 257 - - - | = | Form excellent splints for fractures, &c. |
| Blumea grandis, *D.C.*, (Plant,) p. 128. | = | As a source of Camphor. |

| Indian Products. | | British Officinal Articles. |
|---|---|---|
| Citrus Bergamia, *Risso.*, (Juice of fruit,) p. 46. (*Lime Juice*) - - | = | As a source of Citric Acid. |
| Clitorea ternatea, *Linn.*, (Syrup of the flowers,) p. 80 - - - | = | As a colouring agent. |
| Hibiscus Rosa sinensis, *Linn.*, (Petals,) p. 35 - - - - - | = | Substitute for Litmus as a test. |
| Musa sapientum, *Linn.*, (Leaves,) p. 233. (Plantain leaves) - - | = | Form excellent dressing for blistered or excoriated surfaces, also as an impermeable covering, water-dressing, and shades for the eyes in ophthalmia. |
| Phyllanthus Emblica, *Linn.*, (Wood,) p. 205 - - - - - - | = | As a means of clearing muddy water. |
| Pterocarpus santalinus, *Linn.*, (Wood,) p. 71. (*Red Sandal Wood*) - - | = | As a colouring agent in place of Cochineal. |
| Salicornia Indica, *Willd.*, S. brachiata, *Roxb.*, and other species, (Plant,) p. 183 - - - | = | Yield on incineration large quantities of Barilla. |
| Squalus Carcharias, *Linn.*, (Stearine,) p. 280. (*Squalin.*) - - - | = | Substitute for lard in pharmacy. |
| Strychnos potatorum, *Linn.*, (Seeds,) p. 146. (*Clearing Nut*) - - | = | As a means of clearing muddy water. |

# APPENDIX.

# APPENDIX.

---

### ([1]), p. 1. **Aconitum Napellus (Season of Collection).**

The importance of the direction as to the season of collecting Aconite root is evident from the following statement, based on analyses conducted by Mr. T. Herapath:—The average product of the fresh *root collected after flowering* was 8·58 grains of Aconitia in the pound; in the same, dried, 35·72. In the *root collected before flowering* the yield of Aconitia was only 3·5 grains per pound in the fresh, and 12·13 in the dried root (*Royle's Mat. Med., Ed. Headland*, p. 263). With reference to this subject, Dr. Wight offers the following observations:—"Aconite root," he remarks, "is biennial; "that is, the root of the current season produces at the same time "the plant above ground and one or more laterals below, to perform the same office next year, after the decay of the parent, which "dies with the plant. When dug up towards the end of the "summer it consists of two parts: first, the parent root, dark-coloured, firm, and somewhat wrinkled; and, secondly, the "offshoots or laterals, pale or nearly white, plump, and succulent, "each attached by a short neck to the parent, and terminating "above in a scaly crown or bud, the origin of the next year's vegetation. With these facts before us, it may be inferred, in accordance with the views of Prof. Christison (who first directed "our attention to them), that the old root is the one charged with the "active principle, whilst the laterals are merely stored with the "nourishment required for the next year's vegetation. This view "of the case serves to explain Mr. Herapath's statement given "above. Separate analyses of the old root, and of the young "succulent laterals, are still required to determine the relative "proportion of aconitia in each of these parts. In spring, about "the time the new leaves are appearing above ground, the last "year's root has quite disappeared. Roots dug at that season, "never having borne vegetation, would, we apprehend, be found "on analysis destitute of aconitia."

### ([2]), p. 3. **Bikh** or **Bish (Etymology of).**

The etymology of the word *Bikh* or *Bish* (a Hindústani word, which, used generally, signifies simply poison, but, as applied to the root of this plant, *the* poison *par excellence*), as well as the synonymy of the article, has been elucidated by Dr. Royle (*Illust.*, vol. i. p. 46), Major Madden (*Journ. of Asiat. Soc. of Bengal*, May, 1848, p. 364), and Dr. Birdwood (*Bombay Products*, p. 1). In the neighbourhood of Calcutta, Aconite root is best known by the name of *Kath-Bish;* at Dacca, as *Meetha Bish;* in the North-western Provinces, as *Meetha Teelia;* and in Behar, as *Dakra.*

### ([3]), p. 3. Aconitum ferox (Relative Strength of the two varieties).

Dr. Headland (*Royle, Mat. Med.*, p. 266) found the proportion of aconitia in the white spongy variety, compared with the denser variety, to be about 5 to 3.

### ([4]), p. 3. Aconitum ferox (Medical Properties and Uses of).

Full details of the physiological effects observed by Dr. Pereira in his experiments on animals with this drug, are given in *Wallich's Plant. Asiat. Rar.*, vol. i. p. 35, and in *Edinburgh Journ. of Nat. and Geogr. Science*, July 1850, p. 235. Its uses in medicine are entered into by Sir W. O'Shaughnessy (*Bengal Disp.*, p. 165). The *Taleef Shereef* (pp. 107, 636) contains a full account of its uses in native practice. For some interesting remarks on its toxicology, see Dr. Norman Chevers (*Med. Jurisprudence of Bengal*, p. 81, *et seq.*).

### ([5]), p. 4. Aconitum heterophyllum (Medical Properties of).

Strong evidence in favour of Atís as an antiperiodic is adduced by Mr. Heming, of the Bengal Medical Service (*Journ. Agri.-Hort. Soc. of India*, 1857, vol. ix. App. p. 193). His report is based on upwards of 400 cases of periodical fevers of all types. Dr. J. Forbes Watson regards it as the most promising indigenous antiperiodic of India. Its use in ordinary intermittents, given in twenty-grain doses every morning, or during apyrexia, is favourably reported of by Dr. W. Dymock. Dr. J. Balfour (*Ind. Ann. of Med. Sci.*, 1858, vol. v. p. 548) states that for two years he had Atis in constant use, and found it a most useful febrifuge, given in doses of half a drachm mixed with a little water, every four or six hours during the intermissions, commencing its use during or towards the termination of the sweating stage. Of 66 cases of intermittent fever treated by it, of which notes were kept, it proved fully successful in 37, and comparatively so in 18; in 11 it failed. He points out the necessity of selecting good specimens for use, much that is sold in the bazaar being of very inferior quality. He directs that every root should be broken across, and all which are not pure white, with a short starchy fracture, should be discarded. He adds, "when I mention that for the first three months (from December "1st, 1857) I have not expended one grain of quinine as a febri-"fuge, and that my cases have been treated chiefly with Narcotine "and Atis, it will, I trust, be allowed that these are valuable "remedies; but they require fair play, and judicious use and com-"bination."

Dr. W. J. Moore (*Indian Ann. of Med. Sci.*, 1866, vol. ix. p. 519) also describes Atis and Berberis as the two best bazaar medicines for malarious fevers. Dr. W. Wright and Sub-Assistant Surgeon Oody Chund Dutt regard it as equal in power to Cinchona as an antiperiodic. Dr. Bholanauth Boze reports having found it uncertain in its effects, and not to be relied upon in complicated cases. This, however, applies equally to all antiperiodics.

### ([6]), p. 4. Coptis Teeta (Medical Properties of).

For an account of this drug, and its virtues as a tonic, consult Wallich (*Calcutta Med.-Phys. Trans.*, 1835, vol. viii. p. 85), Twining (*Ibid.*, p. 94), O'Shaughnessy (*Bengal Disp.*, p. 163), Macpherson (*Ind. Ann. of Med. Sci.*, 1856, vol. iii. p. 397), and Capt. Lowther (*Journ. Agri.-Hort. Soc. of India,* 1858, vol. x. App. p. 6). The late Dr. Pereira has identified it with the *Mahmirah* of the ancients (see *Pharm. Journ.*, 1851, vol. xi. p. 294). The reasons which induced the Editor to refer this drug to *Thalictrum foliolosum*, D.C., are given in *Indian Ann. of Med. Sci.*, 1858, vol. v. p. 621. Subsequent research, however, seems to confirm the correctness of Dr. Pereira's views. The root is described and figured by Guibourt (*Hist. des Drogues Simpl.*, vol. ii. p. 526), under the name of *Racine de Chynlen* or *de Mangouste.* It is the *Chynlen* of Murray (*App. Med.*, vol. vi. p. 153), and the *Son-line* or *Chyn-len* of Ainslie (*Mat. Ind.*, vol. ii. p. 400).

### ([7]), p. 10. Tinospora cordifolia (Medical Properties of).

Consult Piddington (*Calcutta Med. Phys. Trans.*, 1829, vol. iv. p. 431), Dr. H. Goodeve (*Ibid.*, vol. vii. P. i. p. 15), and O'Shaughnessy (*Bengal Disp.*, p. 198). The Editor employed Gulancha as an antiperiodic in twenty cases of ordinary quotidian fevers occurring in Burmah. In each case it prevented the accession of the cold stage, but it did not appear to diminish the severity, or prevent the regular return, of the hot stage; a peculiarity not observed by the Editor in the use of any other remedy of the same class. It is more valuable as a bitter tonic than as an antiperiodic. A full detail of its uses in native practice has been published by Dewan Ramcomul Sen (*Calcutta Med.-Phys. Trans.*, vol. iii. p. 294).

### ([8]), p. 12. Berberis Asiatica, &c. (Medical Properties of).

A full account of the medicinal properties and uses of the Indian Barberry, as well as its botanical history and pharmacology, will be found in a paper by Dr. W. S. Stiven (*Indian Ann. of Med. Sci.*, April 1856, p. 416). Further information is contained in papers by Dr. C. R. Francis (*Ibid.*, p. 452), Dr. J. Macpherson (*Ibid.*, p. 389), Dr. L. W. Stewart (*Madras Quart. Med. Journ.*, April 1861, p. 343), and Mr. P. A. Minas (*Indian Ann. of Med. Sci.*, Jan. 1859, p. 180). For a chemical history of Berberine see a paper by Prof. J. E. Meyer (*Madras Quart. Med. Journ.*, 1863, vol. vi. p. 1).

### ([9]), p. 12. Berberis Asiatica (as an Antiperiodic).

The mode of treatment of intermittent and other forms of paroxysmal fevers by this remedy pursued by Dr. Stiven, which appears to have been eminently successful, is as follows. After the operation of a purgative, and on the accession of the cold stage, from four to six drachms of the tincture (of the strength named in the text) are administered, and the patient is well covered with blankets. The immediate effect of this in general was found to be great discomfort, with an urgent thirst, and longing for fresh air. The wishes of the patient, however, if gratified, were found prejudicial to the treatment. In the course of an hour or so, the body becomes hot, and gradually covered with a gentle exudation from the skin, which increases till it terminates in profuse sweating. This in due course wears off, and the body is left cool and free from all uneasiness except weakness, which is felt to a great degree. A little thin sago or arrowroot is now given, and the patient generally falls into a comfortable sleep and awakes quite well, and no second attack comes on. A little infusion of Chiretta, with a mild aperient, is all the subsequent treatment required in most cases. The effects produced by this remedy, given as above, so closely resemble those which are observed in the use of Warburg's Drops, that Dr. Stiven is inclined to believe that the latter is mainly a preparation of Berberis.

### (10), p. 13. **Rusot (in Diseases of the Eye).**

Rusot, as an application to the eye in diseases of that organ, is of very ancient origin. Prof. Royle (*Linnean Trans.*, vol. xvii. p. 83) was the first to identify it with the *Lycium Indicum* of the ancients; and the subsequent researches of Prof. Sir J. Y. Simpson (*Pharm. Journ.*, 1854, vol. xiii. p. 413) leave no room to justify a doubt as to their identity. By the ancients, as by the native practitioners in India at the present time, it was held in repute in the treatment of eye affections. Trials with it were instituted by Dr. Wise at the Eye Infirmary at Calcutta, and by Mr. Walker at the Edinburgh Eye Dispensary: the results in both instances were communicated to Prof. Simpson, who has embodied them in his paper above alluded to. The cases in which it proved most effectual in Mr. Walker's hands were those of the conjunctiva, such as the simple, catarrhal, and pustular forms of ulceration. The other affections benefited in a minor degree were simple rheumatic or catarrho-rheumatic inflammation, and ophthalmia tarsi. Prof. Simpson in his own practice witnessed, in one or two cases of recent conjunctival ophthalmia, speedy relief and eventual cure by its means. The mode of application in each instance was the same,—that followed out in Bengal, and brought to notice by Dr. Wise. It consists in mixing equal weights of Rusot and burnt alum, and half the weight of opium, with lemon or lime juice, till the mixture has the consistence of cream, and applying it round the eyelids and over the eyebrows of the affected organ, repeating the application twice in the twenty-four hours. Its application is attended with a considerable or even painful sensation of burning. How far the efficacy of the nostrum depends upon the Rusot may admit of a question, since numerous cases of conjunctival ophthalmia have fallen under the observation of the Editor during his residence in India, which yielded to powdered alum and lime juice alone (fused together on a piece of heated iron) applied to the eyebrows in the manner directed above. The latter is a common mode of treatment amongst the people of the Madras Peninsula, and by no means an inefficacious one.

(11), p. 15. **Hill Opium.**

Dr. W. L. Macgregor (*Diseases of North-western Provinces, &c., Calcutta*, 1843) asserts the superiority of "Hill Opium" over the drug prepared on the plains (pp. 232–3). He considers that whilst it produces the full effect as a sedative and narcotic, it causes none of the headache and other disagreeable effects so often observed in the use of the ordinary drug. The dose ranges from three to six grains (p. 240); and under certain circumstances, as in cholera, it may be given safely in larger doses. Examined by Dr. F. Mouat (*loc. cit.*, p. 295), it is described as being of a fine consistence, brownish black colour internally, homogeneous, and possessing little of the smell and bitter taste of ordinary opium. The proportion of morphia, on a hurried and rough analysis, was found to be about 3 per cent. An analysis of Dr. Mactier's is cited by Lieut. Pogson (*Journ. Agri.-Hort. Soc. of India*; 1863, vol. xiii. P. ii. p. 9, App.) to the effect that ordinary Hill opium, when free from adulteration, contains more morphia than the best Turkey opium, and twice as much as the Government opium of Benares and Patna; the actual proportions, however, are not given. It would be desirable to know more of this article.

(12), p. 16. **Opium (Adulteration of).**

The adulterations of opium constitute a subject of much importance, but of great obscurity. No method at once trustworthy and easy has yet been suggested for determining its purity. The only sure test, the determination of the amount of morphia, is a complex and delicate operation. Practical druggists rely almost entirely on external characters, such as odour, taste, texture, moisture, and freedom from mechanical admixture. These, in experienced hands, are in general sufficient, but without great practice they constitute fallacious criterions (*Christison*). With special reference to the adulterations practised in India, the following judicious remarks by Dr. Eatwell merit especial notice in this place: "The nature of the adulterations practised by the cultivator is very various. The grosser impurities usually mixed with the drug to increase its weight are mud, sand, powdered charcoal, soot, cow dung, pounded poppy petals, and pounded seeds of various descriptions. All these substances are readily discoverable on breaking up the drug in cold water, removing the soluble and lighter portions of the diffused mass by decantation, and carefully examining the sediment. By this means, impurities of the above nature usually become physically apparent. Flour is a very favourite article of adulteration, but is readily detected. Opium so adulterated, speedily becomes sour; it breaks with a peculiar short rugged fracture, and on squeezing a mass of the drug after immersion in water, the starch may be seen oozing from its surface. The application of the iodine test, however, furnishes conclusive evidence of its presence, or at least of that of some amylaceous compound. The farina of the boiled potato is not unfrequently made use of; ghee (clarified butter) and goor (an impure treacle) are also occasionally used, as being articles at the command of most of the cultivators. Their presence is revealed by the peculiar odour and consistence which they impart to the drug. In addition to the above, a variety of vegetable juices, extracts, pulps, and colouring matters are occasionally fraudulently mixed with the opium; such are the inspissated juice of the common prickly pear (*Cactus Dillenii*), extracts prepared from tobacco, datura, and Indian hemp. The gummy exudations from various plants are frequently used; and of pulps, the most frequently employed are those of the tamarind and of the Bael fruit (*Ægle Marmelos*). To impart colour to the drug various substances are employed, as catechu, turmeric, and the pounded flowers of the Mowha tree (*Bassia latifolia*)." After remarking on the uncertainty of all the tests of the purity of opium, with the exception of morphiometry, Dr. Eatwell continues: "In cold water it breaks down readily into curdy flakes of the colour of pea-soup, which gradually subside, leaving the supernatant liquor of a deep brownish-yellow colour. When broken under water by the hand, the drug adheres moderately to the fingers at first, but is soon entirely diffused. Should it contain gum fraudulently mixed, this latter adheres pertinaceously to the hands, and is with difficulty removed; and in this manner he states that he frequently detected the presence of a substance similar to bird lime, probably the tenacious juice of the Banyan tree (*Ficus Indica*). If, to a portion of the cold watery infusion in a test tube, a few drops of a solution of diacetate of lead be added, a dirty grey precipitate (Meconate of lead) falls, so copious as nearly to equal in bulk the amount of fluid in the tube. Ammonia throws down a very similar and almost equally abundant precipitate, consisting of resin and the alkaloid, which on exposure to the air speedily assumes a black colour. Tincture of iodine throws down a brick-red precipitate, and tincture of the sesquichloride of iron occasions a similar precipitate of somewhat darker colour. These tests may be applied in a few seconds, and the comparative result of the precipitate thrown down may enable us to form a rude estimate of the amount of opium in a given specimen. In very largely adulterated specimens the evidence afforded by the above means is sufficiently marked. A solution of gelatine for the detection of tannic acid, and strong alcohol for the precipitation of gum, form the only other chemical reagents likely to be required. (See an excellent account of the cultivation and preparation of opium, by Dr. Eatwell in *Pharm. Journ.*, 1852, vols. xi. and xii.)

### ([13]), p. 22. **Narcotine (as an Antiperiodic).**

The antiperiodic virtues of Narcotine were first pointed out by Sir W. O'Shaughnessy, who, in addition to his own personal testimony, adduces the experience of Drs. Stewart, Chapman, Goodeve, and numerous other medical men of standing in India, in its favour (*Bengal Ph.*, p. 261). Trials with it in England by Dr. Roots proving unsatisfactory, it fell into comparative disuse, the reason being, according to Sir W. O'Shaughnessy, that it was not properly prepared according to his process given in Bengal Ph. In 1858 it was very favourably reported upon by Dr. J. Balfour (*Ind. Ann. of Med. Sci.*, vol. v. p. 547), who employed it extensively in the fevers of Rohilcund, Rangoon, and Delhi. He prescribed large doses, a scruple in the sweating stage followed by another similar dose 6 or 12 hours afterwards, according to the expected paroxysms. In tertians he gave three doses during the interval, arranging so that the last be taken two or three hours before the period of the next invasion.

Narcotine, according to the experience of Dr. Balfour, evinces none of the discomfort of quinine in large doses, but occasionally a peculiar nervous state, and a sensation of numbness and drowsiness, productive of no permanent mischief. He also found it occasionally cause nausea and vomiting. The most recent and complete evidence in favour of its antiperiodic powers is by Dr. A. Garden (*Indian Ann. of Med. Sci.*, 1861, vol. vii. p. 400). During a severe epidemic at Ghazepore in 1859–60, he prescribed it in 684 cases, in 194 of which he kept accurate notes of the effects of the remedy. The general conclusion which he arrived at was that, though not of equal value with quinine, it has a just claim to the next place in the ranks of antiperiodics, and that there is no other drug (quinine excepted) which cures so rapidly, so surely, and with so little expenditure of the drug itself, at the same time that it is free from disagreeable effects in the majority of cases. The reader is referred to Dr. Garden's excellent paper for statistical data; but it may be mentioned that in 684 cases there were 9 deaths; that in the 194 cases of which notes were kept the remedy failed in 3·6 per cent. of the cases treated; and that the average quantity required to arrest the fever was 22·7 grains, and 16·3 grains during convalescence, being a total expenditure of 39 grains, or about two scruples. The usual dose varied from a grain and a half to three grains, and in rare cases this was increased to six grains, but the larger doses were found in some instances to cause nausea, vomiting, and giddiness. As a general rule a purgative preceded the use of the Narcotine.

The Narcotine employed in the earlier trials with it in India, and with which such good results were obtained, was prepared according to the process given in the Bengal Pharmacopœia (p. 259), which is as follows: "Take of best Bengal Opium, two pounds; Alcohol " at ·835, two gallons. Break down the opium by the hand in one " third of the spirit; when reduced to pulp, add the second; strain " through cloth and press strongly; knead the mass with the last " third of the spirit, and strain and press as before; unite the " liquors. To these add enough of the strongest ammonia to cause " the mixture to restore reddened litmus paper to a blue colour; " distil till two thirds of the alcohol are drawn off. Remove the " still from the fire, and decant the fluid into a glazed basin. Let " this stand for twelve hours. Collect the crystals which have " formed, press them in cloth, and wash them well with distilled " or rain water. The washings may be thrown away. Diffuse the " mass through two quarts of water, and add by degrees one ounce " of muriatic acid. Pour off the liquor, and repeat this process; " mix the liquors, and then add pure ammonia water in slight " excess. Throw the precipitate on calico, wash it with two or " more effusions of soft water, then press into cakes, and dry in the " air stove at 130° till it ceases to lose weight." As Narcotine is almost insoluble in water it is best obtained from the portion of opium which remains undissolved when acted upon by water in the preparation of morphia. The residue should be digested with acetic acid, filtered, and ammonia added in excess. Narcotine mixed with and coloured by organic matter is precipitated. It may be purified by solution in alcohol, and treated with animal charcoal.

### ([14]), p. 22. Argemone Mexicana (Properties of).

See Dr. E. Huggins, of Nevis (*Lond. Med. Bot. Trans.*, Nov. 9, 1827, p. 1), Dr. M. Short (*Ibid.* p. 3), and Dr. W. Hamilton (*Pharm. Journ.*, vol. iv. p. 167, *Ibid.* vol. v. p. 23, *Ibid.* vol. ix. p. 129, *Ibid.* vol. xii. p. 192, and *Ibid.* vol. xiii. p. 642). Attached to the report of Dr. Bonavia received from India, are the opinions of seven Bengal medical officers, viz., Drs. Selons, Whitshaw, Jamieson, Cantor, Condon, Ellis, and Cannon, all of whom, with the exception of the last-named, report favourably of Argemone oil as an aperient, especially in colic. See also a paper by Dr. Bonavia (*Indian Med. Gaz.*, 1866, Aug. 1, p. 206). For a full account of its supposed properties and uses in the West Indies, consult Barham (*Hort. Americanus*, p. 152) and Lunan (*Hort. Jamaicencis*, vol. ii. p. 311). The narcotic properties ascribed to them in their works are probably due to a confusion which apparently existed between the capsules of this plant and those of the Datura, between which there is a general similarity. Sir W. O'Shaughnessy mentions a yellow principle, *Argemonene*, which he discovered in the juice. It would be very desirable to know more of it.

### ([15]), p. 26. Gynocardia odorata.

For an account of the medical properties and uses of Chaulmúgra see Dr. F. Mouat (*Indian Ann. of Med. Sci.*, 1854, vol. i. p. 648), Dr. Hobson (*Edin. Med. Journ.*, *July* 1855, p. 50, and *Bengal Disp.*, p. 207). Dr. B. N. Bose reports very favourably of it in leprosy, employed both internally and externally. Dr. R. C. Bose states that he has often carried the dose of the oil to half a drachm and a drachm without observing any ill effects.

### ([16]), p. 23. Garcinia morella, *Desrous*, Var. pedicellata.

The long disputed question of the botanical source of the Gamboge of Siam has been determined by Mr. Daniel Hanbury, F.R.S. (*Linnean Trans.*, 1864, vol. xxiv. P. iii. p. 487) in favour of this tree. Garcinia Morella, the *Hebradendron Cambogioides* of Graham (*Hooker, Comp. to Bot. Mag.*, vol. ii. t. 27), yields a good gamboge, which might easily be collected.

### ([17]), p. 30. Garcinia pictoria (Medical Properties of).

The medicinal properties of Indian or Mysore Gamboge have been examined by Drs. Kellie, Arthur, and Cleghorn (*Madras Med. Reports*, 1855, p. 432 *et seq.*) and by Dr. J. Kirkpatrick (*Cat. of Mysore Drugs*, No. 478). The general result arrived at was that it is a safe and efficient hydragogue purgative, though not so powerful in its action as the Gamboge of Siam. For a full account, together with an analysis of this drug, see a paper by Prof. Christison (*Pharm. Journ.*, 1847, vol. vi. p. 60). From a few trials he instituted with it, he observes that it seems to exert the same action, attended with the same inconveniences, as ordinary gamboge. Its action in dropsical affections is favourably reported of by Dr. W. Van Someren, of Madras.

### ([18]), p. 31. Garcinia purpurea.

For details of preparation, properties, and uses of the concrete oil (*Kokum Butter*) consult *Journ. of Asiat. Soc. of Bengal*, 1833, vol. ii. p. 592, and Dr. Pereira, *Pharm. Journ.*, 1852, vol. vi. p. 65.

### ([19]), p. 32. Dipterocarpus lævis (Medical Properties and Uses of).

The value of Gurjun Balsam or Wood Oil, as a substitute for copaiba in the treatment of gonorrhœa, was first pointed out in 1838 by Sir W. O'Shaughnessy (*Bengal Disp.*, p. 222), and its efficacy was tested in 1852 in a few cases by the Editor, with satisfactory results. These have since been confirmed by Dr. T. B. Henderson, of Glasgow, who states that he employed it only in cases where copaiba had been fully tried and had failed, and that it proved uniformly successful, its action being unattended with any unpleasant symptoms. He prescribed it in doses of a teaspoonful uncombined, twice or thrice daily (*Glasgow Med. Journ.*, 1865). Dr. Rean, after extensive experience in its use, pronounces it equal to copaiba in the treatment of gonorrhœa, after the subsidence of the acute stage. According to Sub-Assistant Surgeon Kanny Loll Dey, it is more efficacious than copaiba in gleet. He mentions likewise that it has been used externally as a stimulant application to indolent ulcers. Dr. H. B. Montgomery (*Madras Quart. Journ. of Med.*, 1862, vol. v. p. 114), remarks that it is apt to produce an eruption of a character similar to that occasionally following the use of copaiba; and he mentions a case of this which fell under his own observation. An essential oil of Gurjun was officinal in the Bengal Ph. ; but every good effect which may be expected from it, is more readily obtainable from the balsam in its crude state. Some interesting remarks on the physical characters of this balsam, especially in its relation to copaiba, have been published by Mr. C. Lowe (*Pharm. Journ.*, vol. xiv. p. 65), Mr. D. Hanbury (*Ibid.*, vol. xv. p. 321), M. Guibourt (*Ibid.*, vol. xvi. p. 332), and Dr. De Vry (*Ibid.*, vol. xvi. p. 373).

### ([20]), p. 46. Ægle Marmelos (Analysis of).

See Prof. Macnamara, of Calcutta (*Indian Ann. of Med. Sci.*, vol. ii. p. 233), and Mr. Pollock (*Lancet*, July 1853).

### ([21]), p. 46. Ægle Marmelos (Medical Properties and Uses of).

The value of Bael in intestinal affections, though noticed by Rheede (*Hort. Malab.*, vol. iii. p. 37), Burman (*Flor. Ind.*, Ed. 1768, p. 109), and other old writers, attracted little notice till 1853, when Sir Ranald Martin (*Lancet*, 1853, vol. ii. p. 53) called the attention of the Profession to it. Dr. J. Shortt and Dr. J. Newton, as the result of their respective personal experience, report very favourably of its action in dysentery. According to Dr. J. A. Green, a sherbet of the ripe fruit, taken every morning, proves serviceable in the dyspepsia of Europeans, when accompanied by obstinate constipation and flatulence. He adds that the unripe fruit baked for six hours is a powerful astringent, and as such is used by the natives in dysentery. Dr. B. Bose advocates the daily use of a sherbet of this fruit during cholera epidemics as a prophylatic. At such seasons it is doubtless of service to regulate the bowels carefully, avoiding either constipation or purgation. Dr. G. Bidie (*Madras Quart. Journ. of Med.*, 1862, vol. v. p. 44) states that the fruit of *Feronia elephantum*, or Wood-apple, which bears a general resemblance to Bael, is often substituted for it in hospital supplies, and being comparatively useless has induced many to treat the Bael with neglect. The fullest account of its properties and uses is by Dr. A. Grant (*Indian Ann. of Med. Sci.*, 1854, vol. ii. p. 224). Other papers containing much interesting information on this drug have been published by Dr. Hugh Cleghorn (*Ibid.*, p. 222), Baboo Ramcomol Shan (*Calcutta Med. Phys. Trans.*, vol. iv. p. 110), Dr. Pereira (*Pharm. Journ.*, vol. x. p. 165).—(*Technologist*, April 1st, 1866, vol. vi. p. 396), and Lieut. Pogson (*Journ. Agri.-Hort. Soc. of India*, 1858, vol. x. P. ii. p. 157).

### ([22]), p. 48. Toddalia aculeata.

Strong testimony to the value of Toddalia root is borne by Dr. G. Bidie, who states that though he has not employed it as a febrifuge, he can speak with confidence of its great value as a stimulant and tonic. Every part of the plant, he remarks, has a pungent bitter taste and a pleasant aroma, but these qualities are most marked in the root. The dried root-bark is of a yellowish-brown colour, and retains its pungency and bitterness for a long time. The whole plant possesses active stimulant, carminative, and tonic properties; and he adds that he knows of no single remedy in which all these three qualities are so happily combined. This article possesses additional interest from having been identified by M. Guibourt (*Hist. des Drogues Simpl.*, vol. ii. p. 530) with *Lopez Root* (*Racine de Jean Lopez, Radix Lopeziana*), which formerly enjoyed considerable repute in Europe as a remedy in diarrhœa. Mr. Daniel Hanbury, from examination of genuine specimens of the root, confirms M. Guibourt's views. A full account of Lopez Root, its properties and uses, is furnished by Murray (*Apparatus Medicaminum*, Ed. 1792, vol. vi. p. 164).

### ([23]), p. 52. Olibanum (Medical Uses of).

Attention has recently been called to the medicinal uses of Olibanum, by Dr. Delioux (*Brit. and For. Med. Chir. Rev.*, Jan. 1862, p. 242), who considers that it has fallen into unmerited disuse, and that it possesses virtues equal to the Balsams of Tolu and Peru, for which it may be advantageously substituted in hospital practice, on account of its comparative cheapness, and from the fact that as an internal remedy it is generally more agreeable to the stomach. He places the medium dose at about fifteen grains, in the form of pill or emulsion. He reports very favourably of olibanum fumes, generated by placing the gum resin on burning coals, in the treatment of the chronic forms of bronchitis and laryngitis; he found that they moderated the morbid secretions, and alleviated the cough and dyspnœa. Attention has also been called by Dr. Romei to the value of Olibanum as a local application to carbuncle (anthrax), on which he considers it exercises a specific influence. The good effects ascribed to it by Dr. Romei have been further confirmed by Dr. Caifassi (*Rev. Thêrap. du Midi*, 28th Feb. 1853), and M. Desmartins (*Ibid.*, and *Chemist*, 1854, p. 506). It is hoped that it will meet with trials in India. where it can be obtained of good quality at a small cost. Dr. J. Newton reports having frequently used it as a local stimulant to "blind boils," so common at certain seasons in many parts of India. He regards it as the best application, bringing them to a head sooner than any other remedy. He likewise states that it is given in ten-grain doses in gonorrhœa.

### ([24]), p. 54. Azadirachta Indica (Analysis of).

According to the analysis of Dr. Cornish (*Indian Ann. of Med. Sci.*, 1857, vol. iv. p. 109), this bark contains a volatile oil, a bitter resin, gum, starch, saccharine matter, an astringent substance (*catechin*), and a bitter crystallizable principle named by him *Margosine*, which is probably identical with that previously obtained by Mr. Piddington (*Calcutta Med. Phys. Trans.*, vol. iii. p. 430), and named by him *Sulphate of Azederine*. It was found most abundantly in the inner bark, the external layers being more rich in astringent principle. Dr. Cornish likewise examined the oil of the seeds, and found it to contain an alkaloid, and a bitter substance having all the characters of an acid, which he designates *Margosic Acid*.

### ([25]), p. 54. Azadirachta Indica (Medical Properties and Uses of).

The value of Nim or Margosa Bark in the treatment of periodical fevers is noticed by Fra Bartolomeo (*Voyage to the East Indies*, pp. 410, 413), Sonnerat (*Voyage*, Ed. 1787, vol. ii. p. 151), and other old writers; but it was first brought prominently forward, in 1813, by Dr. D. White (*Ainslie, Mat. Med. of Hindoostan*, p. 123), who stated that he had witnessed success from its employment fully equal to what might have been expected from Cinchona. Its claims to the character of an antiperiodic have been carefully examined by Dr. W. R. Cornish (*Indian Ann. of Med. Sci.*, 1857, vol. iv. p. 104), and Dr. Wyndowe (*Ibid.*, p. 112); and the result, based on statistical data, as expressed by the former, is to the effect that Margosa bark is nearly as effective in the treatment of intermittents as the old-established remedies, cinchona and arsenic. A similar conclusion was arrived at by Dr. Foulis (*Madras Med. Reports*, 1855, p. 89). He employed the powdered bark in drachm doses, repeated every three or four hours. An extract of the bark is favourably reported of by Mr. Jadubchunder Sett, of Bareilly (*Indian Ann. of Med. Sci.*, April 1856, p. 394). The general tenor of the reports received from India tends to show that it is effectual as an antiperiodic chiefly in the milder forms of periodical fever; but that as a tonic in convalesence after febrile and inflammatory affections, it is very valuable. Dr. C. Macnamara advocates the use of the watery extract of the dry leaves in cases of leprosy (*Mr. Kanny Loll Dey*). Further information on the properties and uses of various parts of this tree will be found in Dr. Cornish's paper, and in one by the Editor (*Indian Ann. of Med. Sci.*, 1857, vol. iv. p. 448). A full account of its uses in native practice is given in the *Taleef Shereef*, p. 170, No. 1,015.

### (26), p. 54. **Azadirachta Indica (Nim Poultice).**

Dr. J. P. Grant (*Madras Med. Journ.*, 1839, vol. i. p. 420), and Dr. D. Dunbar (*Ibid.*, 1842, vol. iv. p. 80), speak highly of Nim poultices in ill-conditioned and sloughing ulcerations. The Editor has elsewhere recorded his opinion of the value of these applications (*Indian Ann. of Med. Sci.*, 1857, vol. iv. p. 454).

### (27), p. 55. **Soymida febrifuga (Analysis of).**

See analysis of the bark by Dr. A. Overbeck (*Archiv. der Pharm.*, 1851, and *Pharm. Journ.*, vol. xi. p. 420). He failed to detect in it any crystallizable principle or alkaloid, and he even doubts if the bitter amorphous principle which he discovered is a peculiar principle of the bark. Mr. Piddington (*Calcutta Med. Phys. Trans.*, vol. iv.) described a bitter crystallizable principle obtained from this bark; but it was found that he had been experimenting on Nux Vomica bark, which is often sold in the bazaars under the same Hindústani name (*Rohun*), and that his supposed Sulphate of Rohuna was in fact a salt of Strychnia! (See *Corbyn's Indian Rev.*, 1837, vol. i. p. 287.)

### (28), p. 55. **Soymida febrifuga (Medical Properties and Uses of).**

The medicinal properties and uses of Rohun bark, especially its claims to the character of an antiperiodic, have been examined by Roxburgh (*Flor. Ind.*, vol. ii. p. 398), Dr. Duncan (*Tentamen Inaug. de Swietenià Soymidà, Edin.*, 1794), Dr. Breton (*Med.-Chir. Trans.*,

1820, vol. xi. p. 310), and Dr. Spilsbury (*Calcutta Med.-Phys. Trans.*, 1831, vol. v. p. 430). The last-named gentleman found that, in large doses, it produced vertigo, similar to that produced by quinine. This is in accordance with the statement in the Madras Report, quoted by Dr. J. Macpherson (*Indian Ann. of Med. Sci.*, vol. iii. p. 391), in which it is stated that, when taken internally beyond the quantity of five or six drachms daily, it produces vertigo and other head symptoms. Sir W. O'Shaughnessy (*Bengal Disp.*, p. 249) speaks slightingly of its powers as an antiperiodic, but his opinion is apparently based rather on theoretical grounds than on actual trials with it. Dr. Breton speaks well of an extract prepared from the bark, which he employed with advantage in several obstinate cases of diarrhœa.

### ([29]), p. 64. **Tamarindus Indica.**

The Tamarind seed, deprived of its testa, is held in considerable repute by the natives as an astringent in bowel affections (*Ainslie, Mat. Ind.*, vol. ii. p. 327). Dr. J. Shortt regards it as a valuable remedy in bad cases of diarrhœa and dysentery, having seen some good cures effected by it. A decoction of tamarind leaves is a popular application in ophthalmia.

### ([30]), p. 63. **Catechu (Medical Uses of).**

In intermittent fevers Catechu was employed in 175 cases by Dr. C. Timins (*Madras Med. Reports*, 1855, p. 239). He administered it in doses of grs. x. to grs. xii., in conjunction with infusion of Chiretta. Further trials were made with it by Dr. W. R. Cornish (*Indian Ann. of Med. Sci.*, 1857, vol. iv. p. 119), which tend to confirm Dr. Timins' views. He points out the necessity of ascertaining the quality of the catechu employed, as much of that sold in the bazaars is worthless. As an antiperiodic it may be ranked with galls. Dr. Æ. Ross reports, after repeated trials, that Catechu exercises a beneficial influence on scurvy, not only in its local effect on the gums, but on the constitution generally. Mr. Moodeen Sheriff speaks highly of the value of an ointment containing a drachm of finely powdered catechu and one ounce of simple ointment, in the treatment of various forms of ulceration. In obstinate cases he adds sixteen grains of powdered sulphate of copper to each ounce. With these he reports having treated with success syphilitic, leprous, indurated, and other ulcerations, after the failure of all ordinary remedies.

### ([31]), p. 68. **Cæsalpinia Bonducella (Analysis of).**

See Mr. Piddington's analysis of these seeds in *Calcutta Med-Phys. Trans.*, vol. iv. p. 429. A more complete examination is a desideratum.

(32), p. 68. **Cæsalpinia Bonducella (Medical Properties and Uses of).**

Amongst the numerous testimonies in favour of the antiperiodic and tonic properties of Bonduc nut, we may cite Dr. Royle (*Illust.*, vol. i. p. 85), Dr. Ludlow (*Calcutta Med.-Phys. Trans.*, vol. iii. p. 59), Mr. J. Hutchinson (*Ibid.*, vol. v. p. 42), Dr. Stewart (*Ibid.*, vol. iv. p. 437), Mr. Twining (*Diseases of Bengal*, vol. ii. p. 217), Dr. Elderton (*Outlines of the Practice of Physic*, p. 204), and Assistant-Surgeon Bholanauth Doss (*Indian Ann. of Med. Sci.*, vol. iii. p. 393). In some cases in which this remedy was tried by the Editor the results were unsatisfactory, and Dr. Kirkpatrick (*Cat. of Mysore Drugs*, No. 468) found its operation uncertain. In some cases it seemed to cure intermittents as rapidly as quinine, whereas in others it had no effect. The general tenor of the reports received from India, especially from Dr. Æ. Ross, Dr. Oswald, Dr. J. Shortt, Dr. J. Newton, Dr. Bholanauth Bose, and Sub-Assistant Surgeon Odoy Chund Dutt, is in favour of the antiperiodic and tonic powers of this remedy. According to Dr. Kirkpatrick, the root in ten-grain doses is superior to the seed as a tonic and antiperiodic. Most of the reports notice the use of the bruised seeds as an application in orchitis, but no one appears to have witnessed benefit from it. Further remarks on this drug will be found in a paper by the Editor (*Indian Ann. of Med. Sci.*, 1858, vol. v. p. 616).

(33), p. 74. **Butea frondosa (Inspissated Juice of).**

For a fuller account of this drug (Bengal or Butea Kino), consult O'Shaughnessy (*Bengal Disp.*, p. 296), Pereira (*Mat. Med.*, vol. ii. P. ii. p. 329), Royle (*Mat. Med.*, p. 398), Christison (*Disp.*, p. 577), Guibourt (*Hist. des Drogues Simpl.*, vol. iii. p. 394), *Journ. of Agri.-Hort. Soc. of India*, 1852, vol. viii. p. 24, and *Proceedings of Royal Asiat. Soc.*, May 1838.

(34), p. 74. **Abrus precatorius (Medical Properties of).**

Brief notices of the properties of this root, especially with reference to its employment as a substitute for Liquorice, are given by Dr. J. Fleming (*Asiat. Researches*, vol. xi.), Sir W. O'Shaughnessy (*Bengal Disp.*, p. 297), Drury (*Useful Plants of India*, p. 3), Dalzell and Gibson (*Bombay Flora*, p. 76), and Bouton (*Med. Plants of Mauritius*, p. 43). The demulcent properties of this and other parts of the plant have been noticed by the Editor elsewhere (*Madras Quart. Med. Journ.*, 1860, vol. i. p. 61).

(35), p. 74. **Arachis hypogæa (Oil of).**

The following note on Ground-nut Oil prepared at the Government garden at Hewrah, in the Deccan, is supplied by Dr. J. Winchester, late Medical Storekeeper at Bombay: "This oil is uni-

"formly used in Western India instead of Olive Oil. It is of a pale-
"straw colour, without smell, and so pure in taste that fish can
"be cooked with it, and rendered quite as agreeable to the palate
"as with ghee or clarified butter. Tested with alcohol and ether,
"it was found perfectly free from adulteration. The annual supply
"received from Hewrah varied from 1,000 to 3,000 lbs. It was
"prepared by hydraulic pressure, and accepted by the whole
"medical department as a complete substitute for Olive Oil."

(36), p. 93. **Punica granatum (Cortex Granati).**

Dr. Kirkpatrick (*Cat. of Mysore Drugs*, No. 474) informs us that he has found the rind of the fruit a valuable tonic and astringent, and that in decoction with cloves it is the best remedy he knows for the chronic forms of dysentery under which the native poor of India so often suffer. Its value as an astringent has long been acknowledged. The Editor has repeatedly used it with the best effect.

(37), p. 94. **Compound Extract of Colocynth.**

This Extract has been prepared with great success in India. It was supplied to the medical stores at Bombay from the Government manufactory at Hewra, to the extent of 150 or 200 lbs. annually. Dr. Winchester, late Medical Storekeeper at Bombay, on whose authority this is stated, remarks: "By those who know the profusion in
"which the Cucurbitaceæ grow all over the plains of Western India,
"it would naturally be expected that this medicine should be amply
"supplied, not only for the medical use of the army, but for export."
That sent to the stores was of the finest quality; and as the Medical Storekeeper supplied the scammony and the soap, the one purchased in the bazaar and the other received from England, the Compound Extract of Colocynth was quite equal to any imported.

(38), p. 99. **Carum (Ptychotis) Ajowan (Seeds of).**

These seeds, under the name of *Ajava seeds*, were brought to the notice of the Profession in England, about the middle of the last century, by Dr. Percival (*Essays*, vol. ii. p. 226, and *Med. Comment.*, 1773, vol. i. p. 276); but they never appear to have come much into use. That they possess valuable properties as a carminative is beyond a doubt. Dr. G. Bidie, who has called the special attention of the Committee to this drug, remarks, "In moderate quantities
"it increases the flow of saliva, augments the secretion of gastric
"juice, and acts as a stimulant, carminative, and tonic. As a topical
"remedy it may be used with advantage, along with astringents, in
"cases of relaxed sore throats. For disguising the taste of disagree-
"able drugs, and obviating their tendency to cause nausea and grip-
"ing, I know of no remedy of equal power." Testimony of a similar

character is borne by Mr. J. J. Wood (*Madras Quart. Med. Journ.*, 1862, vol. v. p. 293), who considers that it combines the stimulant quality of capsicum or mustard with the bitter property of chiretta, and the antispasmodic virtues of assafœtida. The oil, diluted with soap liniment or any bland oil, is reported to prove valuable as a stimulant embrocation in chronic rheumatism. Mr. Wood considers the proportion of seed ordinarily employed in preparing the distilled water to be far too small. On the authority of Mr. H. H. Lynsdale, he advises 3 lbs. of the bruised seeds to six quart bottles of water, and distil over four.

(39), p. 107. **Hydrocotyle Asiatica (Medical Properties of, &c.)**

An interesting account of the introduction, in 1852, of this plant, in the treatment of leprosy by Dr. Boileau, is furnished by M. Bouton (*Med. Plants of Mauritius*, p. 74). See also the memoir of Dr. Alexander Hunter (*Madras Med. Reports*, 1855, p. 356), which, in addition to a detail of his trials with the remedy at the Leper Hospital at Madras, contains the analysis of the plant by M. Lépine, and other particulars relating to its botany, pharmacology, &c. Dr. J. Shortt reports favourably of it, regarding it as a capital alterative and tonic in all leprous affections. The Editor's trials with this remedy are given in *Indian Ann. of Med. Sci.*, 1858, vol. v. p. 597.

(40), p. 109. **Cinchona. Introduction of, into India.**

The introduction of the quinine yielding Cinchonas into British India was suggested by Dr. Royle as early as 1835, and was persistently urged by him on the Court of Directors at every favourable opportunity.

The Dutch naturalists had also for a long time made similar attempts to induce their government to introduce these trees into Java, but without effect, till 1852, when M. Hasskarl was sent to South America for the purpose. He brought back with him to Java living plants of several species of Cinchona, but, it is said, for the most part, of inferior sorts.

In 1852, and several times after, the Government of India called the attention of the authorities at home to the great cost of quinine, and the consequent desirability of their cultivating the plant for themselves.

In the year 1854, Dr. Royle sent to India six young Cinchona plants obtained from the Gardens at Kew and the Horticultural Society. These plants were the produce of seeds collected in 1847 by the distinguished French botanist and traveller, M. Weddell, to whom mainly we owe our present exact knowledge of the species of Cinchona. They were taken to Calcutta by Mr. Fortune, and thence forwarded to Darjiling by Dr. Falconer, where they did not survive the first winter.

Notwithstanding the failure of this first small attempt, Dr. Royle continued confident of success, and pressed the importance of sending a skilled person direct to the Cinchona districts. At that time the Indian Government was spending about 7,000*l*. a year on bark and quinine. Soon after the cost rose to 12,000*l*. a year, and after 1857, in which year there was a considerable increase of European troops, the annual outlay became proportionally increased.

The matter thus at length acquired sufficient importance in the eyes of the authorities both in India and at home, and in 1859 Lord Stanley, then Secretary of State for India, resolved to despatch an expedition to the Cinchona countries. He selected for its organization, Mr. Clements Markham, whose previous knowledge of the country well fitted him for the purpose. Mr. Markham determined to proceed himself to the Calisaya region of Bolivia, and after consultation with Sir W. Hooker, the Director of Kew Gardens, who took a lively interest in the success of the experiment, he directed Mr. Spruce, a naturalist at that time exploring the Upper Amazons, to proceed to the red-bark forests of Equador. Mr. Pritchett was at the same time sent to the grey bark districts of Peru, and forcinghouses were prepared at Kew for the reception of plants and seeds.

Mr. Markham left England in December 1859, and returned viâ Panama with a collection of live plants. He proceeded at once overland to Bombay, and thence to the Neilgherries, where he arrived safely in the autumn of 1860. Large quantities of plants and seeds collected by Mr. Spruce and Mr. Pritchett arrived early in 1861. Sites for the cultivation were selected by Mr. Markham, with the assistance of Mr. MacIvor, to whose charge their culture was entrusted.

As a matter of precaution, a part of the plants and many seeds were left at Kew, where they germinated well and grew vigorously. As soon as the stock was sufficient, the experiment was extended to other parts of India. Plants and seeds were forwarded to Mr. Thwaites, the Director of the Ceylon Botanic Garden, and to Dr. Anderson, the Superintendent of the Calcutta Botanic Garden. Dr. Anderson was also sent to Java to get information as to the Dutch culture. Mr. Thwaites established his plantations on the slopes of the mountains of the central province of Ceylon, and Dr. Anderson chose for the purpose various sites in Sikkim. The culture was everywhere successful, Vast numbers of plants have been raised from seeds and cuttings; the trees have attained a considerable size, have flowered and ripened seeds, and the yield of alkalis is as great or greater than in the native country of the plant. The success of this most important experiment is thus placed beyond a doubt.

For the following facts relative to the present state of Cinchona cultivation in India, the Committee are indebted to Mr. Markham.

According to the latest reports, there were in January 1867 1,785,303 Cinchona plants in the Government plantations on the Neilgherry hills, of which 401,211 were permanently planted out. The total area under actual cultivation was 673 acres, and 125,747 plants have been issued to the public.

Private plantations have been formed on the Neilgherries and Koondahs, in Wynaad and Coorg; and the Rajah of Travancore has caused a small Cinchona garden to be established at Peermède.

In March 1862, Cinchona plants were first sent up to Darjeeling, and the experiment was commenced there in the following June, with 211 plants. The plantations are at Libong and Rungbi, on well protected spurs below Darjiling. In January 1867 there were 625,408 plants, and 67,280 were permanently planted out. At Kangra, in the Punjab, Major Nassau Lees has formed a Cinchona Plantation at a place which he has called 'New Quito;' and the Government of Bombay have established a small experimental garden at Lingmulla, on the Mahabaleshwur hills.

It was considered to be very important that all the species of known value should be introduced from South America into India; and the results of their cultivation, up to 1867, have been as follows :—

I. **C. Calisaya** (*Yellow bark*). Up to last year the shrubby variety alone had been obtained; but in the autumn of 1866 a large supply of seeds of the tree variety (*C. vera* of Weddell) was received, which germinated freely. In January 1867 there were 40,000 plants of *C. Calisaya* in the Neilgherry plantations. Most important results may be expected from their cultivation, which will be ascertained in the course of a few years.

II. **C. succirubra** (*Red bark*). The trees of this species are now so large as to interlace, although 12 feet apart. They are growing at 4,000 to 6,000 feet above the sea. Mr. McIvor's method of mossing the stems has increased the thickness of the bark, and, according to Mr. Howard's analysis, doubled the yield of febrifuge alkaloids. A third crop of bark off the same tree, renewed under moss, has given the following unprecedented yield of quinine and kindred alkaloids:

| | | |
|---|---|---|
| Crystallized sulphates - - - | 8·45 | per cent. |
| Alkaloids soluble in ether* (cinchonidine and quinine) - - - | 1·14 | „ |
| Cinchonicine - - - - - | 0·20 | „ |
| | 9·79 | |

Original bark, 6 months under moss, yielded 9·26 per cent. of alkaloids; while unmossed bark gave 6·95 per cent. These specimens were all from the Neilgherries. Red bark, about two years old, from Darjeeling, has given 3½ per cent.

III. **C. officinalis** (*Crown bark*). The plants of this species rank next in luxuriance to the red barks, and are much more hardy, growing as well upon grass as upon forest land, and flourishing even on the highest ridges of the Neilgherries, when sheltered from the full force of the monsoon. A specimen of crown bark from the Neilgherries, being a second crop from the same tree renewed under moss, gave the following results:

| | | |
|---|---|---|
| Crystallized sulphates - - - | 6·52 | per cent. |
| Alkaloids soluble in ether (quinine and cinchonidine) - - - | 1·35 | „ |
| Cinchonicine - - - - - | 0·15 | „ |
| | 8·02 | |

---

* i.e., quinine and cinchonidine. The progressive increase in the yield, in red barks grown on the Neilgherries, is as follows :—

| | | |
|---|---|---|
| 1863 (18 months growth) - | 4·10 | p.c. |
| 1864 (2 years and 5 months) | 5·20 | „ |
| 1865 (3 years and 5 months) | 5·44 | „ |
| 1866 (third time renewed) | 7·64 | „ |
| 1867 (4 years) - - | 9·79 | „ |

Original bark of this species, nine months under moss, yielded 7·37 per cent. of alkaloids, and small quill bark 4·73 per cent.

IV. **C. micrantha, C. nitida, C. Peruviana,** &c., (*Grey barks*). These species grow luxuriantly with the red bark plants. A very remarkable result of their cultivation has been that, whereas in their native Peruvian forests near Huanuco they yield nothing but the comparatively useless alkaloid called cinchonine, an analysis of specimens of their bark from the Neilgherries shows that the cinchonine has almost disappeared, and that a very large per-centage of the valuable alkaloid, Quinidine, has taken its place.

V. **C. lancifolia** (*New Granada barks*). There are 304 plants of this species growing on the Neilgherries, derived from a plant received from Java, and originally from seeds gathered by Dr. Karsten, near Pasto. But this is not the most valuable New Granada species, and the Secretary of State for India has sanctioned the despatch of a collector to attempt once more to obtain plants or seeds of the exceedingly valuable kind that is known to grow near Popeyan and Pitayo.

VI. **C. Pahudiana.** This is the worthless Java species, of which there are 425 plants on the Neilgherries; but they are not propagated; and an analysis of bark, nine months under moss, only gave 0·761 per cent. of alkaloids.

In 1866 the Secretary of State for India in Council appointed an experienced chemist, Mr. Broughton, to conduct investigations and analyses at the Neilgherry plantations. From his first report a few of the more interesting passages are appended:

### *Abridged Extract from Mr. Broughton's First Report,* dated April 12th, 1867.

Attention has been chiefly directed to an examination of *Cinchona succirubra.* Of all the species yet naturalized in India this exhibits the most vigorous growth. It is numerically the most important; and it is, moreover, the one which will first find its way into actual consumption.

C. succirubra.

An inspection of the more advanced portions of the plantations reveals considerable differences in the habit and appearances of the individual Red Bark trees. This has already been remarked by Mr. Markham, who suggested that these variations might probably be connected with differences in their yield of alkaloids. The accuracy of this conjecture is rendered evident by the results of the analysis of the trunk bark of four trees, which are calcutated in per-centages of dry bark, as given below:—

| —— | I. | II. | III. | IV. |
|---|---|---|---|---|
| Total alkaloids (hydrated) - - - - | 4·85 | 7·00 | 6·40 | 6·4 |
| Alkaloid soluble in ether (Quinine) - - | 3·25 | 4·25 | 4·75 | 1·7 |
| Cinchonidine and Cinchonine - - - | 1·60 | 2·75 | 1·65 | 4·7 |
| Sulphate of Quinine obtained crystallized - | 3·00 | 4·00 | 4·55 | 1·7 |

In the above analyses, as well as in those given subsequently, the Sulphate of Quinine has been obtained in as pure a state as possible.

Of No I., it may be remarked that, though the poorest specimen that has come under my notice, it gives at least an equal yield to the best Ecuador Red Barks. Nos, II., III., and IV. are considerably richer. Seven per cent. of alkaloids in the natural (unmossed) bark appeared to me so large an amount that I was led to repeat the analysis by a different method, which, however, closely corroborated the former results. The richness of their barks in alkaloids, though entitling them to the first place amongst our Indian barks, is not in many respects a true measure of their intrinsic value for manufacturing purposes. Their value depends also on the readiness with which the alkaloid can be obtained in a pure and crystalline form. in this respect the natural "unmossed" Succirubra bark is at some disadvantage, since its alkaloids are more difficult to obtain In a pure form than those yielded by some other kinds.

Bark of branches.

The above analyses were made with the bark of the trunk, which is much richer than that of the branches yielding "quill bark." Some of the latter yielded but three per cent. of alkaloids, from which 1·4 per cent. of crystalline sulphates was obtained.

Root bark.

An examination of the root bark of *C. succirubra* corroborated the statement of Dr. De Vrij, that it contains a large per-centage of alkaloids, viz., 2·15 of Quinine, and 3·85 of Cinchonidiue and Cinchonine, giving a total percentage of 6·0 of alkaloids. In no case, however, could the roots be a remunerative source of alkaloids, since the bark is thin, contains 74 per cent. of water, and is laborious to procure.

Leaves.

From four pounds weight of the leaves were obtained 3·1 grains of alkaloids, of which about one grain was soluble in ether, and gave a faint indication of Quinine when tested with chlorine water and ammonia. No crystalline salt could be obtained. The leaves appear rich in Quinovin.

C. officinalis

Next to C. succirubra, the most important species we at present possess in India is *C. officinalis,* whose varieties yield the Crown barks. Of these varieties, *C. Bonplandiana* holds the first place. The trunk-bark of a tree of this variety yielded in one instance 3·6 per cent. of alkaloids (Quinine 2·8, and Cinchonine and Cinchonidine 0·8), and in another 3·8 per cent. (Quinine 3·0 and Cinchonine 0·8); the yield of Sulphate of Quinine being in the first instance 2·8, and in the other 2·9 per cent. This bark possesses, for manufacturing purposes, certain advantages over the Red Bark, that in some measure compensate for the smaller yield and slower growth of the tree producing it. The Crown Bark yields its alkaloids with greater ease, owing to the small amount of resin and coloring matter with which they are associated. The bark yielded by this variety is of admirable quality, and nearly equal to the fine Calisaya Bark of Bolivia.

C. micrantha.

An analysis of the trunk-bark of *C. micrantha,* four years and a half growth, yielded 7·1 per cent of alkaloids, of which only 0·3 was Quinine, whilst the remaining 6·8 was Cinchonine, which crystallized from solution in alcohol with great readiness and purity, forming splendid crystals 0·18 inch long. Huanuco Bark contains usually about 2·0 per cent. of alkaloid. Should Cinchonine come into use as a febrifuge, the Micrantha bark will furnish the most easy and abundant source.

Effects of "mossing."

The results of the observations on the plan of "mossing," introduced by Mr. McIvor on the Neilgherries, were on the whole corroborative of Mr. Howard's previous statements, demonstrating that under this treatment there was a marked increase in the yield of alkaloids. Facts and experiments render it highly probable that the exposure of the *living* bark to direct sun-light has the effect of diminishing the yield of alkaloids, and hence the advantage of direct protection.

### ([41]), p. 110. Cinchona Leaves (Medical Properties of).

The leaves of *Cinchona Succirubra*, grown in India, have been examined by Mr. J. E. Howard (*Gov. Record, Madras Quart. Med. Journ.*, 1863, vol. vii. p. 425), who obtained from them, in the first instance, alkaloid to the extent of 0·11 per cent., of which part was soluble in ether, the remainder in spirits of wine, and afterwards 0·19 per cent. of precipitate still more combined with astringent matter. "From these data," Mr. Howard observes, "it seems to " follow that the leaves will not supply a material for the extraction " of Quinine, but that they will nevertheless be very useful, when " used fresh, or in recently prepared decoction or infusion, for the " cure of the fevers of the country. To this end the abundance of " Kinovic acid they contain, equal (weighed in the rough state) to " 4·20 per cent., may also conduce." Trials with them have been made by Dr. W. N. Chipperfield (*Madras Quart. Med. Journ.*, 1866, vol. x. p. 85), and Dr. Collins, Civil Surgeon, Darjeeling (*Journ. Agri.-Hort. Soc. of India*, 1863, vol. xiii. P. 1. p. 6), and the result has been, on the whole, favourable. In mild uncomplicated cases it proved useful, like many other astringent tonics, but it is evidently in no way comparable to Quinine as an antiperiodic. Dr. Chipperfield employed three formula: (1.) Cinchona Leaves, 1½ oz.; Dilute Sulphuric Acid, 2 fl. drs.; Cold Water, 20 oz. (2.) Cinchona Leaves, 1½ oz.; Dilute Sulphuric Acid, 2 fl. drs.; Water, 20 oz.; boil for ten minutes, and strain. (3.) Cinchona Leaves, 1 oz.; Water, 6 oz.; boil for ten minutes, and strain. Dose of each, 3 oz. to 4 oz. thrice daily. He observed no difference between leaves of *C. succirubra* and those of *C. condaminea*.

### ([41a]), p. 115. Cinchona Alkaloids (Antiperiodic powers of).

A Commission having, in 1866, been appointed in the Madras Presidency to examine the antiperiodic powers of Cinchonine, Cinchonidine, and Quinidine, supplies of these alkaloids were placed at the disposal of medical officers at "notedly malarious stations," and were tested in 1145 cases of paroxysmal fevers of all types; 410 by Sulphate of Cinchonine, 359 by Sulphate of Cinchonidine, and 376 by Sulphate of Quinidine. Of the 1145 cases treated, there were 4 deaths (all at Goodaloor in the Wynaad District, the fever being complicated with pneumonia or diarrhœa), and 27 failures, the latter presenting a per-centage of just over 2 per cent. This result must be considered as very satisfactory. The following abridged quotations from the report will serve to place the subject in a clearer light. The doses and mode of administration varied a good deal. Some medical officers used large doses (grs. xv. to xx), others medium doses (grs. viii. to x.), and some small doses (grs. ii. to v.) As a general rule it appears that those experiments were most successful in which medium doses were administered in a single dose daily, the cases recovering more expeditiously than when larger or smaller quantities were employed. Large doses of either of these alkaloids produce effects very similar to those of Quinine. Disagreeable noises in the head, singing in the ears, deafness, and giddiness, were the most noticeable symptoms. Vomiting, nausea, and purging were also occasionally noticed to follow their use. Small or moderate doses produced none of these effects, while they improved the appetite, strengthened the digestion, and in many cases appeared to have a marked effect in reducing the size of congested spleens, The evidence adduced does not show any particular superiority of one alkaloid over the other. The average dose of each is apparently about ten grains. The Sulphate of Quinidine is, perhaps, the one regarding which there is the least difference of opinion as to its merits; all three are undoubtedly antiperiodic, and capable of controlling paroxysmal fevers. The Sulphate of Cinchonine in large doses, perhaps, causes more unpleasant symptoms than the others, but on this point further evidence is wanting. In some cases, larger quantities were exhibited than were necessary to check the fever. "The main conclusion "which the members of the Commission have derived from the "data before them is, that these alkaloids, hitherto little valued in "medicine, are scarcely, if at all, inferior as therapeutical agents "to Quinine."

### ([42]), p. 115. Ipecacuanha in Dysentery.

The re-introduction of Ipecacuanha in large doses in the treatment of acute dysentery, is due to Mr. E. J. Docker (*Lancet, July and August*, 1858). Much valuable information on this mode of treatment, drawn mainly from facts supplied by the medical officers of the Madras army, is furnished by Dr. W. R. Cornish (*Madras Quart. Med. Journ., Jan.* 1861, p. 41). A full resumé of the subject has been published by Dr. J. Ewart (*Indian Ann. of Med. Sci.*, 1863, vol. viii. p. 396). The results, on the whole, have been of the most satisfactory description.

### ([43]), p. 124. Extract of Taraxacum.

Extract of Taraxacum, prepared from the fresh plant cultivated at the Government garden at Hewra, in the Deccan, is favourably reported of by Dr. Winchester, late Medical Storekeeper at Bombay. It is supplied, he remarks, in the form of a powdered Extract, sun dried, and forwarded in air-tight boxes to the extent annually of at least 50 or 60 lbs., in supplies of 10 or 15 lbs. at a time, thus ensuring its perfect freshness.

(44), p. 132. **Extract of Diospyros.**

The value of this Extract as an astringent rests mainly on the testimony of Sir W. O'Shaughnessy (*Bengal Disp.*, p. 488, and *Bengal Ph.*, p. 290). It is favourably spoken of by Sub-Assistant Surgeon Odoy Chund Dutt. Dr. J. Short mentions that the astringent juice of the fruit is used by the natives as a local application to bruises and sprains, the swelling attendant on which it relieves. There is little doubt that it possesses powerfully astringent properties, and is deserving of a high place amongst indigenous remedies of this class.

(45), p. 137. **Alstonia scholaris (Medical Properties of).**

See a paper by Dr. A. Gibson in *Pharm. Journ.*, 1853, vol. xii. p. 422, which contains a short but interesting account of this drug. Mr. Nimmo, in 1839, called attention to it as a powerful tonic, and suggested its use as an antiperiodic (*Graham's Bombay Plants*, p. 115). It is a remedy of considerable promise. See remarks on its botanical characters in Art. Holarrhena antidysenterica (*infra*).

(46), p. 138. **Holarrhena antidysenterica (Botanical History of).**

With reference to the confusion which has so long existed between the different species of *Holarrhena* and *Wrightia*, Dr. Wight supplies the following interesting remarks:—" Linnæus, while preparing " his Flora Zeylanica, found in Herman's Herbarium a plant corre" sponding with Burman's *Nerium Indicum siliquis angustis, &c.* " (*Thesaur. Zeylan.*, tab. 77); to that plant he subjoined as a synonym " Rheede's *Codaga pala* (*Hort. Mal.* 1, 47), a continental and widely " different plant, reported by Rheede to be possessed of great medi" cinal virtues, especially in the cure of bowel affections; and appa" rently on the strength of that report, he subsequently gave this " double or spurious species the name of *Nerium antidysentericum*, " though no such virtues were ever attributed to the Ceylon plant, " which still retains the name. So far all is clear, the real confusion " only commencing when it was long after ascertained that two " distinct genera were combined under one specific name.

" In 1809 Mr. Brown published (*Wern. Trans.*) an admirable revi" sion of the Natural Order *Apocyneæ*. In that memoir Linnæus's " Ceylon half of *N. antidysentericum* formed the type of Brown's " new genus *Wrightia*, while the Malabar half fell into another new " genus, *Holarrhena*.

" About the same time, Roxburgh was engaged in preparing his " MSS. Flora Indica, and a noble series of drawings representing " almost every species described. In that collection are figures of " three *Apocynous* trees, all having a general resemblance to each other, " but each referrible to a distinct genus. One was a new species of " *Wrightia* (*W. tinctoria*, Br., *Nerium*, Roxb.); another of *Holarrhena*, " in fact, the true *Codaga pala*, which he referred to *Echites* (*E. anti-* " *dysenterica*, Roxb.); and the third, *Alstonia*, which als he referred " to *Echites*, *E. scholaris*, Roxb. 'Of the two first,' he remarks in " his Flora, 'they are both natives of the mountains which bound "'the Rajamundry Circars on the north side, and are so much alike "'in most respects (the nectarium excepted), that without a tolerable "'knowledge of both, the one may be mistaken for the other; and "'I have no doubt but the bark of the *Nerium* may have been "'gathered and sold for the *Conessi*, to which I attribute the dis- "'repute that has fallen on *Conessi* bark in Europe; for with the "'natives of most parts of India it is deemed a specific in most "'complaints of the bowels; and I am inclined to think it deserves "'a better name than it has hitherto acquired amongst Europeans.' " Of the third all we know from him is the name, written on the draw- " ing, the description being apparently lost. It, however, has the " character of possessing virtues similar to those of *Conessi*, and is " about as likely to be mistaken for the *Conessi* as the *Wrightia*, but " less injuriously, if it possess the properties attributed to it by the " natives.

" From this history it would appear that, to some extent at least, " the mistakes are fairly attributable to two allied and somewhat " similar genera having each a species bearing a therapeutical name, " while the one best known, and probably oftenest heard of, possesses " no therapeutic virtue. The first and most obvious remedy is for us, " as far as we can, to make known that the Ceylon *Wrightia anti-* " *dysenterica* and *W. Zeylanica* are but one species (a fact we have " ascertained by examination of the original specimens), and ought " both to be included under the latter name, thus removing the prin- " cipal source of the confusion, by suppressing the misleading " name *antidysenterica* in connexion with *Wrightia*.

" Then as to the distinction of the three plants named, we think " that, without going into the minutiæ of exact botanical description, " characters sufficiently precise for their ready discrimination by " collectors might easily be found, the more so as they belong to " three separate genera, nay, sections of the order.

" As regards habit, they are all arboreous. The bark in all is " milky; hence the native name *Pala*. The flowers in all are white, " clustered, either terminal or on short axillary branchlets. The " fruit in all are long, slender, pendulous follicles in pairs, usually " adhering at the points. The seeds in all are furnished with tufts " of white silky hairs. The two first have opposite ovate leaves, " rounded at the base, pointed or acuminated at the point, while the " last has them obovate; that is, broad, rounded at the apex, and " tapering towards the base, and whorled on the branches. From " these particulars it will be seen they all agree in general aspect; " the points on which they differ are more minute, but at the same " time more precise, demanding greater care for their accurate dis- " crimination.

" The first and most certain distinctions are found in the seeds, " when these are procurable.

" In *Wrightia*, Br. (*Nerium*, Linn. and Roxb.), they are furnished " at the lower end, that next the footstalk of the follicle, with a tuft " of delicate white silky hairs.

" In *Holarrhena*, Br. (*Echites*, Roxb.), they are furnished with a " tuft of hairs on the upper end, that most remote from the foot- " stalk:

" Whilst in *Alstonia*, Br. (*Echites*, Linn. and Roxb.), they are " flattened and have a tuft at both ends, being attached to the follicle " by the middle.

" As regards the corolla, the distinctions are equally precise, and " more conspicuous, at least between *Wrightia* and *Holarrhena*, " the two most likely to be mistaken for each other.

"In *Wrightia tinctoria* the tube of the corolla is about twice the "length of the calyx; the limb five-lobed; lobes before expansion "twisted towards the *right;* stamens inserted within the mouth of the "corolla; anthers arrow-shaped, adhering round the stigma, and "protruding in the form of a cone from the orifice; surrounded by a "filamentous crown (*Nectarium*, Roxb.), the velvetty fimbriæ of which "are about half the length of the lobes. Here the conically projecting "anthers and fimbriately crowned orifice of the tube of the corolla "form the prominently distinctive marks derivable from the flowers "of this species.

"In *Holarrhena antidysenterica* the tube is slender, three or four "times the length of the calyx, dilated at the base, contracted above; "limb five-lobed; lobes twisted to the *left* before expansion; orifice "of the tube, naked or without appendages; stamens inserted at the "bottom of the tube within the dilated portion. In this case, the "absence of appendages about the orifice of the tube, and the hidden "position of the stamens at the bottom of it, most readily distin-"guish this from the preceding.

"*Alstonia Scholaris* is best distinguished from the other two by the "leaves, which form whorls or rings round the branches, and are "broad, obovate, rounded above, tapering below; tube of the corolla "short, hairy within, limb five-lobed; lobes twisted towards the "*right;* stamens inserted about the middle, not projecting. The "follicles in this are long and pendulous, resembling a scourge of "small cords, whence, perhaps, the specific name."

A cursory examination of the specimens of *Holarrhena* in the Banksian, Indian, and Kew Herbaria, leads us to suspect that *H. antidysenterica*, *H. Codaga*, *H. pubescens*, and *H. Malaccensis* are all only varieties of the same species, and are endowed with similar, if not identical medicinal properties.

### ([47]), p. 140. **Hemidesmine.**

Professor Christison is of opinion that this so-called crystallizable principle, described first by Mr. Garden (*Lond. Med. Gazette*, vol. xx. p. 800), (and named by him, from an erroneous view of the botanical source of the root, *Smilasperic acid*), and subsequently by Dr. A. J. Scott, of Madras (*Indian Ann. of Med. Sci.*, 1856, vol. iii. p. 336), is in reality only a stearopten, and he mentions having long since obtained it by simple distillation of the root with water. A further examination of this substance is desirable.

### ([48]), p. 141. **Mudar.**

Much difference of opinion has existed as to which species of Calotropis is the true Mudar. The subject has been carefully examined by Dr. Wight (*Madras Lit. and Sci. Journ.*, 1835, vol. ii. p. 70); and although he decides in favour of *C. procera*, there appears little doubt that the closely allied species, *C. gigantea*, is possessed of considerable activity as an emetic and diaphoretic.

### ([49]), p. 141. **Mudarine.**

This principle was first discovered by Dr. Duncan (*Edinburgh Med. and Surg. Journ.*, July 1st, 1829) in the dried root bark. He found that it acted as an emetic, and regarded it as the active principle of the root. Its watery solution has the remarkable property of coagulating or gelatinising by the application of heat, and of becoming fluid again as the solution cools. Dr. Duncan, in addition to analysis, supplies in his paper much valuable information with regard to the medicinal properties of Mudar. It is probably to this principle that Dr. Van Someren alludes in his report; he states that he has used "an alkaloid" educed from this plant, as an emetic, and found it very successful.

### ([50]), p. 141. Mudar (Therapeutic Uses of).

For testimony in favour of the employment of Mudar in leprosy, see Dr. Robinson (*Med. Chir. Trans.*, vol. x. p. 27), Dr. Playfair (*Calcutta Med. Phys. Trans.*, vol. i. p. 77), Dr. J. R. Voss (*Ibid.*, vol. ii. p. 409), Dr. Ainslie (*Royal Asiat. Soc. Trans.*, 1826, vol. i.), Dr. S. Rogers (*Madras Med. Journ.*, 1843, vol. v. p. 391), and Dr. Irvine (*Med. Topog. of Ajmeer*, p. 126.) It failed, either wholly or partially, in the hands of Dr. D. Young (*Calcutta Med. Phys. Trans.*, vol. ii. p. 334), Dr. J. Kirkpatrick (*Cat. of Mysore Drugs*, No. 463), and Dr. Waring (*Indian Ann. of Med. Sci.*, 1858, vol. v. p. 588). For a summary of its uses in syphilitic affections, obstinate ulcerations, &c., see the last-named paper. Consult also a monograph by Dr. Casanova, "*Essai sur le Mudar (Calotropis Mudarii), contenant l'histoire naturelle de cette plante, ses propriétés physiques, chimiques, et médicinales,*" an English translation of which was published by Dr. Richy, at Calcutta, in 1833. Its uses in native practice are given at considerable length in the Taleef Shereef, p. 5, and in *Corbyn's Ind. Med. Journ.* 1838, p. 32. As a remedy in the dysentery of the natives, it is very favourably reported on by Assistant-Surgeon J. J. Durant (*India Med. Gaz.*, May 1st, 1866, p. 112). He regards it in those cases as a perfect substitute for ipecacuanha. For adults, he commences with a large dose, never less than a scruple, and seldom going beyond a drachm. In ordinary cases, the smaller dose is preferable. For children he prescribes it in a dose of one or two grains for every year of age, three or four times a day. He found its physiological effects precisely similar to those of ipecacuanha, like which also it may be given variously combined as individual circumstances may require. He has had no experience with this remedy amongst Europeans.

### ([51]), p. 142. Tylophora asthmatica (Emetic properties of).

Dr. J. Kirkpatrick's observations on this subject (*Cat. of Mysore Drugs*, No. 470) are conclusive. After remarking that the powdered root and juice are used by the people of Mysore as an emetic, he adds, "I have administered this medicine in at least a thousand "cases, and found it most valuable. In dysentery, and as a simple "emetic, it is in every way comparable with Ipecacuanha. The dose "is from 20 to 30 grains, with half a grain or a grain of Tartar Emetic, "if strong emesis is required. If the dysentery distinctly arise from "intermittent disease, Quinine is conjoined. The form of the medi-"cine I use is the powder of the dry leaf. If the root were used, "the supply would soon be exhausted; besides I have found it less "certain than the leaf. The preparation of the juice would at all "times be troublesome and tedious. In catarrhal and chronic coughs "it seems to act well. Its efficacy as a substitute for Ipecacuanha, "not only as a simple emetic but as a remedy in dysentery, asthma, "and catarrhal affections, is confirmed by the report of Dr. Oswald, "Mr. Moodeen Sheriff, and others. According to the latter, the "best treatment of snake bites consists in producing free emesis "by the express juice of this plant, and following up its use with "diffusible stimulants." These views are further confirmed by Dr. G. Bidie in a note with which he favoured the Committee; he considers that, like Ipecacuanha and Tartar Emetic, it acts as a specific emetic, exciting vomiting after absorption, by its action on the vagus.

### ([52]), p. 148. **Chiretta (Varieties of).**

See an excellent paper "On the Varieties of Chiretta used in the Hospitals of Southern India," by Dr. Hugh Cleghorn (*Indian Ann. of Med. Sci.*, 1856, vol. iii. p. 270). It contains three good illustrations.

### ([53]), p. 155. **Kaladana (Purgative Properties of).**

See Sir W. O'Shaughnessy, Drs. Chapman, Leckie, Green, Martin, Stewart, and Goodeve (*Bengal Disp.*, pp. 525–6), Dr. Kirkpatrick (*Cat. of Mysore Drugs*, No. 467), Report of the Madras Drug Committee (*Madras Med. Reports*, 1855, p. 423), and Dr. Waring (*Pharm. Journ.*, 1866, vol. vii. p. 496.) Dr. G. Bidie, in a note addressed to the Editor, bears testimony to its value as a purgative, and he has furnished specimens of the resin *Pharbitisin* prepared by himself. From the above testimonies, and from reports of other medical officers, it appears certain that Kaladana is a safe and manageable purgative. Dr. W. Dymock, of Bombay, however, reports having on one occasion seen excessive purgation in an adult produced by one seed. This should apparently be regarded as an exceptional case. This seed is the *Hub-ul-nil* of Arabian authors.

### ([54]), p. 161. **Andrographis paniculata (Medical Properties of).**

For notices of the medical properties and uses of this plant see Fleming (*Asiat. Researches*, vol. xi.), Ainslie (*Mat. Ind.*, vol. i. p. 96), Drury (*Useful Plants of India*, p. 36), and Waring (*Indian Ann. of Med. Sci.*, vol. v. p. 618). Roxburgh (*Flor. Ind.*, vol. i. p. 117), who furnishes its botanical characters at length, remarks that one of its Hindústani names, *Maha-tita*, signifies *King of bitters*, adding, "and a very powerful and much esteemed one it is."

### ([55]), p. 166. **Oil of Peppermint, in Puerperal Fever.**

See an interesting paper by Mr. Dove, of Norwich (*Brit. Med. Journ.*, April 9th, 1859). He proposes it as a substitute for the nauseous oil of Turpentine in this class of cases. He prescribes it to the extent of from thirty to forty drops, in divided doses in the twenty-four hours, preceding its use by a stimulating aperient. The effects of this simple treatment were on the whole satisfactory. He considers that probably all volatile oils would act as well as that of Turpentine.

### ([56]), p. 175. Datura (Poisoning by, in India).

For an interesting account of professional poisoners, or *Dhatureeas* as they are commonly called from the use they make of this drug, see Dr. Norman Chevers (*Med. Jurisp. of Bengal, &c.*, pp. 104, 108, 121.) The whole subject of poisoning by Dhatura, as far as India is concerned, will be found carefully stated in the above work. See also some interesting remarks on the same subject by Mr. W. J. Palmer (*Indian Med. Gaz.*, 1866, vol. i. pp. 176, 292 and 319), and Dr. J. Irving (*Indian Ann. of Med. Sci.*, 1864, vol. ix. p. 1 *et seq.*)

### ([57]), p. 177. Extract of Henbane.

Henbane has been introduced into India, and thrives well at moderate altitudes. Dr. Winchester speaks highly of the Extract prepared at the Government garden at Hewra, in the Deccan, whence from 150 to 200 lbs. were supplied annually for the use of the Bombay army. Large supplies also have been prepared at Húnsúr, in Mysore, by Dr. Hilbers, and this, tested at the Civil Dispensaries in the Madras Presidency, was pronounced equally efficacious with the European article (*Indian Ann. of Med. Sci.*, vol. iii. p. 337). The importance of encouraging the manufacture of this and other allied drugs in India cannot be overrated.

### ([58]), p. 179. Nicotiana Tabacum, in Tetanus.

Dr. W. Dymock calls attention to the use of poultices of tobacco leaves to the spine in tetanus. This practice was first introduced by Dr. Leith into the European General Hospital, Bombay, and Dr. Dymock states that he has seen decidedly good effects from it. It is worthy of a trial.

### ([59]), p. 196. Cinnamomum iners. (As a Source of Cassia bark.)

Dr. Æ. Ross states that this tree is very abundant in the Balaghât jungles of North Canara, and that it was from this locality that the cassia bark, once so largely exported from that district, was obtained. The smaller branches, when carefully prepared, he pronounces to be nearly equal to that of *C. Zeylanicum*. At his recommendation, Dr. Ross states, the Bombay Government now farms out these trees, and by this means a very considerable addition has been made to the revenue. It may be used as a substitute for Cinnamon, to which, adds Dr. Ross, it can hardly be reckoned inferior. Its Canarese name is *Cuddoo-Lavanga.*

### ([59]), p. 197. Santalum album.

The following memorandum by Dr. G. Bidie on Sandal Wood, and the mode of extraction of its volatile oil, is of especial interest and value as being the result of personal observation. We give the statement without abridgment.—"This (*Santalum album*, Linn.) is " a small tree, rarely exceeding 25 feet in height, and very limited " in its range, being most abundant in the Mysore country, where " it grows on the eastern slopes of the Western Ghats, just beyond " the limits of the Mulnaad or rain country. It is carefully pro- " tected by Government, and only the trees that have reached ma- " turity, which they do in from 18 to 25 years, are cut down. The " felling takes place in the end of the year, and the trees are then " stripped of their bark and conveyed to various depôts, where they " are cut into billets, which are carefully dressed and sorted ac- " cording to the quality of the wood. These billets form the sandal- " wood of commerce, and are sold by weight at an annual auction, " native merchants congregating from all parts of India to make " purchases. The pieces that are straight, and have most heart " wood, fetch the highest price, as the fragrance for which they are " so much prized depends on the presence of an essential oil, which " is chiefly situated in the dark central wood of the tree. The " Mysore Government has long had establishments for extracting " the oil, which is sold at the annual auctions along with the wood, " and chiefly bought up for exportation to China and Arabia. It is " procured from the wood by distillation, the roots yielding the " largest quantity and finest quality of oil. The body of the still " is a large globular clay pot with a circular mouth, and is about " $2\frac{1}{2}$ feet deep by about $6\frac{1}{2}$ feet circumference at the bilge. No " capital is used, but the mouth of the still when charged is closed " with a clay lid, having a small hole in its centre, through which " a bent copper tube, about $5\frac{1}{2}$ feet long, is passed for the escape of " the vapour. The lower end of the tube is conveyed inside a " copper receiver, placed in a large porous vessel containing cold " water. When preparing the sandal for distillation the white or " sap wood is rejected, and the heart wood is cut into small chips, " of which about 2 maunds or 50 lbs. are put into the still. As " much water is then added as will just cover the chips, and distil- " lation is slowly carried on for 10 days and nights, by which time " the whole of the oil is extracted. As the water from time to time " gets low in the still, fresh supplies are added from the heated " contents of the refrigeratory. The quantity of oil yielded by " wood of good quality is at the rate of 10 oz. per maund, or 2·5 per " cent. It is transparent and of a pale yellow colour, and has a " resinous taste and sweet peculiar smell, which is best appreciated " by rubbing a few drops of the oil on the warm hand. Its sp. " grav. is about 0·980. The wood is used in various ways as a per- " fume by the natives, and also as a medicine, being supposed to " possess cooling properties, although, from the presence and nature " of the essential oil just referred to, it must be more or less of a " stimulant character."

### ([60]), p. 199. Aristolochia Indica, in Snake Bites.

The importance of the subject of remedies for snake bites can only be duly appreciated by those who have resided in localities where accidents from this cause are rife. In some districts in India deaths from snake bites are far from uncommon; thus, Dr. Imlach, Civil Surgeon at Shikapore (*Bombay Med. Phys Trans.*, 1856, vol. iii. p. 80), states that in one season, in one collectorate, Shikapore, no less than 306 cases of snake bites were officially reported, the mortality being 63, or about 20·58 per cent. Reports from other districts, which may be set down as comprising about one-fifth of Scinde, are furnished by Dr. Imlach, from which it may be concluded that the deaths from this cause alone, in the whole province, in one season were not less than 300. Another example, taken from an interesting paper by Colonel Munro (*Journ. of Agri.-Hort. Soc. of India*, vol. vi. P. i. p. 1), may be cited; viz., the Zillah of Midnapore, where official returns show that during a period of twenty-one months (from January 1845 to October 1846) no less than 402 deaths had occurred in that Zillah alone from snake bites. The Editor has elsewhere (*Madras Quart. Med. Journ.*, 1861, vol. iii. p. 340) shown his reasons for believing that if an antidote exist in the vegetable kingdom, it will most probably be found in the Natural Order Aristolochiaceæ. As far as is at present known, no remedy has superior claims to Liquor Ammoniæ, the efficacy of which is often striking.

### ([61]), p. 200. **Croton Seeds, as a stimulant.**

Dr. Erasmus Wilson (*Diseases of the Skin*, p. 177, *et seq.*) speaks highly of a Tincture (bruised Croton Seeds ℥i, Rectified Spirit ℥iv) as a stimulant application in cutaneous affections, especially in eczema, lichen, ichthyosis, and erythema. He employed it in a diluted form as follows: Tincture of Croton Seeds f. ℥i., Spirit of Rosemary ℥i., Rose Water ℥iii. A remedy so easily procurable in India is worthy of a trial in obstinate skin diseases, so common amongst the natives.

### ([62]), p. 201. **Ricinus communis.**

Two varieties of Castor Oil seeds are met with in India; the one large, and the other small. Popular opinion is in favour of the superiority of the latter, but Dr. G. Bidie states that he has been enabled to prove that they possess equal powers as a purgative. Most of the Castor Oil met with in the bazaars of India, prepared by the combined action of boiling, exposing to the sun, and pressure, is of a brownish colour, and thick. It is much more active in its operation than the ordinary oil obtained from the Government stores. This Dr. Winchester ascribes to the admixture of the seeds of the Croton Oil plant, which he states is grown indiscriminately with the Castor Oil plant. Castor Oil, of excellent quality, is prepared, by simple pressure, at the different depôts in India.

### ([63]), p. 202. **Kamala (Anthelmintic Properties of).**

See Dr. C. Mackinnon (*Indian Ann. of Med. Sci.*, 1853, vol. i. p. 286), to whom is due the credit of first bringing this remedy to the notice of the Profession; also Dr. T. Anderson (*Ibid.*, 1856, vol. iii p. 82), Dr. C. A. Gordon (*Med. Times and Gaz.*, Nov. 1856, p. 538, and May 1857, p. 429), Dr. Ramskill (*Lancet*, 1858. vol. i. p. 476),

Dr. Leared (*Ibid.*, p. 541), and Dr. Peacock (*Med. Times and Gaz.*, Nov. 6th, 1858). Dr. Anderson enters fully into the history of the drug generally. A new variety of Kamala has recently been brought to notice by Dr. Flückiger, of Bern (*Pharm. Journ.* Dec. 1867, p. 279). Apart from its dissimilar structure, when examined under the microscope, the new Kamala differs most obviously from the old, in its darker colour, larger grains, and freedom from earthy impurities. There is little doubt that it is the produce of another species of Mallotus.

### ([64]), p. 210. **Nut-Galls, as an Antiperiodic.**

The employment of Galls in the treatment of intermittent fevers is of old date (see *Murray, Apparatus Med.*, 1792, vol. vi. p. 9, and *Cullen's Mat. Med.*, 1789, vol. ii. p 46); but the attention of the Profession in India has recently been directed to them for this purpose, by Dr. C. Timins, of Madras (*Madras Med. Reports*, 1855, p. 236), who reported very favourably of their efficacy when given in doses of grs. x. to xii., in conjunction with the infusion of Chiretta. Further trials with it have been made by Dr. W. R. Cornish (*Indian Ann. of Med. Sci.*, 1857, vol. iv. p. 115), which tend to confirm Dr. Timins' views. In about half his cases (101) he prescribed it in powder, in doses of from twenty to thirty grains, three or four times a day; in the remainder he employed a strong infusion, half an ounce to a pint of water, in doses of one and a half to three fluid ounces. Dr. J. Macpherson (*Indian Ann. of Med. Sci.*, 1856, vol. iii. p. 381), however, states that Dr. Timins' formula was tried extensively in the dispensaries of Bengal, and that the general result was unfavourable, conveying the impression that the mixture was not equal to the common country febrifuges. It appears to be only adapted for the mildest form of the disease, which generally yields to a purgative, followed by any mild astringent bitter, aided by a few days' residence in hospital.

### ([65]), p. 216. **Cannabis Sativa (Medical Properties of, &c).**

With reference to the therapeutic applications of Indian Hemp, Professor Christison offers the following valuable remarks, derived from his personal experience with this drug: "I have for some " years," he observes, "used a very good alcoholic Extract, sent " to me from Calcutta twenty years ago, and still as powerful as " ever to subdue pain, obtain sleep, and put an end to spasm in " circumstances under which Morphia either did not suit or was " objected to by the patient; and after wide experience with it, I " am quite satisfied that it is an excellent substitute for it, if given " in sufficient doses. The difficulty is, to be always sure of the " quality of the Extract, or rather of the Gunjah, from which the " Extract is obtained. I have known two grains of my alcoholic " Extract, given in the form of Tincture, put an end, promptly and " permanently, to the agonizing pain caused by biliary calculus " impacted in the ducts; and there can be no more unequivocal " test than this of the potency of an anodyne. I have long been " convinced, and new experience confirms the conviction, that for " energy, certainty, and convenience, Indian Hemp is the next

" anodyne, hypnotic, and antispasmodic, to opium and its deriva- " tives, and often equal to it." He considers that a well prepared alcoholic Extract is the best of all forms for use, but it requires to be prepared from Gunjah, not too old, collected in the right district, and at the right season. The ordinary resin (*Churrus*) is generally very impure and untrustworthy. The fullest account of the history and physiological effects of Indian Hemp is furnished by Sir W. O'Shaughnessy (*Bengal Disp.*, pp. 579–604), who first brought it to the notice of the Profession. For its claims as a hypnotic, see Dr. Fromuller (*Brit. and For. Med. Chir. Rev.*, Jan. 1861, p. 248); as a parturifacient, consult Professor Sir J. Y. Simpson (*Monthly Journal of Med. Science*, July 1852, p. 91), Professor Christison (*Ibid*, 1851, pp. 39, 117), and Dr. J. Grigor (*Ibid.*, August 1852, p. 125). Dr. J. Laurence (*Madras Med. Journ.*, 1844, vol. vi. p. 274) has published an interesting paper on the prevalence and ill effects of the use of Bhang in the native army.

(66) p. 228. **Ginger, as a local application in affections of the Eye.**

See some remarks on this subject by Dr. Turnbull (*Med. Gaz.* Nov. 15th, 1851), It is doubtful if Ginger possesses any *special* stimulant influence in these cases.

(67), p. 255. **Grass Oils (Botanical Source of).**

In determining the various species of *Andropogon* which yield the different kinds of Lemon Grass Oil, the Committee have received much valuable assistance from Colonel W. Munro, C.B., who has made the Gramineæ his peculiar study.

(68), p. 255. **Andropogon citratum (Medical Properties of).**

From several trials with Lemon Grass Oil, the Editor feels justified in speaking highly of it, not only as an external application in rheumatism and other painful affections, but as a stimulant and diaphoretic when administered internally. Amongst the natives and Indo-Britons of Southern India, it is one of their most highly esteemed remedies in Cholera; and the Editor has witnessed cases in which it certainly seemed to moderate and check the vomiting, whilst it served to raise the depressed state of the constitution. It is well worthy of future trials, especially in the earlier stages of the disease. Dr. Æneas Ross reports very favourably of a warm infusion prepared by macerating about four ounces of the leaves in a pint of hot water. He states that he has used it very successfully as a diaphoretic in febrile affections, especially in weakly subjects, or when the fever is of a typhoid type. It is much used, and proves a valuable remedy, according to the same authority, in dropsical affections consequent on prolonged attacks of fevers so prevalent in malarious countries.

(69), p. 256. **Rúsa ka tel, as a rubefacient.**

This Oil, occasionally called also *Oil of Namur*, was first brought to notice in 1825 by Dr. N. Maxwell (*Calcutta Med. Phys. Trans.*, vol. i. p. 367), and it was further described in 1827 by Dr. Forsyth (*Ibid.*, vol. iii. p. 213). From a series of trials instituted with it at Madras, by Drs. Cole, Kellie, and Hunter, it appears that as an application in rheumatism its efficacy is chiefly limited to recent cases. In the severer forms and in the chronic stage, the oil, even when undiluted, afforded only slight relief (*see Madras Medical Reports*, 1855, p. 431, *seq.*) Favourable reports of it have been received from Dr. W. Dymock, Dr. L. W. Stewart, Dr. Æ. Ross, &c. Examined by Dr. J. Stenhouse, it was found to consist of a mixture of a pure volatile oil ($C^4 H^5$) and a fluid resin, the latter being probably a product of the oxidation of the oil (*see Pharm. Journ.*, 1845, vol. iv. p. 276).

(70), p. 261. **Ceylon Moss.**

See analyses by O'Shaughnessy, Bley, and Riegel, quoted by Pereira (*Mat. Med.*, vol. ii. P. i. p. 15), who furnishes likewise the most complete account we possess of the properties and uses of this article.

(71), p. 274. **Leeches (Amount of blood drawn by them).**

The blood-drawing power of the Indian leech has been carefully examined by Dr. A. H. Leith (*Bombay Med. Phys. Trans.*, 1841, vol. iv. p. 50, and *Ibid.*, 1860, vol. v. N.S. p. 94). As stated in the text, he ascertained that, as a general rule, leeches draw from four to five times their weight of blood, the fluctuation being apparently attributable partly to the state of the leeches, and partly to the state of the cutaneous circulation of the patient. In order to obtain four or five ounces of blood, he orders one ounce of leeches to be weighed and applied; if ten or twelve ounces, he orders two and a half ounces of leeches, and so on. Local depletion, he remarks, is thus practised with a precision equal to that of cupping by an expert operator, and far exceeding that of ordinary cuppers. Although the size of the leeches was not found materially to affect the quantity of blood drawn, yet it is a matter of some importance that large ones should be used, as by thus lessening the number of bites the patient is saved from unnecessary pain, and the indefinite small oozing of blood after their application is lessened. The leeches commonly used in Bombay, adds Dr. Leith, are so small that he has known fifteen dozen of them weigh but three ounces, and it is difficult to obtain leeches of such size that twelve or even eighteen will weigh an ounce, unless by previous arrangement with the leechman. In hospitals, however, where the leechman is paid by the month, it is most easy to obtain large leeches, as it is merely by their repeated application that they attain their large capacity. As a check on the leechman, and in order to prevent the use of leeches before they have recovered from their last repletion and disgorgement, which requires about three weeks, Dr. Leith practised the precaution of having the weight of those ordered ascertained, after they have filled themselves, as well as before they were applied. As a commentary on these practical observations of Dr. Leith with regard to leeches in India, it may be interesting to add the conclusions arrived at by M. Moquin-Tandon with reference to the European leech. Small leeches will abstract two and a half times, the small middle-sized four times, the large middle-sized five and a half times, and the large five times and one eleventh part of their own weight of blood (*Med. Zoology*, p. 146). The average of these results tends to confirm Dr. Leith's observations.

### ([72]), p. 274. **Hirudiniculture in India.**

Interesting accounts of the modes of leech breeding pursued by the natives of India are furnished by Dr. Gibson (*Bombay Med. Phys. Trans.*, vol. i. p. 312) and Lieut. R. M. Johnstone (*Ibid.*, 1846, vol. viii. p. 93); but a far simpler, and it is believed more effectual, plan, is the use of the apparatus proposed by M. Vayson, of Bordeaux, and called after him a *Vaysonier*. It is so simple in its construction as to be as easily applicable in India as elsewhere. The apparatus simply consists of a common earthen vessel, having the form of a truncated cone reversed; the lower part is perforated by a number of holes, but not so large as to allow of the leeches passing through them. The vessel is then filled with peat or bog earth, and a number of leeches are placed upon it, which embed themselves in the earth. The upper opening of the vessel is then covered up with a piece of coarse canvas. When it is desired to send the leeches to a distance, the earth is made as damp as possible, and the vessel is packed in a box or wicker basket. When it is wanted only to preserve the animals, the lower part of the vessel is placed in water to the depth of about four inches, and the creatures are left to themselves. In consequence of the infiltration, the lower layers of the earth are soon saturated with water, while the upper portion remains almost dry. The leeches know perfectly well how to choose between these two extremes the layer which is best adapted for them, and form in it galleries in which they live, grow, and produce their cocoons. This *Vaysonier* answers equally well for the preservation, conveyance, and reproduction of the leeches (*Moquin-Tandon, Med. Zoology*, p. 147).

### ([73]), p. 274. **Medicinal Leech of Western India, (Description of.)**

Dr. H. J. Carter furnishes the following description of the medicinal leech of Western India:—"It is lacustrine, from two to three inches "long in a state of rest after having been used, but less previously. "It is uniformly granulated or studded with minute papillæ all over "the surface; of a dark olive-green on the back, and a lighter one "on the belly; with seven regularly interrupted lines running "down the back, of which the central one is more continuous "than the rest; no spots on the belly; a yellow line divides the "dorsal from the ventral surface; and the head is provided with "twelve eyes, which are arranged as follows:—Two in front of "the first segment, median, approximated, and transverse; four "on the first segment, two of which are immediately behind and "in a line with the foregoing, and two others situated laterally; "two on the fourth segment laterally, and the other two on the "seventh segment laterally. The margin of the lip is uneven, "and slightly notched on the median line in front." This corresponds, in a degree, as pointed out by Dr. Carter, with *Hirudo granulosa, Savigny*, described by MM. Gervais and Van Beneden (*Zoologie Médicale*, 1859, p. 175), who states that it is employed medically at Pondicherry.

(74), p. 277. **Mylabris Cichorii as a substitute for Cantharides.**

See Reports by Drs. D. S. Young, A. Walker, T. Key, and W. Mortimer (*Madras Med. Journ.*, 1841, vol. iii. p. 96); Ainslie, (*Mat. Ind.*, vol. ii. p. 417); and O'Shaughnessy (*Bengal Disp.*, p. 683). It was first brought to notice, in 1809, by General Hardwicke (*Asiat. Researches*, vol. v.), and excellent accounts of it were soon after published by Dr. A. Burt and Dr. W. Hunter (*Ibid.*, vol. v. p. 423). See also Dr. J. Fleming (*Cat. of Indian Drugs, &c.*, p. 58), who advises that the insect should be collected in the morning or evening, killed by the steam of boiling vinegar, subsequently dried thoroughly in the sun, and preserved in well-stoppered bottles. Dr. G. Bidie (*Madras Quart. Med. Journ.*, 1862, vol. v. p. 261) speaks of September (before the setting in of the monsoon, Ed.) as the best time for collecting them.

(75), p. 279. **Indian Isinglass.**

Isinglass, regarded however, commercially, as of inferior quality, is prepared in many parts of India. That from Bengal, analysed by Mr. E. Solly (*Pharm. Journ.*, vol. i. p. 145), and found to contain from 86 to 92 per cent. of gelatine, has been supposed to be obtained from *Polynemus teria*, Buchanan; but Dr. F. Day states that this species has no air bladder; hence it cannot be a source of Isinglass. That from the western coast of the Peninsula is obtained from various fish. Dr. F. Day (*Fishes of Malabar*, 4to, 1865) enumerates the following: 1. an undetermined species of *Siluroid*, of the sub-group *Arii*, known to the natives by the name of *Yeta;* 2. *Polynemus Indicus*, Shaw; 3. *Lobotes Surinamensis*, Cuv. et Val.; 4. *Otolithus argenteus*, Cuv. et Val.; and 5. *Osteogeniosus militaris*, Bleeker. Much interesting information on the subject will be found in Dr. Royle's pamphlet "*On the Production of Isinglass along the Coasts of India.*" London, 1842.

(76), p. 346. **Hartal as an antiperiodic.**

Under the name of *Hartal*, Mr. S. Clark, of the Bengal Medical Service (*Med. Times and Gazette*, 11th June 1859) found a white impalpable powder held in high esteem in some parts of Northern India as an antiperiodic. On chemical examination it proved to be, not arsenic, as its name would imply, but Selenite in a calcined form. It is prepared by the natives by placing equal parts of selenite and fresh aloe juice in two small earthen pots luted together, and subjected to the heat of a fire for about twelve hours. Mr. Clark prescribed this substance in doses of from five to ten grains for adults, and from one to three grains for children, in intermittent fevers and other cases requiring tonics; and he states that he found it an excellent substitute for quinine, both alone and in combination with other remedies. Considering the similarity between the names of this substance and some forms of arsenic, the greatest caution should be exercised in seeing that the latter, actively poisonous, is not substituted for the former, which there is reason to suppose is almost inert.

# INDEX.

Synonyms and native names are printed in Italics.
Natural orders are printed in small capitals.

# ERRATA.

Page 34. For "Collodion" read "Collodium."

" 80. For "Cicerarietinum" read "Cicer arietinum."

" 96. For "CURCUBITA" read "CUCURBITA."

" 155. Insert ([53]).

" 202. For "Philippiensis" read "Philippinensis."

" 235. For "*scapifolia*" read "*scapiflora*."

" 261. For "Gracilaræ" read "Gracilariæ."

" 313. For "Hevar" read "*Hepar* Sulphuris."

" 315. For "Chlorates" read "Chloratis."

" 360. For "Lythargyrum" read "Lithargyrum."